T0336696

Information and Communication Technologies, Society and Human Beings:
Theory and Framework

Darek M. Haftor
Linnaeus University, Sweden

Anita Mirijamdotter
Linnaeus University, Sweden

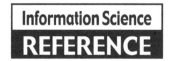

INFORMATION SCIENCE REFERENCE
Hershey · New York

Director of Editorial Content:	Kristin Klinger
Director of Book Publications:	Julia Mosemann
Acquisitions Editor:	Lindsay Johnston
Development Editor:	Christine Bufton
Publishing Assistant:	Keith Glazewski; Travis Gundrum
Typesetter:	Keith Glazewski
Production Editor:	Jamie Snavely
Cover Design:	Lisa Tosheff

Published in the United States of America by
Information Science Reference (an imprint of IGI Global)
701 E. Chocolate Avenue
Hershey PA 17033
Tel: 717-533-8845
Fax: 717-533-8661
E-mail: cust@igi-global.com
Web site: http://www.igi-global.com

Library of Congress Cataloging-in-Publication Data

Information and communication technologies, society and human beings : theory and framework / Darek M. Haftor and Anita Mirijamdotter, editors.   p. cm.
  "To honour Professor Bradley, more than forty well established scholars, within various related disciplines, have contributed with leading edge essays"--Preface. Includes bibliographical references and index.
  Summary: "This book offers contributions that articulate a set of aspects of information and communication technologies in human and social contexts, such as the individuals, groups, organizations and their management - addressing both descriptive and normative questions. It gives a unique presentation of the field understood as Social Informatics"--Provided by publisher.
  ISBN 978-1-60960-057-0 (hardcover) -- ISBN 978-1-60960-059-4 (ebook) 1. Information society--Social aspects. 2. Information technology--Social aspects. 3. Computers and civilization. I. Haftor, Darek M., 1969- II. Mirijamdotter, Anita, 1955- III. Bradley, Gunilla.   HM851.I529 2011
   303.48'33092--dc22
                     2010018444

British Cataloguing in Publication Data
A Cataloguing in Publication record for this book is available from the British Library.

All work contributed to this book is new, previously-unpublished material. The views expressed in this book are those of the authors, but not necessarily of the publisher.

Editorial Advisory Board

Tabula Gratulatoria

The following people and institutions listed below, expressed their congratulations to Professor Emerita Gunilla Bradley:

Aaron Marcus, USA
Afzal Sher, Sweden
Agneta Olerup, Sweden
Alexander Grishin, Sweden
Alladi Venkatesch, USA
Alvaro Taveira, USA
Ana Isabel B. B. Paraguay, Brasil
Ana Rusu, Romania
Anders Flodström, Sweden
Anders Nilsson, Sweden
Andy Imada, USA
Andy Sloane, UK
Ann Bishop, USA
Ann Hägerfors, Sweden
Ann Lantz, Sweden
Anna Croon Fors, Sweden
Annika Vänje Rosell, Sweden
Ari-Veikko Anttiroiko, Finland
Barbara Cohen, USA
Barbara Craig, New Zealand
Bengt Sandblad, Sweden
Bernt Ericson, Sweden
BG Wennersten, Sweden
Birger Rapp, Sweden
Birgit Erngren, Sweden
Björn Pehrson, Sweden
Brian Loader, UK
Brian Kleiner, USA
Börje Ahlström, Sweden
Carl Gustaf Jansson, Sweden

Cecilia Schelin Seidegård, Sweden
Celina Raffl, Austria
Charlotte Wiberg, Sweden
Chris Zielinski, UK
Chrisanthi Avgerou, UK
Christian Fuchs, Austria
Christina Neumayer, Denmark/Austria
Claire Dormann, Canada
Colin Beardon, New Zealand
Constantine Stephanidis, Greece
David Haken, USA
Department of Informatics, Umeå University, Sweden
Dick Scott, USA
Don Schauder, Australia
d'Udekem-Gevers Marie, Belgium
Eduard Aibar, Spain
Elisabeth Davenport, UK
Enda Fallon, Ireland
Erland Hjelmquist, Sweden
Eva Jansson, Sweden
Eva Lindh Waterworth, Sweden
Felix Van Rijn, The Netherlands
Franci Pivec, Slovenia
Louise Yngström, Sweden
Geoff Busby, UK
Georg Aichholzer, Austria
Gerald Maguire, Sweden
Gordon B. Davis, USA
Graeme Johanson, Australia
Gudrun Wicander, Sweden
Gunnar Karlsson, Sweden
Gunnar Landgren, Sweden
Gunnela Westlander, Sweden
Gunhild Agnér Sigbo, Sweden
Gustavo Cardoso, Portugal
Görel Strömqvist, Sweden
Henry M. Levin, USA
Hiroshi Tamura, Japan
Homa Bahrami, USA
Ingrid Melinder, Sweden
Ingegerd Palmér, Sweden
James G. March, USA
Jan Gulliksen, Sweden
Janne Carlsson, Sweden

Janne Elvelid, Sweden
Jenny Persson, Sweden
Jens Zander, Sweden
Johanna Sefyrin, Sweden
Jonny Holmstrom, Sweden
Kai K. Kimppa, Finland
Kajsa Ellegård, Sweden
Karin Hedström, Sweden
Karine Barzilai-Nahon, USA
Karl W Sandberg, Sweden
Karolyn Snyder, USA
Katarina Lindblad-Gidlund, Sweden
Kathy Buckner, UK
Kay Fielden, New Zealand
Kenneth Abrahamsson, Sweden
Klaus Brunnstein, Germany
Kiyoshi Murata, Japan
Kristina Höök, Sweden
Kåre Bremer, Sweden
Lars Ilshammar, Sweden
Lars Qvortrup, Danmark
Lars W. Nord, Sweden
Lazar Rusu, Romania
Leah Lievrouw, USA
Leif Bloch Rasmussen, Denmark
Lena Martensson, Sweden
Lennart Bergström, Sweden
Leopoldina Fortunati, Italy
Liam Bannon, Ireland
Louise Yngström, Sweden
Love Ekenberg, Sweden
Madeleine Leijonhufvud, Sweden
Madelene Sandström, Sweden
Maja Andjelkovic, UK
Maggie McPherson, UK
Mandi Axmann, Australia
Manfred Tscheligi, Austria
Manuel Castells, USA
Margareta Norell, Sweden
Ma. Theresa Mendoza-Rivera, Philippines
Marie Gevers, Belgium
Marie-Louise von Bergmann-Winberg, Sweden
Mark Kramer, Austria
Markku Mattila, Finland

Markku I. Nurminen, Finland
Martin Carnoy, USA
Marvin J. Dainoff, USA
Mats Edenius, Sweden
Matthias Schaffranek, Austria
Michael Gurstein,Canada
Mikael Östling, Sweden
Mikael Söderström, Sweden
Mikael Wiberg, Sweden
Nils Enlund, Finland/Sweden
Ola Henfridsson, Sweden
Olov Östberg, Sweden
Paschal Preston, Ireland
Patrick Rau, China
Per Gudmundson, Sweden
Per Levén, Sweden
Pernilla Gripenberg, Finland
Pertti Järvinen, Finland
Peter Day, UK
Peter Fleissner, Austria
Peter Nilsson, Sweden
Peter Revay, Sweden
Peter van den Besselaar, The Netherlands
Peter Vink, The Netherlands
Peter Arnfalk, Sweden
Piet Kommers, The Netherlands
Rafael Capurro, Germany
Rasmus Klocker Larsen, Sweden
Rinzou Ebukuro, Japan
Robert Bichler, Austria
Robert Pinter, Hungary
Robin Mansell, UK
Rudi Schmiede, Germany
Sara Eriksén, Sweden
Sheila Zimic, Sweden
Sigbrit Franke, Sweden
Sonja Buchegger, Sweden
Stefan Blachfellner, Austria
Steve Whittaker, UK
Stig Hagstrom, USA
Sture Hagglund, Sweden
Thomas Sjöland, Sweden
Tazu Togo, Japan
Terry Winograd, USA

Theresa Rivera, Philippines
Thomas Sjöland, Sweden
Tomas Ohlin, Sweden
Tone Bratteteig, Norway
Toomas Timpka, Sweden
Ulf Hedestig, Sweden
Ulf P Lundgren, Sweden
Ulrica Löfstedt, Sweden
Ursula Maier-Rabler, Austria
Vassilios Laopodis,Greece
Victor Kaptelinin, Sweden
Vincent Duffy, USA
Viveca Asproth, Sweden
Vivian Vimarlund, Sweden
Vivianne and BG Wennersten, Sweden
William Dutton, UK
William Petersson, Sweden
Åke Grönlund, Sweden
Åsa Rudström, Sweden
Åsa Smedberg, Sweden

Table of Contents

Section 1
Gunilla Bradley's Research Journey

Chapter 1

Geraldine Pratchett-Hultkrantz, Independent Scholar, Sweden

Chapter 2

Annagreta Dyring, Independent Scholar, Sweden

Section 2
The Convergence Theory on ICT, Society, and Human Beings

Chapter 3

Gunilla Bradley, Royal Institute of Technology (KTH,) Sweden

Chapter 4

William Mciver, Jr., National Research Council, Institute for Information Technology, Canada

Section 3
Psychological & Usability Aspects of ICT

Section 4
ICT in Work Life and Private Life: Organisational and Psychosocial Aspects

Section 7
Ethical Aspects on ICT

Section 8
Trans-Disciplinary Studies

Section 9
The Emerging Message

Foreword

It is a great honour for Linnaeus University to host the anniversary ceremony for Professor Gunilla Bradley.

On the 1st of January 2010 Linnaeus University opened its doors for the first time as the newest university of Sweden, the result of a merger between University of Kalmar and Växjö University. Linnaeus University is a modern, international university in Småland. Although Gunilla never worked at Linnaeus University, she represents its fundamental ideas in an excellent manner. Gunilla's research has been modern and international in the sense that she analyses the relationship between people, ICT, society and the environment. She proposes research questions for the future, and presents actions to achieve a good ICT society. Last but not least, Gunilla was born in Småland. Curiosity, creativity, companionship and utility – these are the terms by which we interpret Carl Linnaeus' achievements. This mission is also very much relevant for Gunilla's research. Linnaeus University would like to thank Gunilla for her significant research efforts and hope that she will continue to support researchers in informatics and media technology at our university.

Stephen Hwang
Rector

Lena Fritzén
Prorector

Preface

In 1970's there were not many people that inquired about the psychological and social effects of this thing we today label '*Information and Communication Technology*'. Professor Emerita Dr Gunilla Bradley did this; and this is the key reason for the design and writing of this unique volume!

Recently, Professor Bradley celebrated happily her 70th birthday while continuing to astonish us with her formulation of new, yet not heard of, quests for knowledge – just as she started to do this nearly four decades ago...

To honour Professor Bradley, more than forty well established scholars, within various related disciplines, have contributed with leading edge essays. Each contribution articulates a set of aspects of information and communication technologies in human and social contexts, such as the individuals, groups, organisations and their management – addressing both descriptive and normative questions. In that manner, as a collection of research essays this volume represents a unique presentation of the field understood here as *Social Informatics*.

However, unlike most of available assembled volumes, this book offers its reader two additional contributions. Firstly, the included essays conceived together as a whole give rise to an emergent message, that none of the essay presents itself. The working assumption here is that the identified emergent message articulates the hidden structure of the intellectual field of Social Informatics.

Secondly, colourful biographical notes of Professor Gunilla Bradley are presented in a fashion that communicates some central characteristics of a pioneering scholar. Being recognised as one of the leading developers and proponents of Social Informatics, these biographical notes serve as a source of inspiration and role model for younger researchers.

We warmly welcome the reader into a journey of intellectual rigour, novelty, curiosity, drama, and futurology...

INTRODUCTION

Information and Communication technology (ICT) and its effects on human beings and society is the theme of this book. By that, this book addresses the interaction between the ICT, the Individual, the Organizations, and the Society. Analyses of interactions, human effects and the interrelations are important since these result in reciprocal effects which may reinforce each other in both positive and negative ways. Changes in behaviour, perspectives, values, competencies, social and psychological aspects, etc. are all of human concern. This means that we need to critically reflect on how behaviour, values, competencies, etc. are influenced, shaped and directed by ICT use and thus, are being extended to the human and social conditions of mankind.

This recognition is by now established. Computer Science and ICT related disciplines work more and more together with behavioural and social sciences to contribute to studies of cognitive effects and changes, psychosocial changes, motivational and emotional changes, organisational and institutional changes, societal changes, value changes and new lifestyles; all these are examples of this extensive research area that addresses interrelations of ICT, Society, and Human Beings.

This book includes a unique presentation of the field of ICT and Social Change, which is an area of immense attention in contemporary life, both private and professional. The developments in computer technology, telecommunication technology, and media technology have led to, the so-called, converging technologies, which also converge our private and professional lives, and our private and professional roles. Professor Emerita Gunilla Bradley, to whom this book is dedicated, holds close to forty years of pioneering research in this field. A succinct extraction of her lifelong research is illustrated in the Bradley Convergence Model, which is presented in Section 2. The model as such is in principle a graphical illustration of ongoing changes in the Information Society, also called the Net Society. It syntheses theoretical frameworks in Bradley's research on psychosocial work environment and computerization based on experience from research programs starting in the 1970's and carried out during various phases of the history of computerization. The main message of the model is its articulation of key generative mechanism that ICT brings into our social world, which in turn transforms this social world. The Net Society is the emerging result driven by this generative and transformative mechanism. The Convergence Model, and Dr Bradley's research, has influenced and continues to influence and inspire scholars around the world.

This book is based on forty-three contributions mostly written by senior researchers, of which a majority have a lifelong research experience within the field of ICT and Social Change. The book also contains contributions from younger researchers who grew up with the new technology. Most of the contributions in the book are novel essays that represent contemporary international research. Yet, the book also embraces a historical perspective through some contributions written more than twenty years ago. In what follows, these essays are introduced and grouped in eight parts. These parts are all related to the life long pioneering research of Professor Emerita Gunilla Bradley and the influence and inspiration her work has had on scholars around the world.

The reader may also find this book as a guide that includes fruitful exploratory research orientations. These may serve as a point of reference for further research on what remains a profound challenge for our human endeavours: the future interconnected global society and economy, all by technology.

SECTION 1: GUNILLA BRADLEY'S RESEARCH JOURNEY

The innovative nature of the research discussed in this book has been very stimulating for a long time, changing the world profoundly. With current technological developments, human actions have become more diligent, challenging the design of new technologies with an unprecedented scope.

Positively, the technological revolution has deeply affected many aspects of human lives, e.g., making it easier to communicate, socialize and develop relation over distances. To put forward this remarkable change, this part begins by presenting the colourful biography of Gunilla Bradley. This biography precisely presents innovative exploratory research, in relation to psychosocial and technological aspects, which are Gunilla's substantial and constructive contributions in her life-long pioneering research. It brings the context of many ideas where psychological, sociological and technological issues have engaged Gunilla for some time now, and inspired researchers across the world.

This part also contains two special essays written by Annagreta Dyring who has a long professional relationship to Gunilla and Geraldine Pratchett-Hultkrantz, Gunilla's best friend. Both have deep insights in the academic world. Annagreta gives a presentation of Gunilla's passion, strength and knowledge in the field of Information and Communication Technology. She illustrates in a very melodic manner the engagement of Gunilla's outstanding work and research in this field. She has remarkably described Gunilla's intuition and interests, especially with her role of stimulating women to contribute to areas of research, such as technological developments, which traditionally have been seen to belong to men. Geraldine's, essay continues to bring up marvellous achievements and qualities of Gunilla's experience for many decades. She describes in a very tranquil way all of Gunilla's different challenges that have followed her life. Even more, Geraldine develops her essay by continuously presenting Gunilla's unique professionalism and fruitful contributions in the area of ICT to the whole world.

SECTION 2: THE CONVERGENCE THEORY ON ICT, SOCIETY, AND HUMAN BEINGS

This part sets off by Gunilla Bradley's summarising overview of her Convergence Model and illustrations on ongoing changes in the Net Society. The description of the model is kept short and structured with reference to the concepts Globalization, ICT, Life Environment, Life Role, and Effects on Humans. For interested readers, the essay includes references to other publications where the theoretical framework, which this model builds on, is elaborated more.

The subsequent essays elaborate on parts of the Convergence Model. The first is William McIver's analogy to the science of 'Ekistics', i.e., human settlements, which include regional, city, community planning and residential design. He points at the comprehensive and systemic view of the Convergence Model which has provided a framework that enables understanding of the relation between previously studied disparate phenomena. He also put forward the model as a conceptual device for elaborating on advancing societal transformation toward improved human quality.

Larry Stillman and Tom Denison, in the next essay, make some comparisons between the convergence theory and Anthony Gidden´s structuration theory. They suggest linking to Gidden's Structuration Theory and state that the model has the opportunity to mediate the agency-structure dichotomy. They underline that ICT mediates the constitution of both agency and structure and, simultaneously, the two create ICT. This perspective implies that ICT is both a product and a process of human intentionality and choices, and of social structures and impositions.

Kristina Orth-Gomér continues. Her contribution is an elaboration on the Convergence Model's contribution for the development of human well-being and this is done from a medical and public health perspective. Orth-Gomér recalls the variety of independent research that sends the same signal: the quantity and quality of human interaction in social settings is needed for human wellbeing! In this, the Convergence Model characterizes the societal dynamic of such human interactions, as induced and transformed by ICT. Moreover, Bradley's advancement of the so-called concept "Smart-homes" offers a future human environment that can enable such social interactions and, thus, contribute to the human well-being.

In the final essay of Section 2, Alice Robbin addresses a particular aspect of social interaction that is ICT mediated, namely the induced multi-tasking. Thus, the introduction of ICT in the various human and social context, work or private, exposes humans for constant and dynamic interruptions with changes of attention and meaning, hence changes in mental or cognitive activities. In this context, the technological convergence as well as the convergence of conventional social roles and life environments may produce an increased opportunity for multi-tasking. This, in turn, may pose an opportunity and a challenge, in the latter leading to a cognitive burden, stress and failure. Therefore, there is a need for normative considerations of the design, introduction and utilisation of ICT, all aimed at Bradley's visions of a "people-centred perspective" in order to achieve "the good society".

To sum up the overall message of this part, Bradley's Convergence Model offers an understanding of the relation of converging ICT and globalization to the human and societal forces which are involved in societal transformations. This understanding, in turn, may guide us to directing the transformation towards the achievement of human well-being and control, rather than becoming its victims or products.

SECTION 3: PSYCHOLOGICAL & USABILITY ASPECTS OF ICT

The contributions of Michael J.H. Smith and colleagues introduce section 3. Prof. Smith looks back at more than thirty years of acquaintance with Gunilla Bradley and her research. He acknowledges the inspiration and insight that he and many others around the world has gained through Bradley's research on how ICT transforms our daily lives and through her promotion of quality of life issues. The two subsequent articles are reprints of Human Factors and Ergonomics Society publications in honour of Gunilla Bradley, to illustrate her influence on their work. One article deals with how electronically monitoring worker performance may lead to psychosocial stress and related somatic symptoms. The second article hypothesizes that the psychosocial stress encountered in the working conditions, created by computer technology, may lead to musculoskeletal symptoms in workers independently from the physical ergonomic considerations of their work.

Michelle Robertson advances the relation between ICT, psychosocial work environment and health, including family life and leisure time. She points to research results that illustrate the complexity surrounding computer use and impact of ICT on knowledge workers. Her findings show that an individual's success of interaction with ICT, particularly the elimination of stress, is conditioned both by micro-aspect of the terminal, such as information and system design, and even more by macro-aspects, such as organisational structures, culture, leadership, role or job design, education and communication structures and processes.

Holger Luczak and colleagues are analysing their experimental evaluations of human-computer interaction among elderly people in terms of various input devices. Physical and cognitive deficiencies, which emerge in humans due to aging, limit the ability to interact with ICT. The findings based on their experiments support and emphasize that the technology have to be designed in a manner that compensates these deficiencies and, thus, facilitates effective ICT interaction.

The contribution of Vladimir Munipov illustrates the influence of Bradley's work on the development of social and psychological aspects of ergonomics in the former Soviet Union and Russia. Munipov suggests that the human-centred design of ICT, as advocated by Bradley, requires that human mental processes must be mediated by ICT in a comprehensive manner, so that human meaning is enabled and mediated. By that Munipov, drawing on Bradley's research, departs from the Russian prevailing model of cognitive processes as forms of activity.

Hal Hendrick's exploration of man's various cognitive styles – e.g. conformist or creative – shows that this does not only determine the way man cognises his or her problem situations at hand, but also the way man interacts with his or her organisational context and with the ICT-mediated information. Hendrick found that in the latter context, cognitively concrete people want their information presented in a clear, unambiguous, step-by-step approach and are less concerned about the underlying rational, principles, or conceptual basis of the material. In contrast, cognitively complex people prefer to have the material presented in a manner that enables them to grasp the underlying concepts and principles.

Sebastiano Bagnara and Simone Pozzi advocate that in ICT design, including interfaces and mode of human interaction, the conventional approach of studying the average users, on which to base design decisions, should be given up. They argue for a HCI movement from a nomothetic research mode, that focus on the identification of general and universal mechanisms of human behaviour, to an idiographic mode, which looks upon the individual as a unique personality. The latter approach focuses on a personalised design, whic adapts the mode of interaction to particular users needs and cognitive styles.

Linked to personalized design are approaches aimed at privacy-enhancing identity management as put forward by Simone Fischer-Hübner and John Sören Pettersson. They point to challenges in relation to HCI design for managing privacy in human and social affairs. The authors note that privacy-enhancing identity management implies that users can make informed choices about releases of personal data, selections of credentials for proving personal properties, and about their privacy and trust policy settings.

The final contribution of section 3 is Birgitta Bergvall-Kåreborn and Anna Ståhlbröst who elaborate the phenomenon of Living Lab. This is the term for a development and test milieu, where ICT may be shaped in a participatory and human-centred manner. The notion of Living Lab implies a real-life milieu where actual or natural human conditions and situations are part of the development process. This is a long step from conventional IS development approaches, which has little or no chance to account for human actual situations. In addition, the ultimate idea for the Living Lab milieu and approach is to offer new ways of managing innovation processes.

SECTION 4: ICT IN WORK LIFE AND PRIVATE LIFE – ORGANISATIONAL AND PSYCHOSOCIAL ASPECTS

Eila Järvenpää and Stina Immonen address how ICT as a tool in the workplace has transformed the conduct of work. In this transition – from old-fashioned, paper and pen based office work, to contemporary knowledge-based and ICT enabled work profiles – they argue that little research is produced regarding the work, stress and well-being in the context of ICT enabling knowledge based work. Their study ranges from 1970's and onwards, studying the use of ICT applications for office work. They conclude that even though applications have become more advanced, the nature of (knowledge) work and user needs may not have been appropriately taken into account. The key focus of the published research seems to be put into visual display units!

Peter Hoonakker et.al. continue on this theme in their essay on work environment in intensive care units and the introduction of telemedicine. Although promising, research is needed in a number of issues, e.g., how tele-intensive-care-units affect communication and trust in the work team, how the technological environment affects staff work load, quality of care and patient safety. The authors set out to examine some of these issues from a socio-technical perspective including key factors related to work in virtual teams.

In the next essay Jacques Steyn argues that contemporary design of ICT and the employment of ICT in various contexts – also other than workplace – mimics the industrial work-place. He suggests that the work-oriented design should be replaced by human-needs centred design, which will help to reduce task load, effort and stress, and open up for increased human satisfaction and well-being. Steyn exemplifies his ideas of this non work-space design approach through the function of social media, such as Facebook, that manage to satisfy the human need of social belonging.

Ulrika Danielsson and Karin Danielsson Öberg review research that addresses the blurring of the boarders between workspace and leisure space, as induced by ICT. Today, being physically away from the workplace does not mean that we are necessarily changing to another environment or leaving our work tasks behind in psychological terms. The authors identify a set of challenges for humans, such as overload, stress and fatigue. Their suggestion to promote human well-being is to design ICT in a manner that articulates and communicates the distinctions between leisure and work. The design challenges are thus to attend to the borderlines between different life roles and life environments.

Hans-Erik Nissen, finally, elaborates on the design of ICT to enable human centred communication and action. He suggests that ICT design from a human-oriented perspective, should be broadened from ICT as a tool for control – of a machine or human being – to ICT incorporated as a means to facilitate sense-making, understanding and critical argumentation. Enabling juxtaposition of competing facts and values is a particular requirement for various democratic processes and empowerment of people dominated by unwanted structures, whether in the work-place or society. Nissen ponders on Web 2.0 enabled e-conferences as such means.

SECTION 5: E-CONFERENCES & E-LEARNING

The essays of section 5 contribute to what Bradley refers to as Global Spaces, in this case, in the field of academic events and higher education. New possibilities and dimensions for teaching, learning and interaction are proposed. Pedro Isaías discusses using Web 2.0 to combine real and on-line conferences. Virve Siirak argues for instructional design, which blends ICT mediated and face-to-face communication and has a base in social constructivist learning theory, for developing both efficient learning and a learning culture. Finally, Elspeth McKay bases her argument in awareness of different cognitive styles when designing courses and courseware. For effective learning design her advice is attention to the human-dimension of human-computer interaction (HCI) as reinforced by Gunilla Bradley's Convergence Model. Professor Bradley's research into interactive effects of ICT tools taps right into some of the issues faced by people who utilize their right for information access. As illustrated in this part, the theory related to Bradley's psychosocial life environment and quality of life and well-being, has been an inspiration for researchers also in the field of e-conferences and e-learning.

SECTION 6: THE INFORMATION AND COMMUNICATION SOCIETY

The Information and Communication Society provides us with unique challenges - opportunities as well as risks. This is the theme of the included contributions in section 6. Simon Rogerson looks afresh on the current potentials of the so-called Information Age, which has stimulated people across the world to communicate across the giant network, forming a new global society, the Information Society. Looking back at Gunilla's good society, the Information Society is seen as a potential to practice ethical considerations that are of great value, composing a good global society. Furthermore, Rogerson addresses the very subject matter of ICT-devices: the information. He highlights that the central matter of ICT is the trustworthiness of the information provided by our tools rather than its quantity and frequency. He argues that the rapid development and integration of various kinds of ICT threatens the quality of provided information. Further, according to Rogerson, the dramatic consequences of unreliable information imply that we have a moral obligation to address information integrity. ICT allows us to blend forms, such as prose, poetry, music and pictures, and deliver them using, for example, writing and singing in either a serious or humorous fashion. We need to learn how to benefit from this varied diet of fit-for-purpose information and how to judge trustworthy information.

Peter Crowley continues in this theme by addressing the role of ICT for the continuous establishment and re-establishment of our civil societies. He stresses the need of mindfulness to avoid merely 'technology push' approaches where ICT is introduced as such, for the sake of itself, or only for commercial reasons. Crowley suggests engaging in the matter by converging a top down and a bottom up approach. By top down he proposes that governments and international organisations provide adequate literacy enabling structures, as well as affordable and accessible technology infrastructures. By the bottom up approach he proposes to include a self-organising civil society, both local and global. He argues that the bottom up is both desirable and necessary to complement the top down for reaching sustainable development and global justice. Challenges he points out, include avoiding permanently locked society into the divide of information-rich and information-poor, thus creating information feudalism or the 'digital divide'.

The growth of ICT support for a variety of social and community networks has allowed for a rich and complex range of interactions and methods of participation. Barrett Caldwell argues that the use of such networks can be considered as enabling technologies to support previously difficult social interactions, e.g., when being separated by time or distance, or experiencing complications due to social dynamics. To study social interactions in ICTs he suggests some quantitative analytical tools based on engineering and measures of efficiency and effort required to sustain connections between entities. These measures are referred to as mathematical properties of coupling, persistence and work functions. The belief is that our understanding of social and technological dynamics, and ultimately social networks behaviour in the Information Society, will progress and will be enhanced through applying the suggested tools.

Sarai Lastra addresses the ICT use and social factors for supporting democratic processes in communities. She proposes a participatory design approach for understanding the essence and ethos of a community. Her finding is that community events are assets that represent collective knowledge. These assets are formed by an emerging collective belief system that influences community actions and relationships. Lastra's proposed design approach aims for a high degree of participation by the community members with the purpose of aligning the ICT being designed with the community ethos.

The subsequent essay by Sangeeta Sharma addresses the focal research problem of how ICT can help in formation of socio-ethically inclusive societies with universal ethics as the epicentre. The process of globalization is unifying various cultures leading to the creation of Multiculturalists society. As an effect various ethnic groups are expanding their boundaries to form larger social structures. Although social mixing, ethnic groups have own social spaces where the concept of spatial management can contribute. Spaces of various ethno-cultural formations are merged into single social unit. The merging can be facilitated by building up mutual trust and respect for each other, which in turn can be reinforced by communicating with the help of Information and Communication Technologies. Hence, the role of ICT in enhancing the process of unification is crucial to develop social reconfiguration and new identities as it penetrates the tightened boundaries of ethnic groups.

Margaret Tan puts attention to the Information Society from the perspective of interconnectivity of fast evolving digital technologies that enable individuals and communities to express, communicate, interact and to share their creative works and knowledge, leading to a so called 'co-space'. Tan argues that this collaborative space provides a new paradigm shift to the economic and social ecology of information and knowledge creation. The new co-space can facilitate profound networks of relationships that not only constitute a valuable conduit for the conduct of social affairs but also the social production of intellectual capital. She states that the key to today's innovations may be to develop the organisational ability to harness social production efforts so as to use them in the formulation of competitive actions at the individual, organisational as well as national level.

Natalie Pang argues in a similar vein as Tan that collective processes in both virtual and physical communities contain multiplier effects. One of these effects lies in the subtractability of resources, i.e., whether or not one person's appropriation of a resource reduces the availability of that resource for others. Pang maintains, throughout the paper, that it is essential to see all of these collective processes of interactions as two-way, dialogical relationships, that is, they never occur in isolation and are constantly in negotiation (and renegotiation) with structural forces such as their institutional frameworks and contemporary environments. She shows that "knowledge commons" have become popular for denoting public spaces that support the creation, use, and storage of public resources. These are free from market constraints, and are accessible to everyone in the community.

In the area of ICT, the abundance of development agendas and plans for developing information/knowledge societies is quite significant. Eduardo Villanueva Mansilla states that the agendas have taken the route towards economic and industrial development, infrastructure building, educational reform, basic social services, e-government, etc. He points out the need to shift from institutional focus of policy making to societal considerations, which include the potential for cultural development, with emphasis in the need for digital independence, not just in terms of infrastructure, but also of production and consumption of media products based on a dynamic and participatory community of users.

Lorenz M. Hilty discusses the potential contribution of ICT to Sustainable Development. The necessary conditions are a reduction of the input of natural resources into industrial production and consumption. Hilty introduces a conceptual framework, which accounts for positive and negative impacts of ICT on physical flows. This framework addresses three levels: the ICT life cycle itself, life cycles of other products influenced by ICT applications, and patterns of production and consumption. Hilty concludes that what we need is a deep structural change towards an economic system in which value-creation is mainly based on information processing, while keeping the physical properties of material within some limits that ensure that it can be recycled. In such sustainable information society, the open technological standards will play a crucial role.

Social and cultural sustainability in relation to an e-commerce application used in the kitchen of a Swedish public school is the focus of the essay by Christina Mörtberg et al. They illustrate how an e-commerce application complicated the daily routines in the school kitchen rather than making the ordering of food stuff easier or more flexible. They show how small things that were vital in the staff's day-to-day activities illuminated the e-commerce application's problems and weaknesses. These problems highlight social and cultural sustainability including consequences of design, which lacks involvement of users in design and implementation of IT systems and services.

Wolfgang Hofkirchner, the last essay of section 6, has entitled his contribution "ICTs for the Good Society". His vision for a global information society builds on the idea of ICTs and society as a transdisciplinary research field, which orients toward the fulfilment of values that are against the rule of domination. The main argument is that not only a society that exploits nature, as was found with reduced notions of sustainability, but also a society that does not meet the criterion of social compatibility, or a society that does not abide by technology assessment, would in the long run break down and not qualify for being sustainable. In this context we notice the lifework of Gunilla Bradley, which has been intrinsically motivated towards safeguarding human well-being and the search for societal conditions that enable individual self-fulfilment, given the rapid development and deployment of converging digital technologies. Hofkirchner's conclusion is that Bradley's focus on the Individual in the network age is crucial to the vision of the good society. The vision he considers necessary is that of a Global Sustainable Information Society.

SECTION 7: ETHICAL ASPECTS ON ICT

In what way should we program computers to control human beings, Jacob Palme discusses in his contribution. He brings up a critical question that reflects today's astronomic technological advancements, on which mankind act. How to program and how to control computers not to become judges? This is the main question that Palme elaborates by introducing examples related to human rules and laws. He argues that such rules and laws, interpreted by humans, are more acceptable than rules interpreted by computers. Diane Whitehouse and Penny Duquenoy continue on this theme by discussing what is the right manner to use ICT for eHealth. They have observed that many ICT practitioners find it hard to associate the topic of ethics with their training about technologies and therefore provide us with ways in which teaching and practice for ICT professionals and trainees can be enhanced and extended to increase the awareness of ethical issues in eHealth.

Jacques Berleur addresses the normative question of who is governing the Internet, and then, how is it governed? If Internet is not regarded only in technological terms, but as a social phenomenon, and an inherent part of the Information Society, the notion of self-governance or self-regulation assumes a central position. This implies that all involved actors, whether users or developers, constitute the governors. Berleur therefore puts forward some guidelines for the self-governing which builds on equality and respect for humankind.

Darek Haftor continues in this vein by proposing a conceptual framework, aimed to guide normative considerations and decisions in the course of the development of ICT. The advanced proposal aims towards careful and self-critical reflections on the normative decisions made when developing ICT, and also the consequences of these decisions for human and social affairs.

The contribution by Kristo Ivanov concludes this part. Ivanov investigates two distinct approaches for the development of ICT – a culturally minded and a politically and ethically minded approach. He concludes that the praxis of ethically sound ICT development presupposes the existence of an ethically sound social structure – or, in other words, the ethical characteristics of ICT are the products of the ethical properties of the social systems that produce this ICT.

SECTION 8: TRANS-DISCIPLINARY STUDIES

The final part that includes contributed essays is devoted to trans-disciplinary studies. Susan M. Dray addresses the relation and therein the gap, between the academic endeavour and the practice. She suggests that this gaps can be simplified in terms of 'academics don't do practitioner relevant research, since they focus more on rigor and isolating variables rather than dealing with 'real and complex problems'. However, practitioners have the tendency to suppress skepticism and critical thinking as a team, who always try to reach consensus and move forward. Dray states that it is crucial to bridge this gap for a "better" future for the field of Human Computer Interaction and suggests more joint collaboration fronted by a professional association that brings people together form a variety of disciplines and geographical locations.

However, trans-disciplinary and multidisciplinary engagement is a difficult and complex endeavour. Myra Strober has studied multidisciplinary seminars and the experience of the involved seminar participants. Her research provides a set of heuristic recommendations for how to succeed with interdisciplinary settings, particularly in terms of the research process. This includes making it clear for the participants that interdisciplinary research is challenging both in terms of the content and in terms of the process. The various roles and hierarchies within academic context may easily hinder open communication, hence must be recognised explicitly; this includes also respect for each other's ideas and contributions. Additionally, the purpose of interdisciplinary dialogues must be very clear for all involved and criteria for its success.

The extraordinary complexity of knowledge in today's world creates a paradox, Strober observes. On the one hand, the complexity of knowledge induces narrower and narrow specialisations of experts. On the other hand, the real-life complexities can not be fully understood in terms of small chunks only: there is a need for a holistic comprehension of human challenges, where the various disciplinary subdomains are interrelated in a meaningful manner. We conclude that most of the chapters in this volume strive towards this holistic comprehension.

SECTION 9: THE EMERGING MESSAGE

The essay in part 9, written by the editors, put attention to the message that emerges out of the contributions in the previous parts. People's use of ICTs give rise to new kinds of societies, new forms of organising, new ways of interacting. This also leads to the emergence of a new social order with inherent formal and informal inter-human power structures, which need to be governed. The unifying value among the contributors is that ICT should contribute to human well-being and some guidelines drawn out of these are summarized towards the end. The final message we wish to convey is that ICTs, like all technologies, are a human intervention produced by ideas and aspirations to control the environment. So, following Gunilla Bradley's words, let us use this opportunity for redesigning society towards peace, democracy, welfare and life quality for all.

Darek M. Haftor
Linnaeus University, Sweden

Anita Mirijamdotter
Linnaeus University, Sweden

Acknowledgment

The editors of this Volume would like to express our gratitude to the numerous people who have been involved in putting together this book. First of all we wish to thank all the distinguished contributing scholars who have provided us with so many hours of interesting reading and thought provocations. An additional thanks to the members of the Local Editorial Board, who have supported reviews of the contributions. We are also grateful to Linnaeus University who have afforded necessary support for carrying through this work. In this aspect we are deeply grateful to Miranda Kajtazi and Gunn Jensen who have worked so hard with the tedious work of reviewing and editing to get everything into the same format and see to that all details are there and in appropriate order. Finally, we also wish to thank IGI Global for their support and guidance.

Darek M. Haftor
Linnaeus University, Sweden

Anita Mirijamdotter
Linnaeus University, Sweden

Section 1
Gunilla Bradley's Research Journey

Curriculum Vitae (CV) for Gunilla Bradley (GB)

CONTENT OF THE CV

- Short biography
- Previous positions
- Summary of research
- Ongoing research
- Pedagogical activities and experiences
- Key note speaker, committees, boards etc
- Awards

SHORT BIOGRAPHY

Gunilla Bradley (GB) is since 2002 Professor in Informatics at Royal Institute of Technology (KTH) - IT university and School of Information and Communication Technology (ICT) - since 2005 professor emerita. 1997 she was appointed Professor of Informatics at Umeå University and worked for Umeå University and Mid Sweden University during five years. In 1984 she got the competency as full professor in Technology and Social Change at Linköping University.

She has a background in the behavioural sciences and is an authorized psychologist. Her research concerns the interplay between Information and Communication Technology (ICT), Human Beings, and Society. Beginning in 1973, she initiated and led cross-disciplinary research programs on computerisation and working life at Department of Sociology at Stockholm University, during twenty years. She has two years been a visiting scholar at Stanford University and Professor of Technology and Social Change at the Royal Institute of Technology, Stockholm.

GB has authored thirteen books (mainly in Swedish) and numerous articles in international scientific journals, also contributed extensively to the popular science press. In 1992-94 she served as General Chair of the world conference on "Organisational Design and Management" (ODAM) with the subtitle "New Technology – Challenges for Human Organisation and Human Resource Development in a Changing World (see below). In 1997 GB received the Namur Award from the International Federation for Information Processing (IFIP) for her pioneering research to increase the social awareness of the impact of ICT. In 2008 she was guest professor at Paris Lodron University in Salzburg and the ICT &

Society Center. Since 2008 she is Chair of an annual international IADIS conference that she designed and entitled "ICT, Society and Human Beings". IADIS= International Association for Developing the Information Society (NGO org.).

Selected Books

- "Social and Community Informatics: Humans on the Net" (Routledge, 2006)
- "Humans on the Net: Information and Communication Technology (ICT) Work Organization and Human Beings" (Stockholm, SE: Prevent, 2001)
- "Human Factors in Organisational Design and Management" subtitled "New Technology: Challenges for Human Organisation and Human Resource Development in a Changing World" (Bradley and Hendrick [Eds.], North Holland, Elsevier, 1994)
- "Computers and the Psychosocial Work Environment" (Taylor and Francis, 1989)
- "Computer Technology, Work Life, and Communication." (The Swedish Delegation for Long Term Research. Stockholm, Liber, 1977). (in Swedish)

For details see Bibliography.

Educational Background

- Competency for full professorship in Technology and Social Change, Linköping University, 1984
- Competency as associate professor, Gothenburg University, 1973
- Ph.D. in Educational Psychology, Gothenburg University, 1972
- Authorized Psychologist, 1972
- Medical studies Karolinska Institute, Stockholm
- Bachelor´s degree in Psychology, Sociology, Ethnography, and Pedagogics (1961)

PREVIOUS POSITIONS

- **2008-2009:** Guest professor at Paris-Lodron University, Salzburg, ICT & Society Centre
- **2002:** Professor Informatics, Royal Institute of Technology (KTH), School of ICT, Stockholm.
- **1997-2001:** Professor in Informatics, Umeå University and Mid Sweden University
- **1995-1997:** Professor Technology and Social Change, Royal Institute of Technology, Stockholm.
- **1994-1995:** Stockholm University (Sweden), Program Manager for Crosscultural and Crossdiciplinary Research on Information Technology, Organisational Change, and Human Behavior
- **1992-1994:** International Ergonomics Association, General Chair of the 4th International Conference on Organizational Design and Management (ODAM-IV)
- **1991-1992:** Stanford University (USA), Visiting research professor
- **1988-1992:** Stockholm University, Institute for International Education, Program Manager for the research on "Computer Technology and Working Life: Knowledge based systems—Organizational and Psychosocial aspects of their Introduction and Use"
- **1987-1988:** Stanford University (USA), Visiting research professor
- **1981-1987:** Stockholm University, Department of Sociology, Program Manager for the research program "Computerization and Impact on the Psychosocial Work Environment".
- **1973-1981:** Stockholm University, Department of Sociology, Project Manager for "Computerization and its impact on Work Environment for Salaried Employees in Sweden" (RAM-project)

Figure 1. Research program on interplay between ICT—humans—society

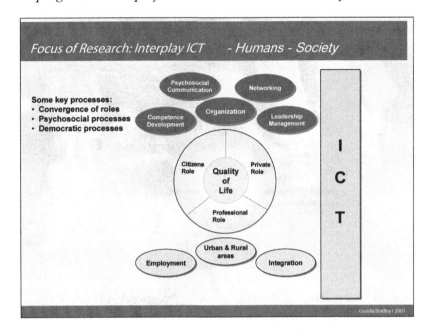

SUMMARY OF RESEARCH

Research in the 2000th at School of ICT, Royal Institute of Technology (KTH), Stockholm

1. Research Overview: Social Informatics

A research program on **Social Informatics** (SI) was elaborated in 1997 by Bradley and entitled: "Research on Interplay ICT - Humans - Society". It also inspired other universities in Sweden and abroad and themes/tracks at international scientific conferences in IT-related disciplines.
Figure 1 is an overview of the research areas in the program:

Social Informatics (SI) refers to research and study that examines societal, social, psychosocial and organisational changes at the development, introduction and use of computers and later what we name ICT. I focus on all the changes that occur at the interplay between ICT, Society, and Human Beings. SI includes research that are labelled as Social impacts of computing, Social analysis of ICT, Studies of Computer-Mediated Communication (CMC), Organizational Design and Management and ICT, Computers and Society, Organizational Informatics, Community Informatics, Media and Communications. There are new terminology contiously.

The following selected books have played a major role in the process of "defining" the social informatics research programs:

- Bradley, G. (2006). *Social and Community Informatics - Humans on the Net*. London/ New York, UK/NY: Routledge.
- Bradley, G. (Ed.) (2001). *Humans on the Net. Information and Communication Technology (ICT) Work Organization and Human Beings*. Stockholm, SE: Prevent.
- Bradley, G. E., & Hendrick, H. W. (Eds.) (1994, May 29-June 1). Human factors in organizational design and management: Development, introduction, and use of new technology challenges for human organization and human resource development in a

Figure 2. The convergence theory on ICT, society and human beings (Bradley 2006)

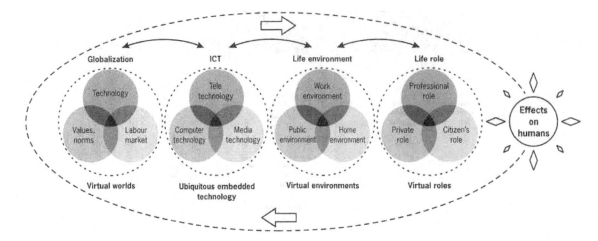

changing world. In *Proceedings of the 4th International Symposium on Organizational Design and Management (ODAMIV)*, Stockholm, Sweden. Amsterdam, London, New York, & Tokyo: Elsevier.

- Bradley, G. (1989). *Computers and the Psychosocial Work Environment*. London/Philadelphia, UK/PA: Taylor & Francis.

A model to capture the broader concepts and the dynamics of their interrelations - "Convergence Model - ICT and Psychosocial Life Environment" is presented in Figure 2 (Source:Bradley 2001 and 2006)

2. Research Projects in Social Informatics

There were five original groups and projects in the research program from 1997 on ICT, Humans, and Society (see below):

- The cross disciplinary research program "Interactive Creative Environments" (ICE-project), that Bradley coordinated at KTH was a strong contribution to "Social Informatics"

- "Networking" (NET)
- "Societal and Psychosocial Challenges and ICT - comparisons between a rural community and a suburban community" (RURBAN)
- "Towards a Global Learning Space - ICT, Learning, and Competence in organisational and societal contexts"
- "Home of the Future - ICT and Changes in human behaviour patterns in the Net Era" (see under "Ongoing Research" below).

3. Network of Excellence: ICT and the Psychosocial Life Environment: Main Changes (Project Coordinator: Gunilla Bradley)

The Network of Excellence was concerned with human organisation and psychosocial work environment related to Information and Communication Technology (ICT), as well as the psychosocial home environment. The purpose was to disseminate and synthesise research with a crossdisciplinary perspective and thereby elaborate on the interaction between ICT and work organisations, human communication, stress, allocation issues, knowledge transfer, and so called "global villages". The purpose was also to contribute to a discussion on desirable actions on various levels and utmost how ICT can be used for deepening human qualities. The participants were distinguished researchers/ professors from Europe and some researchers from USA and South East Asia, about 10 persons. Most of the participants contributed with one chapter in the book "Humans on the Net" subtitled "ICT, Work Organization and Human Beings" (Bradley (Ed.), 2001). The network was established at an EU workshop that I was invited to organise in Brussels 1999.

Research in the 1990´s

In 1991 I returned to Stanford to do the final reporting from the research project on "Knowledge Based Systems and Organisational and Psychosocial aspects" (KBS project) and to develop new research on competence development in 10 high tech companies in Silicon Valley, top ranking in sales, profits and return on sales. Among the companies were both electronic industries and pharmaceutical industries. The focus was on main theories on competence requirements and development as well as strategies for education, in house courses, and on the job training. This study was undertaken in collaboration with the University of Southern California.

In 1991 I was invited to serve as general chair (1992-1994) for the international conference on "Organizational Design and Management (ODAM IV)" with the subtitle "Development, Introduction and Use of New Technology - Challenges for Human Organization and Human Resource Development in a Changing World". Researchers from more than 30 countries in Europe, USA and Asia participated and the proceedings are available in a hardcover book (750 pp) published by Taylor & Francis. I also served as the main editor of the book of proceedings.

In 1989 I received two awards, the "Golden Leaf" for important contributions within research on psychosocial work environment and was elected to the "Professional Woman of the Year" in Sweden.

In 1997 I received the IFIP Namur Award for pioneering crossdisciplinary research on the impact of Information and Communication Technology especially concerning the interaction between Technology, Organization and Humans.

At the Royal Institute of Technology (KTH) starting from 1994, I was involved in extensive research planning, trying to integrate international, national and local research approaches. I thereby served as program manager for the interdisciplinary research on "Interactive Creative Environments" (ICE) with the subtitle "Computers, Networks and Organizational Design Supporting Technology Transfer". The program was coordinated from the Department of Teleinformatics, KTH. I collaborated with Faculty from the following disciplines; Social psychology and Pedagogics; Industrial economy; Regional planning; Social anthropology; Ethnology; Law and Informatics; Teleinformatics. The ICE project was directly associated with the interdisciplinary research and education program between Stanford and Swedish universities (Sweden Silicon Valley Link Program; S-SVL-program.)

In the middle of the 1990s I initiated a regional development and research project supported by the EU programs "Employment" and "Adapt". The project contained the development and implementation of an IT-center to support the upstart and survival of small enterprises in a rural area as well as strengthening the citizen's role in the community. The research part concerned analyses of the development of networks and IT-supported organizational structures, employment rate, various aspects of quality of life, and integration of immigrants into the Swedish work life. This brought me back to my home village in Småland in the rural area in the South of Sweden. A R&D strategy was to integrate my academic, industrial, and local community networks.

Research in the 1970´s and the 1980´s

The very first part of my research focused on women in work life. I made a broad study of employees in a large commercial bank (Svenska Handelsbanken) in 1968. Based on this study I presented my Ph D thesis, entitled "Woman and Career" in 1972. I then specialized in organizational behavior and information technology and initiated and led an interdisciplinary research program on computerization and its effects on structural and psychosocial changes in working life. Researchers in Department of Business Administration, Psychology, Computer Science and Sociology joined my research group at the Department of Sociology, Stockholm University. Initially I developed two theoretical models with two levels of abstraction on the relation between information technology and changes in working life. They were tested empirically in three main companies, representing three main historical phases in computer technology; batch systems with mainframe computers, on line systems with visual display terminals, and systems with micro-computers. The companies included the Swedish post office, an insurance company and an electronic industry.

Within the project on microcomputerization, two professional roles in a multinational electronic industry, were analyzed both historically and in relation to the use of computer support in the work process. The subproject "The Role of Engineers and the New Computer Technology" concerned the most common traditional male profession at the time and the engineers were using CAD systems (computer aided design). The subproject "The Role of Secretaries using Word Processing" deals with the most common traditional female profession at the time.

While a visiting research professor at Stanford university in 1987, I designed a research plan for a project entitled "Knowledge based systems (KBS, applied AI) and the Psychosocial and Organizational Impact". At that time artificial intelligence (AI) was discussed mainly in computer science and philosophy. I made a pilot study in an electronic company close to Stanford and with interviewed AI pioneer scholars at the Stanford and Berkley Universities. Then I formulated a set of hypotheses and carried out the empirical studies in Sweden in three frontline companies; an electronic production industry, an aircraft industry, and a commercial bank – with support of two Swedish research foundations.

ONGOING RESEARCH

In my present role as professor emerita I am mainly serving in the following roles: Chair of one annual international conference; Member of scientific advisory boards of international conferences (IFIP, HCII, IADIS, CIRN, ODAM) and international journals; Reviewer/Referee for full professorships; Key note speaker; Mentor.

Mentorship and "The Third Task of the Universities"

My present research encompasses to a large extent mentorship for junior and senior scientists and contributions to disseminate research information outside the university (the so called "third task" of the Swedish universities). Examples are invitations to serve as key note speaker, presentations of my latest books for various audiences, contributions with chapters in books intended to be used as textbooks. Advocating at School of ICT, KTH and other universities and centres is still another task. The purpose is to bring the behavioural and the social sciences closer to the technical IT related disciplines. The intension is to change the imbalance in R&D between the "technological push" and a "people push" , with the basic purpose to contribute to technology applications from a deeper understanding of the work place, the home and the society. The vision is to move from technology for all to quality of life for all - towards a society where people´s basic needs for belonging, influence, meaningfulness are fulfilled.

The Home of the Future: Information and Communication Technology (ICT) Changes in Society and Human Behaviour Patterns in the Net Era

The overall purpose of the research project concerns ICT and changes in society and human behaviour patterns in the Net Era. The objective is to describe and analyse the ongoing social changes with focus on 'working from home' and 'homing from work' - emphasized by the increased use of ICT-related services and products. The home is considered both as a physical and a virtual space. To obtain an in-depth understanding of the change of peoples' life roles in the Net Era, analyses of human and organizational behaviour related to the professional role, private role and citizen's role are performed.

A crossdisciplinary approach characterizes the research. International comparative analyses between environments in network organizations are used. Three types of field studies were included, covering strategic organizations (homes) - one urban, one suburban and one rural in Sweden. International comparative studies with a cross disciplinary approach were done in US West and East Coast, Singapore & Malaysia, and Japan.

The big challenge in the near future is "intelligent environments" and "intelligent living" in a broad sense. The process of change is both socially driven and technology driven. Driving technology forces are the converging and embedded technologies (ubiquitous and ambient technology).

The following trends are enforcing the home as a communication sphere and the basis for a lot of activities and experiences which are connected

to human needs: The home as the extended family centre; The home as a care centre; The home as a multimedia centre; The home as a centre for democratic dialogue; The home as a market place; The home as a learning centre. These trends are crucial for both many industries in the future e g paper and electronic industries, construction, telecom industries and organisation and new "intermediaries". Analyses from this project are included in my current publications.

Quality of Life in Research at the School of ICT

The aim of the project is to understand how "quality of life and well-being for all" is involved in basic research as well as in the more applied sciences. Interviews are made with most research leaders and professor colleagues at the School of ICT, approaching how they perceive that their research, directly or indirectly, in short term or in long term perspective, will contribute to a larger societal context and to values on various levels of analysis: quality of life, well-being, integrity, security, trust, health, deepening of democracy, personal growth, sustainability and other ethical considerations. Discussions are held on how the chain of reasoning could be described with regard to these concerns, also identifying various actors (driving forces) contributing to the "Good ICT Society". Experiences from this project is valid for my mentoring and advisory role. The key words applied were: Quality of life, research policy, social construction, socioeconomic and environmental impact, technology innovation, sustainability.

Syntheses

A new period in the research process was composing a textbook for international use: Bradley (2006) "Social and Community Informatics – Humans on the Net", (Routledge). I am currently lecturing internationally and in Sweden, thereby contributing to "Social Informatics" and/or "Community

Informatics" which are established as academic disciplines and/or cross disciplinary research centers/institutes at universities in several countries. World conferences in the field are held e g IFIP (International Federation for Information Processing) - conference on"Social Informatics – An Information Society for All" HCC7 in 2006, Maribor (Slovenia) and annual conferences in "Community Informatics" (CIRN) in Prato (Italy). The discipline Informatics has grown to focus the use of ICT in work life, private live and the role as citizen. This broad research field has also become a main concern in many other disciplines and centres.

In 2007 and 2008 I held doctoral courses in Social and Community Informatics, based on my latest book at Helsinki Technical University and Salzburg University, where she served as guest professor in 2008 at Paris Lodron University in Salzburg and the ICT & Society Center.

Since 2008 I am the Chair of the annual IADIS conference on "ICT, Society and Human Beings". The first international conference was held in Amsterdam, and the second took place in Algarve in Portugal, in 2008. IADIS= International Association for Developing the Information Society. Next one will be held in Freiburg, Germany in 2010.

Sustainable Development and ICT is the content of a special issue of the International Journal of Information, Communication Society (iCS) in 2010, where I serve as co-editor.

Figure 2 is the theoretical model on the societal and social changes in the Network Society, further described in a chapter in this Festschrift on request from the Editors.

PEDAGOGICAL ACTIVITIES AND EXPERIENCES: SELECTED LIST

- Advisor for graduate students often with a crossdisciplinary orientation; computer science, educational psychology, sociology, and psychology
- Advisor for doctoral students from Dept. of Informatics, Dept of Computer and System Sciences, Dept of Business Administration and Dept of Educational Psychology, for Universities abroad external advisor and external examiner.
- Author of 13 books, most of which have been or are being used for educational purposes .
- In 1996-1997 I organized a crossdisciplinary "IT-pedagogical" seminar series entitled "Toward a Global Learning Space" within the Sweden-Silicon Valley Link program and with invited lecturers with deep and broad knowledge in the field. The purpose was to create a meeting place for researchers and doctoral students from mainly three academic areas; organizational and social psychology, pedagogics and IT-related disciplines within KTH. The seminars discussed and identified important research areas in the interface between IT research and the behavioral sciences.
- In 1998- 1999, I organized a seminar series in Informatics with invited international researchers open to all teachers and doctoral students.
- In 1998 -1999, I organized a doctoral course "ICT and Worklife2000" for informatic students in the north of Sweden: Luleå Technical University, Umeå University, Mid-Sweden university. This course was a strong start for NIRS (Nordic Informatics Research School).
- In 2000 – 2009 advisor for doctoral students and mentor for senior researchers in Sweden and internationally
- In 2004 and 2005 lectures at the international master student course at KTH "ICT and Global Management"
- In 2007 Doctorial Courses in Social and Community Informatics at Helsinki Tech-

nical University, Finland and in 2008 at Salzburg University, ICT & Society Center

- Invited key note speaker – see under "Key Note Speaker, Committees, Boards and other functions" in the CV.

KEY NOTE SPEAKER, COMMITTEES, BOARDS AND OTHER FUNCTIONS

Invited Key Note Speaker

- *International Ergonomics Association* IEA 2000 Congress San Diego July 30– Aug 4.
- Nordic delegate and speaker at *World Information Technology Forum (WITFOR)*, Vilnius 2003. Organizer: IFIP under the auspices of UNESCO and hosted by the Government of Lithuania.
- International conference on *Risk and Safety Management in Industry, Logistics, Transport and Military Service: New Solutions for the 21st Century*. Tallinn Technical University, March 2003.
- *IFIP Summer School on Risks and Challenges of the Network Society* Karlstad, August 4 – 8, 2003.
- *The International Conference on Assistive Technology (ICAT 2003)*, organised by the British Computer Society. London, December 2-3, 2003.
- *8ᵗʰ International Conference on Human Aspects of Advanced Manufacturing Agility & Hybrid Automation (Haamaha 2003)*. Rome, May 26-30, 2003.
- *9ᵗʰ International Conference on Human Aspects of Advanced Manufacturing Agility & Hybrid Automation, Haamaha 2004)*. Galway, Ireland, August 25-27, 2004.
- *International Association for Development of the Information Society (IADIS) Inter-*

national Conference E-society 2004, Avila Spain, July 16-19, 2004.

- *International Association for Development of the Information Society (IADIS) Conference on Web Based Communities*. Algarve, Portugal February 23-25, 2005
- *VIS 2005 Visions of the Information Society Conference*, EMPA, Technology and Society Laboratory, Empa -ETH, St. Gallen, Switzerland, November 3–4, 2005
- *The 8ᵗʰ International Scientific Conference on Human Factors in Organizational Design and Management (ODAM VIII)*. Maui, USA June 22-25, 2005.
- *CIRN (Community Informatics Research Network) conference on "Community Informatics – Prospects for Communities and Action"*, Prato, Italy, November 5-7, 2007
- *CIRN (Community Informatics Research Network) conference "ICTs for Social Inclusion: What is the Reality"*, Prato, Italy, October 27-30, 2008
- *IFIP Converging Technology Conference – "The Convergence Theory on ICT and Psychosocial Life Environment". IFIP WG 9.2 Computers and Social Accountability. Maribour, Slovenia, May 17-18, 2010.*

Committees and Boards

- Expert evaluator on professorships: Stanford University, School of Education; University of Wisconsin, School of Engineering; University of Southern California, Dept of Human Factors and Systems Sciences; Umeå University, Dept of Informatics; Växjö University, Institution of Mathematics and System Technology, Informatics Department; Luleå Technical University.
- Expert evaluator on docent competency: Lund University, Dept. of Informatics; Umeå University, Dept. of Informatics, Uppsala

University, Dept of Computer and Information Science.

- Numerous doctoral thesis committee memberships e g at Royal Institute of Technology (KTH), Dept of Industrial Economy and Organization, Stockholm University (SU), Dept of Business Administration, SU/KTH Dept of Computer and Systems Science, Technical University of Luleå, Dept of Work Science, Umeå University Dept. of Informatics, Gothenburg University, Dept. of Informatics, Linköping University, Dept of Computer and Information Science, external reviewer at Helsinki Technical University Finland and Monash University Australia.
- Opponent on Ph D theses at various departments and universities.
- Chair of IEA-ODAM Technical Group 1992-1994 (IEA=International Ergonomics Association, ODAM= Organizational Design and Management)
- Board member of the - Swedish Center for Working Life. Appointed by the Swedish government
- Member of The Swedish National Committee of Psychology, associated with International Council of Scientific Union (ICSU), appointed by the Swedish Academy of Sciences
- Member of the Committee for Research Information in the Swedish Council for Planning and Coordination of research (FRN)
- Member of the program committee for HCII conference, from 1987 to 2009, International Conferences (HCII = Human Computer Interaction International)
- Faculty member of Nordic Interactive Network Organisation
- Board member for the Conference on Visions of the Information Society (VSIS), EMPA, St. Gallen, Switzerland 2005
- Expert in the Swedish Governmental Committee on Electronic Communication 2004

- Member of international advisory committee for "ICT & Society Center", University of Salzburg, Austria

Advisory Boards and Programme Committees in 2010

- Member of editorial board of the journal "Information and Communication Society", iCS (Routledge)
- Honorary member of the editorial board of "Triple C-cognition, ommunication, cooperation". Open Access Journal for a Global Sustainable Information Society.
- Member of the program committee for HCII Conferences (HCII = Human Computer Interaction International
- Member of the Scientific Advisory Board for Human Computer Interaction International (HCII)
- Member of the International Ergonomics Association (IEA) and the Cmmittee on Organisational Design and Management (ODAM) within IEA.
- International Federation of Information Processing (IFIP): Board member of IFIP work groups: WG 9.1 Computers and Work, WG 9.3 Home Oriented Informatics and Telematics, WG 9.9 CT and Sustainable Development
- Chair of the annual IADIS conference on "ICT, Society and Human Beings" IADIS - International Association for Developing the Information Society (NGO org.)
- Member of the organisation committee of the annual Community Informatics conferences, at the Monash Centre, Prato, Italy
- Member of Community Informatics Research Network (CIRN)

Figure 3. A family photo of Gunilla Bradley (the photo has been created by Adobe Photoshop support).

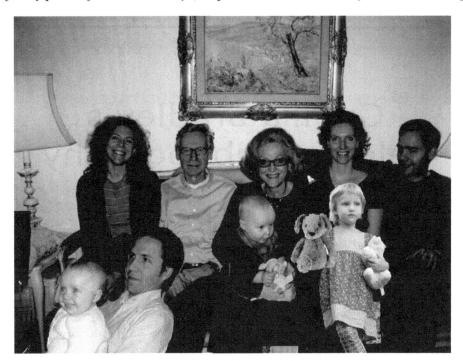

CV > AWARDS

- The "Namur Award" from International Federation for Information Processing (IFIP) for pioneering research to increase the awareness of the social and psychological impact of ICT.
- The "Golden Leaf" award for important contributions and for special contribution and research in the field of psychosocial work environment, from the Professional Association for Psychologists in Sweden.
- "Professional Woman of the Year" in Sweden, by the Association for Business and Professional Women, BPW Sweden.
- Received the "Honors Lectureship Award", University of Central Florida, USA.
- Three grandchildren, born 2006 (Lydia), 2009 (Nadja), 2009 (Cate) (see Figure 3).

Gunilla Bradley's Selected Bibliography

Figure 1. Professor emerita Gunilla Bradley (Photo: Janne Åhman)

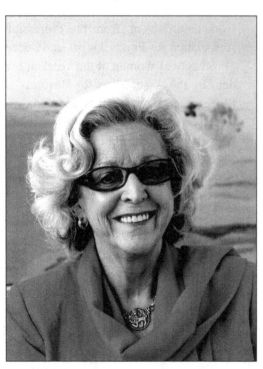

BOOKS

Bradley, G. (2006). *Social and Community Informatics - Humans on the Net*. London/New York, UK/NY: Routledge.

Bradley, G. (Ed.) (2001). *Humans on the Net. Information and Communication Technology (ICT) Work Organization and Human Beings*. Stockholm, SE: Prevent. ISBN 91-7522-701-0.

Bradley, G. E., & Hendrick, H. W. (Eds.) (1994, May 29-June 1). Human factors in organizational design and management: Development, introduction, and use of new technology challenges for human organization and human resource development in a changing world. In *Proceedings of the 4th International Symposium on Organizational Design and Management (ODAM IV)*, Stockholm, Sweden. Amsterdam, London, New York, & Tokyo: Elsevier.

Bradley, G. (1989). *Computers and the Psychosocial Work Environment*. London/Philadelphia, UK/PA: Taylor & Francis.

Bradley, G., Bergström, C., & Lindeberg, S. (1988). *The Role of Engineers and The New Computer Technology* (In Swedish: *Ingenjörsrollen och den framtida datatekniken*. Stockholm, SE: Carlssons.

Bradley, G. (1986). *Psykosocial arbetsmiljö och datorer* (1st edition). Stockholm, SE: Akademiliteratur. Natur & Kultur 1988, (2ed edition).

Bradley, G. Bergström, C., & Sundberg, L. (1984). *The Role of Secretaries and Word Processing Systems – Office Work in Transition (In Swedish: Sekreterarrollen vid ord- och textbehandling - kontorsyrke i förändring)*. Stockholm, SE: University.

Bradley, G. (1981). *Work Environment and Display terminals – social psychological aspects of the work environment. (In Swedish: "Arbetsmiljö och Bildskärmsterminaler - socialpsykologiska aspekter av arbetsmiljön)*. Arbetsmiljöfonden, Stockholm, SE: Liber förlag/Allmänna förlaget.

Bradley, G. (1979). *Professional Roles and Quality of Life, (In Swedish: Yrkesroller och Livsmiljö)*. Stockholm, SE: Wahlström, & Widstrands vardagspsykologiserie.

Bradley, G. (1977). *Computer technology, Work life and Communication (In Swedish: Datateknik, arbetsliv och kommunikation*. The Swedish Delegation for long term motivated research. (Swedish: Samarbetskommittén för långsiktsmotiverad forskning - Forskningsrådsnämnden (FRN). Stockholm, SE: Liber förlag.

Bradley, G., Börjesson, K., Lundgren, M. (1974). *Salaried Employees and Work Environment (in Swedish Tjänstemän och Arbetsmiljö)*. Presented at the TCO congress in 1972. Stockholm: TCO report (Central Federation of Salaried Employees in Sweden).

Bradley, G. (1972). *Women and Carrear. A study on womens interest in promotion in relation to work satisfaction, home environment and edutional background. (In Swedish: Kvinnan och karriären. En studie om kvinnors befordringsintresse i relation till arbetstillfredsställelse, hemmiljö och skolutbildning)*. Doctorial thesis at Depatment of Educational Psychology, Gothenburg university. Published as a book. Stockhom, SE: PA-rådet.

Bradley, G. (1970). *Work Attitudes and Interest in Promotion with Female Bank Employees. (In Swedish: Arbetsattityder och befordringsintresse hos kvinnliga bankanställda)*. Licentiat thesis at the Department of Educational Psychology. Gothenberg University. Published as a book. Stockholm, SE: PA-Rådet.

PUBLICATIONS 2003 AND LATER

Bradley, G. (2003). Människan i IT- samhälle (Humans in the ICT society). *Book chapter in the anthology Friskfaktorer (Factors for Good Health)*. Stockhom, SE: Prevent (Management and Labour Improving Work Environment).

Bradley, G. (2003). ICT for Deepening Human and Societal Qualities. (Invited presentation) at the World Information Technology Forum (WITFOR), Vilnius 2003. Organizer: IFIP under the auspices of UNESCO and hosted by the Government of Lithuania. In WITFOR 2003 White Book (Dipak Khakhar (Ed.). *IFIP World Information Technology Forum*. Laxenburg, AU: IFIP Press.

Bradley, G. (2003). Humans on the Net - Psychosocial Life Environment in the E-society (key note speech). In *Risk and Safety Management in Industry, Logistics, Transport and Military Service: New Solutions for the 21st Century*. Tallinn Technical University.

Bradley, G. (2003). Theories on the impact of information and communication technology on the psychosocial life environment. In D. Harris, V. Duffy, M. Smith, & C. Stephanidis (Eds.), *Human - Centred Computing - Cognitive, Social and Ergonomic Aspects, Vol.3*, Proceedings of HCI International 2003 in Crete, Greece. London, UK: Lawrence Erlbaum Associates, Publishers.

Bradley, G. (2004). Humans on the Net - Psychosocial Life Environment in the E-society (key note speech). At the 8´th *International Conference on Human Aspects of Advanced Manufacturing Agility & Hybrid Automation* (Haamaha 2004), May. Rome, Italy.

Bradley, G. (2004). Humans on the Net - Risks and Opportunities in the Net Era. (Key not speech). At the *IFIP Summer School*, Karlstad, August 4 - 8, 2003. In P. Duquenoy, S. Fischer Hubner, J. Holvast, & A. Zuccato (Eds.), *Risks and Challenges of the Network Society*. Karlstad Universtiy Studies.

Jansson, E., & Bradley, G. (2005). Sustainability in Collaborative Network Structures - with focus on the Psychosocial Work Environment in Distributed Teams. *Proceedings of the CIRN conference on Sustainability and Community Technology: What does this mean for Community Informatics?* Monash Centre, Prato, Italy.

Bradley, G. (2005). Towards Global Villages - Networks in action. *Proceedings of the CIRN conference on Sustainability and Community Technology: What does this mean for Community Informatics?* Monash Centre. Centre for Community Networking Research School of Information Management & Systems, Prato: Monash University and Community Informatics Research Network (CIRN).

Bradley, G. (2005). The Convergence Theory on Information and Communication Technology (ICT) and the Psychosocial Life Environment - The Connected Home. In G. Smith, & G. Salvendy (Eds.), *Proceedings of the HCI International 2005 conference*. Mahwah, NJ: Lawrence Erlbaum Associates, Inc.

Bradley, G. (2005). Sustainability in the E-society workplace - Theory and reflection on ICT and Psychosocial Communication. In G. Smith, & G. Salvendy (Eds.), *Proceedings of the HCI International 2005 conference*. Mahwah, NJ: Lawrence Erlbaum Associates, Inc.

Bradley, G. (2005). *Information and Communication Technology (ICT) for Deepening Human and Societal Qualities.* Invited key note speech. In P. Carayon, M. Robertson, B. Kleiner, & P. Hoonakker (Eds.), *Human Factors in Organizational Design and Management - VIII. Proceedings of the The 8th International Scientific Conference on Human Factors in Organizational Design and Management.* Maui, USA June 22-25. Santa Monica: IEA Press.

Bradley, G. (2005). Towards Global Villages - Networks in action. *Community Informatics Research Network (CIRN) -, Colloquium and Conference Proceedings 2005.* Centre for Community Networking Research School of Information Management & Systems, Monash University and Community Informatics Research Network.

Bradley, G. (2005). The Convergence Theory on Information and Communication Technology (ICT) and the Psychosocial Life Environment – The Connected Home. In G. Salvendy (Ed). *Proceedings of the HCI International 2005 conference*. Mahwah, NJ: Lawrence Erlbaum Associates, Inc.

Bradley, G. (2005). Sustainability in the E-society workplace – Theory and reflection on ICT and Psychosocial Communication. In G. Salvendy (Ed). *Proceedings of the HCI International 2005 conference.* Mahwah, NJ: Lawrence Erlbaum Associates, Inc.

Bradley, G. (2005). Information and Communication Technology (ICT) for Deepening Human and Societal Qualities. In P. Carayon, M. Robertson, B. Kleiner, & P. Hoonakker (Eds.), *Human Factors in Organizational Design and Management - VIII. Proceedings of the The 8th International Scientific Conference on Human Factors in Organizational Design and Management.* Maui, USA June 22-25. Santa Monica: IEA Press.

Bradley, G. (2005). *Social and Community Informatics – Humans on the Net.* Invited key note speech at IADIS (International Association for Development of the Information Society) 2005 on "Web Based Communities", Algarve, Portugal, February 23-25, 2005.

Bradley, G. (2005). *Social Informatics – Humans in the Network Society.* Invited key note speech at the international conference "Visions of the Information Society Conference (VIS)", Empa, Swiss Federal Laboratories for Materials Testing and Research. St Gallen, Switzerland, November 3-4, 2005.

Bradley, G. (2005). *Information and Communication Technology (ICT) for Deepening Human and Societal Qualities.* Invited key note speech at Human Factors in Organizational Design and Management – *VIII*, Maui, Hawaii, USA, June 22-25, 2005. (Also in book of proceedings). IEA Press.

Bradley, G. (2006). *Social and Community Informatics – Humans on the Net.* London/New York, UK/NY: Routledge.

Bradley, G. (2006). Social Informatics – From Theory to Actions for the Good ICT Society. In J. Berleur, M. Nurminen, & J. Impagliazzo (Eds.), *Social Informatics: An Information Society for All? In Remembrance of Rob Kling* (pp. 383-394). UK: Springer.

Bradley, G. (2007). *Collaboration between people for Sustainability in the ICT Society.* In M.J. Smith, G. Salvendy (Eds.), Human Interface, Part II, Proceedings *at the HCI International 2007* (pp. 703-712). Berlin Heidelberg: Springer-Verlag.

Bradley, G. (2007). *Is there a theory in Community Informatics*? Invited talk at CIRN (Community Informatics Research Network) conference on "Community Informatics – Prospects for Communities and Action", Prato, Italy, November 5-7, 2007. Wikipedia.

Bradley, G. (Ed.) (2008*). ICT, Society and Human Beings.* Proceedings of IADIS Multi Conferencce on Computer Science and Information Systems. Amsterdam, NL: IADIS Press.

Bradley, G. (2009). From a Rural Village to a High Tech Urban Environment - Research and some Reflections from a Community Informatics Perspective. *Key note speech at the 5th Prato Community Informatics & Development Informatics Conference 2008: ICTs for Social Inclusion: What is the Reality?* 27 October-30 October, Monash Centre, Prato Italy.

Bichler, R. M., Bradley, G., Hofkirchner, W. (2010). Editorial Comment. Sustainable Development and ICTs. *Information, Communication & Society,* 13(1). London, UK: Routledge.

PUBLICATIONS 1994-2002

Bradley, G. E. & Hendrick, H. W. (Eds.) (1994). *Human Factors in Organizational Design and Management subtitle "Development, Introduction and Use of New Technology- Challenges for Human Organization and Human Resource Development in a Changing World"*. Proceedings from The 4ᵗʰ International Symposium on Organizational Design and Management (ODAM IV). Amsterdam/London/NY/Tokyo: North Holland, Elsevier.

Bradley, G. (1995). Macroergonomic Approaches to Creating Real Change. Symposium overview. *Proceedings of the Human Factors and Ergonomics Society Annual Meeting*, October 9-13, 1995. San Diego, USA.

Bradley, G. (1995, March). Datorn - En dörr för visioner (Computers - a Door for Visions). *Digitalen*, 9-11.

Bradley, G. (1996). Implementing Virtual Organizations - Challenges for rural areas. In *Proceedings from the 1ˢᵗ International Conference on Applied Ergonomics (ICAE '96)*. Istanbul, Turkey.

Bradley, G., & Bradley, W. (1996). Computers in the Bakery - From Theory to Action. In O. Brown, & H. W. Hendrick (Eds.), *Human Factors in Organizational Design and Management-V*, *Proceedings from ODAM V*, Amsterdam: Elsevier Science.

Bradley, G., & Bradley, W. (1997). Teleinformatics in a Global Village - From Baking to IT, In G. Salvendy, M. J. Smith, & R. J. Koubek (Eds.), *Design of Computing Systems. Proceedings of the Seventh International Conference on Human-Computer Interaction.* Amsterdam/Lausanne/New York/Oxford/Shannan/Tokyo: Elsevier.

Bradley, G. (1997). Interactive Creative Environments (ICE) - strategic organizational and psychosocial factors. In G. Salvendy, M. J. Smith, & R. J. Koubek (Eds.), *Design of Computing Systems. Proceedings of the Seventh International Conference on Human-Computer Interaction.* Amsterdam/Lausanne/New York/Oxford/Shannan/Tokyo: Elsevier.

Robertson, M., & Bradley, G. (1997). Competence development in ten high tech companies in Silicon Valley. In G. Salvendy, M. J. Smith, & R. J. Koubek (Eds.), *Design of Computing Systems. Proceedings of the Seventh International Conference on Human-Computer Interaction.* Amsterdam/Lausanne/New York/Oxford/Shannan/Tokyo: Elsevier.

Bradley, G., & Bradley, W. (1997). Rural and suburban settlements as teleinformatic organizations - some comparisons and some challenges from Ekistic Macroergonomics. In P. Seppälä et.al. (Eds.), *From Experience to Innovation. Proceedings of the 13th Triennial Congress of the International Ergonomics Association.* Tampere: Finnish Institute of Occupational Health.

Bradley, G., & Bradley, W. (1997). Humans in the information society - from batch processing to network computers ", In P. Seppälä et.al. (Eds.), *From Experience to Innovation. Proceedings of the 13th Triennial Congress of the International Ergonomics Association.* Tampere: Finnish Institute of Occupational Health.

Bradley, G. (1998). Humans in the Information and Communication Society - how we will live, learn, and work" *IFIP Namur Award speech*, electronically published http://www.info.fundp.ac.be/~jbl/IFIP/NALectures.html

Bradley, G., & Bradley W. (1998). Towards Global Villages - Networks in action. In P. Vink, E.A.P. Konigsveld, & S. Dhondt (Eds.), *Human Factors in Organizational Design and Management-VI. Proceedings from ODAM VI.* Amsterdam: Elsevier Science.

Bradley, G. (1998). To Live, to Learn and to Work in the IT society, (In Swedish: Leva, lära och arbeta i IT-samhället). *The journal of Miljön på jobbet.* Stockholm, SE: Arbetarskyddsstyrelsen.

Bradley, G. (1998). Information Technology and Human Communication (In Swedish Informationsteknik och mänsklig kommunikation). In the journal of *Blickpunkten*, 1. Stockholm, SE: Inrikesdepartementet.

Bradley, G. (1999). Networks in Action. In *Proceedings from the 9th European Congress on Work and Organizational Psychology*, Espoo-Helsinki, Finland.

Bradley, L., Andersson, N., & Bradley, G. (2000). *Home of the Future - Information and Communication Technology (ICT) - changes in society and human behavior patterns in the net era.* FSCN Report R00-1. Mid Sweden.

Bradley, L., & Bradley, G. (2000). Home of the Future and ICT - Integration of professional and private roles. *Special issue of "Ergonomics", Vol. 43, No. 6 and included in the congress CD-ROM proceedings at the IEA/HFES 2000 Congress*, San Diego, USA.

Bradley, G. (2000).The Information and Communication Society: How people will live and work in the new millennium. *Special issue of "Ergonomics", Vol. 43, No. 6 and included in the congress CD-ROM proceedings at the IEA/ HFES 2000 Congress*, San Diego, USA. London: Taylor & Francis.

Bradley, L., & Bradley, G. (2000). Home of the Future- integration of professional and private roles. *Proceedings of IEA2000/HFES2000 Congress.* London: Taylor&Francis.

Bradley, G. (Ed.) (2001). Humans on the Net. Information and Communication Technology (ICT) Work Organization and Human Beings. Stockholm, SE: Prevent.

Bradley, G. (2001). Theoretical Perspective on the Impact of Information and Communication Technology (ICT) on our Psychosocial Life Environment". In M. J. Smith & G. Salvendy (Eds.), *Systems, Social and Internationalization Design Aspects of Human-Computer Interaction* (pp. 76-80). Mahwah, NJ: Lawrence Erlbaum Ass. Inc., Publishers.

Bradley, L., & Bradley, G. (2001). The Home as a Virtual and Physical Space - Experiences from USA and South-East Asia". In M. J. Smith & G. Salvendy (Eds.), *Systems, Social and Internationalization Design Aspects of Human - Computer Interaction* (pp. 81-85). Mahwah, NJ:Lawrence Erlbaum Ass. Inc., Publishers.

Bradley, G. (2001). Information and Communication Technology (ICT) and Humans: how we will live, learn and work. In G. Bradley (Ed.), *Humans on the Net* (pp. 22-44). Stockholm, SE: Prevent.

Bradley, G., & Bradley, L. (2001). Home of the Future and ICT - Integration of professional and private roles". In G. Bradley (Ed.), *Humans on the Net* (pp. 197 -222). Stockholm, SE: Prevent.

Bradley, G. (2002). Theoretical Perspective on the Interplay Between ICT and Quality of Life. In K. Brunnstein & J. Berleur (Eds.), *Human Choice and Computers: Issues of Choice and Quality of Life in the Information Society* (pp. 31- 41). Boston / Dordrecht / London: Kluver Academic Publishers.

Bradley, G. (2002). Human needs in the IT society. In *Proceedings of the 6th International Scientific Conference on Work With Display Units - WWDU 2002* (pp 40-41). Berlin: Egonomic Institut fur Arbeits- und Sozialforschung.

Bradley, G. (2002). Information and Communication Technology (ICT) and Changes in Work Life: Macroergonomic Considerations. In H. W. Hendrick & B. M. Kleiner (Eds.) *Macroergonomics Theory, Methods, and Applications* (pp. 173 – 178). Mahwah, NJ: Lawrence Erlbaum Ass. Inc., Publishers.

Bradley, G. (2002). *The Brave New World – Interview with Gunilla Bradley. (In Swedish Du Sköna Nya Värld).* In the book Scenes from a Work Life – 60 Years with Arbetarskyddsnämnden (now Prevent). Prevent: Collaborative Organisation for Workers Health and Safety Stockholm, SE: Prevent.

PUBLICATIONS 1970-1993

Research Reports and Books (1970-1993)

Bradley, G. (1970). *Work Attitudes and Interest in Promotion with Female Bank Employees. (In Swedish: Arbetsattityder och befordringsintresse hos kvinnliga bankanställda).* Licentiat thesis at the Department of Educational Psychology. Gothenberg University. Published as a book. Stockholm, SE: PA-Rådet.

Bradley, G. (1972). *Women and Carrear. A study on womens interest in promotion in relation to work satisfaction, home environment and edutional background. (In Swedish: Kvinnan och karriären. En studie om kvinnors befordringsintresse i relation till arbetstillfredsställelse, hemmiljö och skolutbildning).* Doctorial thesis at Depatment of Educational Psychology, Gothenburg university. Published as a book. Stockhom, SE: PA-rådet.

Bradley, G. (1972). *Women's interest in promotion in relation to job satisfaction and home and school background.* Rapport från Pedagogiska Institutionen. Göteborg (Sammanläggningsdel av doktorsavhandling, (nr 1+2 ovan).

Bradley, G.. & Patkai, P. (1974). *Shift Work at Mechanized Logging in the Forest – Social psychological and Psycho-physiological aspects.* (In Swedish: *Skiftarbete vid mekaniserad avverkning i skogsbruket - socialpsykologiska och psykofysiologiska aspekter).* Garpenberg: Skogshögskolan, Institutionen för skogsteknik. Report no 66.

Bradley, G, Börjesson, K, Lundgren, M (1974). *Salaried Employees and Work Environment (in Swedish Tjänstemän och Arbetsmiljö).* Presented at the TCO congress in 1972. Stockholm: TCO report (Central Federation of Salaried Employees in Sweden).

Bradley, G., & Nilsson, I. (1977). *Arbetsmiljö och datorisering. En sammanfattning av delrapport I oh II.* Stockholms universitet. RAM- research report no 4.

Bradley, G. (1977). *Computer technology, Work life and Communication (In Swedish: Datateknik, arbetsliv och kommunikation.* The Swedish Delegation for long term motivated research. (Swedish: Samarbetskommittén för långsiktsmotiverad forskning - Forskningsrådsnämnden (FRN). Stockholm, SE: Liber förlag.

Bradley, G. (1979). *Samspelet mellan datateknik - arbets- miljö - fysiska och psykiska symptom.* Stockholms universitet. RAM-research report no 6.

Bradley, G. (1981). *Work Environment and Display terminals – social psychological aspects of the work environment. (In Swedish: "Arbetsmiljö och Bildskärmsterminaler - socialpsykologiska aspekter av arbetsmiljön).* Arbetsmiljöfonden, Stockholm, SE: Liber förlag/Allmänna förlaget.

Bradley, G., Bergström, C., & Lindeberg, S. (1988). *The Role of Engineers and The New Computer Technology* (In Swedish: *Ingenjörsrollen och den framtida datatekniken*. Stockholm, SE: Carlssons.

Bradley, G. (1989). *Computers and the Psychosocial Work Environment*. London/Philadelphia: Taylor & Francis (254 s.) Även i svensk version "Psykosocial arbetsmiljö och datorer". Stockholm: Akademiliteratur 1986, första upplagan, Natur & Kultur 1988, andra upplagan.

Bradley, G. (1988). *Computer Technology and Work Life -Knowledge Based Computer Systems - Organizational and Psychological Aspects of their Introduction and Use*. Research application to the Swedish Work Environment Fund. (In English and in Swedish).

Bradley, G. (1989). Knowledge based systems and Work Design. In C. M. Haslegrave, J. R. Wilson, E. N. Corlett, & I. Manenica (Eds.), *Work Design in Practice*. London/Philadelphia: Taylor & Francis.

Bradley, G. (1990). *Communication between People in the Future Office* (In Swedish: *Kommunikation mellan människor i framtidens kontor*. In the journal of *Morgondagens kontor - arbetsliv och teknologi*. Stockholm: Byggnadsstyrelsen - tekniska byråns information.

Bradley, G., & Holm, P. (1990). *Knowledge based systems – Organizational and psychosocial aspects – Early experiences from the Swedish Car Industry*. (In Swedish: *Kunskapsbaserade datorsystem - organisatoriska och psykosociala aspekter. Tidiga erfarenheter från en svensk bilindustri)*. Research report in the KBS- project. Department of International Education, Stockholm University.

Bradley, G., & Holm, P. (1991). *Knowledge based systems – Organisational and psychosocial aspects – Early experiences from a Swedish Commercial Bank* (In Swedish: *Kunskapsbaserade datorsystem -organisatoriska och psykosociala aspekter. Tidiga erfarenheter från en svensk affärsbank)*. Research report in the KBS- project. Department of International Education, Stockholm University.

Bradley, G., & Bradley, L. (1991). *Knowledge based systems – Organisational and psychosocial aspects Early experiences from a Swedish Electronic Industry* (In Swedish: *Kunskapsbaserade datorsystem - organisatoriska och psykosociala aspekter - tidiga erfarenheter från ett elektronikföretag.)* Research report in the KBS- project. Department of International Education, Stockholm University.

Bradley, G., & Holm, P. (1992). *Knowledge based systems – Organisational and psychosocial aspects. Interviews with Experts in AI and KBS in USA and Sweden* (In Swedish: *Kunskapsbaserade datorsystem - organisatoriska och psykosociala aspekter. Intervjuer med experter i USA och Sverige.* Research report in the KBS- project. Department of International Education, Stockholm University.

Bradley, G., & Strömqvist G. (1991). Weaving the Technological and Social Fabric for the Future. *Report from an international conference on Telematics in the Pacific Rim, with special emphasis on Telework and Distance Learning*.

Bradley, G. (1993). *Computer Technology and Work Life – A studie on Knowledge based computer systems – A summary* (In Swedish: *Datateknik och arbetsliv - en studie av kunskapsbaserade datorsystem. Sammanfattning nr 1588)*. Stockholm, SE: Arbetsmiljöfonden.

Popular Science (1970-1993)

Bradley, G. (1979). *Professional Roles and Quality of Life, (In Swedish: Yrkesroller och Livsmiljö).* Stockholm, SE: Wahlström, & Widstrands vardagspsykologiserie.

Bradley, G. (1980). *Datorn och arbetsmiljön. Rapport till TCO-konferensen "Datorutvecklingen - styra eller styras",* okt 1980. RAM-rapport 8.

Bradley, G. (1980). *Computerization and Working Life from a Psychosocial Point of View.* RAM-rapport 9.

Bradley, G., Bergström, C., & Sundberg, L. (1984). *The Role of Secretaries and Word Processing Systems – Office Work in Transition (In Swedish: Sekreterarrollen vid ord- och textbehandling - kontorsyrke i förändring).* Stockholm, SE: University.

Bradley, G. (1986). *Stress and Office Automation (in Swedish: Stress och kontorsautomation).* Stockholm, SE: Teldok.

International Conference Proceedings And International Scientific Articles (1970-1993)

Bradley, G. (1979). Computerization and some Psychosocial factors in the Work Environment. *Proceedings of the conference Reducing Occupational Stress, New York, 1977. NIOSH Publication* (pp. 78-140), (s.30-40). U.S. Department of Health, Education, and Welfare.

Bradley, G. (1983). *Computers and their psychosocial impact especially with regard to women.* Report presented at the International Women's Seminar in Salzburg 1982. RAM-rapport 11.

Bradley, G. (1985). Computers and Work Content, Work Load and Stress - Analyses and Women's participation Strategies. In A. Olerup, L. Schneider & E. Monod (Eds.), *Women, Work and Computerization: Opportunities and Disadvantages. Proceedings of an IFIP conference 1984* (pp. 249-263). Amsterdam, NL: Elsevier Science Publishers B.V. (North Holland).

Bradley, G. (1987). Use of Visual Display Terminals and Psychosocial Work Environment - from Theoretical Model to Action. In B. Knave & P. G. Widebäck (Eds.), *Work with Display Units 86 (WWDU)* (pp. 78-90). Amsterdam, NL: Elsevier Science Publishers B.V. (North Holland).

Bradley, G. (1987). Changing Roles in an Electronic Industry - Engineers Using CAD System and Secretaries Using Word-processing System. In G. Salvendy, S. L. Sauter, & J. J. Hurell, Jr. (Eds.), *The 2nd International Conference on Human-Computer Interaction (HCI). Social Ergonomic and Stress aspects of Work with Computers* (pp. 295-302). Amsterdam, NL: Elsevier Science Publishers B.V. (North-Holland).

Bradley, G. (1988). Women, Work and Computers. In G. Westlander & J. M. Stellman (Eds.), *Government Policy and Women's Health Care. The Swedish Alternative* (pp. 112-132). New York/ London, NY/UK: The Haworth Press.

Bradley, G. (1989). Knowledge based systems - organizational and psychosocial aspects of their introduction and use. In M. J. Smith & G. Salvendy (Eds.). *Work with Computers: Organizational, Mangement, Stress and Health Aspects.* Amsterdam, NL: Elsevier Science Publishers B.V. (North Holland).

Bradley, G. (1989). Knowledge based systems and Work Design. In C. M. Haslegrave, J. R. Wilson, E. N. Corlett, & I. Manenica (Eds.), *Work Design in Practice.* London/Philadelphia: Taylor & Francis.

Bradley, G., & Strömqvist, G. (1990). Computerization and Telecommunications - Future challenges for education-Power, Knowledge and Influence. *The 12ᵗʰ Annual Conference "Pacific Telecommunications: Weaving the Technological and Social Fabric" PTC.* Honolulu, USA.

Bradley, G. (1990). Knowledge-based systems - Swedish experiences of the Social and Psychosocial Impact. In K. Noro, & O. Brown Jr. (Eds.), *Human Factors in the Organizational Design and Management - III.* Amsterdam, NL: Elsevier Science Publishers B.V. (North-Holland).

Bradley, G., Steere, M., & Strömqvist, G. (1991). Engineers Using Computer - Aided Design and Knowledge-based systems: Changing Professional roles. *International Journal of Human Factors in Manufacturing,* 1(3) 221-232.

Bradley, G. (1991, August). *Work Environment and Computers. New Technology Work Organization and Professional Roles.* Paper presented at People Productivity Computers, a seminar about how modern computer support and robot support should be organized. Organized by LO, SFO and PTK. Uppsala, Sweden.

Bradley, G. (1991, July). Psychosocial Environment and the Information Age. Paper presented at the IFIP WG 9.2 International Summer School on Social Citizenship in the Information Age (see no C20), Brighton.

Bradley, G. (1991). *The Changing Role of Engineers: from Traditional Technology to Knowledge Based Systems.* Participation in a panel "Facilitating crosscultural diversity in the technology change process", at the 11'th Congress International Ergonomics Association (IEA). Paris 15-20 July, 1991.

Bradley, G. (1991). Organizational Communication and Computer Technology - Empirical research findings and future trends. Special plenary session on "Macroergonmics: contemporary issues and applications" at the 11'th IEA Congress. Paris 15-20 July, 1991.

Bradley, G., & Robertson, M. (1991, July). *Computers, Psychosocial Work Environment, and Stress. A comparative theoretical analyses or organizations and action strategies. Plenary presentation at the 11ᵗʰ Congress International Ergonomics Association.* Paris, France.

Bradley, G. (1991). Changing Roles of Engineers and Knowledge Based Systems. In D. F. Kocaoglu, & K. D. Niwa (Eds.), *Technology Management. The New International Language. Proceedings of Portland "International Conference on Management of Engineering and Technology.* Portland: IEEE Engineering Management Society and Japan Society for Science Policy and Research Management.

Bradley, G., Holm, P., Steere, M., & Strömqvist, G. (1992). Psychosocial communication and computerization. *Invited article for the journal Computers in Human Behavior.* In B. Lindström (Ed.), *Special issue entitled "Swedish research on learning and instruction with computers.*

Bradley, G. (1993). Psychosocial Environment and the information age. In P. Beardon, & D. Whitehouse (Eds.), *Computers and Society* (pp. 27-45). London/New York, UK/NY: Taylor & Francis.

Bradley, G. (1993). Knowledge-Based Systems - Experiences of the organizational and psychosocial impact. In O. Brown, Jr., & V. Kobzev (Eds.), *Ergonomics in Russia, the other independent states and around the world. Past present and future. Proceedings at the first ergonomic conference.* St. Petersburg, RU: Russian Egonomics Association.

Bradley, G. (1993). Macroergonomic consider-ations in the computerization of complex organi-zations - What happens to the work organization? In W. S. Marras, W. Karwowski, J. Smith, & L. Pacholski (Eds.), *The Ergonomics of Manual Work*. London/New York, UK/NY: Taylor and Francis.

Bradley, G. (1993). Toward a Knowledge Shar-ing Organization. In M. J. Smith, & G. Salvendy (Eds.), *Human-Computer Interaction: Applica-tions and Case Studies". Proceedings of the Fifth International Conference on Human-Computer Interaction*. Amsterdam/London/New York: Elsevier.

Holm, P., & Bradley, G. (1993). Human Compe-tence, Work Organization, and Knowledge based system. In M. J. Smith, & G. Salvendy (Eds.), *Human-Computer Interaction: Applications and Case Studies". Proceedings of the Fifth Interna-tional Conference on Human-Computer Interac-tion*. Amsterdam/London/New York: Elsevier.

Chapter 1
Gunilla Bradley:
A Personal Glimpse

Geraldine Pratchett-Hultkrantz
Independent Scholar, Sweden

Gunilla Bradley first breezed into my life over 30 years ago. She came as strong spring breeze with her great personality wafting around her. Her children have attended my English Kindergarten School and since then we have been close and firm friends who have undertaken many journeys together and have experienced LIFE in a way that I haven't experienced with any other friends. It is a great privilege for me to be able to present some excerpts of her life and deeds.

She has her roots in a small village, Högsby, in the southern province of Småland. It was from Småland that great numbers of people emigrated to the U.S.A. in the 19th and 20th centuries and founded successful businesses and farming communities. Inhabitants from this province are well-

known for their great tenacity, pioneering spirit, entrepreneurship, economic ability and kindness to others. Gunilla has all these qualities in abundance. She started at the local school and after showing that she was a very capable and intelligent pupil her original plan was to become a teacher and specialise in French and Russian but instead she found herself studying psychology at Uppsala University. The drive and ambition in Gunilla must, amongst others, come from her maternal grandmother who drove a very successful bakery in Högsby together with other family members.

As far as I understand Gunilla was a very shy and timid youngster when she left Högsby but she had great support and encouragement from her parents and grandmother and with a scholarship in her rucksack she started off her new life at Uppsala University. Already at the age of eleven

DOI: 10.4018/978-1-60960-057-0.ch001

she had started to suffer from regular migraine headaches. This was of course very troublesome but being Gunilla she turned this suffering into something positive. This condition forced her to plan ahead and always be prepared with the work at hand. It taught her self-discipline.

She took her Bachelor's degree in psychology and behavioural sciences, but also spent some time on medical studies, marketing consultancy and sociology. However, she felt dissatisfied with her choice of psychology and as she explains after the devastating suicide of her father: "how could I help others when I couldn't even help my father!" Another factor was that at the beginning of the '60's the labour market for psychologists in Sweden was minimal. Her thoughts turned to becoming a physician and she applied to the prestigious Karolinska Institute in Stockholm, but after attending a year of studies there she was thwarted in that choice of career due to a very serious inflammation of the kidneys. After missing several exams due to her health one of the teachers said to her: "You will probably be a professor one day because you have failed this!" How right he was!

Gunilla's father had been an electrician and sometimes as a youngster she had accompanied him when he installed electricity in outlying farms – both in the farmhouses but especially in the cow sheds. Here she observed the enormous impact on every day tasks that the electricity made. A seed for the future had been sown!

At the end of the 1960's Gunilla was surrounded by many computer scientists and computer professionals, e.g. her husband, sister and sister-in-law. What they were doing was intriguing and an opening into that world came when Gunilla was invited to lead an investigation into the work environment for the Swedish Central Federation for Salaried Employees (TCO) in Sweden and the results were presented at a congress in 1972. Her explorative study showed that especial attention should be paid to the impact that computerisation was making. The same year she applied for a cross-disciplinary programme on Computerisation and Changes in the Work life for salaried employees and for many years she led this programme at the University of Stockholm.

In 1969 her husband was struck down with a very severe type of rheumatoid arthritis which seriously handicapped him. Gunilla tried to work from home during the initial stages of his illness but in those days it was much more difficult without the communication tools that we have today. It is just not comparable! However, with her indomitable spirit she proceeded to write her doctor's thesis "Women and Career," and received her degree in Educational Psychology at Gothenburg University in 1972. As we have seen women's role in the workplace was dear to her heart. She had taken note of how her own mother had had no opportunity to follow her desire to study art and art history. Her expected role had been to stay at home and take care of the family.

During the years 1973-1997 the question of her salary was very precarious. She had to apply every year for research money for her own salary as well as for remuneration for her research team. This was in spite of her being an Associate Professor. Tenure wasn't an option as every time she applied for tenure others in the pipeline were given priority. Being a woman in a man-dominated science was a liability.

In the 1970's there was "computer anxiety." Would the computers take over from workers and clerks and how would the social and professional life of those categories be affected? Gunilla carried on with her research on "Computers and Work Environment," but met a good deal of criticism and opposition. Male colleagues felt threatened and were anxious about their own careers. Here was this woman encroaching on their territory! Not only that but she was expecting a baby! How could they possibly take her seriously? She did get support and encouragement though from the Trade Unions and Employer Organisations.

In the late 1970's efforts by the government were made to conduct research tied to a new professional education programme for Personal and Work Life Issues in Sweden. A new Professorship entitled "The Computer Society" was suggested by the governmental committee, to be hosted by the Department of Sociology at the University of Stockholm. This was frowned upon by the academic world. Computers were not considered worthy of research in social and behavioural sciences. They were only good for statistics! This viewpoint made life very difficult for Gunilla and she was thwarted at every turn. She was passed over in favour of male colleagues time and time again when she applied for various positions and the future looked gloomy. However, being the strong character that she is she became all the more determined. By now she had two beautiful daughters and a very supportive husband in spite of his grave illness.

Her great hobby and delight has been painting – both landscapes and portraits. She had started painting at the age of seven when an aunt from the Province of Dalecarlia brought her some oil paints and a piece of hardboard. This hobby has perhaps allowed her to use her hands and brain in another way and flee into the world of art – a truly beautiful and stimulating world thereby enabling her to keep her equilibrium at all times.

In 1985 out of the blue came a grant from the Swedish Work Environment Fund which made it possible for her to spend a year as visiting professor at Stanford University in California. What a wonderful chance this was to get away from the doom and gloom here in her field. This proved to be a very fulfilling time for the whole family and Gunilla was appreciated there for her great knowledge and research experience. By this time she had many publications to her name and was recognised as a full professor in Technology and Social Change at Linköping University.

Before leaving for America two faculty meetings at the University of Stockholm had prioritised a Professorship in the field of Computer Technology and Work-Life tied to a new cross-disciplinary centre under the auspices of the Department of Computer and System Sciences. However, on her return to Sweden she found that she had been sacked from the University of Stockholm due to lack of funds! It turned out that the whole project that she had been involved in had been scrapped. Hence, at the end of the 1980's back in Stockholm it was once again doom and gloom and Gunilla suffered a deep depression as a consequence of treacherous deeds both in her private and professional life and she spent some time in therapy.

Again she pulled through and showed her tenacity. She was presented with two awards that brightened up her life considerably. One was the "Golden Leaf" from the Swedish Association of psychologists and the other was "Professional Woman of the Year."

A new area in computer technology appeared and Gunilla conducted pioneering research in this field, a field that was under hard debate and was perceived as frightening - Artificial Intelligence (AI) and Knowledge Based Systems (KBS). This time she received adequate funding from three Foundations. Field studies were performed in front line companies in Sweden applying advanced applications – KBS. However Stanford University was the right place at that time for both the theoretical and empirical work.

In 1991 she returned to Stanford and another fruitful and positive sejour there working on various projects with American colleagues. These years in Stanford were very stimulating for the whole family, and Gunilla's daughters Linda and Karin have definitely been positively affected in their choice of careers because of the enriching time they spent in Stanford. She continued working on an earlier project and initiated a new project with studies of 10 high tech. companies in Silicon Valley. She was given a very fine welcome and had, of course with her warm, generous and winning way a very wide network of friends and colleagues with whom she could pick up life almost as though she had never been away. Life was smiling again!

Whilst in California she received an invitation from the executive committee of the world organisation International Ergonomics Association to serve as general chair for the International Conference on Organisational Design and Management that was to be held in Stockholm in 1994. Would she be crazy to take on an enormous world conference like that? Of course there were many who said 'don't do it, it will be a terrific task.' But being an intrepid fighter and finding the challenge stimulating she agreed to take it on.

Gunilla came to me with her address and opening speech and we went through it together, and had several rehearsals with my husband and myself acting as the congress audience. Of course the Congress was a great success even though there was an ongoing power game with one person acting on a national level and another on an international level. However, Gunilla gained respect from the official bodies in Sweden and her international network was established.

From 1994-1997 she taught and researched as guest Professor at the Royal Institute of Technology (KTH) in Stockholm working closely with IT research in Kista., Sweden's equivalent to Silicon Valley. Her grandmother's bakery was, on her initiative turned into a Computer Learning Centre for that geographically rural area to combat unemployment. So, as always, her great community spirit shined through.

Throughout all these years we had been neighbours and whenever we could we took our morning walks and ventilated all our problems – both personal and professional. In this way I believe that we helped each other enormously as I was also involved in academic life and knew all the back-biting that went on. A problem aired is a problem shared, and I, for one, have had great help from Gunilla on our walking sessions.

In 1997 she received the IFIP Namur Award for pioneering cross disciplinary research on the social and organisational impact of Information and Communication Technology. Following that she joined the staff of Umeå University as Professor and in that capacity she was able to start up research in Informatics at the new Mid-Sweden University. These were fruitful years also taking in congresses in the U.S.A. and Europe.

2002 found Gunilla back in Stockholm to take up the chair at the new IT University in Kista, campus of the Royal Institute of Technology. She was the only female professor out of 25 professors. Many interesting projects came to the fore – among them for example 'The Home of the Future.'

Throughout her career Gunilla has focussed on 'humans,' – how does all this new technology affect humans, women and men. What impact does it have on our lives? She has really tried to do her utmost for people.

She rang me up one day in 2007 and said, 'will you come with me to the Human Computer Interaction International (HCII) Congress in Peking in July?' Of course, without any hesitation I accepted and we had such an interesting and stimulating time. I also feel that we touched the lives of some of the other delegates in a very positive way. For me, a humanist, it was an insight into the many ways that new technology can help people.

Now when Gunilla is emerita there is slightly, and I stress slightly, more time for walks and journeys together. She has also now been blessed with three grandchildren. We are still airing our feelings and problems and her visions for the future, where once again the focus is on people. That everyone should have access to the Net. That it should enrich our lives and well-being as well as empowering us. Democracy should increase because of it and peace should ensue.

Gunilla is now reaping the harvest after all the years of tilling and ploughing. May she continue to do so. I am certainly a richer person for having her as a dear friend.

Lidingö, 2009

Chapter 2
A Butterfly of Masterly Adroitness

Annagreta Dyring
Independent Scholar, Sweden

Intelligence is a refined form of an insect's antennae.

Horace Engdahl

The Aurora butterfly has elegant antennae. This butterfly was discovered by the botanist Carl Linnaeus from the Swedish Province of Småland. The Latin name is *Anthocharis* meaning beautiful flower.

It should be said that women view the world differently from men. In general a woman has other premises, other experiences, maybe even other values. Therefore science needs women.

In addition they are needed statistically as an expression of our renowned equality.

Gunilla Bradley, whom we can liken to the Aurora butterfly, is as sharp as her male colleagues, but she has partially different values and her own particular feelers. She chose to study the role of humans and their opportunities in the modern machinations of society. Humans as an increasingly effective cog in a computerised society is indeed infected territory. The subject is sometimes politically uncomfortable. In such cases she has temporarily closed her wings and waited for morning. Sensibly she soon saw the welcoming biotope in the west, in sun-drenched California.

Working life is ruled by traditions, power structures and economic prerequisites and the adaptation of people to these conditions is under

DOI: 10.4018/978-1-60960-057-0.ch002

severe strain. To conduct research on these structures and under these premises is to open up one's visor and perspectives.

If one is to analyse the development of society one must focus on the softer human factors. New research methods need to be applied and tested from a perspective of equity. Personal experiences of everyday life outside the academic world are an asset in such research. Gunilla Bradley's background from the forested landscape in Småland has provided a solid ground to stand on. Respect for the various 'roles' of people is not always learnt at school, but comes from our early environment.

To develop technology and control its possibilities has traditionally been the field of men. Today Information and Communication Technology (ICT) steers more and more people's reality, directly or indirectly. The participation of women and their opportunities in this development has always interested Gunilla Bradley. Using welfare as the utmost goal she has also studied many branches, life environment, and roles in the upheaval within technological development. Terms such as quality of life, welfare for all and peace are here of the utmost importance. Gunilla Bradley has impressed us with her conscious struggle for the wide usage of high-quality accomplishment within ICT research. She has also created many successful forms of international collaboration and networks. This has not been achieved overnight. It has had to be built brick by brick where the highest quality of her research has been the best aid.

In the turmoil of technological development popular science is also needed as a bridge-builder, but not least also for paving the way for democracy. In Sweden contacts between research and the surrounding society has moved in waves. In the 1980's Public Understanding of Science was on the way up in Sweden and Internationally. Gunilla Bradley was one of those people who worked early on to promote open science. Her perspective was concentrated on the "human factor" and its conditions in the work environment and in everyday life. Initially this view was looked upon as "Science Light" by the traditionalists. In reality it concerned important analyses for the future of modern society.

There is a great need of researchers who go their own way. Reality is not constant, values vary and the academic balance is not always well calibrated. Gunilla Bradley's consistent perusal of the individual's meeting with the IT society has not been main-stream. Therefore it gives me great pleasure to see that Gunilla owns such a prominent position in the international community of researchers. There her contributions are highly valued. Today she inspires many young scientists all over the world. Her questions and results carry much weight and purpose internationally. They are of fundamental importance irrespective of national boundaries.

Finally, a personal reflection - when Gunilla and I talk on the telephone it takes time before we are finished. She talks a long time when she is passionate about a subject, and she is nearly always passionate. On many occasions she is very open, unprotected in conversation. She acts the same way with her research. It absorbs her completely. She gives of herself without thinking that she is a butterfly.

Section 2
The Convergence Theory on ICT, Society, and Human Beings

Chapter 3
The Convergence Theory on ICT, Society, and Human Beings:
Towards the Good ICT Society

Gunilla Bradley
Royal Institute of Technology (KTH,) Sweden

ABSTRACT

The convergence model illustrates ongoing changes in the Net Society. The theoretical model synthesises the theoretical framework in the author's research on the psychosocial work environment and computerization. Interdisciplinary research programs were initiated by the author in the 1970s, leading to analysis of societal changes related to various periods in 'the history' of ICT. The description of the convergence model is structured with reference to the core concepts of Globalisation, ICT, Life Environment, Life Role, and Effects on Humans. Convergence and Interactions are important features of the model that organizes analysis at the individual, organisational, community, and societal levels.

INTRODUCTION

When I celebrated my 70th birthday we arranged a huge party for friends and relatives in a former palace in the centre of Stockholm. Old school-mates also attended. A family orchestra played and people danced. There were many speeches. Dr Darek Haftor informed us that he and Professor Anita Mirijamdotter, with the support of the newly established Linnaeus University, planned a *Festschrift* and a *Fest* to honour me. I was delighted by this wonderful initiative; to my mind this initiative usually occurs after you have died. So why not!

Early on the editors had asked me to contribute a chapter about the development of my convergence theory. Should I write a paper in my own *Festschrift*? Nonetheless, I went ahead and submitted an outline. I later learned that many chapter authors had referred to my convergence model. So when the editors elaborated a structure for the *Festschrift* chapters, they created a section on the 'Convergence theory on ICT, Society, and Human Beings', insisting that there were good reasons to get a concise description of the model 'from the horse's mouth'.

DOI: 10.4018/978-1-60960-057-0.ch003

Let me begin with some history of how the Convergence Model and its conceptual components developed. For this, we need to return to the 1970s, when countries like Sweden were attempting to build political, economic, and social structures that would shape a sustainable democratic society but also provide a balance between the main political systems of capitalism and socialism. This was a great challenge for a small country geographically located between the super powers that represented these political systems. In 1977, the Act on Employee Participation in Decision-Making (MBL) was signed. The concept of a psychosocial work environment was integrated in Swedish laws and in agreements between the labour market parties. Over the next 20 years, Sweden was on its way to introducing economic democracy through distributed citizen ownership of production. By the beginning of the 1990s, however, public anxiety grew that subsequently led to the election of a liberal government and many of the structures shaped during the former governments were dissolved. The evolution of societal structures and their representations in political action at the time were later described for international readers in my 1989 book *Computers and the Psychosocial Work Environment*.

During those 20 years, in the 1970s and 1980s, advanced studies examined the corresponding structures in work life that were facilitated by available superstructures at the societal level. The focus of information and communication technology (ICT)-related research was on participation in the development of computerised information systems. Some research programs also addressed the broader work life structures (illustrated later in my discussion of 'Objective (Structural) Work Environment' concepts in Figures 2 and 3). The focus was on monotonous and repetitive work that was by and large found in the industrial sector but also in the service sector. 'Alienation among workers' was the title of many articles during the 1970s, often with reference to Marx and to Blauner's book *Alienation and Freedom*. Along

with the change in governance philosophy that took place during the early 1990s, this dimension of the psychosocial work environment is no longer on the agenda of labour unions or is found in work life studies.

For many years theories, methods, and results from my research were published only in the Swedish language. *Psychosocial Work Environment and Computers* was my first international book (1986 in Swedish; 1989 in English). The research programs I initiated and led dealt with the four principal historical periods of computerisation and ICT: from the mainframe period with the use of batch processing systems; to the online period and use of display terminals; later to micro-computerization at the appearance of microchips; and to the net period where communication technologies have played a dominant role in the convergence of computer, tele-technology, and media technologies.

During these many years I worked and developed my theoretical framework independently of other theorists who have contributed to thinking about the Information Society. To exclude them from my personal history would neglect how their thinking helps locate the evolution of my own thinking about the complexity of interactions with technology and its effects on the individual, work life, and society; thus a section of this chapter briefly summarises their major theoretical contributions. The reference list at the end of the chapter provides some of the sources where I describe the model in detail and how it was developed as a result of the interaction between theory and the more than 30 years of empirical research that I have been involved in.

The convergence model has become kind of 'life partner' when I reflect on my personal history as an academic and when I look at the world around me. My focus has always been on analysing problems in the world that I have perceived as important, not defined in a disciplinary way as a sociologist, psychologist, computer scientist, or informatician. Nearly every day I get 'confirmation' of hypotheses tied to the model when I read and listen to the mass media.

Definition and then operationalisation of theoretical concepts are permanent tasks for research in the field because the basic structures are changing and new ones are identified. I exemplify this process with some figures from a program in the 1970s and 1980s and refer to various chapters in my book *Social and Community Informatics - Humans on the Net* where the entire process of the interaction between theory and empirical work is presented with special focus on studying the introduction, development, and use of ICT.

Nonetheless, empirical work has become more difficult because of the increasing rate of change. That is why the model's former elliptical form has been transformed into a wheel that runs faster and faster. It calls for forward action! And for global collaboration! We need visionary goals for the society, for the people in the society, and for future generations. By transferring to action the reasoning that led to the Convergence Model, we can influence our life environment through our professional, private, and citizen's roles.

THE CONVERGENCE THEORY ON ICT, SOCIETY, AND HUMAN BEINGS

Structures in Interaction with Human Beings

The Convergence Model can be seen as the evolution of my initial theoretical models. I have often subtitled it 'ICT and the Psychosocial Life Environment'.[1] It synthesises the theoretical framework of my research on the psychosocial work environment and computerization that originated in the 1970s and in the research programs during various phases of the history of computerization. Hence, my discussion of the historical evolution of the development of this model begins at the fourth period of computerisation (end) and ends at the first period of computerisation (beginning) of the development of my theoretical models.

The model is primarily a graphical representation of ongoing changes in the Net Society whose important features are Convergence and Interactions. Here *Convergence* means a move towards a common content. *Interaction* means that technology interacts in the social world with values and beliefs. The *psychosocial environment* refers to the process involving the interaction between the objective structural and subjective perceived environments.[2]

The important key processes in the model are Convergence, Interaction, Participation, Psychosocial processes, Globalization, and Democratic processes. Complexity characterises these processes. There are four levels of analysis: individual, organisational, communal, and societal Converging circles graphically reflect the ongoing processes. There is ongoing interaction between the 'clusters of circles'. Structures impact on human beings but human beings also impact structures.[3]

The overall dynamics are illustrated by the arrows and symbols and are partly described under each bolded sub-headline in the figure. The thin double-directed arrows in the outer part of the big circle represent interaction between the clusters of circles and the broad arrows represent the main direction for the movement and the process described in the circle. The main direction (broad arrow) is emphasised by an increasing change in the society due to globalisation and the accelerated rate of ICT research and development.

The principal constituents of convergence theory are presented in Figure 1. The description of its components is organized with reference to concepts in the outer circle: Globalization, ICT, Life Environment, Life Role, and Effects on Humans (in the middle).

1. Globalisation (lower left in the circle in Figure 1): This component represents what many theorists define as societal structural factors. A convergence entitled *Globalisation* is occurring

Figure 1. Convergence model on ICT and the psychosocial life environment (Bradley 2005, 2006)

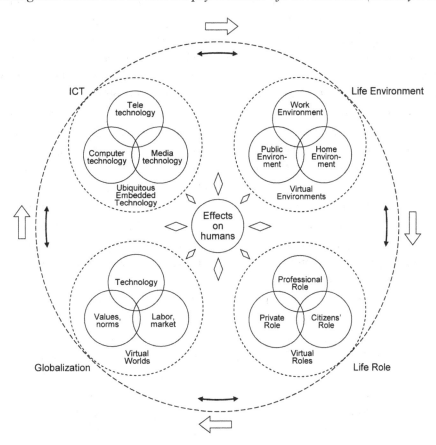

between Technology, Norms/Values (Economy), and Labour Market. Values related to the economic system are a strong driver. Values related to culture and religion may operate independently or support an economic system. Collaborative structures and international collaboration including access to new markets (in economic terms) are expanding geographically. Electronic commerce and electronic market places are changing the structure of work life. At present our work life is principally based on national and international trade which have become more global. Indeed, the geographical space of the future will be both global and beyond, including applications of virtual reality (VR). The dotted line around the converging circles illustrates the Virtual Worlds.

2. ICT (upper left): Computer technology, telecommunication technology, and media tech-

nology have converged to be defined as ICT. Processes have become integrated at various levels of analysis. The convergence process is always (re) enforced by smaller, cheaper and more powerful technical components. ICT is increasingly being used in almost every activity and increasingly embedded in every day life (ubiquitous computing). The borders between software and hardware have already been 'blurred' for a long time. Convergence between ICT and Bioscience and Nanotechnology has contributed to invisible convergences. Knowledge companies and knowledge workers are increasing and knowledge is being managed in new ways. In the twenty-first century multiple communication channels are available. Meta-level channels, e.g., meta-media of virtual reality (VR) and controlled reality environments (environments that we manipulate and manage in VR) are increasingly available. ICT have the capability of influencing governance structures and processes. The dotted line around the three circles illustrates embedded (pervasive, ubiquitous) technology.

The interaction between the 'ICT' and 'Globalisation' clusters give a powerful push to the main direction of the speed of the 'wheel'.

3. Life Environment (upper right): The Work Environment, Home Environment, and Public Environment are converging into a Life Environment where work and public environments move into our homes. A new emphasis on certain dimensions in the current psychosocial environment as well as identifying new dimensions in the psychosocial environment is important. We have to be open for unanticipated implications. The dotted line around the three circles illustrates the Virtual Environments.

In Media research the term 'environment' is often replaced by 'spheres' and the discourse is about the work sphere, the public sphere, and the private spheres. The concept of 'landscape' is coming into use.

4. Life Role (lower right): The Professional Role, the Private Role, and the Citizen's Role converge to become a Life Role. A Role is the position, task, or function a person has in a particular context and the norms and expectations associated with this position or task. Every person has a set of roles played in various contexts; role conflict takes place when various roles are difficult to integrate. Role appears where psychology and sociology meet; social psychology emphasises the corresponding interaction between the levels of analysis of social structures and the individual. In democracies people can create and influence their roles; they are not solely a 'victim' of socieal structures.

Changes are taking place in the home and home environment where professional, private, citizen, and learning roles have begun to converge and convergence is increasing. The home

can be regarded as a communication sphere that encompasses an extended family centre, a care centre, a multimedia centre, a centre for democratic dialogue, a market place, a learning centre, and an entertainment centre. The home is moving towards encompassing both virtual and physical space. Technologies like ICT have become embedded and have already altered behavioural patterns in the home and home environments on several continents (Bradley 2000; Bradley & Bradley 2001; Bradley 2005; Danielsson 2007; Jansson 2005).

5. Effects on Humans (in the middle): The Effects on Humans is represented by the circle in the middle with arrows pointing in two directions similar to a flower or a compass to illustrate interactions. The individual is affected by ICT, by the Life Environment with its three sub-environments, by the Life Role with its three sub-roles, and by Globalisation with its three components of values, technology, and labour market. Individuals influence and are influenced by technology, the environment, their own roles, and phenomena at the organisational and societal level and by the new virtual reality with its subparts. The individual can influence and is influenced by the clusters of circles or single circles as illustrated by the double direct arrows between the inner circle 'Effects on Humans' and the clusters of circles around it. Effects on the individual have become more multi-faceted and complex. How humans react to their situations can be roughly categorized as either active or passive, which is represented in the box on the right hand side in Figure 3. Examples of active reactions are involvement, creative behaviour, and protest. Examples of passive reactions are alienation and certain psycho-physiological symptoms.

6. Virtual Reality (VR) as a summarizing concept is illustrated by the four circles marked with dotted lines that surround the four clusters of converging circles represent our participation in cyberspace at various levels. In the lower left section we can talk about *Virtual Worlds* at the global level. Within the concept of ICT the phrase *Embedded (Pervasive, Ubiquitous)* makes the technology less obvious to the individual and to society as a whole; the tempo of the embedded processes is accelerating. *Virtual Environments* in the upper right part of the figure has been a common concept for some time; other names are online communities and virtual communities.

Virtual Human Roles (lower right section) are emerging. The main tools are the internet and web technologies, mobile phones, and new software applications known as social media (Facebook, Twitter, etc.) that are transforming work, private, and citizen roles. More time is spent on the net. The professional role has both real and virtual components. The private role is increasingly dominated by one's presence in cyberspace. In a more extreme form, VR is expressed by another person/personality that people take on, for example, avatars in various online games. VR is also a significant factor in reshaping the power balance between authority and the grassroots and strengthening civil society

Convergence Theory and the Effects on Humans

Regarding Effects on Humans in the middle of Figure 1, we can conclude that the use of ICT has thus far changed the human qualities of identity and self-perception, social competence, creativity, integrity, trust, dependency, and vulnerability. For example, the identity of humans has acquired new and additional bases through participation in various virtual and online communities. Each of those qualities can be either strengthened or weakened. In stress-theoretical terms we often talk about the importance of balance. ICT contributes to a balance or imbalance between, for example, the emotional and rational components of life, between female and male aspects, and between involvement and alienation.

Research indicates an accelerated tempo in the (post) industrialised world. Certain types of

'ICT stress' are related to increased dependency on computers and networks and to an increased expectation that these technologies are functioning well. Stress phenomena in the internet world are information overload, contact overload, demands for availability, lack of organisational filters, and difficulty in separating 'noise' from essentials. Changing levels of expectations by others and ourselves and altered perceptions of time and space are basic factors that contribute to ICT-related stress.

Tasks, roles, and environments that expose people to one of the two poles of over-stimulation and under-stimulation should be avoided due to: the risk of stress (the individual level); the risk of a fragmented labour force (group/organisation levels); the risk of a digital divide in nation-states; and the risk of marginalisation and exclusion from the mainstream of society (individual, group, and societal levels) (Bradley 1979, 1989).

More attention needs to be given at the individual level with respect to interaction between ICT–Society–Individual. There are both positive and negative impacts on the individual. In the current flexible network organisation too much responsibility is placed on the individual who loses permanent employment. In the current highly competitive market place, knowledge workers have become members of a 'peripheral work force', wholly responsible for their competency development and for marketing themselves. Although this may be seen as freedom from paid work in a traditional sense and freedom to choose your life, nonetheless, we all need a basic security as employees and citizens. There needs to be balance between a strong society and strong individuals. Most people are not 'strong' throughout life. We need to think in terms of sustainability in both the physical and social environment and to develop ways to create sustainable human beings. The increasing number of courses in mindfulness, preventive stress, cognitive behaviour therapy, provide sources for reflection.

Convergence Theory and Allocation Issues

Despite the observable process of convergence in the ICT society, there are also counter-movements, a process of divergence. Regions, nations, and subgroups in the world strive towards separation, self-government, autonomy, and sometimes self-determined isolation.

The allocation issue is related in a broad sense. It has always been possible to make huge profits as society became computerised. The question of allocating profits should have been a key issue at an early stage in policy programs. But not until recently—even if a global economy could have been anticipated, has the allocation issue come into focus for action at national and global levels, to address a needed balance in many domains. This balance includes: between work and leisure time, paid and unpaid services of citizen, production and reproduction, cities and rural areas; and profits between sectors within a country, industrialised countries, and industrialised and industrially-developing countries.

The often used 'Digital divide' is an analytical term, whereas 'Allocation issue' (allocation of resources) is a political term. The potential of balancing deep divides in resources is inherent in ICT. But both short-term and long-term action plans are needed. Otherwise, the risk increases for conflict and aggression.

How do the Convergence Theory of ICT and the Psychosocial Life Environment Relate to Other Theories about the Information Society?

Here I provide an abbreviated summary of classical theories in the area of the information society and several perspectives of the work life environment. [4]

Classical Theories of the Information Society

In answer the question posed in the title of this section, I want to refer to Frank Webster's (1995) *Theories of the Information Society* that is an interrogative and skeptical view of the concept of an 'Information Society'. He presents five definitions of the information society that represent criteria for the new society (technology, economy, occupation, space, and culture) and analyses contemporary social theories rather than the social impacts of technology. A 'pro-Information Society perspective' means that the theory offers hypotheses that posit a clear shift to something new, to a quite different type of society. An 'anti-Information Society perspective' are a group of theories that argue that structures and processes have been maintained and that there is no need talk about a new era of 'Information Society'. Frameworks and terminologies associated with pro-Information Society perspectives are post-industrialism, postmodernism, flexible specialisation, and the information mode of development. Frameworks and terminologies regarded as anti-Information Society theories include: neo-Marxism, regulation theory, flexible accumulation, the nation-state and violence, and the public sphere. I briefly summarise the main content of these five theories according to Webster.

Giddens (2000) argues that the origins of today's 'information societies' are to be found in surveillance activities driven principally by the requirements of a world organised into nation-states. The modern world consists of nations that are 'information societies' and have always been so, but need even more to maintain allocative resources such as planning and administration, authoritative resources such as power and control, and information which is the core of modern military affairs.

Giddens recognizes that information per se has great importance in society, but contends that the significant character of society is continuity, that patterns and structures in society reappear, and that ICT does not challenge those patterns and structures.

According to Schiller's (1993) Critical Theory, labeled neo-Marxism, ICT is essential for the stability and health of the economic system. He concludes that ICT is controlled by corporate capitalism and international empires, market criteria, and consumerism, which means that it is necessary to sell a global life style. Information is a commodity. Consequently, he asks: For whose benefit and under whose control is ICT implemented? The strength of Schiller's argument lies in his presentation of alternative ways of organising society and in his contention that the information society has a real human history developed by social forces.

Habermas (1989) fears that the public sphere—the independent arena where public opinion was formed over a period of about 100 years and of major importance to the proper conduct of democraciesis—is being diminished. The quality of information determines the health of the participants. ICT emphasises commercial principles and systems of mass communication. Information content is characterised by actions, adventure, trivia, and sensations.

The 'Regulation School' addresses theories about how a capitalist system achieves stability. Fordism (Keynesianism of the industrial society) has evolved to post-Fordism which is characterised by globalisation of markets, production, finance, and communication; corporate restructuring (e.g., downsizing, outsourcing, ICT infrastructure, less mass production); flexible specialisation; and effects on labour (e.g., flexibility of employees, wage flexibility, time flexibility).

Postmodernism posits a new type of society; a paradigm shift has taken place. According to Barthes, reality is primarily a matter of language and discourse; hence, the world is informational. For Baudrillard, culture is one important sign of the Information Society; however, the signs are simulations not representations and there is no distinction between the real and unreal or the true and false. Vatimo believes that the expansion of media creates multi-perspectivism. Lyotard argues that knowledge and information is treated as a commodity; truth is replaced by a plurality of truths; requirements for new skills emerge; and life-long education becomes necessary.

Webster argues that, nonetheless, characteristics of capitalist continuity in the society remain. At the same time, however, there is a shift in orientation to a novel form of work organisation and to changes in occupational patterns. He concludes that there has been no system break.

Finally, a summary of theories of the Information Society must mention the possibly most comprehensive contribution in the last decade, Castells´s (1996-1998) triology *The Information Age: Economy, Society, and Culture*. These volumes represent a 'life work' that is comparable to Marx´s *Das Kapital*. Not only is the trilogy deeply theoretical, it presents empirical data to support all the reasons to dicuss a Net society. Nor can we ignore Jensen's (1999) discussion of the Dream Society which represents the end of humankind´s multimillenium epoch of material domination and he predicts the beginning of the first post-materialistic era. He organizes the most important raw materials of the twenty-first century into four eras: agricultural (soil, fields, livestock); industrial (coal, oil, steel); information (data, information, knowledge); and dream (pictures, stories, myths, legends). He emphasises that the raw materials that dominate in the dream era are also available in less-developed countries like African countries, India, along the Polar Circle, and the Pacific Islands.

My own perspective on this complex issue is an integration of both 'pro-Information Society' and 'anti-Information Society' theories. In the short run, the development of the society may appear as a continuation according to Giddens. But in a market-driven globalised world there will be an antithesis, a stage where a paradigm shift occurs that results in a deeper rethinking in order to ensure the survival of society. The network society in its various shapes alters the basis for individual and societal identities. Web communities are bringing together people across new dimensions. The prerequisites for informal power are growing and power will not be associated with capital to the same degree as it currently is. The costs of empowering people with knowledge capital are gradually being reduced. The economic crisis in 2009 has increased awareness of societal vulnerability (the speed of the recession process was ICT-related).

Another general comment on the relationship between Convergence Theory and the more macro-level theories summarised above is that the introduction and use of ICT in the home environment should not be left to governance steering factors that have been present in work life. A cross-disciplinary research program is called for and should be integrated with full-scale models for various applications. Basic human needs and 'people push' technology not 'technology push' should be guiding principles.

Theories of Working Life

Theories that more directly relate to the corporate world and working life in a broad sense come from many academic disciplines and academic communities, cultures that have different perspectives and focuses. What are the contributions from the information systems community? For many years the focus was on the *development and design* of information systems and later on the *introduction and use* of information systems. The tele-technology and media technology parts of the ICT concept were not addressed for many years. Some contributions after 2000 are the following:

Melville, Kraemer and Gurbaxani (2004) developed a model of IT business value and thereby chose a resource-based view of the firm, which is often used in management literature and international business. They applied their integrative model to synthesise research about IT business value and developed propositions for future research in the field. Their conceptual model is comprehensive and shows the complexity of the field. Although integrative, it is, however, not interactive in the sense that interaction between theoretical levels of analysis is discussed. The main concepts are resources in the form of technological IT resources, human IT resources, and complementary organizational resources. The other concepts are business processes and performance with a focus on the competitive environment: industry characteristics, trading partner resources, and business processes. Within a macro environment are country characteristics and similar concepts.

Schulze and Orlikowski (2001) explored the discourse on virtual organising and identified a number of metaphors that characterise various aspects of virtuality. They examined the various metaphors in the practitioner-directed literature on virtual organizing and concluded that the discourse contained a multiplicity of different metaphors, such as virtual organizing as a platform, existing in space, composed of bits, operating as a community and engaging in a network of relationships. They suggest that, due to the absence of experiences to guide practice, these images shape people's views of and actions towards virtual organizing. They then analyzed these metaphors with regard to type of organizing, meaning, source, examples, affordance, and challenge. Their conclusion that metaphors are powerful tools of social construction suggests that researchers and practitioners must be aware of their critical implications and unintended consequences.

Another strand of research in the information systems literature is user acceptance theory (Davis, Bagozzi, & Warshaw 1989). Van der Heijden (2004) discusses the differences in user acceptance models for productivity-oriented and pleasure-oriented information systems, hence emphasizing various values.

Values focused research can also be found in the formation of world-wide networks of various ICT-related academic schools that share some common perspective (e.g., Network for Value Sensitive Design; Community Informatics Research; The International Conference on the Social and Ethical Impacts of Information and Communication Technologies; International Association for Developing the Information Society; and the ICTs and Society Network).

Critical research has been more common outside the information systems community but this is changing. According to Walsham (2005), a critical approach is a perspective that includes, for example, the social construction of 'truth', historical and cultural contingency, and power relations. He argues that there is a need for information systems research that is critical and is aimed at creating a 'better world' with technology. He draws implications for action in terms of a research agenda, teaching activities, publishing, and institution building. A 'better' world with ICT should not mean better in purely economic terms but also related globally to social and spiritual welfare. He concludes that global futures in general and the information systems field in particular are not pre-determined but result from our own efforts and actions.

FROM THEORY TO ACTION

Visions are shared about well-being, democracy, and the quality of life for all as well as social, economic, and ecological sustainability, as illustrated with the convergence of circles in Figure 1. We can all be actors in this process: in nongovernmental organizations and as researchers, teachers, IT professionals, and individuals.

Official bodies at the international and national levels such as the World Summit on the Information Society (WSIS) and national ICT programs are actors as we move to a global ICT society. During the last few years critical questions have been formulated by international agencies about how to focus attention on human beings and their social and societal environments and how to create an 'Information Society for All' when developing increasingly complex information and communication technology (ICT) systems that take account of their complex contexts (UNESCO 2002; e-Europe 2002). The first official statement of goals for the ICT society was formulated at the World IT Forum (WITFOR 2003). Goals articulated in the Vilnius Declaration had important implications for the involvement of the developing countries, such as bridging the digital divide between rich and poor, urban and rural societies, men and women, and generations. Another central concern was reducing poverty through the use of education and ICT. In 2006, the United Nations began a review of the issue of Human Rights; global use of ICT has made the need of this review clear. Europe has a similar agenda.

Research on ICT, society, and the individual and associated psychosocial processes have addressed goals and visions of the ICT society that can be formulated as policy statements (Bradley 2001). These goals are: information access for all, well-being and quality of life for all, enriched social contact between people, integration and respect for diversity, greater autonomy for the individual, prevention of various types of overload and stress, deepening of true human qualities, deepening and broadening of democracy, e-cooperation and peace; and sustainability in a broad sense, including the environment, economy, and human side.

Sustainability has sometimes been used as the principal criterion for a Good Information and Communication Society (Bichler, Bradley, & Hofkirchner 2010; Jansson & Bradley 2004). Sustainability and the use of ICT are closely connected. Important theoretical approaches are system dynamics, holism, human aspects, bottom-up, common good, equality and equity. Many of the concepts overlap and may be analysed from

Figure 2. Computer technology and work environment (Bradley 1977)

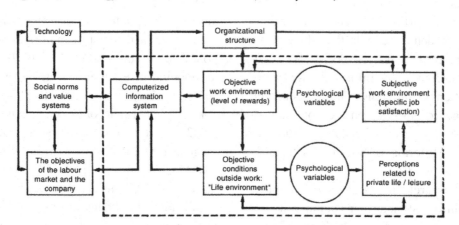

various perspectives. Action-oriented and value-oriented research is coming to the fore.

Many academic communities are addressing the complex issue of 'ICT, Work Organization, and Society. These include the organisational design and management section of the International Ergonomics Association, the ETHICOMP conference for ethical and social issues related to ICT, the Community Informatics Research Network, the computer supported cooperative work society, sub-tracks of Human Computer Interaction International, and working groups of the International Federation of Information Processing. The European Conference on Information Systems and the correspondent International Conference on Information Systems have recently become more open to these issues. Relevant research is, consequently, fragmented and difficult to locate. However, new journals are appearing with a broad cross-disciplinary perspective. New interdisciplinary centres have been established and definitions of what constitutes a discipline are taking place in parallel with growing specialization, especially within electronics and hardware.

Social Informatics is increasingly a mandatory part in education and training in ICT-related disciplines. How can Social Informatics be defined? I have found that definitions sometimes create divisions due to the labyrinth of academic

language. So, what should I do? As a university emerita one of my priorities was to develop a textbook on 'Social and Community Informatics' for international use. The book contains theory, empirical studies in various spheres of life (industry, community, and home), methodology and action for developing the 'Good Information and Communication Society'. I have used this book to teach doctoral and master courses and to inspire junior scientists.

SUMMARY OF THE EVOLUTION OF THE CONVERGENCE MODEL

Figures one through four can be used to summarise the development of the convergence theory on 'ICT, Society and Human Beings'. The figures are interrelated; concepts in one figure are mirrored in the other figures. For a deeper understanding about that interplay I have to refer to my latest book (2006).

Figure 2 is the original theoretical model developed in the 1970s for applying for research funding. The main concepts were furthered defined (see figure 3) and then operationalised in empirical measures in a series of research projects. Of course, the concepts in Figure 2 could be updated and renamed: for example, 'Computerized

Information System' as 'ICT' and 'Organizational Structure' as 'Network Organisations'. The model in Figure 2 was also the basis for defining the 'psychosocial work environment', which was so important in the early 1970s when Sweden created the governance structures that made a work life democracy possible. The core perspective is, however, found in the convergence model represented in Figures 1 and 4.

The broad concepts in the original model described in Figure 2 were refined and brought to empirical studies through various forms of methods for collecting and analysing the empirical evidence. A correspondent model for analysis with focus on Stress was applied later and is described in my 1989 and 2006 books. Stress is one of the 'Reactions' in the box to the right in Figure 3.

The convergence model in Figure 4 implies that cross-disciplinary research is crucial. Disciplines represented in the components of the model are, from left to right: political science and economy; ICT-related disciplines; sociology, ethnography, urban/rural planning, and architecture; and social psychology and psychology.

A tree can summarize the actions on various levels. The tree in Figure 5 was derived during the first phases of computerisation and characterises how the technology was introduced in a country like Sweden (the so-called Swedish Model). Some special concerns are mentioned below that are valid for ICT and the network period of technological development in the twenty-first century.

Some additions and changes should be inserted.

- The trunk of the tree could represent 'Global level'.
- An 'International level' branch should be added.
- A 'Community level' branch should be added that represents 'Virtual Reality' and 'Life Role'.

- The branch entitled 'Technology' should be divided into sub-branches of tele-technology, computer technology, media technology, and ubiquitous (embedded) technology; however, the integration and convergence of the technologies could be illustrated.
- Regarding the branch 'Company level' many factors have lost their governance functions in the new flexible companies that are more often organised in networks. Trade unions are no longer active in the same way in the fields of technology or the work environment but must assume new forms of strategies and collaborative structures.

New branches and new sub-branches should be added. Other branches have lost their relevance.

CONCLUSION

In a field of research whose empirical world is one of accelerated rate of change and complexity, there needs to be much stronger international support for cross-disciplinary, cross-cultural, and action-oriented research on the topic 'ICT for Deepening of Humane and Societal Qualities'.

Central questions about the role of ICT and human rights have a high priority: How can Human Rights be more deeply understood, exemplified, and applied in the ICT society? How can we use various components of ICT such as the internet, web, and social media for dialogue between cultures to foster mutual understanding and enrich us all?

Within disciplines like Informatics, research and development need to address work processes and management connected to the sphere of production life and to people's life environment and patterns of psychosocial communication. Analysis and design of ICT and social systems at both the local and global levels are needed because dis-

Figure 3. The relationship between objective and subjective work environments (Source Bradley 1979, 1989)

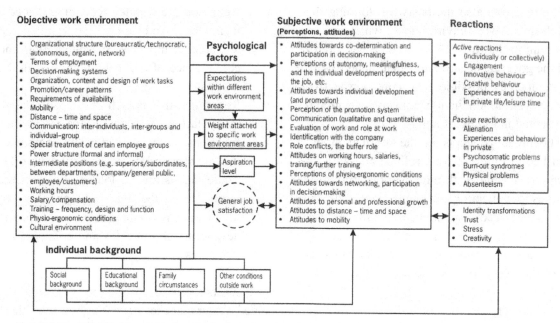

Figure 2.2 The relationship between objective and subjective work environments

Figure 4. The convergence model

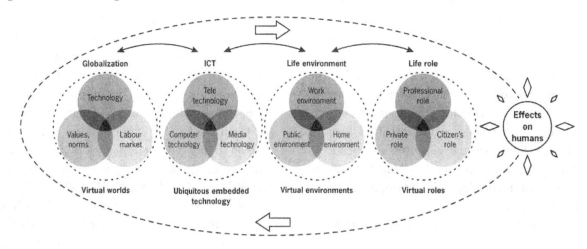

tributed computer power, strong telecommunications, and mobile equipment create opportunities for deepening democracy and strengthening the individual and her influence on society but also increase the risk of government centralization and the misuse of power.

There are many ways to illustrate desirable goals for a Good ICT Society. I have already mentioned in an earlier section that the first official international statement of goals for the ICT society was formulated at the 2003 World IT Forum and that the policy goals of the Vilnius Declaration

Figure 5. Action strategies in Sweden in the 1970s (Bradley 1989)

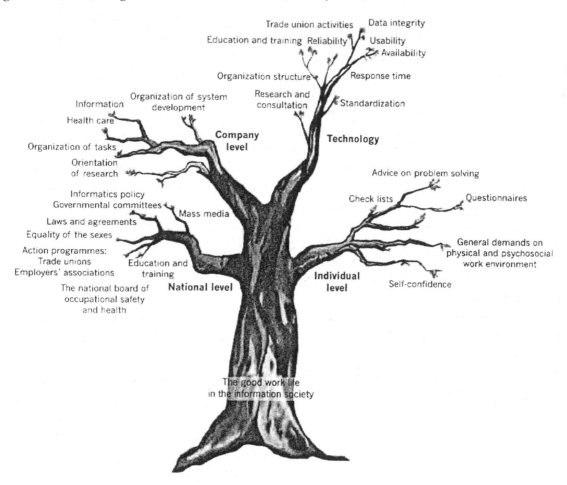

had important implications for the global society and especially for developing nations. The goals that ICT should contribute to that were articulated by the Vilnius Declaration are:

- Bridging the digital divide between rich and poor in the world; urban and rural societies; men and women; and different generations
- Ensuring the freedom of expression enshrined in Article 19 of the universal declaration of human rights and other such instruments
- Reducing poverty through the use of education and Information and Communications Technology (ICT)

- Facilitating the social integration of excluded segments of societies
- Respecting linguistic and cultural diversity
- Fostering the creation of public domains with full respect of intellectual property rights
- Supporting communities in fighting illiteracy
- Encouraging e-governance and e-democracy initiatives
- Improving the quality of life through effective health service systems
- Protecting the local and global environment for future generations

Academic discourses on most of the concepts are embedded in these goals. Theories and empirical research must, however, be balanced with action-oriented and value-oriented research. All of us have a role to play, especially because we ourselves have experienced profound changes in our professional, citizen, and private sphere roles.

The visions and goals for the Good ICT society for Human Beings need stronger recognition and action strategies that provide for a deeper and broader integration of ICT in society. We need to move from a 'technology for all' philosophy to a 'well-being and quality of life for all' philosophy. The World Summit on the Information Society offers us an opportunity for a wide range of actors to develop principles and prioritise actions that lead to democratic, inclusive, participatory, and development-oriented CT societies at the local, national, and international levels. Towards a society where people's basic physical needs as well as the needs for social belonging, influence, learning and growth, confidence, and meaningfulness are fulfilled.

ACKNOWLEDGMENT

I want to thank Alice Robbin for her valuable comments on an earlier draft of this chapter.

REFERENCES

Bichler, R. M., Bradley, G., & Hofkirchner, W. (2010). Editorial Comment. Sustainable Development and ICTs. *Information Communication and Society, 13*(1).

Bradley, G. (1977). *Datateknik, Arbetsliv och Kommunikation. (Computer Technology, Work Life, and Communication)*. The Swedish delegation for long term research. FRN. Stockholm, SE: Liber (in Swedish).

Bradley, G. (1979). Computerization and some Psychosocial Factors in the Work Environment. In *Proceedings of the conference Reducing Occupational Stress* (pp. 30-40). New York, 1977. U.S. Department of Health, Education, and Welfare, NIOSH Publication No. 78-140.

Bradley, G. (1986). *Psykosocial arbetsmiljö och datorer*. Stockholm, SE: Akademilitteratur.

Bradley, G. (1989). *Computers and the Psychosocial Work Environment*. London/Philadelphia, UK/PA: Taylor & Francis.

Bradley, G. (Ed.). (2001). *Humans on the Net. Information and Communication Technology (ICT) Work Organisation and Human Beings*. Stockholm, SE: Prevent.

Bradley, G. (2003). ICT for deepening human and societal qualities. In *Proceedings of WITFOR 2003. Humans on the Net*. London, UK: Routledge.

Bradley, G. (2005). The Convergence Theory on Information and Communication Technology (ICT) and the Psychosocial Life Environment – The Connected Home. In Salvendy, G. (Ed.). *Proceedings of the HCI International 2005 conference*, 22-27 July 2005, Las Vegas, USA. (CD). Mahwah, NJ: Lawrence Erlbaum Associates.

Bradley, G. (2006). *Social and Community Informatics - Humans on the Net*. London, UK: Routledge.

Bradley, G. (2007). ICT, Work Organisations, and Society. In Anttiroiko, A-V. & Mälkiä, M. (Eds,) *Encyclopedia of Digital Government*. Hershey, PA: Idea Group Inc.

Bradley, G., Börjesson, K., & Lundgren, M. (1974). Arbetsmiljö och tjänstemän (Work Environment and Salaried Employees). Report to the Swedish Central Federation of Salaried Employees. Stockholm, SE: TCO.

Bradley, L. (2005). *Home of the Future Japan – Information and Communication Technology (ICT) and Changes in Society and Human Patterns of Behavior in the Network Era.* KTH Research report ISBN 91-7178-052-1. Stockholm: Royal Institute of Technology (KTH).

Bradley, L., & Bradley, G. (2001). The Home as a Virtual and Physical Space – Experiences from USA and South- East Asia . In Smith, M., & Salvendy, G. (Eds.), *Systems, Social and Internationalization Design Aspects of Human-Computer Interaction* (pp. 81–85). Mahwah, NJ: Lawrence Erlbaum Associates.

Castells, M. (2000). Trilogy on *The Information Age. Economy, Society and Culture.* 1996-97 in English. Daidalos Publisher 2000 (in Swedish).

Castells, M. (2001). *The Internet galaxy.* Oxford, UK: Oxford University Press.

Danielsson, U. (2007). *Relationships Between Information Communication Technology and Psychosocial Life Environment. Students and Young Urban Knowledge Workers in the ICT-Era.* Sundsvall: Mid Sweden University. Doctoral Thesis no 41, 2007.

Davis, F. D., Bagozzi, R. P., & Warshaw, P. R. (1989). User acceptance of computer technology: A comparison of two theoretical models. *Management Science, 35*(8), 983–1003. doi:10.1287/mnsc.35.8.982

Giddens, A. (1990). *The consequences of modernity.* Cambridge, UK: Polity.

Giddens, A. (2000). *Runaway world.* London, UK: Routledge.

Habermas, J. (1989). *The structural transformation of the public sphere.* Cambridge, UK: Polity.

Heylighen, F., & Joslyn, C. (2001). Cybernetics and second order cybernetics. In *Encyclopaedia of Physical Science & Technology* (3rd ed., pp. 155-170), 4.

Jansson, E. (2005). *Working Together when Being Apart. An analysis of distributed Collaborative Work through ICT from Psychosocial and Organisational Perspective.* Doctoral dissertation at Department of Computer and System Sciences, IT University, Royal Institute of Technology, Stockholm.

Jansson, E., & Bradley, G. (2004). Sustainability in Collaborative Network Structures – with focus on the Psychosocial Work Environment in Distributed Teams. In *Proceedings of the CIRN conference on Sustainability and Technology: What does this Mean for Community Informatics, 1* (pp. 271-283). Prato, Italy, 29 September–1 October Community, 2004.

Jensen, R. (1999). *The dream society.* New York/London, NY/UK: McGraw-Hill.

Khakhar, D. (Ed.). (2004). *WITFOR 2003 (WORLD IT FORUM) White Book.* Key note contributions and panel discussions from the 8 commissions. Luxemburg: IFIP Press.

Melville, N., Kraemer, K., & Gurbaxani, V. (2004). Information technology and organisational performance: An integrative model of IT business value. *Management Information Systems Quarterly, 45*(2), 283–322.

Schiller, H. (1993). Public way of private road? *Nation (New York, N.Y.), 12,* 64–66.

ENDNOTES

[1] The convergence model is presented in detail in two chapters of my 2006 book *Social and Community Informatics - Humans on the Net*. The first chapter focuses on the emergence of the theoretical conceptual framework and successive models developed out of the interaction between theory and empirical studies. The second chapter goes one step further. Entitled 'From Theory to Actions – How to Achieve the Good ICT Society – a Tree of Action', it describes the organic model—a tree with its truck, branches, and sub-branches—that was applied to illustrate action on structural changes at various levels of society (see Figure 5).

[2] Essential concepts in the psychosocial work environment include factors such as contact patterns and communication, organisational structure and design, work content and workload, participation in decision-making, promotional and development patterns, and salary conditions and working hours (Bradley, Börjeson, & Lundgren 1972).

[3] This interaction is basic knowledge in most behavioural and social sciences. This is valid for economic, cultural, and political structures at the societal level and, for example, organisational structures and ICT infrastructure at another level. But the process of interaction is expected to differ, for example, for authoritarian and democratic regimes.

[4] These topics are more fully addressed in the second chapter of *Social and Community Informatics – Humans on the Net*.

Chapter 4
An 'Ekistics' for Information and Communication Technologies

William McIver Jr.

National Research Council, Institute for Information Technology, Canada

ABSTRACT

This chapter attempts to draw parallels between Professor Gunilla Bradley's Convergence Model and the body of work by a now seemingly obscure architect and urban planner, Constantinos A. Doxiadis. Doxiadis developed the theory of 'Ekistics' as an attempt to systematize the analysis of 'human settlements', his general term for intentional habitats of any scale organized by humans. Ekistics is not seen by this author as necessarily the sole nor ideal perspective from which to evaluate Bradley's work. It is, nonetheless, seen as relevant, useful, and intriguing for several reasons, the most compelling of which is that Doxiadis offered clear ideas for the practice of Ekistics that could be used as a template for future work in operationalising Bradley's Convergence Model.

REFLECTIONS ON BRADLEY'S CONVERGENCE MODEL

The Convergence Model in Perspective

A field of study comes into its own when it becomes capable of explaining and reflecting upon itself at a systemic level. That is, from a perspective that is broad enough to see at different levels of abstraction how phenomena that were once studied

independently are related. Most scientific fields have undergone this epistemological evolution. Bradley's Convergence Model (2006) has brought social and community informatics to this stage. For this we are grateful to our colleague and friend.

The Convergence Model has given us a comprehensive framework and a process-view of social and communicate informatics where none existed. This systemic view has enabled us to understand the many, disparate phenomena that have been studied and documented within these two connected fields. It has often been the case that vastly different methodologies have

DOI: 10.4018/978-1-60960-057-0.ch004

been used to perform social and community informatics research, often without awareness of other approaches or, if awareness exists, without intention to relate a chosen methodology to those used by others. Arguably, there has also not been a sense for what the research roadmap for community informatics is or should be. A systemic view allows the results of different approaches to be normalized and mapped on to each other to produce new knowledge. A systemic view allows seemingly unrelated terms to be resolved into coherent definitions. A systemic view also allows the scientific production of knowledge to fully begin within a field.

A clear example of the importance of developing a systemic view of a field of study can be seen in mathematics with the independent efforts in the late nineteenth and early twentieth centuries by David Hilbert, Alfred North Whitehead with Bertrand Russell, the Bourbaki group, and others to ground mathematics to some unified system. Hilbert's "23 Problems" -- presented in a now famous speech in 1900 -- listed key unsolved problems and influenced the focus of much of the field of mathematics to this day (Rowe & Gray, 2000). The legacy of Hilbert's challenge can be seen in the nature of Andrew Wile's solution of Fermat's Last Theorem, which is related to the tenth problem in Hilbert's list and which took over 350 years for the field to solve. Wile's approach drew upon disparate areas of mathematics, the linking of which would likely not have been arrived at without the 'roadmap' set out by Hilbert or the development of a systemic view of the discipline that has evolved out of the work Hilbert and the others (c.f. Kolata, 1993).

Kristen Nygaard and Ingar Roggen of Norway were pioneers in the study of social impacts of computer technology (Liskov, 1981; Førstelektor and Godejord, 2009). Ingar Roggen is believed to have originated the term 'sosioinformatikk'(Førstelektor and Godejord, 2009). A common definition of social informatics is "the interdisciplinary study of the design,

uses and consequences of information technologies that takes into account their interaction with institutional and cultural contexts" (Kling, 1999). This study occurs along three principal dimensions: theories and models, methodologies, and philosophical and ethical issues. The Convergence Model is mainly representative of the first category, but it draws deeply from the other two. Community informatics is seen in relation to social informatics as an interdisciplinary field concerned with the development, deployment, and management of information systems designed with and by communities to solve their own problems. Other areas of focus related to social and community informatics have arisen. The most prominent among these is 'development informatics', which is concerned with ICT within developing countries.

The Convergence Model has not been the only important model within the broad scope of research related to social and community informatics. Dervin's (1983) three decade research on sense-making and the resulting Sense-Making methodology is a another example of systemic model on the scale of Bradley's. The Convergence Model is, however, among the first, if not the first, to propose a systemic explanation of the dynamics and interrelationships between a comprehensive set of objects of study within social and community informatics.

A casual reader of Bradley might view her work as solely the result of an exhaustive scientific exercise. For those who have read her more deeply -- and surely for those of us who have been fortunate to be in her presence -- the Convergence Model is clearly the product of an attempt to improve the quality of life within human society. She has stated that an initial motivation for her work was to find out what computer scientists were working on and whether they were contributing to society (2006:6). Her life work represents an assertion that we cannot make appropriate scientific contributions without understanding human needs nor without a comprehensive understanding of how society is affected by the information and communication technologies that we create.

The usefulness of the Convergence Model is critical in this respect and for this period in human development: we confronting multiple global crises, each of which threatens humanity and technology is at the same time implicated in all of them and is seen as offering solutions. It is for this reason that the Convergence Model must be operationalized. A key site for reflecting on the Convergence Model and how it might be extended and operationalised is the renewed interest in cities and a little-known or largely forgotten attempt to model the city-as-system in the way that is analogous to how Bradley has tried to model the relationships between ICT and society.

We are in an era of the pursuit of the 'smart city', where long-standing, mainstream desires for automated and networked communities are now being reified. Once discrete areas of automation and data communication like policing, traffic management, telecommunication, and public transport are now being integrated across the ICT architectures of cities, not to mention integration on other geo-political scales. The economic and political models of cities of all sizes now depend not only on operating in a manner that is technologically 'smart', but on offering their residents and businesses advanced ICT infrastructures. ICT are also being viewed as an essential part of proposed solutions to our crises, most especially climate change as we will discuss below.

Cities can only be studied as a systems, or as convergences of subsystems, whether in terms of their economic impact, physical evolution, consequences of policy, or the social dynamics they foster. Sassen (1991) presented an empirically-derived conception of a global city in *The Global City: London, Tokyo, New York* in which she showed through extensive analyses how such cities can be viewed as interconnected systems, particularly in the context of global economic forces. Castells (2004: 90), among others, has described the need for a complex system of requirements

in urban planning in this age, which recognizes the 'social and functional diversity' of human settlements and the need to respond to changes in social norms in identifying requirements. The Benton Foundation (2004) has, among others, documented systemic gaps in the technologies that exist within cities.

Given the city as a site for reflecting on and applying the Convergence Model, this chapter attempts to draw parallels between Bradley's work and the body of work by a now seemingly obscure architect and urban planner, Constantinos A. Doxiadis. Doxiadis developed the theory of 'Ekistics' as an attempt to systematize the analysis of 'human settlements', his general term for intentional habitats of any scale organized by humans (1968). Ekistics is not seen by this author as necessarily the sole nor ideal perspective from which to evaluate Bradley's work. It is, nonetheless, seen as relevant, useful, and intriguing for four reasons:

1. the motivations for Doxiadis's work were similar to Bradley's;
2. Doxiadis's theory was, like Bradley's, based on extensive empirical research;
3. the scope of Doxiadis's model was comparable to that of the Convergence Model; and
4. Doxiadis offered clear ideas for the practice of Ekistics that could be used as a template for future work in operationalising the Convergence Model.

Through Ekistics, Doxiadis pursued the abstract idea of 'anthropolis' (1974:XIII), a city that satisfies the needs of its inhabitants, its environment, and its own evolution through a systematic and empirical analysis of how 'human settlements' evolve and the problems that they cause.[1] He predicted before widespread awareness of the potential impacts of global networks of communication and commerce that human settlements would converge along many dimensions into an 'ecumenopolis' or global city (1974:10). Sassen

(1991) and others have later arrived independently at related perspectives.

The Convergence Model is based on a fitting metaphor for our time. One could argue that we are at least approaching the creation of an 'ecumennet': a virtual analog of ecumenopolis resulting from the global convergences of data and communication networks; software services; and, recursively, the social, economic, and political dynamics these convergences enable.

THE CITY AS SOLUTION

Rachel Carson in "A Fable for Tomorrow", the opening chapter of her influential book *Silent Spring,* conceptualizes the ideal "town" as part of nature. She wrote that it is "in harmony with its surroundings" and it "lays in the midst of a checkerboard of prosperous farms" (1962:1). She went on, as we know, to describe a situation where a "strange blight [began to creep] over the area and everything began to change" (2).

The basis for Carson's critique was technological: "Only within the moment of time represented by the present century has one species – man – acquired significant power to alter the nature of his world" (6). Ultimately, she argues that "the public must decide." In this case, of course, the decisions she alluded to would be focused on environmental contaminants, or "elixirs of death" as she called them (13). The implication of Carson's work for this discussion is that her principle has been extended in social and community informatics to say that communities must decide how technologies are to be used and to what extent they are allowed to impact their environments. The term 'environment' in this context includes not only the Carsonian natural environment, but various other domains, including science, law, technology, psychology, sociology, politics, and economics. This type of decision-making can occur only through the development of conceptual models and research programs of the nature proposed by

Bradley in her Convergence Model. This must also take place in an ongoing review of impacts.

Concern over the impact of humanity's technology on its habitat has steadily increased over the past century. Doxiadis examined human settlements in this context. Still the popular notion of being "environmental" was and has arguably meant "going back to nature" or in other words to go away from human settlements, most especially the city. This notion has been embedded in many popular socio-economic movements over the years. Back-to-the-land movements of the 1960s and 1970s reinforced the rejection of the city and, thereby to a certain extent, human settlements in general, in their quest for ways of living that were less harmful to both natural environments and humans themselves.

Times have changed, however. The environmental movement has in its maturity evolved a more sophisticated view of the role of human settlements in creating a more environmentally-sustainable future. The *2006 Annual Report of the Cities Alliance* – an organization affiliated with the United Nations Human Settlements Programme (UN-HABITAT, 2006) – pointed to the city as a major solution to our environmental, climate, and resource problems. The report states (3-4):

Cities occupy just 2 percent of the Earth's surface, yet their inhabitants already consume 75 percent of the planet's natural resources for goods and services, and 80 percent of global carbon dioxide emissions originate in towns and cities. Although it has become conventional wisdom for some that cities are threats to both the global and the local environment, the world's urban areas may actually offer the best hope for a sustainable future. ... Cities are already the world's economic engines, accounting for almost 80 percent of total economic growth. Cities are also proven poverty fighters. Urban dwellers have higher incomes than their rural counterparts and consume less energy per unit of economic output.

The recent period has seen these reconceptualizations of the human settlement as solutions to some of the crises facing human society. We have seen this most recently with a rising interest in local agriculture models and, more generally, local economic models.

Whatever the focus, it is increasing difficult, though not impossible, to contemplate these futures without information and communication technologies. An example of this reconceptualization has been the pursuit over the past decade and a half of the so-called 'smart city' or 'intelligent city'. While attractive to many, the smart city is problematic in many ways that must be addressed through social and community informatics research and praxis.

SMART CITIES

The concept of the 'smart city' or 'intelligent city' has been discussed for some time (c.f. Droege, 1997; Dutton, 1987). Part of Graham's characterization of the interest in "smart cities" has been as a ""'post-urban' fantasy" that includes four elements: a move away from materiality, the elimination of distance, electronic forms of democratic transformation, and the 'infinite city'" (2004b:4 – 9). Several formal definitions of the smart city have been derived by organizations that have had as their mandates the evaluation of smart cities. Their definitions each imply subsets of Graham's elements and are invariably and inextricably-linked with the use of advanced information and communication technologies.

The Centre of Regional Science at the Vienna University of Technology; the OTB Research Institute for Housing, Urban and Mobility Studies at the Delft University of Technology; and the Department of Geography at University of Ljubljana have collaborated to produce rankings of smart cities within the European Union. "A Smart City" according to them is "a city well performing in a forward-looking way in [...] six characteristics,

built on the 'smart' combination of endowments and activities of self-decisive, independent and aware citizens" (Centre of Regional Science, Vienna UT, 2007:11). The six characteristics pertain to economy, people, governance, mobility, environment, and living.

Industry Canada oversaw a "Smart Communities" initiative as part of the Government of Canada's portfolio of on-line initiatives, which included other related areas such as eGovernment and healthcare. The Industry Canada initiative selected twelve communities and provided them with funding to support further development of their smart community visions. Smart communities were defined in this Canadian initiative as those having "a vision of the future that involves using information and communication technologies in new and innovative ways to empower their residents, institutions and regions as a whole" (Government of Canada. Industry Canada, 2000:8).

The influential Intelligent Community Forum (ICF) emphasizes the deployment of broadband. It sees broadband as a "fertilizer" for innovation (Intelligent Community Forum, 2008). Intelligent communities are seen as those which are focused on innovation and those which market their community so as to attract globally-competitive businesses and the workforce necessary to maintain them. The ICF defined five indicators of an intelligent community in 2002: (1) significant broadband communications, (2) programs that develop a labour force for "knowledge work", (3) programs to reduce the digital divide, (4) availability of "risk capital" to fund new businesses, and (5) programs for marketing economic development by leveraging the local broadband and knowledge work resources of the community. The ICF's set of current indicators have evolved somewhat. By 2008, the category of "risk capital" had been removed. That indicator seems to have been replaced with "innovation", which is defined as efforts by local governments to build innovation capacity as well as investment in improving e-government efficiencies.

Examples of the types of 'smarts' defined above that can be seen in the cities or projects identified using the criteria in the definitions above. The cities of Seoul and Calgary were cited for their aggressive broadband deployment projects. Fredericton was the first city in North America to deploy a free public WiFi network in its core areas. Areas such as Florida's High Tech Corridor and Sunderland, Tyne & Wear have implemented comprehensive advanced technology infrastructure and policy projects to enhance economic development. Singapore is known for its implementation of comprehensive eGovernment Web services platforms for its citizens, in addition to its wide-spread deployment of broadband. Among European countries, Luxembourg has ranked above average in all of the EU's Smart Cities criteria, including in areas of the intelligence, diversity, and creativity of its people; its economy; lifestyle; and mobility. Montpellier, Maribor, and Ljubljana ranked the highest in terms of "smart environment."

There are many other examples of smart city efforts. Melbourne's CityLink was designed to use electronic tolls and vehicle tracking to reduce traffic congestion. CityLink's approach was to reduce 'start-stop' modes of driving, thereby increasing fuel efficiency and reducing congestion (Homes, 2004). Perhaps the most intriguing example of a smart city because of its scale and its ground-up approach is the new city of Masdar in Abu Dhabi. The Emirate is building what they claim will be "a zero carbon, zero waste city, investing in a range of new energy technologies, establishing a post-graduate research institution and developing a carbon management unit" (Abu Dhabi Future Energy Company, 2009).

There exists a strong counter current in popular discourse to the visions of smart cities implied by the definitions above. Research results reported in the academic literature on the use of information and communication technologies in cities have also raised significant concerns about smart cities. These concerns include issues involving impacts of ICT on urban planning, physical and electronic barriers to access for certain populations, transportation, and the restoration and preservation of social interactions in what many see as the depersonalized metropole.

New York Times columnist Timothy Egan (2009) wrote a lament recently about the changing nature of cities in the context of advanced information and communication technologies. He cited examples where cities are using technologies as the basis for money-saving strategies that have potentially dangerous consequences. The Virginia Transportation Research Council showed in a report that the use of cameras to identify drivers who run red lights – the cause of over 800 deaths and 200,000 injuries in the U.S. -- actually caused the number of accidents to increase (Kassebaum et al., 2007). In the interest of improving work-life balance and work day efficiency, some governments (and businesses) around the world have started to ban employees from initiating work-related e-mail discussions during off hours and have banned the use of personal communication devices within meetings (CBC News, 2008). Indeed it is not clear if there is room for non-ICT ways of being "smart" within the parameters defined above for being a smart city, or at least ways of being smart that involve only a minimum or modest amount of ICT.

Graham and Marvin have pointed out that urban planning is evolving to take into account the interrelationships between ICT and various facets of cities, but that a "coherent new paradigm" has not yet been developed (2004:342). Electronic villages within cities are among what Graham identifies as being within the evolution of a sort of integrative urban planning. In developing such a paradigm, we must consider what Castells (2004:90) described as a complex of requirements in urban planning in this age, which recognizes the 'social and functional diversity' of human settlements and the need to respond to changes in social norms in identifying requirements.

Advanced information and communication technologies and transport provide what Graham terms 'complementarities' (2004a:154). Campanella (2004) and other have seen the concurrent advances in transportation and information and communication technologies as playing a role in reducing 'distance' barriers in human interaction and work. Graham (2004a) and many others have, however, pointed out that complete 'substitution' does not exist. Physical presence is still required for certain types of social processes to be effective. This claim has been supported by a range of studies in cognitive processes and human-computer interaction (c.f. Hollan and Stornetta, 1992; Hollan, Hutchins, & Kirsh, 2000).

Software is also being used or proposed in the transport sector to control entry into certain areas within a city based on the mode of transportation. The goals of these schemes include reduction in traffic congestion and improvements in environmental impacts. Mayor Bloomberg of New York tried to implement a scheme whereby drivers of taxis and private automobiles would be required to pay a premium for driving within certain parts of his city – locations in city centres prone to congestion (Chan, 2007). London has already implemented such a scheme. These schemes are seen as introducing potential barriers for those less able to afford entry but who might have critical needs for entry (Graham, 2004c). Similarly, Castells (2004:84) has identified a paradox involving the virtual linkage and expansion of human settlements via information and communication technologies while at the same time many affluent settlements have raised physical barriers to access.

Social and community informatics has a role in guiding the implementation of smart city visions with respect to the appropriate use of information and communication technologies, as well as in an ongoing monitoring of technology's impacts on society. The range and complexity of the issues involved, as briefly surveyed above, require a model of the scope of the Convergence Model.

THE CONVERGENCE MODEL

Bradley's Convergence Model (2006:52-57) represents the results of her fourth period of research. Her fourth period takes into account the pervasiveness of network technologies and services. Bradley developed, validated, and refined several models over her career based on careful field-based empirical research. Her work culminated in the Convergence Model, which represents the confluence of information and communication technologies and all facets of society (53). The Convergence model has five principle elements (in this author's ordering):

- *Element 1*: human environments, including work and home;
- *Element 2*: characteristics of information, communication, and media technologies;
- *Element 3*: simultaneous life roles of people as a private persons, professionals, and citizens;
- *Element 4*: processes of globalization of values, labour, and technologies through networks; and
- *Element 5*: the resulting impacts on humans of the multidimensional interactions between all of these elements, including this element.

The Convergence model is characterized further in terms of six perspectives:

- *Perspective 1*: it represents four levels of analysis: individuals, organizations, communities, and society(ies);
- *Perspective 2*: it recognizes that human environments may be viewed both objectively and subjectively;
- *Perspective 3*: there may be interactions between the four levels of analysis (*Perspective 1*);

- *Perspective 4*: there may be interactions between the objective and subjective perspectives of human environments.
- *Perspective 5*: there may be interactions between life roles (*Element 3*); and
- *Perspective 6*: all of the elements and perspectives in the Convergence Model are part of a life cycle that causes them to change and evolve.

Bradley's stated goal has been to contribute to "a deeper understanding of the relationship between information and communication technologies and changes in the social and psychological environment (psychosocial life environment)" (2006:1, sec 1.1.1). The comprehensiveness of her model is no doubt due to her multidisciplinary background in psychology, sociology, educational psychology, and ethnography. She has stated that her "theoretical basis" is aligned mainly with social psychology and organizational behaviour (6).

Bradley's focus on community was arguably influenced by the process of electrification in rural Sweden that took place while she was growing up. She has recounted how she accompanied her father while he worked on that effort (5). Her *Computers in the Bakery* project was an example of community-oriented praxis defined by her theoretical work (1996).

The parallels between the processes of development and the current forms of the Convergence Model and the theory Ekistics are, as we will see, remarkable and useful.

EKISTICS

Ekistics was defined by Doxiadis as the "science of human settlements" where the term 'human settlement' represents a community of people, or an 'ekistic unit' (1974:10). Ekistics was Doxiadis's response to what he saw as the need to "arrive at a proper conception and implementation of the facts, concepts and ideas related to [the problems

with] human settlements, and the attempt to re-examine all principles and theories and to readjust the disciplines and professions connected with settlements..." (1968:15). Doxiadis was concerned with the reality that people were most often not happy with their cities or villages (1968:5). He and his research associates sought to predict possible courses of evolution for human settlements by examining the possible evolution of the various dimensions of human society that give rise to and enable the functioning of cities (1974:xv). They exhaustively catalogued and analysed the wide variety of structural elements, patterns, and life cycle processes involved in human settlements around the world; and the ways in which humans corrupt these environments in ways that make them uninhabitable. Doxiadis believed that the development of Ekistics could not occur in the "laboratory" (1968:16). He felt that Ekistics required the study of both the archaeological record of human settlements of the past as well as field studies of existing settlements. He sought to draw the resulting knowledge together into a coherent organization for the field of Ekistics.

Doxiadis defined five basic elements of analysis for human settlements within Ekistics (1968: 21): (1) The characteristics of the natural environmental foundation upon which human settlements are built, (2) humans, (3) society, (4) shells, and (5) networks. The term 'shell' was Doxiadis's generalization of the concept of structures that provide physical covers for functions within the human settlement. A house would be an obvious shell for many human functions, but electrical conduits, airports, and stadiums might also be seen as shells for other types of functions. The term 'network' was Doxiadis's generalization of the concept of arteries through which functions for human settlements are delivered such as people, goods, vehicles, and communications. Roads, postal services, power distribution systems, and shipping routes would all be considered networks.

Doxiadis also defined the 'ekistic unit' as an element of analysis corresponding to the ranges of size and complexity of human settlements (Doxiadis and Papaioannou, 1974:10): (1) people (anthropos), (2) room, (3) house, (4) house group, (5) village, (6) neighborhood, (7) town, (8) city, (9) small metropolis, (10) metropolis, (11) small megalopolis, (12) megalopolis, (13) small continent-spanning city, (14) continent-spanning city, and (15) a global city or an *Ecumenopolis*.

Doxiadis (1968: 109-286) organized Ekistics into four main areas of study and praxis: (1) Ekistic analysis, (2) Ekistic evolution, (3) Ekistic pathology, and (4) Ekistic diagnosis. Ekistic analysis involved the systematic examination of different facets of human settlements, including its basic elements, its ekistic units, and its demographics. Ekistic evolution involved the examination of the processes and forces for the evolution of human settlements, as well as the development of techniques for planning to accommodate this evolution. Doxiadis used the metaphor human diseases as the basis for Ekistics pathology, which examines the types and causes of problems with human settlements. This includes a categorization of "basic diseases" of human settlements including disorderly changes and patterns, and abnormal three dimensional growth (265-277). Doxiadis asked if "Ekistics were an act of medicine or one of creation?" He answered that "the truth is that it is both" (278).

Doxiadis's ultimate objective in developing Ekistics was to articulate a theory and a set of laws for governing human settlements. These included laws of development, laws of extinction of settlements, laws of internal balance between elements within settlements; laws of physical characteristics of elements of settlements, including size, location, functions, structure, and form (1968:287-316). The following are arguably the most important laws of Ekistics, particularly in terms of their parallels with Bradley's Convergence Model:

- *Law 1*: "A human settlement is created in order to satisfy certain needs expressed by different forces, needs of both its own inhabitants and of others" (1968: 288).
- *Law 2*: "Following the creation and operation of a settlement new functions are added which had not been foreseen, and consequently the settlement has to satisfy the initial as well as the additional needs. The more it grows the more important these additional needs may become" (1968:289).
- *Law 3*: "The ultimate goal of a human settlement is to satisfy the needs of its inhabitants, and of the others it serves – particularly those needs leading to happiness and safety" (1968:289).
- *Law 4*: "The satisfaction of the inhabitants cannot be ensured unless all their needs – economic, social, political, technological and cultural – are largely satisfied. There is a unity of purpose in the creation of a settlement; it cannot fulfill *Law 1* if it covers only a few of Man's needs" (1968:289).
- *Law 22*: "... the balance among the elements of a settlement is dynamic" (1968:298).

AN 'EKISTICS' FOR TECHNOLOGIES OF INFORMATION AND COMMUNICATION

Bradley's Convergence Model offers us an invaluable framework for carrying social and community informatics forward. The critical question for her fellow colleagues is 'how do we build upon her research in useful ways?' Bradley has outlined a plan for us (2006:197-236). What should be considered now is a rigorous process to develop specifications for operationalising her plan and to identify new territory that the Convergence Model might cover. Again, the development of the theory of Ekistics offers close parallels in this respect: both the Convergence Model and Ekistics sought to do the following:

- identify and characterize a comprehensive set of objects under study;
- identify and characterize the comprehensive sets of processes or dynamic forces that impact on those objects under study;
- identify and characterize the full range of environments in which these processes and objects under study exist; and,
- account for the multidimensional interactions between the objects and processes under study.

Ekistics differs from the Convergence Model with respect to the level of operationalisation that was performed with the former. Doxiadis's massive work, *Ekistics: An introduction to the science of human settlements,* is an example of this. It and subsequent books documented not only his theory, but provided documentation for the systematic analyses of the many human settlements that Doxiadis and his associates performed using the laws and units of analysis that he defined within the theory.

There is a critical need for this type of systematic pursuit in social and community informatics. Many scientific disciplines have matured through this type of pursuit. Practitioners within certain disciplines like physics and mathematics usually have clear notions of the research 'road map' that identifies their discipline's direction and the research problems that are of prime importance. Practitioners within such disciplines can clearly define their own work in terms of its principle areas of study and praxis in the context of their road map. This is the stage to which we must take community informatics and the Convergence Model.

REFERENCES

Abu Dhabi Future Energy Company (Masdar). (2009). The Masdar Initiative. http://www.masdar. ae/en/Menu/index.aspx?&MenuID=42&CatID= 12&mnu=Cat

Benevolo, L. (1980). *The History of the City* (Culverwell, G., Trans.). Cambridge, MA: The MIT Press.

Benton Foundation. (2004). Defining the Technology Gap: from Losing Ground Bit by Bit: Low-Income Communities in the Information Age . In Stephen, G. (Ed.), *The Cybercities Reader* (pp. 306–308). London, UK: Routledge.

Bradley, G. (2006). *Social and community informatics: humans on the net.* London: Routledge.

Bradley, G., & Bradley, W. (1996). Computers in the Bakery - From Theory to Action. In O. Brown & H. W. Hendrick (Eds.), *Human Factors in Organizational Design and Management-V.* Amsterdam, NL: Elsevier Science. Proceedings from ODAM V, Breckenridge, Colorado, July 31- August 3, 1996.

Campanella, Th. J. (2004). *Webcameras and the Telepresent Landscape. The Cybercities Reader* (pp. 57–63). London, UK: Routledge.

Carson, R. (1962). *Silent Spring.* Boston, MA: Houghton Mifflin.

Castells, M. (2004). Space of Flows, Space of Places: Materials for a Theory of Urbanism in the Information Age . In Stephen, G. (Ed.), *The Cybercities Reader* (pp. 82–93). London: Routledge.

CBC News. (2008, February 1). Federal department's BlackBerry blackout gets mixed reviews. http://www.cbc.ca/news/yourview/2008/02/ federal_departments_blackberry.html

Centre of Regional Science. Vienna UT. (2007, October). Smart cities – Ranking of European medium-sized cities. Retrieved from http://www. smart-cities.eu

Chan, S. (2007, August 14). U.S. Offers New York $354 Million for Congestion Pricing. *New York Times.* Retrieved from http://cityroom.blogs. nytimes.com/2007/08/14/us-will-give-new-york-354-million-for-congestion-pricing/

Dervin, B. (1983, May). *An overview of Sense-Making research: Concepts, methods, and results to date*. Paper presented at the meeting of the International Communication Association, Dallas, TX.

Doxiadis, C. A. (1968). *Ekistics: An introduction to the science of human settlements*. New York: Oxford University Press.

Doxiadis, C. A., & Papaioannou, J. G. (1974). *Ecumenopolis: The Inevitable City of the Future*. London: W.W. Norton & Company, Inc.

Droege, P. (Ed.). (1997). *Intelligent Environments - Spatial Aspect of the Information Revolution*. Elsevier. Retrieved from http://books.google.ca/books?id=zo-iwzll0dIC&dq=Intelligent+Environments+-+Spatial+Aspect+of+the+Information+Revolution&printsec=frontcover&source=bl&ots=M8CGS8IO2Y&sig=yK6q4XIZfcA1ShHScyh7eJ5wdBM&hl=en&ei=Vk9aSuLcNom4M72SsEM&sa=X&oi=book_result&ct=result&resnum=1

Dutton, W. H. (1987). *Wired Cities: Shaping the Future of Communications*. Boston, MA: G. K. Hall & Co.

Egan, T. (2009, June 24). The Self-Service City. *The New York Times, Outposts* (Timothy Egan Blog). Retrieved from http://egan.blogs.nytimes.com/2009/06/24/the-self-service-city/

Godejord, P. A. (2009). GÅ INN I DIN TID – Fra ide til handling. for Informatikk, HiNe. (English: Getting Involved - From Idea to Action (In Norwegian)). Retrieved from http://www.scribd.com/doc/12777702/Getting-Involved-From-Idea-to-Action-In-Norwegian Government of Canada. Industry Canada. (2000). *Smart Communities*. Report of the National Selection Committee. Retrieved from http://smartcommunities.ic.gc.ca

Graham, S. (Ed.). (2004a). *The Cybercities Reader*. London: Routledge.

Graham, S. (2004b). From dreams of transcendence to the remediation of urban life . In Graham, S. (Ed.), *The Cybercities Reader* (pp. 1–29). London: Routledge.

Graham, S. (2004c). The Software-Sorted City: Rethinking the "Digital Divide." . In Graham, S. (Ed.), *The Cybercities Reader* (pp. 324–331). London: Routledge.

Graham, S., & Marvin, S. (2004). Planning Cyber-Cities? Integrating Telecommunications into Urban Planning . In Graham, S. (Ed.), *The Cybercities Reader* (pp. 341–347). London: Routledge.

Hollan, J., Hutchins, E., & Kirsh, D. (2000). Distributed Cognition: Toward a New Foundation for Human-Computer Interaction Research. *ACM Transactions on Computer-Human Interaction, 7*(2), 174–196. doi:10.1145/353485.353487

Hollan, J., & Stornetta, S. (1992). Beyond being there. In *Proceedings of the ACM CHI Conference*. May 3 -7, (pp. 119-125).

Homes, D. (2004). Cybercommuniting on an Information Superhighway: The Case of Melbourne's CityLink . In Graham, S. (Ed.), *The Cybercities Reader* (pp. 341–347). London: Routledge.

Intelligent Community Forum (ICF). (2008). *Intelligent Community Indicators*. Retrieved from http://www.intelligentcommunity.org/index.php?submenu=Research&src=gendocs&ref=Research_Intelligent_Community_Indicators&category=Research

Kassebaum, E. A., Eslambolchi, S., Korukonda, S. K., Garber, N. J., & Miller, J. S. (2007). The impact of red light cameras (photo-red enforcement) on crashes in Virginia. *The Virginia Transportation Research Council*. Retrieved from http://www.virginiadot.org/vtrc/main/online_reports/pdf/07-r2.pdf

Kling, R. (1999). What is Social Informatics and Why Does it Matter? *D-Lib Magazine, 5*(1). doi:10.1045/january99-kling

Kolata, G. (1993, June 29). Scientist at Work: Andrew Wiles; Math Whiz Who Battled 350-Year-Old Problem. *New York Times*. Retrieved from http://www.nytimes.com/1993/06/29/science/scientist-at-work-andrew-wiles-math-whiz-who-battled-350-year-old-problem.html?scp=8&sq=&pagewanted=all

Liskov, B. (1981). Biography of Kristen Nygaard. In R. L. Wexelblat, (Ed.) *History of Programming Languages I*. New York: ACM. Retrieved from http://doi.acm.org/10.1145/800025.1198397

Rowe, D., & Gray, J. J. (2000). *The Hilbert Challenge*. Oxford: Oxford University Press.

Sassen, S. (1991). *The Global City: London, Tokyo, New York*. New Jersey: Princeton University Press.

UN-HABITAT. (2006). *2006 Annual Report of the Cities Alliance*. Retrieved January 5, 2008 from http://www.citiesalliance.org/publications/annual-report/2006-annual-report.html

ENDNOTE

[1]   Doxiadis sometimes referred to this in sociological terms as a state of 'entopia'.

Chapter 5
Gunilla Bradley's 'Good Society' and Structuration Theory:
An Exploratory Excursus

Larry Stillman
Monash University, Australia

Tom Denison
Monash University, Australia

ABSTRACT

This chapter considers Gunilla Bradley's model of technology-in-society as an empirically-focused exercise that reveals psycho-social factors which effect can affect institutional well-being, and that the study of ICTs in society demands a much broader range of understandings of social interaction that has been traditionally associated with Information Systems. Her model also shows that that the study of ICTs in society demands a much broader range of understandings of social interaction that has been traditionally associated with Information Systems. Her model can be enriched by comparison to theories and models, which have emerged from the structuration theory associated with Anthony Giddens, which provides considerable insight about how institutional behaviours are created and transmitted across time and space through the medium of ICTs. This linkage moves the Bradley model from a somewhat functionalist position to one that is more accommodating of human agency, innovation, change, and conflict in different types of social and institutional settings.

INTRODUCTION

In an earlier, short review of Gunilla Bradley's 'Social and community informatics: humans on the net' (Bradley 2006; Stillman 2008), it was suggested that this was a wonderful book, written from the perspective of a Scandinavian woman with a life-time's experience of working with,

and thinking about social-technical issues in work and everyday life. This joint contribution is intended as another acknowledgement to her work and support of others, particularly through the Community Informatics conferences held in Prato, Italy. What struck us in reading her book that it would be worth attempting a study of the relationship between her people-centred theory, and the theory of structuration as developed by originated by the British sociologist Anthony

DOI: 10.4018/978-1-60960-057-0.ch005

Giddens, and then interpreted for ICT research (Bryant and Jary 1991; Jones and Karsten 2003). This task appears particularly worth doing because Gunilla's personal perspective, based on years of field research and presenting a synthesis of many publications (as well has her roots in the Swedish social-democratic tradition, rings a strong chord with Giddens' social-democratic orientation.

This Festschrift contribution represents opportunity to suggest some modifications for further consideration in the model, as well as reflections on its relationship to broader concerns in social theory as a teaching, research, and a practice tool for Community Informatics.

NEW ENGINEERS OR NEW INFORMATION PROFESSIONALS?

Bradley's book was prepared with what she said was 'new kind of engineer in mind' in a society where ICTs were pervasive in augmenting all forms of communication processing (Bradley 2006: 3).

However, given the increasing diversity of people engaged in knowledge and information work that involves questions of design, testing, implementation and theorization about ICT artifacts and relationships, it is not just a question of a 'new type of engineer'. This is an observation that can be drawn from the critical approach developed by Hirschheim and others in their attempt to deconstruct the many complex domains and tasks which cover Information Systems design: no one person, or particular discipline. can be expected to cover the huge range of skills required for the creation of increasingly complex social-technical networks and products in a globalized world (Hirschheim, Klein et al. 1996).

As Bradley observes, broad education and exposure to fundamental social theories and concepts are necessary for the creation a broader cohort of ICT professionals and practitioners, who can think beyond traditional 'engineering' problems.

A broader educational model also indicates the need for a dialogue between non-technical practitioners such as community development workers and those responsible for the design of technical systems, and critically, the engagement of communities themselves in the design process. This is where the perspectives drawn from Community Informatics and the related field of Development Informatics can help to establish richer understandings of what is needed to make more professionals conscious of the complexities of working with social-technologies for social betterment.

For those unfamiliar with the literature and practice of Community Informatics, it is an increasingly well-documented approach to empowering communities with information and communication technologies which brings to bear insights from Information Systems, and Social Informatics (Lamb and Kling 2003). Gurstein, who is widely cited in Community Informatics, recently suggested that Community Informatics involves

... a commitment to universality of technology-enabled opportunity including to the disadvantaged; a recognition that the "lived physical community" is at the very center of individual and family well-being – economic, political, and cultural; a belief that this can be enhanced through the judicious use of ICT; a sophisticated user-focused understanding of Information Technology; and applied social leadership, entrepreneurship and creativity (Gurstein 2007: 12)

That is, Community Informatics is a type of social-technology theorization and practice that promotes social change and human development in conjunction with technology by engaging with local communities and even smaller groupings, such as community organizations, families and informal groups (Stillman and Stoecker 2008). The study of embedded and localised, in situ interactions has led to an increasing number of studies in the IS field, in part because of the failure of traditional, positivist methods of IT research in preference for other forms of theory and research, that 'make visible' what can be so easily missed (Suchman 1995). Technologies can be constructive or disruptive to established ways of doing things, with any combination of effects between, and this is just as much the case in community settings as anywhere else. How to recognise and work with social-technical diversity is also part of the Community Informatics domain of activity. (Avgerou 2002).

From the community development perspective, communities function as locales for 'solidarity and agency', in which solidarity represents deeply held bonds, brought to fruition through human agency (Bhattacharyya 1995), though of course, communities can be disruptive and non-harmonious as well. Despite this restriction, the idea of 'solidarity and agency' at the core of community life also provides a less bounded dimension to the idea of community since it transcends geographic limitations, and can incorporate more dispersed, as well as virtual affiliations. Day and Schuler provide an additional perspective by suggesting that:

Community and voluntary sector groups and organizations form the bedrock of community life through the planning, organization, provision, and support of community activities and services. Although usually under-resourced and over-stretched the community and voluntary sector play a significant role in building and sustaining community. (Schuler and Day 2004: 13)

With its emphasis on empathetic understandings and action being developed with a community's engagement with technology, Community Informatics is part of the interpretive tradition of action research that values and accepts multiple, divergent, and even contradictory 'definitions of the situation', in natural and real world settings (Berger and Luckmann 1966). This orientation is often predicated on theories of social change (Kubisch 1997), and is associated with community development practice in both developed or developing countries (Rothman and Tropman 1970; Heeks 2002).

As an example of this approach, 'technologies of care', that emphasize human communication and personal development predominate in many community settings. Studies have been based upon close studies of the meanings given to technology by workers engaged in face-to-face and sometimes, distributed human services work and community education such as that found in small-scale neighbourhood welfare and educational support organizations (Stillman, Kethers et al. 2009) . Of course, not all community organizations need have the same orientation toward the use of technology (for example, a sports club), but in many situations, there is 'situated use' for people-focussed problem-solving (Suchman 1995; Orlikowski 2000).

Technologies of care can thus be understood as an 'instrumental ensemble' of personal tools and professional techniques, particularly influenced by women's culture and practices in the helping professions. Once again, homage should be paid to Bradley's insights on gender, and this perspective can also be filled out by a growing literature on the feminization of the workforce, including the impact of ICTs on women's work (Wajcman 2001; Huws 2003). ICTs as part of this ensemble influence the shape of communications and action, subject to human intervention and modification. However, as part of the overall technologies of care, ICTs are not pivotal as the vehicle of communication and must be conceived of as part of a process of action and agency for community development and support. They have an adjunct and subsumed function in supporting a cycle of knowledgeable and skilled practices or technologies in the area of community support. However, the *personal meaning* of work is not well explored in Community Informatics writing, and this is where Bradley's model becomes useful.

BRADLEY'S PSYCHOSOCIAL MODEL

Bradley regards work as an activity with deep psychosocial meaning, and the workplace under the impact of modern technology is not inherently degrading to worker interests. Enlightened management practices allow for personal autonomy and human growth. Skilled work, in capitalist societies, like family and leisure, is an important part of human existence and it should allow people to 'achieve a *socio-emotional* balance' by supporting social norms and emotional fulfillment... [these are] major requirements for job satisfaction, psychosocial health and productivity (Bradley 2006: 153).

Sociologically, her views reflect a Durkheimian (Lukes 2004) and structural-functionalist approach (Abercrombie, Turner et al. 2000: supra Functionalism) to workplace order, with an emphasis on what is called 'organic solidarity', through the sharing of values, attitudes, and ways of behaviour. While the details of the differences between Durkheim and other key thinkers such as Weber who took a strong interest in the functional ordering of organizations are beyond the focus of this paper, structural-functionalists emphasize the role of *voluntaristic* belief, ideology and group *socialisation*, rather than the *compulsion* through economic necessity or hegemonic effects that are familiar in various Marxist analyses of power and ideology, drawing on the writings of the Italian theorist Gramsci (Poulantzas 1969; Miliband 1973). This is a viewpoint also developed in critical studies of workplace deskilling via technology(Braverman 1975; Huws 2003).

Her depiction of 'objective' and 'subjective' conditions which are involved in creating socio-emotional balance are addressed in more detail in the discussion below, but at this point, it is sufficient to simply use her terminology to carry forward the discussion. The downside of inappropriate use or implementation of technical systems is manifested in workplace stress, illness,

and industrial chaos, and in the home, with family stress and consequent problems.

As a further step in her integrating approach, Bradley has developed a picture of society as a whole, as ordering through the effects of ICTs. (Bradley 2006: 52ff.). Of particular interest to community informatics is her suggestion that the future home could become 'a multi-purpose... communication centre', which acts as a centre for the democratization of dialogue through communicative interactivity, a marketplace, a learning centre, and as an entertainment centre (Bradley 2006: 128), all of which is dear to the Community Informatics agenda.

Figure 1 summarizes her thinking.

Three key factors underpin her model: the overall technology available in a society, the specific ICT/s being used in an organizational setting, and organizational structure. In the original version of the diagram, based on work published some decades ago, ICTs are referred to as 'Computerized information system', but we suggest that ICTs are a much more contemporary expression of computing power and possibilities.

The tri-partite relationship between technology at a societal level, and organizational structures including ICTs at a meso or micro-level contribute to conditions for the objective and subjective work environment and the objective and subjective conditions outside of work. Organization as a 'structure' includes the legal and formal nature of the enterprise, while the objective work environment consists of the terms and conditions of the work environment. Objective and subjective conditions ('perceptions and attitudes towards the work environment'), are mediated via what Bradley terms 'psychological variables' to create the particular subjective work or outside work and leisure environments.

We suggest that her model is improved by an elucidation of concepts associated with time and space sociology, though she does make an allusion to 'borderless networks' across time and space (Bradley 2006: 157ff.). The ability

Figure 1. Bradley's theoretical model, from Bradley (2006), p. 31 modified (the box 'ICTs' replaces 'Computerized information system')

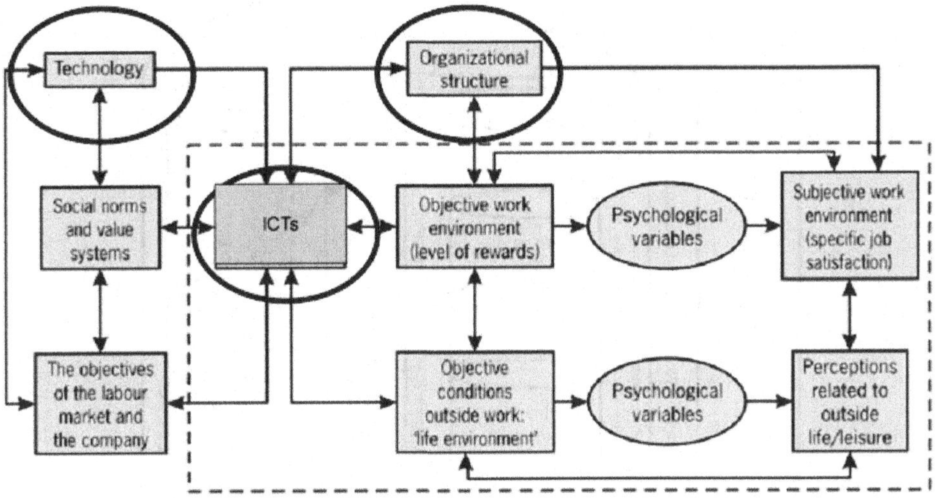

to communicate beyond the physical limits of the body or the building, enhanced by very fast ICTs, is one of the most revolutionary changes that has occurred in the modern area. Thus, hard drives store information that can be accessed at any time or any place and people can work across time-zones and the traditional physical limits of the workplace are broken up and created in new ways provide opportunities for work communication, anywhere, anytime, in any type of enterprise (Giddens 2000).

A model of such 'virtualization' incorporating Bradley's ideas can be developed by the integration of key insights from another Swede, Hagerstrand (1970; 1975). This insight has become of interest to geographers and others interested in tracking daily activity through different technologies and mapping their social effects (Gregory 1986; Gregory 1986) in which the 'friction' of time and space are reduced (Janelle 1969), as incorporated in to structuration theory, as described below. Bradley's schema could be modified to better represent both local and virtual existence.

Another way of representing the scheme, with a certain degree of simplification, taking into account the real effects of time-space activity

is presented below. In this diagram, Bradley's circuit-diagram of social-technical relationship is reworked as series of social technical relationships of 'bundles', using Hagerstrand's language, that are also contained within the dialectic between her so-called objective and psychological work-home conditions. These are overall, structured through social norms and value systems that come to bear in relationship to societal labor market conditions. Significantly however, all this takes place subject to the conditions that time space relationships (the 'wrap around' time-space continuum) offer: the ability to work and communicate through time and space either in situ, or in virtual relationships with others that themselves, leave off into other sets of relationships.

INTEGRATION WITH STRUCTURATION THEORY

Overview

Structuration theory has been enormously influential in Information Systems, with at least 225

Figure 2. Bradley's schema, simplified & modified

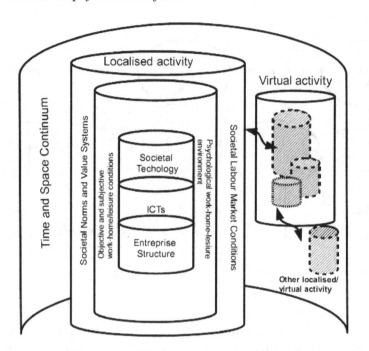

articles identified as of 2003 in relevant journals (Jones and Karsten 2008).

Of particular interest has been the adaptation of Giddens' framework for institutional analysis—or to adopt the language used in the discussion of Bradley— how all sorts of enterprises, large and small (as a kind of durable social institution), are constituted across time and space through knowledgeable human agency and the use of resources (Giddens 1984). The many elements brought together in the theory can be used to develop a rich picture of institutional dynamics and importantly, the relationships between the intersecting values, behaviors, and use of resources in different sorts of organizations, including the use of ICTs.

Thus,

The production or constitution of society is a skilled accomplishment of its members, but one that does not take place under conditions that are either wholly intended or wholly comprehended by them…The key to understanding social order …is not the 'internationalization of values', but

the shifting relations between the production and reproduction of social life by its constituent actors. (Giddens 1976: 102)

There are a number of key ideas that are of particular relevance to institutional analysis, and these provide a systematic way to contextualize Bradley's emphasis on psycho-social factors. Rather than these factors being 'objective' or 'subjective', they are in fact the product of ongoing agency and emergent action by people in their work and home environments. The three key dimensions of structuration—the structures of signification, domination, and legitimation, set in place the institutional character in which people work and live.

1. *Society*—social order—is reproduced though people's constant 'doing' of what they reproduce as ways of behaving.
2. *System,* as generic term, thus refers to the generated, reproduced relations, as well as

institutionally regular social practices which exist across time and place.

3. Critically, the *structural properties of social systems are both medium and outcome of the process of structuration.* Thus, social systems cannot exist outside of what 'structures' exist in society. This is a complex issue subject to long-standing debate in sociological circles, and is beyond the focus of this paper, but the key point is that people have long been puzzled about what is this thing called 'society' and the 'system' which sustains it. It is a theoretical and practical impossibility to have 'objective' 'conditions': as if such 'things' exist as life forms of themselves. In fact, they are, as Giddens suggest, forms of reproduced social practice, subject to the profound influence of access to such things as economic or symbolic power.

Structural properties are primarily communicated and institutionalised through forms of communication, and secondarily, the use of resources as means of control and domination (authoritative and physical), as finally, the use of normative means (the 'rules of the game' in an organization or community via which particular behaviour is acceptable or not).

People take action, using their multiple structural principles or schema (many contradictory) at different levels of tacit or discursive knowledge, commitment, understanding, and social embeddedness (Sewell 1992). Embeddedness and systemness reflect the degrees of reciprocity or integration between actors in either co-presence or across time and space. Specifically, integration refers to the *degree* of interdependence of action, or 'systemness', somewhat similar to Marxist ideas of the hegemony of ideas and ideologies in different institutional settings. Such 'systemness' on a personal level can be gauged through both qualitative means, or quantitative research—the types of things outlined, in the psychosocial dimension, by Bradley.

Lewandowski, in his discussion of embeddedness in Bourdieu, defines the issue as follows:

Embeddedness is both the implicit matrixes of empirical relations in which actors find themselves and the interpretive location from which actors make such implicit ensembles of relations explicit in their everyday practices. The thematization of various forms of embeddedness—linguistic, cultural, economic, political, historical, and so on—is how actors are involved in and appropriate the structured world in which they live. Put in more Bourdieuean terms, thematizing embeddedness is the way we, as context-sensitive bearers of structures, explicitly 'make sense' of and 'play' the social 'games' in which we find ourselves. (Lewandowski 2003: 57)

For example, families (of whatever composition), or organizations of all sorts establish their private practices, languages, symbolic gestures, and understandings of 'what goes', which take time for any visitor to understand, or which are hidden from the public. These, in fact, are Bradley's 'structures' which set the basis for psychosocial factors, which rather than being an external forms, are in fact, based on the interactions of actors in organizations and social systems who 'confront' each other on an ongoing basis, resulting in intricate and endemic negotiations about behaviour and activity.

The same perspective applies to the discussion of conflict and contradiction: we are not speaking of absolutes, but degrees of 'systemness' on both micro and macro-social levels (Giddens 1979: 76ff). These concepts provide a way of describing the specific intersection of signification, domination, and legitimation in organizations, and Giddens also speaks of the 'positioning' of actors in this intersection (Giddens 1984: 83ff).

Furthermore, structural principles, as 'mental' concepts are inherently transportable and transposable, and we constantly move and adapt them from one situation to another. Thus, for example, a person may leave one organization and join another, and, based upon her exposure to day-to-day organizational life, believe she knows how meetings are conducted and particularly, how decisions are made. However, the intersection of her assumptions (structural principles) about meeting protocols with the assumptions in the new organization may not always be a close match and lead to confusion until differences are resolved, or at least, the new assumptions (the structural principles) are absorbed and 'reproduced' by the new player in a way that is acceptable to others. In some cases, of course, the new player's interpretation of meeting and decision-making rules is not accepted and all sorts of difficulties can proceed from that. Thus, one set of assumed 'psychosocial' structures or principles may come into unfortunate conflict with another.

The *study of structuration* is consequently study of how these rules and principles are enacted, reproduced, and transformed using available resources such as ICTs and the degree to which they are embedded in co-present situations (such as the workplace), and across time and space. Bradley's psychosocial measurements provide a way of measuring this embedding in terms of worker or personal 'fit' in particular situations.

RESOURCES IN STRUCTURATION THEORY

In Structuration Theory, resources are of two essential sorts: authority—the capacity to compel someone or something to perform in a particular way, and secondly, of a material sort—things that can be used or manipulated to achieve a goal.

Of particular interest to us are ICTs as a material means, as means of production and transmission of information and knowledge drawn upon by humans to create their organizations and social systems. Power is generated through activity, as actors draw upon particular resources to create particular things within and via the means of

particular time/space locations (for example, computers, are used for teaching, and documents are both accessed and created synchronically and asynchronically at particular locations or 'virtually'), and the resources used to create these activity bundles (such as ICTs) can be stretched over time and space. In fact, Giddens refers to organizations as 'power containers' that can be drawn upon, and by extension, the power—the capacity to use the resources stored in a particular ICT--can also shape the outcome of such activity, for example, through particular software or formatting requirements (Giddens 1984). Thus, time and space are resources which are drawn upon in the creation of social order. For example, the clock has become a device to structure and 'value' time under capitalism and the industrial mode of production (as in work time), and the workplace as a place or locale which is inhabited for many hours a day, subject to the influence of constraining (or liberating) factors becomes imbued with particular characteristics and cultures—the domain of Bradley's psychosocial factors. More recently, and additional transformation has occurred, with the clock (or watch) being absorbed in the mobile phone, linked to calenders and other functions, whether on the mobile itself or a website. Thus time and task are linked even more strongly.

THE OUTCOMES OF STRUCTURATION

Consequently, all forms of social order, including the communities and organizations that are of interest to community informatics practice, consist of people who process and share (or contest) social rules and practice. They function through the interpretive schemes, the stored 'stocks of knowledge' (Giddens 1979: 83), provided by language and other media (such as through ICTs), which provide structure and meaning to communications through time and space (and are shaped by how time and space are constructed by human agents and machines).

Drawing upon particular resources (including the capacity provided by ICTs to achieve goals, these resources can include the possibilities given by ICTs for all forms of communication, including virtual communication. Orlikowski, one of the most influential of Giddens' followers in the study of information systems and the use of ICTs, also suggests the idea of the *duality of technology,* incorporates the view that agency is instantiated through the interaction between human agent and technology. Technological artifacts engage the *interpretive flexibility* of agents: 'technology is created and changed by human action, yet it is also used by humans to accomplish some action'. The technological artifact can be seen as a 'set of features bundled together into an identifiable and bounded package', yet *in use*, it engages user intentions (Orlikowski 1995: 3).

Bradley, with her student Jansson, have highlighted a number of affective issues that are of great relevance to filling out criteria for analysing the different modalities of structuration, and which contribute to a stronger reading of the idea of interpretive flexibility by human agents in conjunction with ICTs. Their argument is quite detailed, but the core is summarized in Table 1, though the focus here is upon workers, rather than

Table 1. Derived from (Bradley 2006: 163-4)

To achieve sustainable communication and collaboration it is vital:
- that the team members get to know each other
- to have fun together
- to trust each other
- to have an organization that supports their work
- to have sufficient ICT support o to learn about team-building
- to learn about conflict-solving
- to have a team space
- to learn communication skills
- to prepare for problems that usually occur in the different stages of a team's life cycle
- that somebody is giving the participants guidance and support to keep them on track
- that somebody keeps the team motivated.

clients in the social-technology relationship. In any case, the risk is that improper management of difficulties associated with affective issues across time and space in the distributed organization or environment can lead to severe disruption of the subjective and objective factors that make for a productive environment.

While Bradley and Jansson were referring in their specific study to distributed working and learning environments, we can reflect again on their argument and its relevance to community informatics environments.

Distributed working and learning environments are becoming more and more common in the world today. Areas that become harder at a distance are building trust and reaching sustainable relationships, since distributed teams do not have the same awareness of each other and receive fewer cues to help them 'read' situations and handle team-building, motivational problems and conflict...it has become essential to analyse how trust-building and psychosocial factors contribute to sustainability in these networks . (Bradley 2006)

'Reading' situations is the task, as they see it, of good management, so that the workplace is happy and productive. From a structurational perspective, this 'reading' is actually the outcome of the negotiation of the dualism and interpretive flexibility of ICTs as the vehicle for multi-dimensional movement of structural principles around communication, norms, and the utilization of resources. Thus, in the world of distributed ICTs that reach across time and space, the kinds of factors that are important for communication and collaboration depend upon the constant reproduction of shared assumptions (most often tacit) about communication and behaviour, using the structural resources that are inherent in any institutional relationship to 'recreate' known patterns and practices on an ongoing basis. This dualistic activity—in which ICTs are not just the means, but also the shaper of message—takes place not just in more traditional organisations such as those studied by Bradley and her colleagues, but in any circumstance in which people come together for purposeful activity in which ICTs are used. This, of course, includes those organisations which we have suggested are bound by a 'technology of care'.

CONCLUSION

Taking Bradley's psychosocial model as a 'reading', for a 'new kind of engineer' it can be considered, first as an empirically-focussed exercise to reveal many psycho-social factors that can affect institutional well-being, and that the study of ICTs in society demands a much broader range of understandings of social interaction that has been traditionally associated with Information Systems.

Second, Bradley's model can also be enriched when linked to the insights provided by structuration theory about how institutional behaviours are created and transmitted across time and space. This linkage moves the Bradley model from a somewhat functionalist position to one that is more accommodating of human agency, innovation, change, and conflict. From this perspective, the 'instrumental ensemble' that comes to constitute an institutional system should be conceived of as a matrix or patterning of psychosocial factors that are both a result of—but also a vehicle—for the key dimensions of structuration, the structures of signification, domination, and legitimation, to set in place the regularly reproduced assumptions and ways of doing things that are recognised as a particular institutional or organizational culture.

From the perspective of Community Informatics, being able to empirically document organizational culture and practice, is critical to changing practices in changes human services work The insight offered by Bradley offers a kind of taxonomy and documentary map for Community Informatics to follow in developing empirically-based responses to situations where the focus of interaction is not so much on the technology, but

'technology of care'. It is these social-technical interactions that are significant forms of social practice that contribute to the good society, the advancement of citizens' rights and community problem solving.

REFERENCES

Abercrombie, N., Turner, B. S., & Hill, S. (2000). *The Penguin Dictionary of Sociology*. London: Penguin.

Avgerou, C. (2002). *Information Systems and Global Diversity*. Oxford: Oxford University Press.

Berger, P. L., & Luckmann, T. (1966). *The Social Construction of Reality; a Treatise in the Sociology of Knowledge*. Garden City, NY: Doubleday.

Bhattacharyya, J. (1995). Solidarity and Agency: Rethinking Community Development. *Human Organization, 54*(1), 60–68.

Bradley, G. (2006). *Social and Community Informatics: Humans on the Net*. London: Routledge.

Braverman, H. (1975). *Labor and Monopoly Capital; the Degradation of Work in the Twentieth Century*. New York: Monthly Review Press.

Bryant, C. G. A., & Jary, D. (1991). *Giddens' Theory of Structuration: A Critical Appreciation*. London: Routledge.

Giddens, A. (1976). *New Rules of Sociological Method: A Positive Critique of Interpretative Sociologies*. London: Hutchinson.

Giddens, A. (1979). *Central Problems in Social Theory: Action, Structure and Contradiction in Social Analysis*. Berkeley, CA: University of California Press.

Giddens, A. (1984). *The Constitution of Society: Outline of the Theory of Structuration*. Berkeley, CA: University of California Press.

Giddens, A. (2000). *Runaway World: How Globalization Is Reshaping Our Lives*. New York: Routledge.

Gregory, D. (1986). Time-Geography. In R. J. Johnston, D. Gregory & D. M. Smith. *The Dictionary of Human Geography* (pp. 485-487). Oxford: Blackwell Reference.

Gregory, D. (1986). Time-Space Distanciation. In R. J. Johnston, D. Gregory & D. M. Smith. *The Dictionary of Human Geography* (pp. 487-492). Oxford: Blackwell Reference.

Gurstein, M. (2007). *What Is Community Informatics (and Why Does It Matter)?* Milan, IT: Polimetrica.

Hagerstrand, T. (1970). What about People in Regional Science? *Papers and Proceedings of the Regional Science Association*, 24, 7-21.

Hagerstrand, T. (1975). Space, Time and Human Conditions. Dynamic Allocation of Urban Space . In Karlqvist, A., Lundqvist, L., & Snickars, F. (Eds.), *Westmead, Hans* (pp. 3–14). Lexington, MA: Lexington Books.

Heeks, R. (2002). Information Systems and Developing Countries: Failure, Success, and Local Improvisations. *The Information Society*, *18*(2), 101–112. doi:10.1080/01972240290075039

Hirschheim, R., Klein, H. K., & Lyytinen, K. (1996). Exploring the Intellectual Structures of Information Systems Development: A Social Action Theoretic Analysis. *Accounting . Management and Information Technologies*, *6*(1-2), 1–64. doi:10.1016/0959-8022(96)00004-5

Huws, U. (2003). *The Making of a Cybertariat: Virtual Work in a Real World*. New York: Monthly Review Press.

Janelle, D. G. (1969). Spatial Reorganization: A Model and Concept. *Annals of the Association of American Geographers. Association of American Geographers*, *59*(2), 348–364. doi:10.1111/j.1467-8306.1969.tb00675.x

Jones, M. R., & Karsten, H. (2003). *Review: Structuration Theory and Information Systems Research*. Judge Institute of Management Working Paper. Cambridge: Cambridge University Press.

Jones, M. R., & Karsten, H. (2008). Giddens's Structuration Theory and Information Systems Research. *Management Information Systems Quarterly*, *32*(1), 125–137.

Kubisch, A. C. (1997). *Voices from the Field: Learning from the Early Work of Comprehensive Community Initiatives*. Washington, DC: Aspen Institute.

Lamb, R., & Kling, R. (2003). Reconceptualising Users as Social Actors in Information Systems Research. *Management Information Systems Quarterly*, *27*(2), 197–235.

Lewandowski, J. D. (2003). Thematizing Embeddedness: Reflexive Sociology as Interpretation. *Philosophy of the Social Sciences*, *30*(1), 49–66. doi:10.1177/004839310003000103

Lukes, S. (2004). Durkheim, Emile (1858–1917). In N. J. Smelser & P. Baltes, *International Encyclopedia of the Social & Behavioral Sciences* (pp. 3897-3903). Oxford, UK: Elsevier Science Ltd.

Miliband (1973). Poulantzas and the Capitalist State. *New Left Review*, I, 82-92.

Orlikowski, W. (1995). *Action and Artifact: The Structuring of Technologies-in-Use*. Retrieved 20 October, 2003, from http://hdl.handle.net/1721.1/2600

Orlikowski, W. J. (2000). Using Technology and Constituting Structures: A Practice Lens for Studying Technology in Organizations. *Organization Science, 11*(4), 404–428. doi:10.1287/orsc.11.4.404.14600

Poulantzas, N. (1969). The Problem of the Capitalist State. *New Left Review, I*(58), 68–78.

Rothman, J., & Tropman, J. E. (1970). Models of Community Organization and Macro Practice Perspectives: Their Mixing and Phasing . In Cox, F. M. (Ed.), *Strategies of Community Organization* (pp. 3–26). Itasca, Ill: FE Peacock.

Schuler, D., & Day, P. (2004). *Community Practice in the Network Society: Local Action/ Global Interaction*. London: Routledge.

Sewell, W. H. (1992). A Theory of Structure: Duality, Agency, and Transformation. *American Journal of Sociology, 98*(1), 1–29. doi:10.1086/229967

Stillman, L. (2008). Gunilla Bradley: Social and Community Informatics: Humans on the Net [Review]. *Information Communication and Society, 11*(3), 433–438.

Stillman, L., Kethers, S., French, R., & Lombard, D. (2009). Adapting Corporate Modelling for Community Informatics. *VINE: The Journal of Information and Knowledge Management Systems, 39*(3), 259–274.

Stillman, L., & Stoecker, R. (2008). Community Informatics . In Garson, G. D., & Khosrow-Pour, M. (Eds.), *Handbook of Research on Public Information Technology* (pp. 50–60). Hershey, PA: Idea Group.

Suchman, L. (1995). Making Work Visible. *Communications of the ACM, 38*(9), 56–61. doi:10.1145/223248.223263

Wajcman, J. (2001). Gender and Technology. In *International Encyclopedia of the Social & Behavioral Sciences* (pp. 5976-5979). Oxford, UK: Elsevier Science Ltd.

Chapter 6

Understanding the Consequences of Technology for Human Interaction and Health:
Gunilla Bradley's Pioneer Scientific Contribution

Kristina Orth-Gomér
Karolinska institutet, Stockholm, Sweden & Charité Universitätsmedizin, Germany

ABSTRACT

Gunilla Bradleys contributions to life sciences are reviewed and explained from a medical and public health perspective. She has developed a research excellence within the field of human interaction and computer technology that has implications that go far beyond her research field. This is because human interaction is crucial for generalized health and welfare of patients and populations. In addition, lack of social human interaction, also referred to as social isolation, is a major risk factor for heart disease, in men as in women. Linking the perspectives of human interaction, technology and health is a formidable task for the research tradition which Gunilla Bradley has created.

INTRODUTION

I shall give a very personal testimony about Gunilla Bradley's work. I will not try to make a well balanced review of Gunilla´s lifelong contribution to science. This is the task of other better positioned colleagues. But it is only natural to be impressed by her formidable list of scientific merits.

With a full background in psychology and computer technology, she has developed a research field around the encounter of human behaviour with computer based technology. She has served as a scientist of excellence in this field for several years, first at the Stockholm University Sociology Department, during which time she also was a guest visiting scientist at Stanford University, USA. She also served at the Universities of Umeå and Växjö. Her present appointment and maybe her most important contribution is with the Royal

DOI: 10.4018/978-1-60960-057-0.ch006

University of Technology as a professor of informatics. She has been a constant creator of cross disciplinary exchange of knowledge between departments within the School of Technology.

When I first met Gunilla Bradley and made her acquaintance, I had learnt that she was an outstanding professor at a Swedish Technical university. But her position and merits were unimportant, in comparison to the impression she made during our conversations.

We met over a dinner buffet at a friend's house. Somebody mentioned her name and started talking about her science, and then someone called me by name. And all of a sudden we were looking at each other realizing we had just met. And then we talked as if we had known each other for years.

Some of the things we talked about are worth mentioning here. They reflected our mutual engagement in what we were doing in our respective scientific areas. But it was also a practical exercise in interactive cross-disciplinary exchange. And because the scientific areas that we represent are very much concerned with each other, and because they depend and benefit from each other, I think they merit being reflected in this Festschrift. I will try and describe our mutual perspectives and merge them into a whole picture (Bradley, G Humans on the Net – Information and Communication Technology (ICT), Work Organisation, and Human Beings)

My own perspective "human interaction and health" is concerned with research and practical experiences around social networks and social support on the one hand and health outcome on the other. Viewing the field from the perspective of "technology and human interaction" Gunilla is concerned with the complex and difficult interface between human minds, human behaviour and human emotions on the one hand and their encounter with technology development on the other. Merging the two perspectives together may result in strategies for using new technology to improve social interaction, improve quality of life and to enhance health.

Gunilla Bradley has been a pioneer in her efforts to create an understanding of what happens with humans when they meet with and adapt to technology, summarized in her book "Social and Community informatics" Routledge 2006). But her contribution to our knowledge goes far beyond behaviour and technology; it also has consequences for the understanding of health effects of social interaction and social ties. For us to better understand the significance of Gunilla Bradley's work in humans, it is important to understand health effects of the social network interactions.

SOCIAL INTERACTION AND HEALTH: QUANTITY OR QUALITY OF INTERACTION?

The significance of social interaction for health has been intensively researched for three decades. A population based study from the Alameda County, California, was the first to show that the more frequent the social contacts, the healthier were the populations.

A burst of reports that more or less confirmed these results followed upon their study, so that in 1988 it was reported in Science about the agreement among researchers that

the number of contacts and their benefit for longevity…are surprisingly similar (House, et al Science 1988).

Two Swedish studies were among the cited ones. The first study was derived from 50 year old men in Göteborg and reported in the Lancet in 1985. The second study was from the adult Swedish population, from which data on social network interaction was obtained as part of the Swedish Survey of Living Conditions, and reported in the J Chronic Diseases, 1987. Both studies had followed their study groups for five years or more and found frequent social contacts to be health promoting (House et al 1988).

But those studies were focussed on number of contacts in defined populations. It was clear that this quantitative knowledge was useful, but it didn't tell the whole story. How come that numerous social contacts were health protective? Which were their nature and their function? Which were their mechanisms?

So, efforts to assess quality of social interaction were made and measures were developed (Undén et al .1991). Such a measure was also developed at the Karolinska laboratory of stress research and analyzed as to its psychometric properties. It consists of two scales, Availability of attachment, (AVAT) and Availability of Social integration (AVSI) .It has been used in many different study groups, from children with deviant behaviour in child psychiatry to coronary artery disease in cardiac patients (Sociala relationer och Hälsa Röda Korset 2008). The AVAT scale describes close emotional ties mainly from family or very close friends; the AVSI scale describes interaction and support from friends, co-workers, relatives, neighbours.

All humans seem to benefit from quantitative aspects of social contacts. Social ties are health protective, regardless of health outcome. The health effects of qualitative social relations are more complex and difficult to demonstrate. Social relations need to satisfy needs that are both 1.emotional, 2. practical and concrete and 3. informational. These are basic human dimensions that characterize human existence and without which we cannot reach full health and wellbeing. It is essential for all members of society to have access to sources of these support dimensions. Emotional support is needed to confirm our deep sense of own worth, yielding an opportunity to reflect our personal identity. It is provided by close family members or friends and based on long term, stable relationships. Tangible and practical support is often provided by more peripheral network members, co-workers, neighbours and so on. It is concerned with tangible help, such as

providing a loan, offering a car ride or helping a colleague at work.

Lastly the importance of access to and provision of informational support cannot be underestimated. To be continuously informed, to share experiences and have the sense of being part of a whole, e.g. at the work site, is essential for good health. These three dimensions of social support are continuously applied in empirical research, in particular research on work environments.

It has been repeatedly demonstrated that all three support dimensions are essential not only for individuals, but also for the health and welfare of a society. In general, studies agree about the basic aspects: the larger the network, the more intense the social interaction, the more favourable the health indices and the better the health. Studies also agree on the role of emotional, tangible and informational support. However, as these aspects are more complex and difficult to measure, results are not as straight forward. Most investigators have found the AVSI scale to be positively associated with better health outcome. Attachment, as measured by the AVAT scale, on the other hand, is not always predictive of good health.

Such an example was seen in middle aged women with coronary heart disease, whose close emotional ties were found to be more stressful than supportive. Consequently, in line with the stress hypothesis, the long term experience of stressful close relationships, marital stress, was a strong predictor of relapse of the heart disease. Women with marital stress had almost three times the risk of a new heart attack, regardless of other risk factors, such as smoking, obesity sedentary life, hypertension and hyperlipidemia (JAMA dec 2000).

Thus there is evidence that social relations may, under unfortunate circumstances, be negative for health and even harmful. The women with heart disease, who had a happy marriage and a good work life, had the best 5 year prognosis. But those women who did not have a relationship, who were living alone, actually fared better than those who experienced severe marital stress. Those women had the worst prognosis. Almost all women had a job at the time of baseline data collection. To many of those women the support from co-workers was important as a buffer against the stresses at both work and at home, suggesting important health benefits of work site network exchange (JAMA okt 2007)

CREATING "SMART HOMES"

In the present network period of ICT profound changes are taking place in human communication - in its structure, quantity and quality.

In 1991 when at Stanford university and before internet was applied deeply and broadly, Gunilla Bradley formulated 7 hypotheses on the relation before ICT and psychosocial communication. Most of the hypotheses were confirmed during the 15 years to come (see Social and Community Informatics, page 82-83 2006: Routledge).

A deep change is also going on in the home environment and I quote from the same source:"The home will become a multipurpose and a communication centre where the nome could be regard as: an extended family centre, a care centre; a multimedia centre; a centre for democratic dialogue, a marketplace; a learning centre; an entertainment centre"

She continues to argue that a so called "smart home" should be service- and not primarily product oriented. It should help the individual to good health, safety and joy and also enable us to deepen human qualities to "give psychological and physical strength to change the society in a humane direction" (Bradley 2006 p 128).

This vision of the future roles and functions of our homes underscores the necessity of manageing and preventing marital and other family related stress.In the Stockholm Study of Women with Heart Disease, women who had experienced longstanding stress and crises in their marital relationships, tripled their risk of a new heart attack (5). In subsequent patient and population studies, from the US (Pittsburgh), Eastern Europe (Hungary) and from Northen Sweden (Umeå) these findings have been confirmed. Furthermore marital discord was found to be risk factor also for the occurrence of a first heart attack.

Thus "smart homes" are essential for family health, both that of patients and that of populations. Gunilla Bradley has foreseen one of the crucial requirements for good population health in the near future. Based on the provisions of welfare and health provided by a strong and innovative technology, her research has implications for building a safe, healthy and creative society for the future.

For these and other reasons the research field of human interaction and computer technology remains crucial and needs further growth and development. We can only hope that Gunilla Bradley will continue her pioneer work for many more years, and that she will provide guidance to all future scholars in this important field of research.

REFERENCES

Bradley, G. (Ed.). (2001). *Humans on the Net - Information and Communication Technology (ICT), Work Organisation and Human Beings.* Stockholm, SE: Prevent.

Bradley, G. (2006). *Social and Community Informatics – Humans on the Net.* London: Routledge.

House, J. S., Landis, K. R., & Umberson, D. (1988). Social Networks and Mortality . *Science, 241*, 540–545. doi:10.1126/science.3399889

Orth-Gomér, K. (Ed.). (2007). *Job strain and risk of recurrent coronary events.* Journal of the American Medical Association.

Orth-Gomér, K., & Perski, A. (Eds.). (2008). *Preventiv medicin – Teori och praktik (Preventive Medicine – Theory and Practice)* (First published in 1999). Stockholm, SE: Studentlitteratur.

Orth-Gomér, K., Wamala, S. P., Horsten, M., Schenck-Gustafsson, K., Schneiderman, N., & Mittleman, M. A. (2000). Marital stress worsens prognosis in women with coronary heart disease . *Journal of the American Medical Association, 284*, 3008–3014. doi:10.1001/jama.284.23.3008

Undén, A.-L., & Orth-Gomér, K. (1991). The measurement of social supports. *Social Science & Medicine, 24*(1), 83–94.

Wenger, N., Chesney, M., & Orth-Gomér, K. (Eds.). (1998). *Women, stress and heart disease.* New Jersey: Erlbaum Association.

Chapter 7
Multitasking:
Some Consequences of the Convergence of Technologies in the Workplace

Alice Robbin
Indiana University Bloomington, Indiana

ABSTRACT

Gunilla Bradley has been an intellectual force for more than forty years. The evolution of her thinking led to a theoretical model that posits the convergence of computer, information, and media technologies and how our work and private lives have been transformed by computerization. This essay examines recent research on this convergence in the context of multitasking, including communicative practices in social and interpersonal interactions at work, effects on the quality of work life and job performance, and the dissolving of the boundaries of work and private lives. Convergence has had both positive and negative effects. It has the potential for improving the quality of social and interpersonal relationships and productivity in the workplace, but, at the same time, substantial evidence shows that multitasking has contributed, sometimes significantly, to increases in stress and cognitive load that have impeded job performance. These effects of computerization were identified very early in Bradley's research investigations, confirming the continued relevance of her research agenda for future work that she proposed more than 20 years ago in her book Computers and the Psychosocial Work Environment.

INTRODUCTION

Forty years of sustained research on the psychosocial aspects of information and communication technologies (ICTs) have resulted in a substantial corpus that is Gunilla Bradley's contribution to understanding how our work and private lives have been transformed by computerization. Her legacy of empirical research on organizational life enriches our understanding of the interdependency and interactions of the social and the technical. Throughout her career she has taken a cross-disciplinary and interdisciplinary path to investigate how computerization affects the physical and psychosocial work environment, as she describes in her 2006 book *Social and*

DOI: 10.4018/978-1-60960-057-0.ch007

Community Informatics: Humans on the Net that summarizes the history of her research and theory-building efforts.[1] This book also reveals her enduring personal commitment to a "people-centered perspective" (p. 2) in order to "achieve the good society" (p. 197). Grounded in theory, rigorous design, carefully specified concepts and their relationships, and empirical methods to test and extend theory, her research has demonstrated that we live in a world where change is a constant and where uncertainty, ambiguity, incomplete information, and unanticipated consequences are the norm. The results of her research are testimony to how ICTs have consequences—both opportunities and risks—for work organizations, human communication, stress, allocation issues, knowledge transfer, and our global village.

Today, we find ourselves in an environment where computer, information, and media technologies have become indispensable and have converged to confound and, indeed, dissolve former distinctions between our public, work, and private lives. Work life is interorganizational, no longer local and for many global; organizational boundaries blur; and new organizational forms have appeared. Where completing our work once depended largely on the constraints of geography and physical location, today it is increasingly at-a-distance (virtual), distributed, portable, and mobile as workers move between, across, and through different physical and social environments and organizational boundaries. Change in work processes has accelerated (Bradley, 2006). Work is increasingly structured as activities, assemblages of tasks "located in a broader organizational setting" (Halverson, 2002, p. 250) that more than ever require explicit cooperative practices, including coordination and collaboration, as workers switch between different projects and tasks and carry out work in-parallel (Fussell et al., 2004; Johnson, May, & Johnson, 2003). Work, at least here in the United States, appears to consume an increasingly larger part of our lives and is no longer bounded by clock time at the office. Activities appear,

Abowd and Mynatt (2000) remark, "continuous in time, a constant ebb and flow of action that has no clear starting or ending point" (p. 31) due to the availability of new computational devices that have "fundamentally change[d] the relationship between humans and computers" (p. 31). Nardi, Whittaker, and Schwarz (2000) point to a significant increase in the "uptake of communications technologies such as email, voicemail, instant messaging, fax, pagers, and cellular telephones, as well as personal digital assistants," contending that "these technologies have led to changes in established work-based communication practices (p. 206). We are seemingly always connected. Thus, as Abowd and Mynatt suggest, "*Continuous* interaction [has] move[d] computing from a localized tool to a constant companion" (p. 31). The single user-to-desktop computer-bound relationship designed for one individual to perform discrete tasks has evolved into a complex web of human-to-human and human-and-nonhuman (tool, object, artifact) relationships that has regulated, intervened in, and modified organizational practices and interpersonal relations at work and in our private lives.

Advances in new digital platforms, the development of innovative applications, the replacement by computers of an array of other technologies, and the convergence of computer, information, and communication technologies have made this possible and in the process are transforming work practices. But has convergence, along with these advances and applications, contributed to or had no effect on different stressors in and outside the workplace? This is the question that this essay addresses in a rather narrow context, that of communication, multitasking, and interruptions.

Part of the story of computerization during the 1970s and 1980s reported in her book *Computers and the Psychosocial Work Environment* concerns communication patterns and work conditions *inside* organizations and the physical and psychological stresses that resulted from the hours *spent in front of* display terminals (Bradley,

1989). The focus on communication is obvious: as Maines (1977) writes, "Through communication processes, people transform themselves and their environment and then respond to those transformations" (p. 242). Bradley (1993) and her colleagues gave special attention to the psychosocial aspects of communication and computerization in what they identified as the "fourth period of computerization," the introduction of knowledge-based systems (KBSs), in an article that appeared in the journal *Computers in Human Behavior*. [2] Worker satisfaction could be explained by the quality of communication with colleagues (human-to-human interaction) and social structural conditions related to the content of work in the organizational environment. Bradley and her colleagues summarized both the advantages and disadvantages associated with replacing personal contact and the qualitative, quantitative, and structural effects of KBS on communication patterns and concluded that "use of computer- and tele-technology deeply interfered with human-to-human interaction, mostly by replacing this human-to-human communication form" (p. 168).

Two other relevant factors contribute to our understanding of the conditions of convergence that Bradley's (1993) long trajectory of research permitted her to observe: First, (different) technologies differ in their effects: they "offer different conditions for the structure of organizations and the psychosocial environment" (p. 482). Second, the evolution of technology is itself a significant variable; change or time matters because we do not study a static system; as Bradley (2000) argues, change is continuous, affecting organizations and their contexts and structures, work roles and processes, and the appearance and disappearance of technology.

My essay follows their recommendation made more than 15 years ago that "the concept of psychosocial communication should be emphasized in the future as an essential part of the psychosocial work environment…and as an essential dimension in organization behavior" (Bradley et al., 1993,

p. 168). I review selected literature on some of the effects of the convergence of computer, information, and media technologies with regard to communication practices and stressors inside the workplace which now extend to the private sphere and family life. [3]

I focus primarily on studies that examine interaction, social context, and the social structure for multitasking and interruptions to illustrate how technologies-in-use intervene in, mediate, and structure social and interpersonal interactions and work life in terms of the psychosocial work environment. [4] The studies described here also underscore that *what* is being communicated—information in human and documentary sources—and task complexity as they affect the psycho-physiological are as important as the specific technologies-in-use for human activity in the work environment and elsewhere.

This recent research also reinforces two other points that Bradley makes concerning discoveries about organizational life: we need to apply multiple theoretical approaches and multiple methodologies for studying organizational life and to address research questions about organizational practices in an interdisciplinary perspective. The various investigations that I describe emphasize the importance of technology for modifying and transforming social behavior, approach technology as a somewhat less instrumental, more humane and user-centered activity, and recognize that technology is as much about cultural practices and a discourse of symbol, metaphor, and rhetorical explanation as it is a tool. Although this review is not about theory, it plays an important part in how this research was conducted, thus warranting a very brief synopsis of the major theoretical underpinnings of the research on the social interactions of multitasking and interruptions in the work place.

The literature that I review focuses on the workplace and is principally carried out by researchers in human-computer interaction (HCI) and computer-supported cooperative work (CSCW); I also refer to a growing literature in psychology, human factors, and ergonomics on the effects of multitasking and interruptions.[5] Thus, as would be expected, a number of theoretical approaches are reflected in the research studies and different conceptual frameworks, theoretical constructs, and different methodological strategies are employed. For example, Halverson (2002, p. 244), who examines HCI and CSCW research, provides us with what she identifies as "a partial list" of the different approaches, which includes activity theory, conversation, coordination theory, distributed cognition theory, grounded theory, situated action, and social/symbolic interactionism.[6] More generally, while understanding that there are significant differences in these theoretical approaches, all are applied to study how technologies and social and human behavior are related, which might be called, writ large, a *social informatics perspective*.[7] Researchers who employ these different approaches emphasize that work practices are *mutually shaped* by the social and technical.[8] Technology shapes work practices but users and their work practices shape technology. As Bradley (2006) comments, "People are products of their social environment, but also have the power to influence and create their environment themselves" (p. 33).

(Inter)action shapes social structure and social structure shapes (inter)action. This perspective further reminds us of another point that Bradley makes and is shared by others of other theoretical and methodological ilk: that outcomes (effects, consequences) of technology-in-use are situationally located, unpredictable, diverse, problematic, complex, inconsistent, paradoxical, disorderly, contradictory, contingent, negotiated, and surprising, evolve over time (emergent), and defy simple conclusions. To put it another way, as Maines writes in his "Forward" to Anselm Strauss's (1993) treatise on a theory of action, "Ambiguity is persistent and persistence is ambiguous" (p. xv).

Moreover, while this literature displays at times structural-functionalist, behaviorist, instrumental means-end, and reductionist biases, this essay mostly reviews a corpus that posits "activity" (or "action") as interactional, temporal, and processual, recognizes the criticality of the structural, and acknowledges the complexity of human experience and the social world.[9] And, finally, as an introduction to the remaining part of this essay, the concept of context becomes essential to an analytical strategy for understanding the complexity of the relationship between the social and the technical. Convergence creates and *is* context (often more than one) for action (activity) in our social world of work; this literature review describes research that examines where multitasking and interruptions are an ordinary part of communicating information in the daily lives of workers where the technologies of computer, information, and media converge.

ENGAGEMENT WITH CONVERGENCE

Media multitasking, writes Li (2009), "has become an increasingly popular phenomenon" as a result of the "development and convergence of many forms of new media and technologies" (p. 15521). He goes on to say that "its inherent mental habits of dividing attention, switching attention, and keeping multiple trains of thought in working memory have significant implications for the way people think, communicate, socialize, learn, and understand the world." Psychologists Ophir and colleagues concur: "In an ever-more saturated media environment, media multitasking—a person's consumption of more than one item or stream of content at the same time—is becoming an increasingly prevalent phenomenon, especially among the young" (Ophir, Nass & Wagner, 2009, p. 15583). Multitasking takes place not just among the young, but also in all aspects of daily life, including the doctor-patient relationship (Chen 2009). No matter the setting, the many available technologies compete for our attention (Adamczyk & Bailey, 2004).

Newspaper articles published in the *New York Times* report serious accidents by adults who multitasked while driving. These include the taxi driver who crashed into an ambulance while talking on his cell phone (Grynbaum, 2009); husbands who insisted on answering their cell phones in the car because it might be an important call from the office or from a client (Richtel, 2009a); blue collar workers who were dependent on computers and cell phones for their next job (Richtel, 2009g); simulations that indicated the consequences of inattention to children crossing the street (Rabin, 2009); and the effects of inattentional blindness (divided attention) of university student pedestrians on cell phones who did not notice a unicycle clown biking on the campus (Parker-Pope, 2009b; Hyman et al., 2009).[10] The number of computer, digital, and media technologies installed in automobiles has led to growing concern about distractions; and the increase in serious traffic accidents in the United States and elsewhere has led to public discussions, legislative hearings, data collection by government agencies, and, in some places, laws to prohibit cell phone use or text messaging while driving (Parker-Pope, 2009a, 2009b; Clifford, 2009; Richtel, 2009b, 2009c, 2009d, 2009e, 2009f; Editors, 2009; U.S. Department of Transportation, 2008).

Li (2009) reflects on the multi-tasking environment that young people have grown up with: the computer which "offers many opportunities for media multitasking" and the Internet which provides a "nonlinear and decentralized structure of information; and on research that has examined the effects of high and low cognitive load on task performance (p. 15523). He suggests that this technological environment is expected to "produce both positive and negative outcomes on cognitive, emotional, and social development." Our knowledge base is currently small with regard to the effects of the convergence of technologies. Nonetheless, we can examine some of the experimental and observational research conducted on multitasking and its consequences by cognitive

psychologists, computer scientists, and human factors researchers who study cognitive control and task-switching performance following interruptions in simulated and actual work settings; and by human-computer interaction researchers who study social behavior in organizations and how people respond to interruptions.

Definitions

"Multitasking" is taken to mean the number of media greater than one that "a person simultaneously consumes when consuming media" (Ophir et al., 2009, p. 15583). I use the definition of "interruptions" employed by Zijstra (1999) and colleagues who conducted a series of experiments to examine "the influence of interruptions on the flow of activities and use of strategies and the psychological and psycho-physiological state of the participants" (p. 170). They defined interruptions as "events which result in the cessation and postponement of an ongoing [main] activity" which is typically resumed after a "certain lapse of time" (pp. 170, 169).

Multiple technologies and multiple tasks with different degrees of familiarity and complexity compete for our attention (Blakeslee, 2009). The brain must allocate attention to multiple environmental stimuli, the stimulus and task representation must be held and manipulated in working memory, and responses must be controlled (Ophir et al., 2009, p. 15583). Multitasking performance requires learning, remembering, planning, and plan-following (Burgess et al., 2000). The individual must be able to filter out irrelevant stimuli due to the increased cognitive load from different mental resources in order to successfully perform tasks (p. 15583). Interruptions have disruptive effects on job performance that are cognitive (mental demand, mental effort) *and* emotional or affect (pleasure, annoyance, frustration, time pressure) (Adamczyk & Bailey, 2004; Bailey & Iqbal, 2008). The physical is also an important component (see Bardram, 2009; Richtel, 2009g for a description of activities inside the automobile and truck). The failure to remember a task in the future after an interruption, known as "prospective memory failure," must be coupled with recall that takes place at the "appropriate moment in time" (Czerwinski, Horvitz & Wilhite, 2004, p. 175).

The emphasis in the two preceding paragraphs has been on activity in the cognitive realm because the work has been carried out by psychologists. However, write McFalane and Latorella (2002, p. 1),

successful job performance also frequently depends on people's abilities to (a) constantly monitor their dynamically changing information environments, (b) collaborate and communicate with other people in the system, and (c) supervise background autonomous services. These critical abilities can require people to simultaneously query a large set of information sources, continuously monitor for important events, and respond to and communicate with other human operators.

Thus, the cognitive acts we describe are about *human engagement* that is *embedded in the social realm* where "social actors experience and manage technologies in their local circumstances" (Knights & Vurdubakis, 2005, p. 182) in collaboration or cooperation with others to get the work done. Interruptions "reveal that the timespace of any individual is not owned and controlled…but can collide and merge with that of another individual" (O'Connaill & Frohlich, 1995). From a social perspective, interruptions constitute "a synchronous interaction which was not initiated by the subject, was unscheduled and resulted in the recipient discontinuing their [sic] current activity" to respond to another person (or object) (O'Connaill & Frohlich, 1995). As such, workers need to be both "self-aligned" with their own work and "in alignment" with others with whom they communicate (Su & Mark, 2008).

Context

A partial list of interactions that workers engage in indicates the complexity of human activities in everyday work life. Bardram (2009) and others (e.g., Saleem et al., 2009; Pennathur et al., 2007; Paoletti, 2009), for example, whose research in the hospital setting provides us with detailed accounts of coordination and collaboration (interacting and communication processes), identify the many human, human-to-human, human-to-nonhuman (the artifact, tool), and human-to-nonhuman-to-human interactions that take place in what is probably one of the most complex and socially structured of work places. These include different paper-based and computer systems; different technologies such as diagnostic machines, fax machines, pagers, and mobile and landline phones; software applications; services; files, data, information, paper and electronic records and other documents; and other workers that reflect the "cooperative nature of real-world human activities" (Bardram, 2009, p. 1012). Engagement in activities that depend on these interactions is context-dependent, constrained by formal and informal rules and routines, and carried out by individuals with a high degree of professionalism and who work in-parallel and independently on their assigned tasks. These activities are mobile, distributed, virtual, and face-to-face as staff meet and move from ward to ward, patient-to-patient, between medicine and patient rooms, between doctors offices and nurses stations, to and from conference rooms, and to and from diagnostic centers.

Also experiencing similar effects of their environment are white collar workers such as those who work at the desktop in call centers (Zuboff, 1988), in air control towers (Weick, 1990), command and control centers (Vaughan, 1996; Neumann, 1995; Perrow, 1998), and the navel ship flight deck (Hutchins, 1996). Blue collar workers, too, are interactants in these relationships: those "truckers, plumbers, delivery drivers, and others [who] are tethered to dispatchers with an array of productivity devices, including on-board computers that send instructions about the next job and keep tabs on drivers' locations" (Richtel, 2009g). University students "sustain a significantly mobile and multitasking system of engagement" at their desktop (Crook & Barrowcliff, 2001, p. 245).

Some might argue that the environment of information and knowledge workers is much simpler than that of the hospital, delivery truck, air control tower, or university dorm room environment. Nonetheless, the descriptions of these environments are essential for making the point that complexity of the task environment (context) is a critical component for understanding the relationship between technology and social behavior. The technologies for multitasking are now widely available, indeed ubiquitous, and interactions with them are both routine and problematic in whatever context that work is carried out. Ophir and colleagues (2009) comment that the "diffusion of larger computing screens supporting multiple windows and browsers, chat, and SMS, and portable media coupled with social and work expectations of immediate responsiveness" are "placing new demands on cognitive processing, and especially on attention allocation" (p. 15585). These are the very same technologies in use by information and knowledge workers and, as such, information processing and cognitive control in their context is as critical an issue for them as for workers in a hospital and for the plumber whose job depends on being first to answer a call. Quan-Haase and Colther's (2005) observational research in a high-technology firm confirms that, indeed, the environment for knowledge workers is equally complex: Multitasking takes place that includes workers who work "interdependently and who perform "three or four operations at the same time, including multiple separate conversations happening in instant messaging and email," with significant pressures of "deadlines for work in process."

Additionally, as Zijstra et al. (1999) remark, whatever the context for those tasks, we need to realize that "the effects of interruptions reach beyond the execution of additional tasks and the change of work strategies" (p. 163). Extending Zijstra et al.'s assessment by employing a more sociological Perrow (1999) conception of what takes place: there are intended effects (first order), unintended and unanticipated consequences (second order), and responses (third order) to the first and second order effects of technology. Rennecker and Godwin (2005) suggest that "Communication technologies…[that] offer the possibility of near-instantaneous access to co-workers through cellular telephony and instant messaging pose the paradoxical consequence of simultaneously decreasing work delays (increased organization, a first-order effect) and increasing work interruptions (increased disorganization, a second-order effect)" (p. 248). They propose the term "third-order effects" to "differentiate between those unintended consequences that stem from the use of the technology and those that represent the creative responses of technology users to the first and second-order effects to achieve both instrumental and symbolic ends" (pp. 254-256).

The next section explores the empirical literature on some of these effects with regard to multitasking and interruptions in the world of work where computer, telecommunication, and media technologies have converged and where they are both the source and solution to organizational and interpersonal problems at and outside work with regard to task completion, communication and interruptions.

Consequences of Mediated Communication Technologies and the Development of Coping Strategies for Multitasking

Although interruptions may be time-consuming and difficult, to the initiator or recipient they may bring personal benefit, interfere with the resumption of a previous task (task switching), or have few effects on task performance. The outcome is a function of a host of factors that can be summarized as the characteristics of the complexity of the task or sub-task performed before the interruption, information processing demands of the current task and task-switching, and timing of the interruption (whether at the beginning, middle, or end of a task or sub-task) (O'Connaill & Frohlich, 1995; Adamczyk & Bailey, 2004; Bailey & Iqbal, 2004; see Rennecker & Godwin, 2005 for an excellent synthesis of the literature). Other relevant factors include the number of interruptions, the duration of an interruption, the familiarity (experience, mastery) with the previous task and new task, and relevance of the new task to the interrupted task.

Two additional psychological factors that affect work performance contribute to how individuals respond to interruptions: need (motivation) for personal control and quality of coping behavior (Rennecker & Godwin, 2005). Personal control motivation and coping behavior will vary along a continuum of low to high and will vary depending on the situation and activity. How people respond to interruptions is a function of their coping behavior; how they manage interruptions, contend Mark et al. (2008) is a function of personality characteristics, including the person's ability to deal with stress, mitigate frustration, maintain flexibility and openness. The technology employed also affects the quality of task performance. Although there is some evidence that interruptions do not result in diminished task performance (Mark, Gudith & Klocke, 2008; Nardi, Whittaker, & Bradner, 2000; Nardi, Whittaker, & Schwarz, 2002; Garrett & Danziger, 2007), overall, the research consistently demonstrates that multitasking results in lower task performance the more complex the task (workload); and interruptions lead to distractions that affect the quality of task effectiveness and increase stress. Interruptions have costs and significant consequences (see Bailey & Iqbal, 2004 and Hyman et al., 2009 for excellent summaries).

Different modes of these communication technologies will have different effects. For example, Hyman et al. (2009) report that students listening to music on an iPod were less likely to experience distractions than students talking on a cell phone. Asynchronous media technology to receive email or a cell phone on vibrate during a meeting suggests greater control and less disruption because a message can be ignored until a task is completed. In contrast, synchronous technology like instant messaging (IM), a beep from the computer to announce the arrival of information, or the ring announcing a telephone call is more likely to be disruptive and may leave the recipient with a sense of less personal control and increased stress related to work performance (see Nagata, 2003). Woerner, Yates, and Orlikowski (2007) discuss the challenges and tensions of maintaining conversational coherence during IM conversations in the geographically distributed workplace setting where they carried out their research. They found that multitasking affected the team's ability to maintain coherence and work together; it was, they found, "distracting and affected both communication and work...because it diverted attention" (pp. 7, 8). Czerwinski et al. (2004) found that the greater the increase in interruptions and the more that needs to be remembered "can wreak havoc with both [communication and work] aspects of prospective memory [remembering and recall] and, hence, can reduce an office worker's daily productivity" (p. 175).

On the other hand, Nardi et al. (2000, 2002) and Garrett and Danziger (2007) present evidence that indicates the positive aspects of IM technology in the pressure-cooker multitasking life of information and knowledge workers. IM was not generally disruptive and the timing of the interactions could be managed and controlled, according to Nardi et al. (2000) and Garrett and Danziger (2007). For Nardi et al.'s (2002) networkers, the multiple communication affordances contributed positively to creating and maintaining personal networks and expanding collaborative networks. For Garrett and Danziger's (2007) information workers IM led to increased computer-mediated personal communication but not an increase in interruptions; these researchers found a technology substitution effect, with IM substituted for other communication technologies.

Communicative practices and technologies-in-use are influenced by the social structure of the organization and norms of its culture (see Alvesson, 2002; Marschall, 2002; Manning, 1996). Contrary to the intentions of designers, implementation of information systems never proceeds according to preconceived plans; that is, how it will be adopted, used, and institutionalized will not conform to original and expected plans made by the designers (Forsythe, 1993; Suchman, 2007). The history of the organization (its biography and how it unfolds, both emergence and enactment), its social structure, and the array of interpersonal relationships that develop between workers will all influence the implementation and use of technologies (see Kling & Scaachi, 1982; Orlikowski, 1992, 2005; Butler & Gray, 2006).

Members of the organization will develop different strategies in the interactions that they have with coworkers depending on established formal and informal relationships (e.g., coworker, subordinate, boss). In other words, responding to interruptions (task-switching) will be influenced by status in the organization's hierarchy of authority. But how the status relationship is mediated by technology may depend on the particular activities and the situation. In any case, the dynamics of a status relationship are expected to greatly influence the motivations and behaviors related to a specific task and how the interruption is perceived. Interruptions made by higher status persons are likely to be accepted more readily than those of equal or lower status. Because the work place is also a resource for friendship, the affective nature of and expectations for (norms of) reciprocity in a relationship with a coworker also influence how the recipient or initiator coworker of an interruption acts (see Rennecker & Godwin, 2005, pp. 258-259). For example, Woermer et al. (2007) found that authority relations of superior-subordinate influenced how IM

conversations were responded to. At the high-tech software firm where they studied IM use, the team manager expected his members to multitask and to be "immediately available and quickly respond to his messages." Although his team members were distracted by his interruptions, they adapted to his "expectations and interaction style" and also acted to control the situation. Quan-Haase, Cothrel and Wellman (2005), who studied IM in a physically co-located group in one high-tech company, found that information provided by IM created connectedness in the work context, enhanced personal relationships, and created opportunities for "unplanned and spontaneous interactions." However, a person's status in the authority hierarchy "played a key role in how their messages were replied to." They found that the "status of the communicator and the urgency of the message [could] be more compelling than the physical presence of someone FTF." Nonetheless, subordinates developed strategies to control the disruptive effects of the IM technology that reduced the social presence of their superiors and IM was effective in individuals who shared strong trusting ties. Quan-Haase and colleagues concluded that how well the technology contributed to effective team work was a function of the influence of social factors such as power, social relationships, and norms within organizations.[11]

Not only information professionals but also young people in high school and college multitask while working. Jeong and Fishbein (2007) found that students spend a "substantial amount of multitasking" using different media (p. 378) while they do their homework, eat, travel, and interact with friends; they listen to audio media, watch TV, and surf the Internet. According to Crook and Barrowcliff (2008), the computer offers "distracting affordances for interaction" for university undergraduates at a university in the United Kingdom for whom computers are "ubiquitously present in their learning environment" (pp. 245, 248). The researchers found that the students were engaged with their computers for long periods of time and that their activities typically involved multitasking. Students had several applications open at once, sound and video played in background while they performed different tasks, and they moved between browsers, text, computer-aided learning packages (CAI) text, games, data, video, graphics, sound, computer-aided learning packages, chat, and email (see Figure 2, p. 251). The opportunities for distraction were considerable and an extensive amount of task-switching took place. Some students who engaged in long sessions moved as often as 79 times between applications; and the ratio between school work and recreational interests was estimated to be 30%:70% (p. 253). The researchers concluded that the "ubiquitous desktop provided in a single interface a rich portfolio of resources relevant to the demands of study," but it was "problematic" because "it created challenges to the "capacity to focus and prioritize activities" (p. 255). It created "obstacles to targeted and productive adoption of available resources" designed for learning: source texts, local course materials, library access, synchronous and asynchronous communications, browsing and downloading tools, computer-supported learning packages, and a wide range of applications for writing, illustrating, transporting, or manipulating data (p. 255).

We take away from their description of the life of undergraduate university students not only insights into the effects of task-switching but how cognitive overload also derives from the nature and quantity of information resources that are available. Technology, task complexity, and information resources cannot be studied independently. This context is emphasized by Mark in research on multitasking that she has conducted with colleagues. Gonzálas and Mark (2004, 2005) conducted research on information workers who work in a fast-paced, constantly changing environment, multitasking in a distributed environment and collaborating on multiple projects. They found that these workers continually switched among "physical and digital artifacts (2004) and between local and global contexts (2005) during the day, but also strategized about how to manage the transitions and cope with their fragmented work lives. In a *New York Times* blog on e-book technology, Mark (2009) comments that reading online and reading text in isolation are not the same because "when you read news, or blogs or fiction, you are reading one document in a networked maze of an unfathomable amount of information." She finds that digital information is a constant distraction. People switch "simple activities an average of every three minutes (e.g. reading email or IM)" and "projects about every 10 and a half minutes." She concludes that "It's just not possible to engage in deep thought about a topic when we're switching so rapidly."

We expect that young people and students of this generation, raised as they are in a multimedia world, would engage in extensive task-switching and use of multiple documents, and, not unexpectedly, researchers would conclude that interruptions had deleterious effects. But to what extent does task-switching and interruptions affect the quality of work of information workers who engage in multiple projects and complex activities and where interruptions are expected to be a common occurrence? O'Connaill and Frohlich (1995) discovered that the information workers they studied responded on average to four interruptions per hour. They found that in most cases 64% of the workers received some benefit from the interruption but that nearly 40% did not immediately resume the work they were doing before the interruption. Czerwinski et al. (2004) examined 11 experienced office software users who were engaged in multitasking in three major projects or tasks in their different work worlds (stock broker, computer science professor, web designer, software development, boat salesman, and network administrator ages 25 to 50 years) who reported an average of 50 task shifts over the period of a week (pp. 176, 179). These Excel user participants believed that the computer improved their productivity, they saw their work as primarily deadline driven, and they were proud of their ability to multitask because "multitasking brought fun and variety to their work" (p. 177). The researchers also analyzed the diary survey that the participants maintained and found that over a six hour day, as many as nine different tasks were identified with an average of 1.75 documents employed in the activity (Figure 2, p. 178).[12] Twelve task events were identified from the diary survey, with the frequency of task-switching ranging from 1% for an application prompt and an emergency, 7% for the return to task, 14% to take a telephone call, 19% for the next task, and 40% for self-initiated task change (Figure 3, p. 178). In sum, the evidence points to the following: The more complex the task (higher mental workload) and the more critical the project, the longer the task lasted, the more documents required, and the more difficult the task-switching (the return to the interrupted task) (p. 178). Research conducted by Iqbal and Bailey (2005, 2006) and colleagues (Iqbal et al., 2005; Iqbal & Horvitz, 2007), who are currently designing interruption reasoning systems, supports these findings but contributes that the task structure needs decomposition because there is also a cost of interruption at subtask boundaries.

In the context of the scientific work place, multitasking with multiple technologies is also a constant. A recent survey of nearly 100,000 scientists about the science workplace about work-life balance and how technology had affected their lives found that scientists experienced high job satisfaction and increased productivity due to their reliance on remote and mobile technologies (Pennock, 2009). However, the survey also found that this "boost in productivity came at a price": more than a third of these science professionals "acknowledged dissatisfaction with their current work-life balance" (p. 1157). Telecommuting has led to erasing the "line between work and home," with scientists working more hours than ever before as a result of the technologies of portable laptops, smart phones, and telecommuting. How to achieve a balance between work and private

lives was the critical issue that needed to be addressed, according to the workforce management firm Kelly Services that had conducted this survey.

Similarly, multitasking is a constant of the social interaction between doctor and patient. In a study of the patient-general practitioner-computer relationship carried out in Australia, researchers found that doctors and patients exhibited different interactions as a result of the computer in the consultation; both patient and doctor engaged each other and the computer which displayed the patient's medical record; and both patient and doctor engaged the computer as a third participant in the interaction (Pearce et al., 2009). Other research indicates that general practitioners, whose interaction relationship with the patient depends on the information content of the visit and the computerized medical record, have learned to modify their behavior. In a study of the National Health Service (United Kingdom), Chan, Stevenson, and McGlade (2008) found that general practitioners altered their communication consulting style depending on the type of problem that the patient presented. Doctors spent considerably less time entering information into their computer and much more time listening to the patient if they had to address a patient's mental or emotional state. Chan et al. concluded that, although the computer was considered a "potentially harmful distraction," they were reassured that doctors were able to "pick up on psychological cues, change their consulting style, and alter the way they used the computer" and that patients were very satisfied with the use of the computer by their doctor during the consultation (p. 537). Likewise, a detailed analysis conducted by Gibson and colleagues (2005) of interactions around a medical decision system of general practitioner multitasking—the management of three "participants" of doctor, patient, and technologies (computer, application software, other documents)—indicated that the doctor intermittently turned his attention away from the computer to the patient and that interactions were coordinated and aligned to each participant's actions" (p. 434).

Finally, in a recent newspaper account one medical doctor reflects on his colleagues and his own work life (Chen 2009): "The demands on our attention have gone, well, viral. Extreme multitasking has invaded the patient-doctor relationship." He recounts an "ever-widening sea of distractions": the "piles of forms to fill, the blinking lights of phone calls on hold, the threads of text messages, columns of e-mails and lists of electronic medical record alerts to attend to." It is "endless multitasking," with doctors suffering high rates of burn-out, "with potentially devastating clinical implications" that include depersonalizing patients, less professionalism, less empathy, and more error prone, becoming depressed, and committing suicide. How to alter the situation? Training doctors to be in the "zone"—to become "mindful"—offers a successful program to "improve a physician's well-being" and also to "sharpen clinical skills." One of the doctors interviewed for the newspaper story comments that "If we can be mindful in the midst of those challenging circumstances, we can derive a greater sense of meaning from even the most demanding situations."

CONCLUSION

Gunilla Bradley's intellectual contributions stimulated this essay that reports on the effects of the convergence of technologies with regard to communicative practices and interactions with multiple technologies. But I come to this *Festschrift* essay with more than an academic's interest in social informatics: Every day my students and I, like everyone else, are personally engaged with multiple technologies. It seemed worthwhile to adopt a "technology-as-practice" perspective to avoid "black-boxing" technology, reinforcing a core principle of her commitment to a science whose goal is investigations that lead

to ameliorating the human condition. Adopting a theoretical tradition that posits a situated technology, one that privileges the "flow of work that takes place over time" and emphasizes that technology is "shaped and managed in actions and interactions with others that contribute to its evolution," directs our attention to "how [technology] is managed collectively" and to a recognition of "open-endedness" (Timmermans 2009, p. 214).

Her research agenda has always represented the scientific humanist's response to the empirical world. And our daily lives affirm the continued relevance of a research agenda for "future work on conditions in a computer society" that Bradley proposed as a series of questions more than 20 years in her book *Computers and the Psychosocial Work Environment*. These questions concern the life conditions that we want, the characteristics of a good work environment and technologies that help us attain our goals, and properties of our social structures, norms, and values systems that promote a positive climate for a society that has been transformed by computerization (pp. 18-19). I wrote at the introduction of this essay about the indispensability of these technologies but also about how they have converged to confound and, indeed, dissolve former distinctions between our public, work, and private lives. Another question that Bradley raised 20 years ago remains more important than ever, as the studies I report confirm: Where, in our work and private life, should we *not* introduce computer technology?

The studies whose findings I summarize above are not definitive, but, certainly, they do not suggest a specter of the end of work as we once knew it that would take place as a result of technology adoption. Yes, we can point to innovations that have been introduced into the workplace, to new forms of organization that have been created, and to the expansion of our horizons from the local to the global. Nonetheless, as these studies demonstrate: we continue to experience fragmented work lives, constant interruptions, increased stress, and a world of work that is now integrated into our private lives.

Thus, our efforts in this new millennium need to be applied to understanding how to leverage these useful affordances and how to adopt positive design technologies that support social and interpersonal processes. The "open-endedness" that I refer to above reflects the optimism about the human condition that has always been part of Gunilla Bradley's stance. There remains much work to do as the research investigations in this essay show. But we get to decide the role we humans play in deciding our condition, Gunilla Bradley tells us.

REFERENCES

Abowd, G., & Mynatt, E. D. (2000). Charting Past, Present, and Future Research in Ubiquitous Computing. *ACM Transactions on Computer-Human Interaction*, *7*(1), 29–58. doi:10.1145/344949.344988

Adamczyk, A., & Bailey, B. P. (2004). If Not Now, When? The Effects of Interruption at Different Moments within Task Execution. *CHI 2004*, Vienna, Austria.

Alvesson, M. (2002). *Understanding Organizational Culture*. London: Sage Publications.

Bailey, B. P., & Iqbal, S. T. (2008). Understanding Changes in Mental Workload during Execution of Goal-directed Tasks and its Application for Interruption Management. *ACM Transactions on Computer-Human Interaction*, *14*(4), 21. Retrieved from http://doi.acm.org/10.1145/1314683.1314689. doi:10.1145/1314683.1314689

Bardram, J. E. (2009). Activity-Based Computing for Medical Work in Hospitals. *ACM Transactions on Computer-Human Interaction*, *16*(2), 1001–1036. doi:10.1145/1534903.1534907

Barthelmess, P., & Anderson, K. M. (2000). A View of Software Development Environments Based on Activity Theory. Retrieved 21 September 2009 from, http://www.ics.uci.edu/~redmiles/activity/final-issue/Anderson/Anderson.pdf

Blakeslee, S. (2001). Car Calls May Leave Brain Short-Handed. *New York Times*, 31 July 2001. Retrieved 17 September 2009 from, http://www.nytimes.com/2001/07/31/science/car-calls-may-leave-brain-short-handed.html

Bradley, G. (1989). *Computers and the Psychosocial Work Environment. Translated from the Swedish by Struan Robertson*. London: Taylor & Francis.

Bradley, G. (1993). What Happens to the Work Organization? In W.S., Marras, W., Karwowski, J.L., Smith, & L. Pacholski (Eds.), *Proceedings of the International Ergonomics Association World Conference on the Ergonomics of Manual Work*, June 14-17, 1993, Warsaw, Poland. Washington/London, DC/UK: Taylor & Francis.

Bradley, G. (2000). The Information and Communication Society: How People Will Live and Work in the New Millennium. *Ergonomics*, *43*(7), 844–857. doi:10.1080/001401300409053

Bradley, G. (2006). *Social and Community Informatics: Humans on the Net*. London: Routledge.

Bradley, G. (2006). Social Informatics: From Theory to Actions for the Good ICT Society. In J Berleur, M.I. Nurminen, & J. Impagliazzo (Eds.), *Social Informatics: An Information Society for All? Proceedings of the Seventh International Conference on Human Choice and Computers (HCC7)* (pp. 183-194), IFIP TC 9. New York: Springer.

Bradley, G., Holm, P., Steere, M., & Strömquist, G. (1993). Psychosocial Communication and Computerization. *Computers in Human Behavior*, *9*(2-3), 157–169. doi:10.1016/0747-5632(93)90004-C

Burgess, P. W., Veitch, E., de Lacy Costello, A., & Shallice, T. (2000). The Cognitive and Neuroanatomical Correlates of Multitasking. *Neuropsychologia, 38*(6), 848–863. doi:10.1016/S0028-3932(99)00134-7

Butler, B. S., & Gray, P. H. (2006). Reliability, Mindfulness, and Information Systems. *Management Information Systems Quarterly, 30*(2), 211–224.

Chan, W.-S., Stevenson, M., & McGlade, K. (2008). Do General Practitioners Change How They Use the Computer During Consultations with Significant Psychological Component? *International Journal of Medical Informatics, 77*(8), 534–538. doi:10.1016/j.ijmedinf.2007.10.005

Chen, P. W. (2009). How Mindfulness Can Make for Better Doctors, *New York Times*. Retrieved 13 October 2009 from, http://www.nytimes.com/2009/10/15/health/15chen.html

Clifford, S. (2009). Doubts about Scare Tactics on Drivers Who Text, *New York Times*. Retrieved 1 September 2009 from, http://www.nytimes.com/2009/09/01/technology/01distracted.html

Crook, C., & Barrowclif, D. (2001). Ubiquitous Computing on Campus: Patterns of Engagement by University Students. *International Journal of Human-Computer Interaction, 31*(2), 234–256.

Czerwinski, M., Horvitz, E., & Wilhite, S. (2004). A Diary Study of Task Switching and Interruptions. In *Proceedings of CHI 2004* (pp. 175-182), April 24-29, 2004, Vienna, Austria.

(Ed.). (2009). Texting to Death (Editorial). *New York Times*. Retrieved 15 September 2009 from, http://www.nytimes.com/2009/09/15/opinion/15tue3.html

Forsythe, D. (1993). The construction of work in artificial intelligence. *Science, Technology & Human Values, 18*(4), 460–479. doi:10.1177/016224399301800404

Fussell, S. R., Kiesler, S., Sctlock, L. D., Scupelli, P., & Weisband, S. (2004). Effects of Instant Messaging on the Management of Multiple Project Trajectories. In *Proceedings of CHI 2004* (pp. 191-198), New York: ACM Publications.

Gibson, M., Jenkings, K. N., Wilson, R., & Purves, I. (2005). Multi-tasking in Practice" Coordinated Activities in the Computer Supported Doctor-Patient Consultation. *International Journal of Medical Informatics, 74*(6), 425–436. doi:10.1016/j.ijmedinf.2005.04.002

Gonzálas, V. M., & Mark, G. (2004). Constant, Constant, Multi-tasking Craziness: Managing Multiple Working Sphere . *CHI, 6*(1), 113–120.

Gonzálas, V. M., & Mark, G. (2005). Managing Currents of Work: Multi-tasking among Multiple Collaborations. In *Proceedings of the 9th European Conference of Computer-supported Cooperative Work (ECSCW '05)* (pp. 143-162), The Netherlands: Springer.

Grint, K., Case, P., & Willcocks, L. (1996). Business Process Reengineering Reappraised: The Politics and Technology of Forgetting. In W.J., Orlikowski, G., Walsham, G., & M. Jones (Eds.), *Proceedings of the IFIP WG8.2 Working Conference on Information Technology and Changes in Organizational Work*, December 1995. London, UK: Chapman & Hall.

Grynbaum, M. M. (2009). Cabbies Stay on Their Phones Despite Ban. *New York Times*. Retrieved August 4, 2009 from http://www.nytimes.com/2009/08/04/nyregion/04taxi.html

Halverson, C. (2002). Activity Theory and Distributed Cognition: Or What Does CSCW Need to Do with Theories? *Computer Supported Cooperative Work, 11*(1/2), 243–267. doi:10.1023/A:1015298005381

Hutchins, E. (1996). *Cognition in the Wild*. Boston, MA: MIT Press.

Hyman, I.E., Boss, S.M., Wise, B.M., McKenzie, K.E., & Caggiano, J.M. (2009). Did You See the Unicycling Clown? Inattentional Blindness while Walking and Talking on a Cell Phone, *Applied Cognitive Psychology*. Published online in Wiley InterScience.doi: 10.1002/acp.1638

Iqbal, S. T., Adamczyk, P. D., Zheng, X. S., & Bailey, B. P. (2005). *Towards an Index of Opportunity: Understanding Changes in Mental Workload during Task Execution. CHI 2005* (pp. 311–320). New York: ACM Publications.

Iqbal, S. T., & Bailey, B. P. (2005). Investigating the Effectiveness of Mental Workload as a Predictor of Opportune Moments for Interruption. In *Proceedings of the CHI 2005* (pp. 311-320). New York: ACM Publications.

Iqbal, S. T., & Bailey, B. P. (2006). Leveraging Characteristics of Task Structure to Predict the Cost of Interruption. In *Proceedings of the CHI 2006* (pp. 741-750). New York: ACM Publications.

Iqbal, S. T., & Horvitz, E. (2007). Disruption and Recovery of Computing Tasks: Field Study, Analysis, and Directions. [New York: ACM Publications.]. *CHI, 2007*, 677–686.

Jeong, S. H., & Fishbein, M. (2007). Predictors of Multitasking with Media: Media Factors and Audience Factors. *Media Psychology, 10*(3), 364–384.

Johnson, P., May, J., & Johnson, H. (2003). Introduction to Multiple and Collaborative Tasks. *ACM Transactions on Computer-Human Interaction, 10*(4), 277–280. doi:10.1145/966930.966931

Kling, R. (1999/2007). What Is Social Informatics and Why Does It Matter? *The Information Society, 23*(4), 205–220. doi:10.1080/01972240701441556

Kling, R., & Scaachi, W. (1982). The Social Web of Computing: Computer Technology as Social Organization. *Advances in Computer, 21*, 2–90.

Knights, D., & McCabe, D. (1998). When "Life is but a Dream": Obliterating Politics through Business Process Reengineering? *Human Relations, 51*(6), 761–798. doi:10.1177/001872679805100604

Knights, D., & Vurdubakis, T. (2005). Information Technology as Organization/Disorganization [Editorial]. *Information and Organization, 15*, 181–184. doi:10.1016/j.infoandorg.2005.06.002

Maines, D. R. (1977). Social Organization and Social Structure in Symbolic Interactionist Thought. *Annual Review of Sociology, 3*, 235–259. doi:10.1146/annurev.so.03.080177.001315

Manning, P. K. (1996). Information Technology in the Police Context: The "Sailor" Phone . *Information Systems Research, 7*(1), 52–62. doi:10.1287/isre.7.1.52

Mark, G. (2009). The Effects of Perpetual Distraction. *New York Times*. Retrieved 22 October 2009 from, http://roomfordebate.blogs.nytimes.com/2009/10/14/does-the-brain-like-e-books/

Mark, G., Gudith, D., & Klocke, U. (2008). The Cost of Interrupted Work: More Speed and Stress. In *Proceedings of the 26th SIGCHI Conference on Human Factors in Computing Systems* (pp. 107-110). New York: ACM Publications.

Marschall, D. (2002). Internet Technologists as an Occupational Community: Ethnographic Evidence. *Information Communication and Society, 5*(1), 51–60. doi:10.1080/13691180110117659

McFarlane, D. C., & Latorella, K. A. (2002). The Scope and Importance of Human Interruption in Human-Computer Interaction Design. *Human-Computer Interaction, 17*(1), 1–61. doi:10.1207/S15327051HCI1701_1

Nagata, S. F. (2003). Multitasking and Interruptions during Mobile Web Tasks. In *Proceedings of the 47th annual meeting of the Human Factors and Ergonomics Society* (pp. 1341-1345). Retrieved 21 September 2009 from, http://interruptions.net/literature/Nagata-HFES03.pdf

Nardi, B., Whittaker, S., & Bradner, E. (2000). Interaction and Outeraction: Instant Messaging in Action. In *Proceedings of the 2000 ACM Conference on Computer Supported Cooperative Work* (pp. 79-88). Philadelphia, PA: ACM Press.

Nardi, B., Whittaker, S., & Schwarz, H. (2002). NetWORKers and their Activity in Intensional Networks. *Computer Supported Cooperative Work, 11*(1-2), 205–242. doi:10.1023/A:1015241914483

Neumann, P. G. (1995). *Computer Related Risks.* New York: ACM Press.

O'Conaill, B., & Frohlich, D. (1995). Timespace in the Workplace: Dealing with Interruptions. In *Proceedings of CHI 1995.* Retrieved from http://old.sigchi.org/chi95/Electronic/documnts/shortppr/boc_bdy.htm

Ophir, R., Nass, C., & Wagner, A. D. (2009). Cognitive Control in Media Multitaskers. *Proceedings of the National Academy of Sciences of the United States of America, 106*(37), 15583–15587. doi:10.1073/pnas.0903620106

Orlikowski, W. J. (1993). Learning from Notes: Organizational Issues in Groupware Implementation. In *Proceedings of the 1992 ACM Conference on Computer-Supported Cooperative Work,* Toronto, Canada.

Orlikowski, W. J. (2005). Material Works: Exploring the Situated Entanglement of Technological Performativity and Human Agency. *Scandinavian Journal of Information Systems, 17*(1), 183–186.

Paoletti, I. (2009). Communication and Diagnostic Work in Medical Emergency Calls in Italy. *Computer Supported Cooperative Work, 18*(2-3), 229–250. doi:10.1007/s10606-009-9091-1

Parker-Pope, T. (2009a, January 13). A Problem of the Brain, Not the Hands: Group Urges Phone Ban for Drivers. *New York Times.* Retrieved 17 August 2009 from, http://www.nytimes.com/2009/01/13/health/13well.html

Parker-Pope, T. (2009b). What Clown on a Unicycle? Studying Cellphone Distraction. *New York Times.* Retrieved 23 October 2009 from http://well.blogs.ytimes.com/2009/10/22/what-clown-on-a-unicycle-studying-cell-phone-distraction/

Pearce, C., Duan, K., Arnold, M., Phillips, C., & Trumble, S. (2009). Doctor, Patient and Computer—A Framework for the New Consultation. *International Journal of Medical Informatics, 78*(1), 32–38. doi:10.1016/j.ijmedinf.2008.07.002

Pennathur, P. R., Bisantz, A. M., Fairbanks, R. J., Perry, S. J., & Wears, R. L. (2007). *Assessing the Impact of Computerization on Work Practice: Information Technology in Emergency Departments.* Presented at the Human Factors and Ergonomics Society 51st Annual Meeting, Baltimore, Maryland, October, 2007.

Pennock, R. (2009). Going Movile. *Nature, 461*(22). Retrieved October 21, 2009 from http://www.nature.com/naturejobs/2009/091022/pdf/nj7267-1157a.pdf

Perrow, C. (1999). *Normal Accidents: Living with High Risk Technologies* (Updated ed.). Princeton, NJ: Princeton University Press.

Quan-Haase, A., & Cothrel, J. (2003). Uses of Information Sources in an Internet-era Firm: Online and Offline. In M.H. Huysman, E. Wenger & V. Wulf (Eds.), *Proceedings of the First International Conference on Communities and Technologies,* Amsterdam, Holland, 19-21 September, Kluwer Academic Publishers, Dordrecht. Retrieved October 3, 2009 from http://www.iisi.de/fileadmin/IISI/upload/C_T/2003/quanhaase-cothrel.pdf

Quan-Haase, A., Cothrel, J., & Wellman, B. (2005). Instant Messaging for Collaboration: A Case Study of a Hightech Firm. *Journal of Computer-Mediated Communication, 10*(4). Retrieved October 3, 2009 from http://jcmc.indiana.edu/vol10/issue4/quan-haase.html

Rabin, R. C. (2009, January 30). When Talking on the Phone May Endanger a Child. *New York Times*. Retrieved September 17, 2009 from http://www.nytimes.com/2009/01/30/health/30phone.html

Rennecker, J., & Godwin, L. (2005). Delays and Interruptions: A Self-Perpetuating Paradox of Communication of Technology Use. *Information and Organization, 15*(3), 247–266. doi:10.1016/j.infoandorg.2005.02.004

Richtel, M. (2009a, September 8). Text Driving Now an Issue in the Back Seat. *New York Times*. Retrieved August 17, 2009 from http://www.nytimes.com/2009/09/09/technology/09distracted.html

Richtel, M. (2009b, August 29). Utah Gets Tough with Texting Drivers. *New York Times*. Retrieved August 17, 2009 from http://www.nytimes.com/2009/08/29/technology/29distracted.html

Richtel, M. (2009c, August 17). Drivers and Legislators Dismiss Cellphone Risks. *New York Times*. Retrieved August 17, 2009 from http://www.nytimes.com/2009/07/19/technology/19distracted.html

Richtel, M. (2009d, August 17). In Study, Texting Lifts Crash Risk by Large Margin. *New York Times*. Retrieved 17 August 2009, http://www.nytimes.com/2009/07/28/technology/28texting.html

Richtel, M. (2009e, July 21). U.S. Withheld Data on Risks of Distracted Driving. *New York Times*. Retrieved September 17, 2009 from http://www.nytimes.com/2009/07/21/technology/21distracted.html

Richtel, M. (2009f, July 29). Senators Seek a Ban on Texting and Driving. *New York Times*. Retrieved September 17, 2009 from http://www.nytimes.com/2009/07/30/technology/30distracted.html

Richtel, M. (2009g, October 1). At 60 M.P.H., Office Work is High Risk. *New York Times*. Retrieved October 1, 2009 from http://www.nytimes.com/2009/10/01/technology/01distracted.html

Robbin, A. (2007). Rob Kling In Search of One Good Theory. *The Information Society, 23*(4), 235–250. doi:10.1080/01972240701444154

Robbin, A. (2010). Theorizing ICT and society: A Preliminary Inquiry into the Methodologies Employed in Research on ICTs and Society: Prologue (An Alternate View of Knowledge Negotiation). *Triple C: Cognition, Communication, Co-operation, 8*(2). Retrieved July 19, 2010, from http://triple-c.at/index.php/tripleC/article/view/171/182

Saleem, J., Russa, A., Justice, C. F., Hagga, H., Ebrighte, P. R., Woodbridge, P. A., & Doebbeling, B. N. (2009). Exploring the Persistence of Paper with the Electronic Health Record. *International Journal of Medical Informatics, 78*(9), 618–628. doi:10.1016/j.ijmedinf.2009.04.001

Strauss, A. L. (1993). *Continual Permutations of Action*. New York: Aldine de Gruyter.

Su, N. M., & Mark, G. (2008). Communication Chains and Multitasking. In *Proceeding of the 26th annual SIGCHI Conference on Human Factors in Computing Systems* (pp. 83-92), New York: ACM Press.

Suchman, L. A. (2007). *Human-Machine Reconfigurations: Plans and Situated Actions* (2nd ed.). Cambridge, UK: Cambridge University Press.

Timmermans, S. (1999). Closed-Chest Cardiac Massage: The Emergence of a Discovery Trajectory. *Science, Technology & Human Values, 24*(2), 213–240. doi:10.1177/016224399902400202

U.S. Department of Transportation. National Safety Board 2008, Driver Electronic Device Use in (2007), Research Note DOT HS 810 963, U.S. Department of Transportation, Washington, DC, June. Retrieved September 17, 2009, http://www-nrd.nhtsa.dot.gov/Pubs/810963.PDF

Vaughan, D. (1996). *The Challenger Launch Decision: Risky Technology, Culture, and Deviance at NASA*. Chicago: University of Chicago Press.

Weeks, J. (2004). *Unpopular Culture: The Ritual of Complaint in a British Bank*. Chicago: University of Chicago Press.

Weick, K. E. (1990). The Vulnerable System: An Analysis of the Tenerife Air Disaster. *Journal of Management, 16*(3), 571–593. doi:10.1177/014920639001600304

Woerner, S. L., Yates, J., & Orlikowski, W. J. (2007). Conversational Coherence in Instant Messaging and Getting Work Done. *40th Annual Hawaii International Conference on System Sciences (HICSS'07)*, 3-6 January, Big Island Hawaii. http://doi.ieeecomputersociety.org/10.1109/HICSS.2007.152

Zijlstra, F. R. H., Roe, R. A., Leonora, A. B., & Krediet, I. (1999). Temporal Factors in Mental Work: Effects of Interrupted Activities. *Journal of Occupational and Organizational Psychology, 72*, 163–185. doi:10.1348/096317999166581

Zuboff, S. (1988). *In the Age of the Smart Machine: The Future of Work and Power*. New York: Basic Books.

ENDNOTES

[1] As I have written elsewhere (Robbin, 2010), my analysis of her corpus found that she has relied on the disciplines of psychology, social psychology, sociology (complex organizations, workplace studies, education, family, professions), health and medicine, and information technology-related disciplines of business administration (management), computer science, and informatics. Reviewing the journals in which she has published, we see that, from early in her career, her disciplinary interests have extended to industrial engineering and design (ergonomics), media studies, communication, and political science (politics, public policy, power, the law, democracy, public administration and management).

[2] Perhaps I could name this the "fifth period of computerization" to distinguish the period from Bradley's "fourth period of computerization" in order to record increased complexity: (i) the move from the relationship of the single individual to the desktop to the relationship of the individual to multiple technologies that increased social interactions; (ii) the increase in the number and "complexity of the many different applications, services, documents, files, users, and other materials involved in achieving the objective of a given activity" (Bardram, 2009, p. 1002); and (iii) the implementation of business process reengineering that was designed to explicitly intervene in traditional social structures of the workplace (see Grint, Case, & Wilcocks, 1996).

[3] This "extending to" acknowledges, as Bradley (2006) has pointed out on many occasions, that we have multiple memberships in social worlds, which increases the complexity of our interactions (see also Strauss, 1993, p. 43).

[4] Bradley (2006) notes that "The term 'psychosocial work environment' is used to signify the course of events or the process that occurs when objective factors in the environment are reflected in the individual's perception (either positive or negative) of work and the conditions of work. The essence [of the psychosocial] is the interaction between the

environment and the individual" (pp. 35-36). The issues of multitasking and how technology influences the quality of work conform to Bradley's "Convergence Model for ICT and Psychosocial Life Environment," and her typology of "objective" and "subjective" factors in the work environment, which also include factors that affect family and leisure time (pp. 40, 48-49, 55). It should be noted that my review does not imply that this is a new domain of study. Indeed, as the references cited by Zijlstra and colleagues (1999) indicate, this topic has been addressed as early as the 1950s with substantial work conducted during the 1970s and 1980s.

5   It is rather surprising (and unfortunate) that during the last 25 years, based on a review of the sociology literature, sociologists of occupations and work appear to have nearly completely ignored the effects of computerization on work life. Most sociological studies are conducted by sociologists marginal to the discipline, in science and technology studies and their research is no longer found in the core journals of sociology.

6   She differentiates between theories, approaches, and methods. She also notes the "cross-pollination of different theoretical approaches."

7   However, and the "however" is very important: there are significant differences in these theories which derive from privileging a particular level or unit of analysis, such as the cognitive, the cultural, or the social, and their relationship(s) with technology (see Halverson, 2002 for an outstanding discussion). Why I hesitate to subsume these different theoretical approaches under "social informatics" is because Kling (2001/2007), who has offered the most elaborated account of social informatics, neglected the cogni-

tive and social psychological properties of the social-cultural-technical system and neglected the transformational processes of artifacts and individuals (see Barthelmess & Anderson, 2000). A particular unit of analysis is privileged over another (e.g., in a Kling perspective, the organization; in activity theory the activity centered around an individual; in distributed cognition the "organizational and social structures, human actors, artifacts on equal footing" nonhuman (Halverson, 2002, pp. 253, 254); and similarly, actor-network theory places the human and non-human network of interactions at the same level. See Robbin (2007) for an analysis of the Kling conception of social informatics.

8   We also use the term "co-constituted": technology and social relations are co-constituted.

9   Were the objective of this essay more expansive, I would also seek out literature that supports historical and symbolical perspectives.

10   Hyman et al. (2009) issue a caution regarding the utility of simulation studies, which is worth reading.

11   Politics is part and parcel of organizational life; however, I do not devote further attention to politics or political processes as they relate to the relationship to technology-in-use (for excellent analyses, see, for example, Weeks [2004] and Knights & McCabe [1998]).

12   The seven largest number of reported tasks were downtime (0.3%), telephone call (8%), routine task (27%, project (18%), personal (5%), meeting (6%), and email (23%). The authors noted that 1.75 documents was a "conservative estimate" (p. 178).

Section 3
Psychological & Usability Aspects of ICT

Prologue to Chapters 8 & 9

Michael J. Smith
University of Wisconsin-Madison, USA

REMINISCENCES ABOUT OUR FRIEND AND SOME OF OUR PAST RESEARCH

I first met Emerita Professor Gunilla Bradley at an international conference on occupational stress sponsored by my former employer, the US National Institute for Occupational Safety and Health (NIOSH), in White Plains, New York in 1977. It was my initial opportunity as a novice researcher in the field of occupational stress to meet many of the top stress researchers in the world. Professor Bradley's research stood out among all of the participants as cutting edge work into the working life issues of the emerging information technologies and how these technologies were transforming the nature of work. I immediately introduced myself to her and asked her to be kind enough to keep me informed of her ideas and research findings. Over the next 30+ years I have been fortunate that Professor Bradley has kept me up to date on her work which has influenced my thinking and research and that of many others around the world. We own a debt of gratitude to her forward thinking and insight about how information technologies have transformed our daily lives and how we work. Her leadership in promoting the need to keep quality of life issues in mind when designing and deploying new technologies has been an inspiration.

My colleagues and I have offered two short articles of our research from the past to this book in honor of Professor Bradley to illustrate her influence on our work. One article deals with how electronically monitoring worker performance can lead to psychosocial stress and related somatic symptoms. The second article hypothesizes that the psychosocial stress encountered in the working conditions created by computer technology may lead to musculoskeletal symptoms in workers independently from the physical ergonomic considerations of their work. These are ideas that grew from the holistic concepts about information technology and quality of working life proposed by Professor Bradley so many years ago. While these studies were published several years ago, the issues presented are still substantial and growing concerns today.

The two studies appear in their original versions as required by US Copyright law and through permission granted by the Human Factors and Ergonomics Society (HFES) solely for this publication. We appreciate the permission granted by the HFES and the willingness of the editors of this book to publish the articles in their original form even though they do not meet the format and space requirements of the book.

We hope that our very good friend and inspiration continues to have a productive and healthy life, and that she will continue to challenge and inspire us for many years to come.

Chapter 8
Electronic Performance Monitoring, Job Design and Psychological Stress

Katherine J.S. Rogers
University of Wisconsin – Madison, USA

Michael J. Smith
University of Wisconsin – Madison, USA

Pascale C. Sainfort
University of Wisconsin – Madison, USA

ABSTRACT

This study helps establish how electronic performance monitoring may influence employee physical strain levels through job design. It identifies job design variables which differ between monitored and non-monitored employees in the telecommunications industry (using discriminant function analysis). These variables' relationships to psychological stress outcomes were examined using multiple regression analysis. A group of 704 employees in three job categories (telephone operator {n=228}, customer service representative {n=230}, and clerk {n=246}) responded to a questionnaire survey mailed to their residence. Four hundred thirty-four of the respondents were monitored and 264 were not. The results indicated that the monitored employees had significantly higher levels of reported psychological stress than the non-monitored employees. The discriminant function analysis of job design variables showed that a variety of job design factors discriminated between monitored and non-monitored employees. High levels of workload, few lulls between periods of high workload, high levels of career/future ambiguity, poor relationships with supervisors, as well as low levels of task meaningfulness and completeness were significant predictors of psychological stress outcomes (tension, anxiety, depression and fatigue).

INTRODUCTION

Electronic performance monitoring has previously been defined as computerized collection,

storage, analysis and reporting of information about employees' productive activities (U.S. Congress, 1987). This definition is used in this study, as it applies to people monitored directly through the use of computers during their work. Previous studies have indicated that the continuous

DOI: 10.4018/978-1-60960-057-0.ch008

monitoring of employee performance is related to psychological stress (Smith et al., 1986; Miezio et al., 1987). However, for the most part, the links between stress and monitoring remain theoretical, although a few papers exist which enumerate the different possible ways monitoring may effect the employee's well- being and performance level through changes in job characteristics, organizational policies and procedures (Smith et al., 1986; Smith and Amick, 1989). The hypothesized differences in job characteristics include: low amounts of control, reduced supervisory support and increased levels of fear of being reprimanded, increased amounts of feedback, increases in performance standards, increased levels of workpressure, increased routinization of work activities, increased pacing, increased workload, reduced peer support, and increased fear of job loss (Smith et al., 1986).

This study helps establish how electronic performance monitoring may influence employee psychological stress levels through changes in job design characteristics. It identifies job design variables whose levels differ between monitored and non-monitored employees, and then examines which of these variables have significant relationships to psychological stress outcomes. However, this study does not address the issue of whether the implementation of monitoring systems actually changes the job design characteristics, or if instead, monitoring systems are more likely to be implemented in existing jobs with these characteristics. If the latter is true, monitoring may magnify or intensify these characteristics (e.g. workload) or the workforce's reaction to them.

METHODS

Sample

In any instructional event it is important to identify the learning domain (the instructional content),

A group of 704 employees in three job categories (telephone operator (n=228}, service representative (n=230), and clerk (n=246}) responded to a questionnaire mailed to their residence. Four hundred thirty-four of the respondents were monitored and 264 were not. Most of the monitored employees are from the positions of operator and service representative, while the vast majority of clerks were not electronically monitored.

The job category of telephone operator includes all types of operators (e.g. directory assistance operators, long distance operators, TOPS operators, TSPS operators). Service representatives include sales, customer, and business representatives. The category of clerk includes employees of the same level of responsibility and classification within the organizations, some of whom work with VDTs. Typical job titles include general clerk, administrative clerk, service clerk and technical clerk.

The sample is overwhelmingly female (90%). The mean age is 39.3 years (std. dev. 9.2), with an average tenure of 13.5 years with the organization.

Analysis

ANOVA and chi-square analyses were used to compare the levels of psychological stress between monitored and non-monitored employees. Discriminant function analysis was performed on the job design characteristics to discern which job design variables had different levels for monitored vs. non-monitored employees. The job design characteristics which discriminated between the two groups were then examined with regard to psychological stress (tension, anxiety, depression and fatigue) using multiple regression analysis.

RESULTS

Analysis of Variance and Chi-Square

The results of ANOVAs and chi-square analyses indicated that the monitored employees had sig-

Figure 1. Levels of psychological stress: Monitored vs. non-monitored employees - Anova and Chi-square results

Stress Outcome Variable	Significance Level
Profile of Mood States	
tension/anxiety	**
depression	**
fatigue	**
NIOSH	
tension	**
anxiety	**
depression	**
fatigue/exhaustion	**

* Significant at the .05 level.
** Significant at the .01 level

NOTE: ANOVA was performed on each of the continuous Profile of Mood States variables. Chi-square analysis was performed on each of the categorical NIOSH variables.

nificantly higher levels of psychological stress than did the non-monitored employees (Figure 1).

Discriminant Analysis

The discriminant analysis of job design variables showed that workload, career/future ambiguity, supervisor feedback, control, workload variability (number of lulls between periods of heavy workload), perceived work standards, traditional supervisor monitoring, client relationships, skill utilization, skill variety, and poor supervisor relationship discriminated between monitored and non-monitored employees in the four job categories (Figure 2).

Regression Analysis

Multiple regression analysis was used to examine the relationships between job characteristics and psychological stress. In addition to the eleven job design variables found to differentiate between the monitored and non-monitored employees, seven demographic variables were also included in the regression analysis (i.e. job category, organization location code, tenure with company, experience in job, age, gender, and a monitored/non-monitored dummy variable). Job category was included in the regression to discern whether there was an effect of job type directly on stress, since the monitored employees are concentrated in the positions of operator and service representative. The organizational location code was included to indicate if the identity of the organization was a predictor of psychological stress.

All of the multiple regressions explained a significant amount of the variance in the seven psychological stress outcomes (p<.01). The only demographic variables that were significant predictors of stress outcomes were gender and organization. Gender was significant in the NIOSH

Figure 2. Job design variables differentiating monitored vs. non-monitored employees - Discriminant function analysis results

Job Design Variable	Weight	Significance Level
control	-.756	**
client relationships	.685	**
workload	.413	**
skill variety	-.390	**
supervisor relationship	.372	**
workload variability	-.291	**
standards	.233	**
skill utilization	-.208	**
task meaningfulness	-.198	**
supervisor feedback	.133	**
task completeness	-.127	*
career/future ambiguity	.102	*
supervisor monitoring	.064	NS
promotions/advancements	-.030	NS

* Significant at the .05 level.
** Significant at the .01 level.

Figure 3. Significant predictors of psychological stress - Multiple regression results

Stress Outcome	Predictor	Beta Coeff.	Significance Level
Profile of Mood States:			
Tension/Anxiety			
(Adj. R2=27.8%)	workload	.237	**
	little workload variability	.127	*
	poor supervisor relationship	.218	**
	career/future ambiguity	.103	*
	task meaningfulness	-.150	**
Depression			
(Adj. R2=16.4%)	workload	.170	**
	poor supervisor relationship	.182	**
	career/future ambiguity	.123	*
	task meaningfulness	-.124	*
	task completeness	-.165	**
Fatigue			
(Adj. R2=24.8%)	organization location	-.112	**
	workload	.302	**
	poor supervisor relationship	.129	*
	career/future ambiguity	.097	*
	task meaningfulness	-.170	**
NIOSH:			
Tension			
(Adj. R2=32.3%)	workload	.270	**
	poor supervisor relationship	.244	**
	career/future ambiguity	.096	*
	task meaningfulness	-.117	*
Anxiety			
(Adj. R2=25.9%)	workload	.294	**
	little workload variability	.163	**
	poor supervisor relationship	.213	**
	task meaningfulness	-.149	**
Depression			
(Adj. R2=20.1%)	workload	.151	*
	little workload variability	.137	*
	poor supervisor relationship	.270	**
	career/future ambiguity	.159	**
	task meaningfulness	-.133	*
Fatigue			
(Adj. R2=22.9%)	gender	-.122	**
	workload	.238	**
	poor supervisor relationship	.183	**

* Significant at the .05 level.
** Significant at the .01 level.

fatigue regression, with women reporting higher levels of fatigue than men, however it was not a predictor for depression, tension or anxiety. The particular organization was a predictor of the POMS fatigue measure, which indicates that organizational policies and cultures may directly affect report of fatigue. High workload, high career/future ambiguity, poor supervisor relationships, low levels of task meaningfulness and low workload variability (having few lulls between high levels of workload) all were significantly related to high levels of stress (Figure 3).

DISCUSSION

The results indicate that although many job design characteristics discriminate between the monitored and non-monitored jobs, the only ones significantly linked to increased levels of psychological stress are high levels of workload, few lulls between periods of heavy workload, a poor relationship with the supervisor, low levels of task meaningfulness, and high career/future ambiguity. (Task completeness was also a predictor in one instance, POMS depression.) Workload and a poor supervisor relationship were significant predictors for all of the stress outcomes, and task meaningfulness was a predictor in all but one instance. The results are relatively consistent, and the regression equations explain anywhere from 16% to 32% of the variance in self-report of psychological stress.

Perceptions of high workload were the most consistent predictor of stress, and were sometimes combined with perceptions of low workload variability (i.e. few lulls between periods of heavy workload in which to think or contemplate). This result may be influenced by the monitoring system itself, or the service standards set by management, based on monitoring performance data. However, perceptions of the standards themselves (fairness, ability to meet standard, etc.) were not linked to psychological stress, although they were discriminators between the monitored and non-monitored employees.

The findings confirm previous research which identified supervisor relationships as a potential source of stress in monitored work (Smith et al., 1986). Supervisory relationships are under the direct control of management, and therefore, in theory, can be changed to alleviate some employee stress. This may reflect the organizational culture and management choices as to how the information collected by the monitoring system is used. (Potentially, the same information could be fed back to the employee in a non- evaluative way by the machine and produce less stress.) That is, the electronically monitored employees have greater fears of being reprimanded than the non-monitored employees, which is associated with higher levels of psychological stress.

Although control and client relationships were the largest contributors to the discriminant function (i.e. have very different levels in the jobs of the monitored and non- monitored jobs), they were not significantly related to psychological stress. The fact that control was not linked to psychological

stress may be due in part to the organizational culture of the workplaces, in that many employees in the telecommunications industry have had jobs with low control for many years. Thus, low control may have ceased to be perceived as a source of stress (Frese and Zapf, 1988). Additionally, the organizational culture may also influence the coping mechanisms associated with contact with hostile clients, since this workforce has also dealt with this stressor for many years.

This study shows that monitored employees report significantly higher levels of psychological stress than do non-monitored employees, in three telecommunications job categories. It cannot, due to its cross-sectional design, show a cause/effect path of electronic monitoring changing job design to create or increase psychological stress. However it does show that many job characteristics differentiate between electronically monitored and non-monitored jobs. Additionally, it identifies which of these job characteristics are linked to self-report of psychological stress. This information is useful to modify existing monitoring systems, and to design new systems for the reduction of job characteristics levels which are associated with psychological stress.

REFERENCES

Frese, M., & Zapf, D. (1988). Methodological Issues in the Study of Work Stress: Objective vs Subjective Measurement of Work Stress and the Question of Longitudinal Studies . In Cooper, C. L., & Payne, R. (Eds.), *Causes, Coping and Consequences of Stress at Work* (pp. 375–411). New York: John Wiley & Sons Ltd.

Miezio, K., Smith, M. J., & Carayon, P. (1987). Electronic Performance Monitoring: Behavioral and Motivational Issues. In S.S. Asfour (Ed.), *Trends in Ergonomics/Human Factors IV*, (pp. 253-257) Amsterdam, NL: North Holland.

Smith, M. J., & Amick, B. C. III. (1989). Electronic Monitoring at the Workplace: Implications for Employee Control and Job Stress . In Sauter, S., & Hurrell, J. (Eds.), *Job Control and Worker Health* (pp. 275–288). Chichester, UK: John Wiley and Sons, Ltd.

Smith, M. J., Carayon, P., & Miezio, K. (1986). Motivational, Behavioral and Psychological Implications of Electronic Monitoring of Worker Performance. *Prepared for the Office of Technology Assessment*. United States Congress. Washington, DC: Office of Technology Assessment, U.S. Congress

U.S. Congress, Office of Technology Assessment. (1987). *The Electronic Supervisor: New Technology, New Tensions. OTA-CIT-333*. Washington, DC: U.S. Government Printing Office.

NOTE

Chapter 9
Psychosocial Considerations in Upper Extremity Cumulative Trauma Disorders

Michael J. Smith
University of Wisconsin-Madison, USA

INTRODUCTION

Current theories of work related cumulative musculoskeletal disorders of the upper extremities indicate that causation is multifactorial (Armstrong et al.,1993; Kuorinka et al., 1995; Smith and Carayon, 1996). Prominently mentioned among the causes are biomechanical exposures which are believed to lead to "micro" trauma to tissues that accumulates over time to produce more serious injury. Also believed to have a role are psychosocial factors that lead to job stress (Smith and Carayon, 1996). There is some debate about the explicit role that these psychosocial factors play. Do they exacerbate the strain due to biomechanical exposures, are they co-causal factors, are they a

DOI: 10.4018/978-1-60960-057-0.ch009

necessary condition for biomechanical exposures to produce problems, or can they produce problems on their own? This paper explores some of the ways that psychosocial factors may affect the risk of upper extremity cumulative trauma disorders (CTD's). For a more detailed discussion see Smith and Carayon (1996) and Moon and Sauter (1996).

TRADITIONAL CTD CAUSATION FACTORS

Traditional risk factors in cumulative trauma disorders (CTD's) of the hand, wrist, arm, shoulder and neck have been tied to the biomechanical aspects of the workplace which lead to tissue strain with repeated exposure, and other factors (Kuorinka et al, 1995). There are eight risk factors that influence the probability of the occurrence of an upper extremity CTD. These are the frequency of motions of the upper extremities (repetition rate and duration of exposure); the posture of the joint, arm, hand, wrist, elbow, shoulder and neck; the force necessary to do a task, or the load that creates forces in the musculature and tissues; vibration; environmental conditions; work organization characteristics; psychosocial conditions; and personal risk factors such as gender. The first four consideration cause direct strain on the joints, muscles, tendons, ligaments, nerves and soft tissue. They have been referred to as biomechanical factors.

It has been postulated that repetitive actions or sets of motions cause "wear and tear" on the joints, rubbing and abrading of the tendons and ligaments, and increased muscular fatigue (Armstrong et al., 1993; Putz-Anderson, 1988; Silverstein et al., 1987; Kuorinka et al., 1995). While there currently is insufficient research evidence to establish the number of movements or the length of exposure that will produce a specific injury or health problem, it is believed that in most situations the higher the number of movements, the greater the potential risk of a CTD problem.

The longer an individual is exposed to a physical stressor, the greater the risk of cumulative trauma (Putz-Anderson, 1988). Duration of exposure can be subdivided into daily actions; extended periods of similar action for weeks, months, and years; and career exposures to action. Continuous daily exposure without breaks for rest can produce local muscle fatigue, general systemic fatigue and possibly micro-damage of muscles, tendons and ligaments. It is suspected that if this exposure is prolonged, over weeks and months, it can lead to a tissue strain; and over a longer duration, it can lead to tissue damage. The extent of career exposure for specific tissues generally defines the potential risk for cumulative trauma. It is believed that the longer the months and years of exposure, the greater the stress accumulation and the higher the risk of permanent injury.

As the upper extremities deviate from the natural or a neutral posture, the risk of a CTO increases (Putz-Anderson, 1988). However, the extent of joint or appendage deviation that produces a health problem has not been specifically quantified through research or experience.

Force can be the result of the effort necessary to complete a task, such as assembling components, twisting wires, picking up washers or lifting a box. Or, force can be influenced by the loading aspects of the materials and tools that are being used such as the weight, weight distribution, size and dimensions of the products or tools. Force can also be influenced by the personal style of the user in carrying out the task. For instance, there can be great variability in the amount of force with which different employees hold a tool or grip the product, or place merchandise onto a conveyor. High force jobs that also have high repetition have been shown to be at a greater risk for certain types of CID's (Silverstein et al., 1987).

Environmental factors such as hot and cold temperatures can make the soft tissues and nerves more susceptible to injury and fatigue (Putz-Anderson, 1988). Some facilities are cold and this can increase the risk of muscle strain and distorts neuro-sensory processes. Hot environments can lead to increased muscle fatigue. Other environmental factors such as vibration can increase upper extremity CID risk.

Personal factors also increase susceptibility to CID. These include, but are not limited to, personal physical conditioning, diseases (such as arthritis, diabetes and gout), prior musculoskeletal injuries, small wrist tunnels, gender, and use of certain hormone treatments such as estrogen. Additionally, some people are more prone to these types of injuries due to their personality and their behavior in carrying out their job.

Workplace ergonomic conditions such as the nature of the work activities, workstation design, and equipment design can contribute to CID problems by affecting the biomechanical factors.

These conditions interact as a system to produce an overall load on the person that can lead to strain.

THE ROLE OF PSYCHOSOCIAL FACTORS

Upper extremity cumulative trauma disorders appear to be more prevalent in occupations that have features that are known to produce job stress, ie, short task cycle, boring, low control, low content and high work pace (Smith and Carayon, 1996). This is logical since many of these same job features lead to an increase in the traditional biomechanical risk factors for CTD's, ie, high repetition, forceful exertions, poor upper extremity posture and long duration of exposure.

There are various ways in which psychosocial factors can increase the risk of a CTD. At the personal level psychosocial factors can create job stress and related psychological and physiological strain. These may increase physiological susceptibility to cm by affecting hormonal responses and circulatory responses that exacerbate the influences of the traditional biomechanical risk factors. Psychological strain can influence personal attitude and behavior which may lead to risky actions.

At the job level, the nature of the task activities (work methods), employee training, availability of assistance and supervisory relations can affect employee exposures, satisfaction, attitude and behavior (techniques). At the organizational level, the policies and procedures of the company can affect exposure through the design of jobs by specifying the length of time engaged in specific activities, establishing work-rest cycles, defining the extent of work pressures and establishing the psychological climate regarding socialization, career and job security. These factors can influence psychological moods that affect motivation, attitude, behavior and health on a holistic basis. Their effects may be to influence the individual's "susceptibility"

for developing a cumulative trauma disorder, or "sensitivity" to pain and discomfort.

STRESS AND CTD'S: A CONCEPTUAL RELATIONSHIP

Biochemical Mechanisms: When an individual is undergoing the psychological and physiological effects of job stress there are changes in body chemistry that may create increased risk of CTD. Cannon (1928) first described this as the "fight or flight" response which was tied to an infusion of adrenaline, and Selye (1956) later refined the medical syndrome associated with this prolonged "arousal" process. Levi (1972) has described the specific mechanisms of the biochemical changes in detail.

The organism's basic reaction to external threat and internal psychological stress is to mobilize energy resources for defensive actions and to "shut down" response mechanisms that could compromise the organism's survival if injured. This reaction is controlled by the autonomic nervous system and is involuntary. That is, there is no thought involved and the person has no control over the responses. When this reaction occurs, there is less blood flow to the extremities, including the muscles and tendons of the extremities. When working requires repeated motions or forceful motions and the person is undergoing stress, then a reduced blood flow will limit the availability of energy resources. It is likely that fatigue will occur sooner and that muscles and tendons could be overworked.

A second biochemical reaction that occurs is an increase in corticosteroids. These, in particular cortisol, can lead to an increase in fluid retention in body tissues. This mechanism may mimic the fluid production and tissue swelling due to repeated friction of the tendon body with the tendon sheath. It may create pressure and pinching of the nerve(s) that can cause the paresthesia and pain in peripheral neuropathy.

According to Selye (1956) at some point in the stress syndrome the organism is unable to continue to respond normally and exhaustion occurs. During this stress induced exhaustion, the immune system is not able to function normally and thus cannot provide the typical resources for repairing damaged tissues. Chronic exposure to cumulative trauma stressors while the organism is undergoing psychological stress may create micro damage that cannot be fully repaired because of reduced immune system capacity.

A fourth biochemical reaction that occurs when an organism is under stress is the increase in peripheral neurotransmitters (in particular norepinepherine) which promotes the capability of the peripheral synapses to respond. This may create a sensitization of the muscles. With increased levels of norepinepherine, the tension in muscles has the potential to be greater as is the amount of force generated by the muscles in performing an activity. This heightened muscle tension may be enhanced by direct "efferent" stimulation due to psychological moods such as anxiety or anger. Thus, when the person is angry or frightened the muscles are typically more tense. These are physiological and psychological processes which can lead to heightened muscle tension that may increase the risk of excessive muscular force when working.

The catecholamines (epinephrine and norepinephrine) also stimulate increases in blood pressure and heart rate. Hypertension has been correlated with carpal tunnel syndrome.

The final biochemical connection is less straightforward. It has been shown that persons suffering from depression and schizophrenia have abnormal patterns in the production of seratonin and endorphins. These natural narcotics are important in influencing mood states, and in promoting sleep and thus a general fatigue burden. A similar pattern of disruption of normal seratonin production has been observed in shiftworkers. Negative mood states such as those prevalent during psychological distress may affect the production of seratonin and endorphins and have negative consequences for muscular fatigue and fatigue recovery.

Psychological Mechanisms. A second major way in which stress can influence the occurrence of CTD's is through its effects on a person's psychological and behavioral reactions. Thus, stress can affect psychological moods, work behavior, coping style and actions, motivation to report injury and motivation to seek treatment.

Upper extremity CTD's are disorders that involve significant pain. Many times, diagnosis of a disorder is based on the nature and extent of pain reported by the person. Stress may serve to increase the frequency of reporting of upper extremity pain because of a general increase in personal sensitivity to pain brought on by negative moods. If the person were not under psychological stress the pain may not be perceived as significant, and could go unreported.

A related issue is a social psychological aspect of illness behavior. It is possible that a person under psychological stress could develop specific physical symptoms (such as sore wrists) that would "legitimate" their general psychological discomfort and pain. Having pains in the wrists and fingers is an acceptable disorder, while feeling depressed may not be acceptable. Thus, the effects of psychological disturbances may be reflected in physical disorders of the musculoskeletal system. This is much like psychosomatic disorders where psychologically induced disturbances lead to physical impairments.

Behavioral Mechanisms. Job stress can influence the behavior of a person in dealing with the work environment. For instance, a person who is stressed may modify work methods that lead to greater biomechanical strain. A person under stress often develops poor attitudes and motivation about the job and about their personal health and well being. They become apathetic. Such a person may not seek medical assistance when early signs of cumulative trauma occur.

Individual behavioral reactions to stress include modified sleeping habits, increased drinking of alcohol, increased smoking, and increased use of drugs. Other behaviors may include increased absenteeism, turnover, and performance deficits. These are all behavioral reactions to stress that serve as maladaptive coping mechanisms.

WORK ORGANIZATION, JOB DESIGN, STRESS AND ETD'S

Smith and Carayon-Sainfort (1989, 1995) have proposed that stress is a result of an imbalance between elements of the work system. This imbalance produces a "load" on the human response mechanisms that can produce adverse reactions, both psychological and physiological. The human responses, which include behavior, physiological reactions and cognition, act as coping mechanisms to bring control over the environmental factors that are creating the imbalance. These efforts, coupled with an inability to achieve balance, produce overloading of the response mechanisms that leads to mental and physical fatigue. Prolonged exposure and fatigue may lead to strain and disease, especially in susceptible persons.

Work load factors, such as quantitative and qualitative overload and overtime have been related to psychological stress (Cooper and Marshall, 1976; Smith, 1987). These same job features can be significant risk factors for CTD's because they affect the level of musculoskeletal effort, the frequency of upper extremity actions, the amount of fatigue and the extent of overall exposure to activity.

Repetitiveness is another psychological job stressor that has been associated with musculoskeletal aches and pains (Salvendy and Smith, 1981; Smith, 1987), mental health disorders (Salvendy and Smith, 1981; Cox, 1985) and behavioral problems such as absenteeism (Cox, 1985). Work pacing affects psychological stress and may create a risk for CTD's. Machine-paced

work tasks are more stressful than non-paced tasks (Salvendy and Smith, 1981). Machine-pacing is particularly stressful because it is often characterized by quantitative overload, high work pressure, repetitiveness and lack of control (Smith, 1985). Ergonomic CTO risk factors, such as the frequency of the repetitive motions and the duration of exposure, can be tied directly to the work pace and work load requirements (work standards) which are established by the organization.

The organizational context for work can influence worker stress and health. Career considerations, status incongruence and lack of job security have been linked to worker stress (Cooper and Marshall, 1976). Other aspects of the organizational context such as role conflict and ambiguity also have negative emotional consequences (Jackson and Schuler, 1985). These conditions may create a working "climate" of distrust, fear and confusion that could lead employees to "perceive" more aches and pains and report more CTD's. In particular, companies that have the potential for reductions in the labor force (lay-off or job loss) may be more susceptible to employees reporting more problems and more serious problems as an economic defense.

Technology may have inherent characteristics that make it stressful, such as physical and mental requirements, software unfriendliness and poor system performance (Carayon-Sainfort, 1992). There is some evidence that shows that video display terminal technology can be a source of physical stress, such as visual and musculoskeletal problems (Smith et al., 1992). Another influence of technology is worker fears of adequate skills to use the technology and fear over job loss due to increased efficiency of technology (Ostberg and Nilsson, 1985; Smith et al., 1987). The way the technology is introduced may also influence worker stress and health, and cm's (Smith and Carayon, 1995). For instance, when workers are not given enough time to get accustomed to the technology, they may develop unhealthy work methods and postures (Smith et al., 1992).

GENERAL CONCLUSION

Much of this discussion has been hypothetical and has been presented to illustrate that there is substantial potential for psychosocial and work organization factors to contribute to upper extremity CTD's. While the research base to know precisely what those roles are and whether they are significant is quite small, it seems very plausible that job stress can have a major influence on the development of upper extremity CTD's.

REFERENCES

Armstrong, T. J., Buckle, P., Fine, L. J., Hagberg, M., Jonsson, B., & Kilborn, A. (1993). A conceptual model for work-related neck and upper limb musculoskeletal disorders. *Scandinavian Journal of Work, Environment & Health, 19,* 73–84.

Cannon, W. B. (1928). The mechanism of emotional disturbance of bodily functions. *The New England Journal of Medicine, 198,* 877–884. doi:10.1056/NEJM192806141981701

Carayon-Sainfort, P. (1992). The use of computer in offices: Impact on task characteristics and worker stress. *International Journal of Human-Computer Interaction, 4*(3), 245–261. doi:10.1080/10447319209526041

Cooper, C. L., & Marshall, J. (1976). Occupational sources of stress: A review of the literature relating to coronary heart disease and mental ill health. *Journal of Occupational Psychology, 49,* 11–28.

Cox, T. (1985). Repetitive work: Occupational stress and health . In Cooper, C. L., & Smith, M. J. (Eds.), *Job Stress and Blue-Collar Work* (pp. 85–112). New York: John Wiley & Sons.

Jackson, S. E., & Schuler, R. S. (1985). A meta-analysis and conceptual critique of research on role ambiguity and role conflict in work settings. *Organizational Behavior and Human Decision Processes, 36,* 16–78. doi:10.1016/0749-5978(85)90020-2

Kuorinka, I., Forcier, L., Hagberg, M., Silverstein, B., & Wells, R. Smith. M., Hendrick, H., Carayon, P., & Perusse, M. (1995). *Work Related Musculoskeletal Disorders (WMDSs): A Reference Book for Prevention.* London: Taylor & Francis.

Levi, L. (1972). *Stress and Distress in Response to Psychosocial Stimuli.* New York: Pergamon Press.

Moon, S., & Sauter, S. (Eds.). (1996). *Beyond Biomechanics: Psychosocial Aspects of Cumulative Trauma Disorders.* London: Taylor & Francis.

Ostberg, O., & Nilsson, C. (1985). Emerging technology and stress . In Cooper, C. L., & Smith, M. I. (Eds.), *Job Stress and Blue-Collar Work* (pp. 149–169). New York: John Wiley & Sons.

Putz-Anderson, V. (Ed.). (1988). *Cumulative Trauma Disorders-A Manual for Musculoskeletal Diseases of the Upper Limbs.* London: Taylor & Francis.

Salvendy, G., & Smith, M. I. (Eds.) (1981). *Machine-Pacing and Occupational Stress.* London: Taylor & Francis.

Selye, J. (1956). *The Stress of Life.* New York: McGraw Hill.

Silverstein, B., Fine, L., & Armstrong, T. (1987). Occupational factors and the carpal tunnel syndrome. *American Journal of Industrial Medicine, 11,* 343–358. doi:10.1002/ajim.4700110310

Smith, M. J. (1985). Machine-paced work and stress . In Cooper, C. L., & Smith, M. J. (Eds.), *Job Stress and Blue- Collar Work* (pp. 51–64). New York: John Wiley & Sons.

Smith, M. J. (1987). Occupational stress . In Salvendy, G. (Ed.), *Handbook of Human Factors* (pp. 844–860). New York: John Wiley & Sons.

Smith, M. J., Carayon, P., Eberts, R., & Salvendy, G. (1992). Human-Computer interaction . In Salvendy, G. (Ed.), *Handbook of Industrial Engineering* (pp. 1107–1144). New York: John Wiley & Sons.

Smith, M. J., & Carayon, P. C. (1995). New technology, automation and work organization: Stress problems and improved technology implementation strategies. *The International Journal of Human Factors in Manufacturing, 5*, 99–116. doi:10.1002/hfm.4530050107

Smith, M. J., & Carayon, P. C. (1996). Work Organization, Stress and Cumulative Trauma Disorders . In Moon, S., & Sauter, S. (Eds.), *Beyond Biomechanics: Psychosocial Aspects of Cumulative Trauma Disorders* (pp. 23–42). London: Taylor & Francis.

Smith, M. J., & Sainfort, P. C. (1989). A balance theory of job design for stress reduction. *International Journal of Industrial Ergonomics, 4*, 67–79. doi:10.1016/0169-8141(89)90051-6

NOTE

Chapter 10

Computers, Psychosocial, Work Environment, and Stress:
A Comparative Theoretical Analysis of Organizations and Action Strategies

Michelle M. Robertson
Liberty Mutual Research Institute for Safety and Health, USA

ABSTRACT

With the rapid rate of new technologies, coupled with telecommunications equipment being introduced into the workplace, further exploration is needed on how to effectively integrate and design these technologies to better support the roles of the individual, organization and society. Occupational roles are expanding along with new patterns of how individuals interact with these evolving technologies and their influences on different levels, that of the individual, organization and society. To more systematically analyze these technology based computerized information systems and their integrations with the physical workplace design, psychosocial issues, work organization and work/family balance factors, two theoretical models are presented and their relationship to workplace stressors and strain. These models highlight the importance of action strategies and applying a system analysis model that incorporates an interdisciplinary and macroergonomics perspective.

PROLOGUE

Professor Gunilla Bradley and I met in 1986 at the ODAM conference (International Symposium on Human Factors in Organizational Design and Management) in Vancouver, where Gunilla served as session chair when I presented some results from my doctoral thesis at the University of Southern California. This led to lifelong col-laboration and friendship. Professor Bradley and I collaborated in the late 1980s to integrate two systems perspectives regarding psychosocial and physiological issues among office and computer workers. Two models and approaches were presented to understand the complexity including the micro and macro ergonomic issues surrounding intensive computer use and the overarching impact of information technology on knowledge workers. We first began by creating system models and building a theoretical approach with the goal of

DOI: 10.4018/978-1-60960-057-0.ch010

focusing on the outcome variable of occupational stress and its effect on the quality of life and well-being of workers. Psychosocial and physiological disturbances, including musculoskeletal and visual disorders were noted in the models. The systems analysis approach allowed us to work through the complexity of the problems and to address strategies and interventions to mitigate these negative effects of computer and information technology on workers. Over the past 30 years, we have used and further developed these models and approaches to guide our respective research fields. Many articles and books have been written and keynote presentations given describing these models and approaches. References to these further works are included in this article. My contribution to this Festschrift summarizes the first article that we published together, which set the foundation for much of my research and at the time influenced research internationally (Bradley & Robertson, 1991). I would like to dedicate this work to Professor Bradley as it reflects our life time commitment to Information Computer Technology as it reflects and acknowledges the strength of her passion and influence in this field and the impact it has made on individuals, organizations and societies.

INTRODUCTION

Integration between computer technology and telecommunications equipment affects the design of occupation roles and our roles as citizens, as well as on new patterns of how these human roles will be combined and balanced. Education and training are essential for the individual's potential to exert influence on her/his work environment and for the quality of life at computerization. This is especially important for preventing or coping with various problems like stress and musculo-skeletal disorders in the information society and minimizing future segmentation of the labor force.

For almost two decades, beginning in the 70s, interdisciplinary research was carried out at Stockholm University on Work Life and Computerization and continued at other universities where Bradley served as professor and research leader. The problems studied are related to a theoretical model developed within a program for analyzing the interplay between computerized information systems <–> psychosocial work environment <–> family life/leisure time/ and health. Building upon this general theoretical model, we focused on one effect variable – stress. We further explored and focused on the formal work organization, work content, communication structure, leadership, role ambiguity and working hours.

Theoretical Analyses

The analyses of stress and working life can be focused on different levels: individual and societal. That is, stress experienced by the individual, fragmentation of the labor force, or marginalization and exclusion from the mainstream of society. Different action strategies must be adopted in order to prevent and counteract stress problems of all these levels. Some types of stress that occur in display terminal work have been counteracted with technical aids that affect response times, availability, screen layout, standardization, etc. However, most stress problems deal with work organization and psychosocial factors, making education and training design/redesign, crucial issues.

Two Theoretical Models

We further developed various strategies by presenting two theoretical models: 1) The model on the relationship between Computer technology, Work Environment and Stress (Bradley, 1989), [See Figure 1], and 2) The seven step-wise Systems Action Model (Robertson & Rahimi, 1990), [See Figure 2]. This proposed model consists of seven steps. They are: 1) defining the problem; 2) developing objectives and activities; 3) developing an evaluation criteria table, 4) modeling

Figure 1. Interplay computer technology, work environment and stress. Source: Bradley, G. (1989) and Bradley G. & Robertson M. (1991)

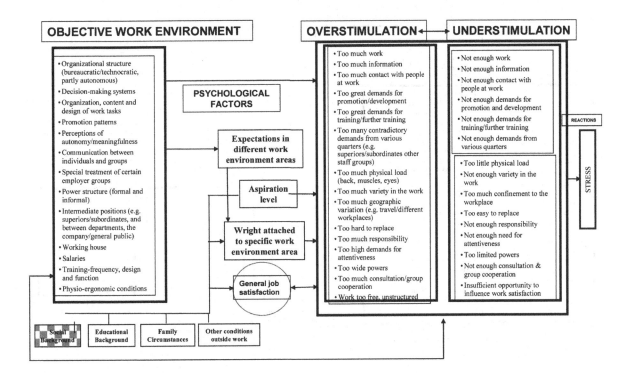

alternatives, 5) evaluate alternatives and select an alternative, 6) planning for implementation and 7) evaluation, feedback and modification process. Each of these analytical steps is represented and explained by a modular graphical diagram or appropriate schematic. Figure 2 presents the Problem Factor Tree, specially created for understanding the complex and systematic causal factors of the psychosocial and physiological strain issues, including musculoskeletal disorders, for computer intensive office workers.

Initial Observations

From our initial observations and comparative analyses between Sweden and USA, we concluded that there is a need for developing a model representing action strategies that incorporate an international perspective. The central concepts found in the Swedish research concerning organizational and psychosocial work environment were initially analyzed and compared with some of the essential main concepts within macro-ergonomics and human factors research in the US. Some of these include: 1) the need to focus on macro-ergonomic principles and definitions of organizational structure incorporating both physical and psychosocial strain issues, 2) action strategies for effective implementation and introduction of computer technology encompassing micro and macro ergonomics considerations, such as workstation design, job content, training and education, organizational structure, organization of professional roles and work tasks, leadership, and communication structures, and 3) consideration for (existing) government or other central

Figure 2. The problem factor on occupational stress. Source: Robertson, M. & Rahimi, M. (1990) and Bradley & Robertson (1991)

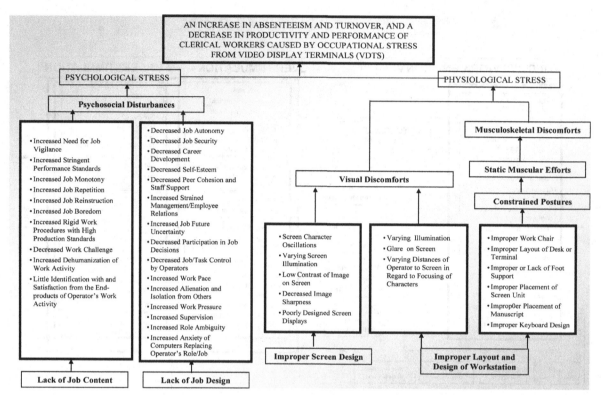

policies in action strategies, addressing important issues such as ethics, democracy, and equality.

FINAL REMARKS

The introduction and use of computer technology and telecommunications on a broad scale brings about new professional roles characterized by various stress symptoms and psychological strain. Computer systems can create work tasks and work situations that fulfill human needs and contribute to both a physically and psychologically healthy environment. This of course, is an individual-subjective-assessment, but research traces causal factors on various levels. Through our participation and collaboration at international conferences (e.g., ODAM Vancouver, 1986 and ODAM Kyoto, 1990), we have recognized a need for comparative analyses of this kind. One indirect effect of these analyses is that our respective Human Factors and Ergonomic societies, and academic societies within Informatics, Computer Science, Telecommunications, and recent Information Technology (IT) related disciplines, may benefit from this cross-fertilization regarding relevant action strategies at the introduction and use of new technologies, especially information and communication technology (ICT). Through these types of international comparative analyses we contributed to the initiation and development of action strategies for the introduction of computer technology. Also, engineers specializing in IT disciplines require education and training that encompasses the role ICT plays in organizations and in society as a whole.

REFERENCES

Bradley, G. (1989). *Computers and the Psychosocial Work Environment.* London: Taylor & Francis.

Bradley, G. (Ed.). (2001). *Humans on the Net. Information and Communication Technology (ICT) Work Organization and Human Beings.* Stockholm, SE: Prevent.

Bradley, G. (2006). *Social and Community Informatics – Humans on the Net.* London: Routledge.

Bradley, G., & Robertson, M. (1991). *Computers, Psychosocial Work Environment, and Stress. A comparative theoretical analyses or organizations and action strategies.* Plenary presentation at the 11th Congress International Ergonomics Association. Paris 15-20 July, 1991.

Robertson, M., & Bradley, G. (1997). Competence development in ten high tech companies in Silicon Valley. In Salvendy, G. & Smith, M. J. & Koubek, R.J. (Eds.). *Design of Computing Systems. Proceedings of the Seventh International Conference on Human-Computer Interaction,* San Francisco, California, USA, August 24-29, 1997. Amsterdam/Lausanne/New York/Oxford/Shannan/Tokyo: Elsevier

Robertson, M., & Rahimi, M. (1990). A systems analysis for implementing video display terminals. *IEEE Transactions on Engineering Management, 37,* 55–62. doi:10.1109/17.45270

Robertson, M. M. (2005). Systems analysis tool (SAT). In Stanton, N. Hedge, A., Brookhuis, K., Salas, Ed., Hendrick, H. (Eds.), *Handbook of Human Factors and Ergonomics methods.* CRC Press.

Robertson, M. M., & Courtney, T. K. (2004). Solving office work systems performance problems- a systems analysis approach. *Theoretical Issues in Ergonomic, 5*(3), 181–197. doi:10.1080/1463922021000032320

Robertson, M. M., & Kleiner, B. (2002). Macroergonomic methods: Assessing work system processes . In Hendrick, H., & Kleiner, B. (Eds.), *Macroergonomics Theory, Methods, and Applications.* New Jersey: Lawrence Erlbaum Associates.

Chapter 11
Touch Screens for the Elderly:
Some Models and Methods, Prototypical Development and Experimental Evaluation of Human–Computer Interaction Concepts for the Elderly

Holger Luczak
Aachen University of Technology, Germany

Christopher M. Schlick
Aachen University of Technology, Germany

Nicole Jochems
Aachen University of Technology, Germany

Sebastian Vetter
Aachen University of Technology, Germany

Bernhard Kausch
Aachen University of Technology, Germany

ABSTRACT

The fast aging of many western and eastern societies and their increasing reliance on information technology create a compelling need to reconsider older users' interactions with computers. Changes in perceptual and motor skill capabilities that often accompany the aging process bring important implications for the design of information input devices. This paper summarizes the results of a laboratory study with different information input device. Three different input devices — mouse, touch screen and eye-gaze — were analyzed concerning efficiency, effectiveness and mental workload with respect to the age group of the computer user. The results derived from data of 90 subjects between 20 and 75 years show that regardless of participant's age group the best performance in terms of short execution time results from touch screen information input. This effect is even more pronounced for the elderly.

DOI: 10.4018/978-1-60960-057-0.ch011

INTRODUCTION

Demographic change requires new ergonomic concepts and methods to support elder working persons, who – due to the prognosed shortage of qualified labor – will be involved in achieve employment for a longer working life until retirement.

Especially "Work With Computing Systems" (WWCS) – formally "Work with Display Units" (WWDU) – will be a major working form that due to automation of working means and a presumably distant attitude of elder employees versus computerized work requires ergonomic attention (Nair et al. 2005, Rogers et al. 1995).

So the use of computers in different contexts may be a barrier of employment for the elder, because a lack of experience and age-dependent changes in performance and strain can be diagnosed which – in itself – is a challenge for ergonomic design efforts in hardware and software (Craik & Salthouse 2008, Czaja & Lee 2002, 2008, Hawthorn 1998, Czaja et al. 1996).

In detail some presumed decreases in sensory as well as motor performance (Craik & Salthouse 2008, Birren & Shaie 2006, Park & Schwarz 2000, Gogging & Stelmach 1990) lead to usability problems in WWCS.

However, models of aging were undergoing some changes in the past (Luczak & Stemann 2008, Luczak & Frenz 2008), especially initiating new views of strategic ergonomic intervention as well as new paths of competency development.

SURVEY

Explanation Models of Aging

Models that cope with changes in the broad picture of performance types and stress forms of aging people have diversified a lot in recent years. In earlier times so called "deficit model" dominated the aging scenarios, which postulates a "graceful" degradation in human information processing and physical functions from the late 20'ies onward (Naegele 2004).

Nowadays the changes that occur with aging are subsumed under the "compensation model" or "sustainable competency model". These models acknowledge that age-dependent changes can be compensated by behavioral strategies, experiences and attitudes, or that the elderly dispose over an alternative performance spectrum as compared to the young (Astor 2006).

However, the decreasing scope is highly individual and depends on the function being considered. A second aspect in the deficit model is the mixture of individual characteristics with age-groups related data sets. The result is an over emphasis of expected slopes, that have almost nothing to do with working periods over lifetime.

However, nobody can escape the fact, that near to death physiological and psychological functions decrease drastically. The superimposition of these decreases, that in individual terms become more frequent the older the persons become, causes the age group related overestimation underlying the deficit model (see Figure 1).

The main message of the "compensation model" is a "win" situation in slopes, when using training incentives for a specific function or when changing in between functions by shifting from the steeper slope to a more even development path function set.

The main message of the "sustainable competency model" is that it is possible to maintain a specific function level or even to improve it over time by respective work demands. The main effect is "winning time" before the expected steep descent occurs.

Both models can respect hindering or improving effects by technology use or technology developments – as the Gehlen thesis of organ projection indicate with "enforcement", "replacement", "substitution" – technology, that can be easily transferred from technology development theory and philosophy to the HCI-practice.

Figure 1. Physiological and psychological functions measurements

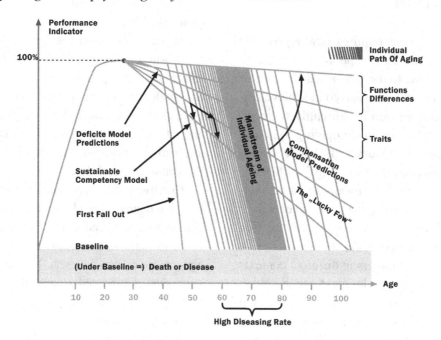

The hypothesis derived from the deficit model are replaced more and more by presumptions of a "differentiated aging process" which postulates physiological and psychological systems' structure and function development to undergo different paths of development with age. Aging – so the hypothesis – is a set of processes with differential development and a complex phenomenon (Czaja 1997).

The considerable interindividual variability of sensory, cognitive and motor systems development as well in the young as in the elderly sets high demands for an ergonomic design of human-computer-interaction, and requires a flexibly adaptive human-computer-interface as oriented for the individual capacities, performance standards and demands. So – by experimental evidence – ergonomics could demonstrate that especially the elderly computer users would be supported in their performance spectrum by ergonomic interventions in the design of hardware and software. That effect was accompanied by lower strain levels and respective postulated improvement of health standards (Czaja & Lee 2008).

Selected Methodological Approaches and Design Variants

Technological Literature Review

In an ergonomic context mainly 3 approaches can be considered, namely technological, organizational and personal, according the so called TOP-design. Consider T-aspects primarily, because they are viewed via personal demands and organizational task related features.

The improvement of input and output devices for HCI requires a view via human individual capacities, skills and preferences, and a view via computing systems, that limits the possibilities of information input and output (Jacob 1993). Technically a differentiation between direct and indirect input devices can be made (Hinckley 2008, Shneidermann 1998). Direct input devices, like touch screen, natural language or ocular fixation inputs make possible a direct, expectation-conforming input, and demand almost no special training when suitably adapted. However indirect input devices, like a mouse, joystick, or trackball, require a transformation of hand movement into cursor movement on the screen, which the users have to be trained for (Greenstein 1997).

Especially regarding elderly users, the age-influenced change in sensori-motor functions leads to problems with the traditional mouse input-device (Vercruyssen 1996). Numerous studies from Iwase and Murata (2003), Smith et al. (1999), Riviere and Thakor (1996), and Walker et al. (1996) identified that effect.

The use of direct input devices to improve the HC interaction denominates a research and design field of utmost importance for elder users (Czaja & Lee 2008, Grandt et al. 2003, Tobias 1987). Various investigations were devoted to alternative input devices and input methods (touch screen, pentablet, trackball) especially to analyze their potentials for elder users when compared to mouse input (Torres 2006, Iwase & Murata 2002, Chaparro et al. 1999a,b, Charness et al. 2004).

The results of these studies permit the conclusion that HCI for elder users can be improved by alternative devices. Especially the touch screen which requires almost no training for novices has considerable advantages for the elder as well (Iwase & Murata 2002, Shneidermann 1998, Pickering 1985). Input with the touch screen is performed directly via the touch-sensible screen itself. Touching the screen surface delivers electric impulses, which determine the coordinates of touch on the screen. In work systems, touch sensitive screens are employed mainly with creative-informatory work, as with product design and architecture (Lin & Chang 2007). The possibility of inputs on large scale touch sensitive screens is interesting in design of other types of work-tasks as well! New application scenarios can be found in human-robot-interaction (Micire et al. 2009) and in production site planning. It demonstrates that large scale touch-sensitive screens enhance the presentation of complex contextual information (Zöllner et al. 2008).

The history of touch screens dates back to the late 1960's. In 1972 the first touch screen terminal

PLATO IV was set in function at the University of Illinois. Since the beginning 80's the technology of identification of multiple touch points (multi-touch) came into the focus of research (Buxton et al. 1985, Nakatani & Rohrlich 1983, Mehta 1982). This technology admits to transfer mouse-related software to the use with touch screens. The parallel identification of multiple touch points can be done by several methods to be analyzed shortly.

Frustrated Total Internal Reflection (FTIR)

This method – introduced in 2006 – is based on high reflexion at the border line of two media with different index of fraction (Kim et al. 2007, Han 2005): Infrared radiation is sent through a pane of acrylic glass, which is reflected at the upper and lower side. The touch causes a declination in the refection angle. The modified angle is measured by infrared cameras and the respective touch coordinates can be calculated. Disadvantages of FTIR –Technology are its sensitivity to daylight and artificial illumination, which sends out infrared and may deteriorated the signal.

Capacitive Sensors

This method seems to admit a very flexible measurement of touch points. The identification is based on the principle of a capacitive interference of a sender and an antenna. A sender-antenna-matrix registers differences in voltage on the surface of the screen and transmits them into touch-coordinates (Rekimoto 2002, Dietz & Leigh 2001). The hardware to identify multiple touch points was developed by MERL – Mitsubishi Research Laboratories – in 2001 and made marketable by presenting the large scale touch sensitive screen named "Diamond-Touch" (Dietz & Leigh 2001). By measuring voltage differences, Diamond Touch is the only system which is able to identify different users, performing touch activities simultaneously. Sony Computer Science

Laboratories – in 2002 – developed "Smartskin", a touch-sensible surface that is based on the technical principles of capacitive interference, but it is mainly used in mobile phones (Hodges et al. 2007, Rekimoto 2002).

The registration of multiple touch points opens new interesting research and design agenda in HCI, especially gesture-based information inputs. So Wu and Balakrishna (2003) investigated the use and the learning curve of different gestures in work with a large scale touch-sensitive display– Diamond Touch – as based on a room planning program and task. Four categories of gestures were distinguished: (1) One-Finger-Gestures, (2) Two-Finger-Gestures, (3) One-Hand-Gestures and (4) Two-Hand-Gestures. The gestures were implemented in software and a study with five subjects assigned with the room planning task was performed, that led to a subjective evaluation.

Based on a newly conceived list of design basics Wu et al. (2006) developed some gesture-based input methods. The following variables were respected: (1) gesture diagnosis (2) gesture execution and (3) universality versus context-related gestures. In a study with ten subjects, between 19-30 years old, their derived gestures were executed in exemplary tasks and classified according to differences with a Likert-scaled questionnaire.

In an explorative study of user-specific gestures by Epps et al. (2006) 20 subjects, between 19-50 years old, should perform 36 exemplary tasks with self-determined gestures. Only restrictions were imposed concerning the use of one versus numerous fingers (1) and the use of one versus two hands (2) respectively. The gestures executed by the subjects were video-taped and consequently characterized according to frequency of use.

A long-term study of work with a large size touch-sensitive screen was performed by Widgor et al. (2007), who – over 13 months – observed a male subject in his WWDU with sequential questioning. The Diamond Touch screen with gesture based mouse (Esenther 2007) was compared to a

standard PC according to the frequency of interactions. The result was convincing, because the subject worked more frequently with the Diamond Touch and evaluated the usability very positively.

In the MERL-Mitsubishi Electric Research Laboratories research was done by Forlines et al. (2007) in a study with 12 subjects, between 22-47 years old, comparing the conventional mouse input with the Diamond Touch use. Based on a combination of a Fitts' task (Fitts 1954) and a displacement task the execution of one finger (1) was compared with mouse-input and (2) the simultaneous execution with two hands was compared to a simultaneous use of two mice. The task determined the priority in performance with input devices: One hand Fitts' task was faster with screen input whereas the displacement task was faster with the mouse-input. In symmetrical execution the touch screen was superior in both tasks considering execution times. At that, the Diamond Touch had better evaluation scores.

Seven gesture-based input methods with one versus two hands execution were compared by Olwal et al. (2008) in a study with 20 subjects, between 19-34 years old. The execution times and failure in a pointing task were determined. Olwal et al. (2008) could demonstrate that their so called "rubbing" and "tapping" techniques could improve the dependent variables.

The analysis of social interaction and the cooperation of several computer users at a touch screen seems to be another research focus. Scott and Carpendale (2006) evaluated in a study with 6 students' couples (three male and three female groups) the suitability of a "storage bin" for co-operative work at a touch screen. The separation of working areas into personal and common was investigated at that.

Morris et al. (2006) implemented 15 different gestures at Diamond Touch, and investigated the suitability of the gestures for cooperative work via a questionnaire. Seven pairs of subjects were involved, three couples of life partners and four couples of colleagues. From users' view all gestures could be easily learned and efficient for individual and cooperative work.

In a rare study with elderly users, Apted et al. (2006) investigated gesture-based input within a cooperative "photo-sharing" application. The subjects were separated into two age groups (six young couples aging 18-24 years, six elderly couples aging 63-84 years). The task was generating a "collage" together from a set of photographs. The photos had to be treated one- or two-handed in displacement, pull-up and pull-down in size, rotation etc. The subjects were video-taped during task execution and observed by one person. A qualitative analysis showed, that the elder subjects had difficulties in performing the 2-hand-operation (downsize, rotation etc.). Total performance time made visible differences in between age groups as well. However, time was not restricted in the DoE, and fractions of time for comments or communication were not separated.

The above mentioned technologically oriented literature analysis – in sum – admits the following conclusions. Focuses of research in "Multitouchscreens" can be identified in software-development and rather simple usability studies. Object of research is mostly executability and effectivity of newly implemented gesture-based input-methods. Most studies follow an explorative DoE with a small sample-size (n<29). The artificial tasks in research frequently lack any relevancy for industrial work systems in production and administration.

A detailed objective performance analysis is mostly missing, as well as stressors and strains analysis. As the demographic becomes more important over the next decades as a parameter of working life, the ergonomic design and experimental evaluation of gesture-based information inputs for touch screens respecting elder users will be of utmost importance. However, we found only one study by Apted et al. (2006) in the context that refers to age. The results are based solely on observation. When the knowledge basis is as weak as identified in this review, experimental efforts are justified.

Age-Related Literature Review

In various experimental studies the problems of elderly computer users when working with the classic mouse as the dominant input device are reported.

In a study involving 12 younger (18-21 years) and 12 older (63-79) participants, Walker et al. (1996) were able to determine that elderly computer users are slower at mouse-based information input and also have a lower degree of accuracy. Smith et al. (1999) came to similar results in their study of 60 participants (20 to 75 years) and determined that elderly participants, particularly in tasks such as "clicking" and "double-clicking", have more usability problems with mouse input than younger participants. Similar studies by Riviere and Thakor (1996) as well as Iwase and Murata (2003) confirmed these differences in execution time as well as accuracy between elderly and younger computer users and concluded that age-induced performance differences are more pronounced for tasks of greater complexity.

Investigating the potentials of alternative input devices improving human-computer interaction is a well-known area of research which is mainly driven by technological progress (see e.g. Czaja & Lee 2008, Grandt et al. 2003, Tobias 1987). In view of the challenges resulting from demographic change, in several studies various alternatives to the common information input by mouse were analyzed and their usability for aging computer users was studied. In this manner, researchers such as Charness et al. (2004, 1995) and Torres (2006) compared the mouse with direct input via pen from an age-specific perspective. Charness et al. (2004, 1995) found a decrease in reaction time affected by the use of a pen. Elderly participants showed, regardless of the input device, a poorer performance than younger participants and the age-specific difference in reaction time was largest for input with the mouse. Furthermore, it was discovered by Torres (2006) that pen-based input was rated "more positive" by the users than information input using a mouse. Chaparro et al. (1999a, 1999b) investigated the mouse compared to a trackball by using both a "point and click" and a "point and drag" task. The ten younger (< 40 years) and ten elderly (> 65 years) participants showed longer response time for the trackball than for the mouse. Subjectively, however, the participants rated the mouse to be more difficult to use. In another age-differentiated study by Iwase and Murata (2002), direct input via a touch screen was compared to mouse input. They measured shorter reaction times and a greater acceptance of the touch screen particularly among elderly participants.

The above-mentioned studies allow the conclusion to be made that human-computer interaction, especially for aging computer users, can be improved through the use of alternative input devices; particularly direct input devices like a pen or touch screen, that do not require a mental transformation of hand movement into cursor movement on the screen are interesting alternatives. Charness et al. (2004) and Tobias (1987) also came to the conclusion that the focus of further investigation should be set on direct input devices that require very little training.

Since their use can be learned quickly and fast reaction times can be achieved especially the touch screen is suitable for aging computer users and a great degree of user satisfaction can be achieved (Shneidermann 1998, Pickering 1985). Potentials for aging computer users, were confirmed in various studies (Rau & Hsu 2005, Umemuro 2004, Pak et al. 2002, Yarnold et al. 1996, Carr et al. 1986).

An additional direct and innovative input device is the so-called eye-gaze input. The control of the cursor position is often based on a head-mounted or contact-free measurement of the viewing position. Compared to interaction by mouse, which requires significant training, eye-gaze controlled input is based on user's "natural behavior" when focusing on visual objects (Jacob 1993). And under certain circumstances it allows an easier and faster processing when compared to traditional input devices (Ware & Mikaelian 1987). There are many studies concerning the use of eye-gaze controlled input methods. The studies of Wobbrock et al. (2008), Kammerer et al. (2008), Huckauf and Urbina (2007), Sibert and Jacob (2000), Jacob (1993), Frey et al. (1990) and Huchinson et al. (1989) do describe the advantages for younger computer users, but do not consider aging users or age-specific differences.

A study by Murata (2006) in which 44 male users were involved had a special focus on aging users. For traditional mouse input, elderly users showed a significantly slower reaction time than younger ones, yet eye-gaze input did not show an age-related difference in reaction times. However, comparisons of the two input devices showed that eye-gaze controlled input leads to a significantly better performance as well as a higher level of acceptance.

Further studies of eye-gaze input specifically dealt with input verification, which plays an important role when using this input technology. Different variants are possible in which information input is, for instance, controlled through set dwell times (Jacob 1993), or in which eye-gaze control is combined with an additional input device. However, it is difficult to determine the optimal duration of dwell times in regard to input verification. A short dwell time can lead to the execution of a command or function simply because the user was performing a quick "look around" ("Midas Touch Problem", Jacob 1991). Alternately, a dwell time that is too long is not compatible with user's natural behavior and works against the advantages of vision-based control, responsiveness and speed. A better alternative are so-called hybrid user interfaces in which eye-gaze input is combined with an additional input device (Sibert & Jacob 2000, Zhai et al. 1999). The combination of the input devices is crucial for good ergonomics. Different hybrid user interfaces, such as the combination with a button on a game pad (Xiao et al. 2005, Ware & Mikaelian 1987), with speech input (Glenn III et al. 1986) and with a mouse (Zhai et al. 1999), have been investigated for younger computer users. The best of our knowledge results for aging computer users in particular, however, have not been published.

These cited studies show that both touch screen and eye-gaze input are promising for aging computer users and that further ergonomic studies should be conducted to explore human performance and workload under different experimental conditions.

COMPARATIVE EXPERIMENTAL STUDY OF INFORMATION INPUT DEVICES

In a laboratory study, different information input devices were compared and analyzed with regard to the age of the users. The focus of the study was the direct comparison of the three input devices—mouse, touch screen and eye-gaze input.

Hypotheses

- Regarding the experimental content of the study it was hypothesized that the younger subjects perform better in terms of shorter execution times as well as fewer errors than the elderly subjects.
- Based on the literature review in the previous sections, a decrease in execution time for the touch screen as well as the eye-gaze input compared to the input by mouse was expected. Concerning the two direct input devices it was hypothesized, that the subjects achieve shorter execution times with the touch screen than with the eye-gaze input.

General Procedure

At the beginning of each trial, user-specific skills and experiences of the participants were recorded. Thus, along with the collection of basic data such as age, gender, education etc., the IST 2000-R "Dice Test" (Liepman et al. 2001) was used to collect data of spatial sense. Additionally, the participants' prior computer experience was determined through questionnaires regarding "computer expertise" (Arning & Ziefle 2008) and "computer literacy" (Sengpiel et al. 2008).

Participants

A total of 90 participants, 36 female and 54 male between 20 and 75 years of age participated in the study (average age: 47.5 years, SD=16.77). For the statistical analysis of the experiment, the participants were divided into three age groups (I: 20-39, II: 40-59, III: 60-75 years). Each age group consisted of 30 participants.

Related to experience with computers, 80 percent of participants indicated daily computer use. Only four participants said that they did not have a PC in their home, whereas two participants had not worked with a computer yet. E-mail programs and the internet were used by more than 70 percent of all test participants on a daily basis.

None of the participants had any experience with the use of an eye-gaze input device.

Age-Differentiated Comparison of Input Devices

The goal of the experimental study was to compare different input devices in regard to age-specific and individual aspects. The three input devices, (1) mouse, (2) touch screen and (3) eye-gaze input, were contrasted with one another by performing a classic two dimensional pointing task according to the study by Murata (2006), see section 3.4.2.

Figure 2. Contact-free eye-based input (right) and touch-based input (left)

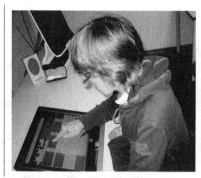 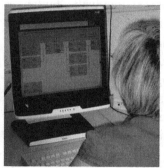

Apparatus

A wireless optical Logitech mouse (model RX650) was used as the reference device for the experiment. The eye-gaze input was based on a Tobii T/X 120 system that, via the integration of eye-tracking equipment in the 17" monitor, allowed a remote, i.e. contact-free, measurement of the point of gaze. In order to stabilize the head and eye position a chin rest was used with eye-gaze input. As a touch input device a 17" touch screen (model 1715; 1280*1024 pixels) manufactured by Elo was used (see Figure 2).

Experimental Task

Based on the investigations by Murata (2006), the three input devices were compared using a two dimensional pointing task. The starting position of the task was presented by a circle in the centre of the screen and the target position was represented by an initially hidden square. The participants' first task was to move the cursor to the starting position. This resulted in the appearance of the target object to which the cursor had to be moved as quickly as possible (see *Figure 3*).

The participants had to complete this task differently, respective to the typical functionality of each device. Using the touch screen, the task consisted of "touching" the starting circle, followed by "touching" the target square with the preferred pointing finger. With the mouse, the cursor had to be positioned in the starting circle first and then in the target square. The reaching of the start and target positions had to be confirmed with a mouse click (start: right, target: left). For the eye-gaze input, the task consisted of fixating on a point within the starting circle first and then within the target square. The duration of fixation on the target object was set to 100 msecs in accordance to Murata (2006).

Independent Variables

Age group (I: 20-39, II: 40-59, III: 60-75 years) and the three input devices (mouse, eye-gaze input,

Figure 3. Description of the two-dimensional pointing task

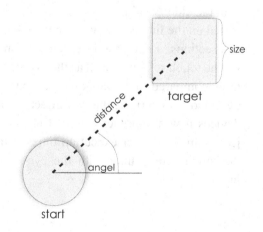

touch screen) were designated as independent variables.

Furthermore, the size of the target object (S) was varied on three levels (40×40 pixels^2, 55×55 pixels^2 and 70×70 pixels^2), the target distance (D) also in three levels (130, 150, and 170 pixels) and the direction of movement in eight angular (A) levels (counterclockwise 0°, 45°, 90°, 135°, 180°, 225°, 270° and 315°) (see Figure 3).

By using the eye gaze input with a constant distance of 70 centimeter to the screen, the smallest target object (40×40 pixel^2) displayed with a distance to the starting point of 130 pixels and a position of 0° will be shown under a visual angle of 25 arc minutes.

Dependent Variables

The execution time required for accomplishing the task was the primary dependent variable. For the touch screen, the time between the first and second touch was measured. And for the mouse, the time between the appearance of the target object and the left-click onto it was measured. For the eye-gaze input, the time between the appearance of the target object and a 100 millisecond (msec) fixation of the target object was calculated.

Because of the different specific characteristics of the input devices the classical approach to evaluate both execution times and error rates was not chosen. When using the mouse or the touch screen, a click/touch far away from the target could be considered as an error. However, when using the eye gaze input, it is hard to say if such an eye movement is not subconsciously controlled. It might as well be caused by shifts of attention, which causes rapid movements of the eye, but not in the hand or arm. Therefore, indirect movements towards the target or off-target clicks/touches were not calculated as errors, but as deviances (Jordan 2002) which lead to longer execution times.

In addition to the execution time, the mental workload was measured with the help of the ZEIS

scale, a two-level intensity scale developed by Pitrella and Käppler (1988). In this computer-based test, a general estimate of the mental workload occurs with the categories "difficult", "medium" or "easy". Then a fine-grained differentiation has to be made using an 11-level extensive rating scale.

Procedure

Before the start of the trials, the Tobii system for the participants' eye movement recording was calibrated. Then the participants had time to practice the task with each input device for about 3 minutes. In the subsequent investigation, the participants had to process three blocks of 72 tasks (corresponding to the number of possible combinations, size*distance*angle) with each of the three input devices. The sequence of the 72 tasks within a block was randomly selected. There was a brief pause (15 secs) between each block. After every three blocks the participants had a longer break (5 mins) in which they rated the most recently used input device with the help of the ZEIS scale. The sequence of input devices was balanced between the participants.

RESULTS

In the following, the results of the three pretests (Dice Test, computer expertise and computer literacy) and the main investigation are described first.

In the main investigation, only the data from the third task block were considered in order to eliminate a training effect.

Due to the fact that our data did not fulfill the preconditions (Soukoreff & MacKenzie 2004) we did not analyze our data by the famous Fitts' law. According to Soukoreff and MacKenzie (2004) the application of Fitts' law requires a large ID-range (2-8 bits) and in the original task definition by Fitts (1954) only one position of the target object (0°) was investigated. Our task definition just models a range of index of difficulty values between 1.51 and 2.39 bits and the position of the target object (angle) has a complex, inconsistent, influence on the execution time.

Statistical Analysis

The statistical analysis was carried out with the help of the statistical software package SPSS Version 14.0. Execution times and mental workload were analyzed by a mixed design ANOVA with age as a between-group factor and input device, width, amplitude and position as within-subjects factors.

The main assumption in ANOVAs with repeated measures is sphericity (see Doncaster & Davey 2007). If the assumption of sphericity was violated, the degrees of freedom were adjusted with Huynh-Feldt respectively Greenhouse-Geisser corrections.

The level of significance for each analysis was set to α=0.05. The Bonferroni post-hoc test was used for multi-level comparisons of the means. Furthermore, the effect size ω² was calculated for significant results (see Field 2005, p. 452). Outliers were eliminated according to the theorem by Tschebyscheff (Sachs 1999). The relationship between the user specific results of the pretests and the results of the main experimental studies was determined by Spearman's correlation coefficient.

Pretest Results

The results of the pretest for determining computer experience (computer literacy, computer expertise) and to determine spatial sense (Dice Test) all showed significant negative correlations with the age group (all p=0.01). The largest negative correlation of r=-.69 was found between the results of the computer expertise test and age group. The correlation between age group and the results of the Dice Test (r=-.55) was also negative but less strong. The complete results are depicted in Table

Table 1. Correlation of the age group with the pretests results

	Computer Literacy	**Computer Expertise**	**Dice test**
Age group	-.63**	-.69**	-.55**
Computer Literacy	1.00	.77**	.48**
Computer Expertise	.77**	1.00	.53**
Dice test	.48**	.53**	1.00

**. Correlation is significant at the 0,01 level

1. If the internal correlations of the pretests results are considered, the redundancy of question from the computer literacy and computer expertise questionnaires are reflected in the high correlation of test results, r=.77.

Execution Time

The analysis of the execution time across all input devices shows a significant main effect in relation to age groups (F=37.236; df=2; p=0.000), with a large effect size of ω²=0.55. Following the post-hoc paired comparisons of means, significant mean differences between the 20 to 39 year-olds and the 40 to 59 year-olds (p=0.000) as well as the 60 to 75 year-olds (p=0.000) age groups were identified. However, the 40 to 59 year-olds unexpectedly did not score significantly better than the 60 to 75 year-olds (see Figure 4). The performance differences in regard to execution time are significantly pronounced between the younger participants (20-39 years) and those in the second and third age groups.

The input device has a significant effect on the execution time (F=95.369; df=1.619; p=0.000) with an effect size of ω²=0.51. As hypothesized the touch screen leads to better performance than the eye-gaze control (p=0.004) and mouse input (p=0.000). A comparison of mouse to eye-gaze input shows that the participants require signifi-

Figure 4. Average execution time and 95% confidence intervals concerning the different age groups

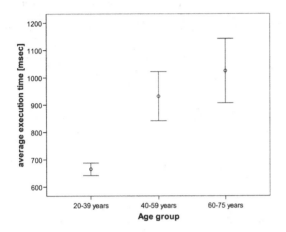

cantly less time for eye-gaze input (p=0.000) (see Figure 5).

Furthermore, a significant interaction between age group and input device occurs (F=7.190; df=3.237; p=0.000). The data show that the average execution times between the 40 to 59 year-olds and the 60 to 75 year-olds differ significantly only for mouse input, while the execution time for the other two input devices, touch screen and eye-gaze

are not significantly different between these age groups (see Figure 5).

Another influencing factor on execution time is the target size (S_1=40×40 pixels^2, S_2=55×55 pixels^2 and S_3=70×70 pixels^2). A significant effect (F=190.100; df=1.943; p=0.000) with an effect size of ω^2=0.44 can be identified for all three sizes. As expected the execution time significantly decreases with increasing target size.

The influence of the target size differs between the age groups (F=2.754; df=3.886; p=0.031) as well as between the input devices (F=31.579; df=2.177; p=0.000). The differences in execution times are less for the 20 to 39 year-old age group than for the 40 to 59 year-olds and 60 to 75 year-old age group and have a greater effect for eye-gaze input than for mouse or touch screen input.

The three different distances to the target position (D_1=130, D_2=150 and D_3=170 pixels) also have a significant effect (F=34.977; df=1.819; p=0,000) (ω^2=0.14) on the execution time. The execution time increases with an increasing target position.

Another significant effect can be found for the eight different angular levels (A_1=0°, A_2=45°, A_3=90°, A_4=135°, A_5=180°, A_6=225°, A_7=270°

Figure 5. Average execution times and 95% confidence intervals concerning the three input devices as well as the age groups

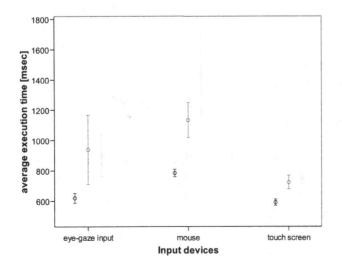

127

and $A_8=315°$) of the target object (F=5.292; df=4.345; p=0.000).

Relationship Between Execution Times and the Pretest Results

The execution times of the main investigation show significant correlations with the pretest results (p=0.000). The correlation coefficients between the pretest results and the execution times during the use of the various input devices (eye-gaze input, mouse, touch screen) are summarized in Table 2. According to this table the age group has the strongest influence on the execution time with the mouse (r=.80). Prior computer experience, measured with the computer literacy and computer expertise questionnaires, is negatively correlated with the execution time for mouse input (r=-.66 and r=-.76). This strong relationship between computer experience, i.e., frequent computer use and thus mouse use, reflects the training the necessity for an efficient use of the input device. In terms of the scores spatial sense (Dice Test), the strongest correlation (r=-.52) with the execution time also exists for the mouse.

Subjective Mental Workload Assessment

The subjective evaluation of mental workload with the help of the ZEIS scale did not differentiate between the age groups; no significant effect regarding age group was found. The elder and younger participants are therefore similar in their evaluation of mental workload when using the three different input devices.

However the results of the ZEIS scale show a significant effect regarding the different input devices (F=103.938; df=1.646; p=0.000), with an effect size of $\omega^2=0.36$. The interaction with the touch screen is thereby seen as "easiest" and the interaction with eye-gaze control as "most difficult" (see Figure 6). Thus, the subjective evaluation by the participants thus does not reflect the objective

Table 2. Relationship between execution times and the pretest results

	Execution time eye-gaze	Execution time mouse	Execution time touch screen
Age group	.37**	.80**	.65**
Dice test	-.23*	-.52**	-.37**
Computer Literacy	-.25*	-.66**	-.46**
Computer Expertise	-.28**	-.76**	-.61**

**. Correlation is significant at the 0.01 level
*. Correlation is significant at the 0.05 level

Figure 6. Average subjective evaluation of mental workload and 95% confidence intervals

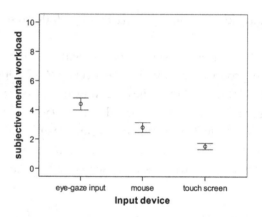

performance data. However, it must generally be noted that all three input devices, on the total scale from 0 to 10 (0-very easy; 10-very difficult), are evaluated as rather easy (see Figure 6).

DISCUSSION

Following a direct comparison of the three input devices investigated in this study, i.e., eye-gaze input, mouse and touch screen, it must be emphasized that, regardless of participants' age, the best performance in terms of short execution time results from touch screen information input. Surprisingly, mouse input showed the poorest average performance among all subjects. However, the effect of the execution time improvement through alternative input devices (touch screen, eye-gaze) varies in strength among the different age groups. The short execution time concerning the touch screen especially for the third age group confirms the empirical results of Iwase and Murata (2002). They showed that especially aging computer users benefit from the use of a touch screen.

The greatest improvement in performance can be achieved for the 60 to 75 year-olds. These participants need on average twice as long as the 20 to 39 year-olds for information input with the mouse. However, when using a touch screen they reach a performance level similar to that of younger people using a mouse (see Figure 5). It is interesting to note that, for eye-gaze control, the 60-75-year-olds performed better, on average, than the 40-59-year-olds. If a comparison is made with the findings of Murata (2006), it can be verified that eye-gaze input leads to a better performance (expressed in execution time) than mouse input. This occurs despite the fact that the age-specific difference for eye-gaze control is less pronounced than for conventional mouse input.

Regarding the pretests results, it can be concluded that a high score in the pretests is corresponding with a shorter execution time for all input devices. Thereby the relationship between prior computer experience (expertise, literacy) and the execution time required is most pronounced for mouse usage. This result can be explained by the training needed in order to use this input device, though.

Despite a convincing "message" of the literature review and the experiment, namely

1. "Use direct input devices!" and
2. "Use touch screens for the elder!" and
3. "Make symbols large and clear!",

it is evident, that we are simply scratching the surface of HCI design for the elderly. Following the semiotical model of Morris (1946), we admit, that with input devices and symbols we act in design of the "physical level". In a design on the "syntactical level", the representation of graphical structures along lifelong experiences with "pictures" and "features of objects" will help the elderly in their perceptual and cognitive efforts of identification of graphics. Structuring the information input along common gestures or by "handwriting" means a considerable enhancement for elderly users with limited motor functions on the syntax-level as well as by implementing motor stereotypes. On the "semantical level" age dependent deficits of working memory could be compensated for by selective presentation of relevant information contents in a mode that respects conceptual compatibility as the principle that minimizes the amount of information to be interpreted and recorded in relation to task-elements under processing.

"Good" software products support this information transmission in a way that considers cultural contexts, individual biographies and such the socialization status of the user - especially the elderly user - in functionality design.

However, experimentally validated concepts with hard data are hardly found in software-ergonomics. So we intend – in a next series of experiments – to investigate variants of a network plan visualization in a project management task setting and to analyze them with regard to age influences. To design a layout of information combining the content information in the network plan with additional structural information in overview maps and simple handling (retrieval, positing, etc.) by gesture-based motor actions on the touch screen may serve as an experimental paradigm for the age-related semantics of software (Schneider et al. 2009).

When it comes to be "pragmatical level" the computer task setting to be performed and its performance supporting functionalities by software components are to be considered. No doubt, that the variety of tasks may be counted in legions and thus the selection of a task that may be age-sensible in itself but with age-compensating software support is the main question in terms of "ecological validity". The task of choice for further experimental investigations was project management together with project management software components, their representation techniques and intervention strategies.

A balance of reasons for this choice demonstrates some "why"s:

- Project planning is a task of information processing, respecting perceptual cognitive and motor functions of the human in a more or less goal development creative surrounding. It condenses important information features of real work into a set of logics.
- Planning is a component of everyday-life and a component of many jobs in gainful employment. Its quality depends on individual intellect and experience (age!) related individual properties and company demands.
- Dozens of software products promise "support". However age-related hints are missing. But a huge market in different company types and company functions is evident.
- The task is limited in extent and time consumption and is thus a useful "laboratory setting" with reproducible components, sequences and logic. It can be designed from "easy" to "difficult" in different representation techniques and support technologies.
- Project planning sets intellectual demands with creative components: It is creative-informatory work and thus a high ranking work form.
- Project planning is the universal approach to develop operations networks, for example in product and service design, in procurement, production, and distribution networks planning, in architecture and administration, in construction and building industries, in military and civil services, and many more application.
- Project planning is easily understood by everybody who's planned a household move, an education sequence, a reservation of a private tour, etc.
- The tasks give room for the elderly persons that formally worked in motor and physically demanding jobs, to develop their expertise into planning of the original work content respecting their competency development in terms of intellectual capabilities, personality traits and especially previous expertise and experiences (Luczak & Frenz 2008).
- The idea of cooperation is implemented in project planning from the beginning on: In this respect we can follow the concepts of the social ICT of Gunilla Bradley (1989, 2006) in DoE and especially as a basis for the development of variables that are hypothetically are affected by or positively influence an age-oriented WWCS.

ACKNOWLEDGMENT

Research was funded by the German National Research Foundation in the Focus Program "Age-differentiated Work Systems" under the code SCHL 1805/1-1 and SCHL 1805/1-2.

REFERENCES

Apted, T., Kay, J., & Quigley, A. (2006). Tabletop sharing of digital photographs for the elderly. In *Proceedings of the 2006 SIGCHI conference on Human Factors in computing systems*. Canada.

Arning, K., & Ziefle, M. (2008). Development and validation of a computer expertise questionnaire for older adults. *Behaviour & Information Technology, 27*(4), 325–329. doi:10.1080/01449290802127153

Astor, M., Koch, C., Klose, G., Reimann, F., Rochhold, S., & Stemann, M. (2006). *Zu alt, um Neues zu lernen? Chancen und Grenzen des gemeinsamen Lernens von älteren und jüngeren Mitarbeitern. QUEM-Materialien der Arbeitsgemeinschaft Betriebliche Weiterbildungsforschung e* (pp. 1–165). V. AWBF.

Birren, J. E., & Schaie, K. W. (2006). *Handbook of the Psychology of Aging.* London: Academic Press.

Bradley, G. (1989). Knowledge based systems and Work Design . In Haslegrave, C. M., Wilson, J. R., Corlett, E. N., & Manenica, I. (Eds.), *Work Design in Practice*. London: Taylor & Francis.

Bradley, G. (2006). *Social and community informatics: humans on the net.* New York: Routledge.

Buxton, W., Hill, R., & Rowley, P. (1985). Issues and Techniques in Touch-Sensitive Tablet Input. *Computer Graphics, 19*(3), 215–224. doi:10.1145/325165.325239

Carr, A. C., Woods, R. T., & Moore, B. J. (1986). Automated Cognitive Assessment of Elderly Patients: A Comparison of Two Types of Response Device. *The British Journal of Clinical Psychology, 25*, 305–306.

Chaparro, A., Bohan, M., Fernandez, J., Choi, S., & Kattel, B. (1999a). The impact of age on computer input devices use: psychophysical and physiological measures. *International Journal of Industrial Ergonomics, 24*, 503–513. doi:10.1016/S0169-8141(98)00077-8

Chaparro, A., Bohan, M., Fernandez, J., Kattel, B., & Choi, S. (1999b). Is the trackball a better input device for the middle-age computer user? *Journal of Occupational Rehabilitation, 9*, 33–43. doi:10.1023/A:1021341415404

Charness, N., Bosmann, E. A., & Elliot, R. G. (1995). Senior-Friendly Input Devices: Is the Pen Mighter than the Mouse? *103rd Annual Convention of the American Psychological Association Meeting*, New York.

Charness, N., Holley, P., Feddon, J., & Jastrzembski, T. (2004). Light pen use and practice minimize age and hand performance differences in pointing tasks. *Human Factors, 46*(3), 373–384. doi:10.1518/hfes.46.3.373.50396

Craik, F. I. M., & Salthouse, T. A. (2008). *The Handbook of Aging and Cognition*. London: Psychology Press.

Czaja, S., & Lee, C. C. (2002). *Designing Computer Systems for older Adults*. New Jersey: Lawrence Erlbaum Associates.

Czaja, S., & Lee, C. C. (2008). Information technology and older adults. In M.G. Hollander, T.K. Landauer, & P.V. Prabhu (Eds.), (pp. 777–792), *Handbook of Human Computer Interaction*.

Czaja, S. J. (1997). Computer technology and the older adult . In Helander, M., & Landauer, T. (Eds.), *Handbook of human - computer interaction* (pp. 797–812). Amsterdam: North-Holland.

Czaja, S. J., Rogers, W. A., Fisk, A. D., & Walker, N. (1996). Aging and acquisition of Computer skills. *Aging and Skilled Performance: Advances in Theory and Applications* (pp. 202-221).

Dietz, P., & Leigh, D. (2001). Diamondtouch: a multi-user touch technology. In *Proceedings of the ACM Symposium on User interface Software and Technology*, USA.

Doncaster, C. P., & Davey, J. H. (2007). *Analysis of Variance and Covariance*. Cambridge: Cambridge University Press. doi:10.1017/CBO9780511611377

Epps, J., Lichman, S., & Wu, M. (2006). A study of hand shape use in tabletop gesture interaction. In *Proceedings of the Computer/Human Interaction CHI*, Canada.

Esenther, A. (2007). *DiamondTouch Mouse Users Manual (Technical Report)*. Cambridge, MA: Mitsubishi Electric Research Laboratories.

Field, A. (2005). *Discovering Statistic using SPSS*. London: Sage Publications.

Fitts, P. M. (1954). The information capacity of the human motor system in controlling the amplitude of movement. *Journal of Experimental Psychology, 47*(6), 381–391. doi:10.1037/h0055392

Forlines, C., Wigdor, D., Shen, C., & Balakrishnan, R. (2007). Direct-touch vs. mouse input for tabletop displays. In *Proceedings of the 2007 SIGCHI conference on human factors in computing systems*, (pp. 647-656) USA

Frey, L. A., White, K. P., & Huchinson, T. E. (1990). Eye-Gaze word processing. *IEEE Transactions on Systems, Man, and Cybernetics, 20*, 944–950. doi:10.1109/21.105094

Glenn, F. A., III, Iavecchia, H. P., Ross, L. V., Stokes, J. M., Weiland, W. J., Weiss, D. Z., & Allen, L. (1986). Eyevoicecontrolled interface. In *Proceedings of the Human Factors Society*, (pp. 322-326).

Gogging, N. L., & Stelmach, G. E. (1990). Age-related Differences in a Kinematic Analysis of Precued Movements. *Canadian Journal on Aging, 9*, 371–385.

Grandt, M., Pfendler, C., & Mooshage, O. (2003). Empirical comparison of five input devices for anti-air warfare operators. In *Proceedings of the 8th International Command and Control Research and Technology Symposium (ICCRTS) on "Information Age Transformation"*, Washington DC.

Greenstein, J. S. (1997). Pointing devices. In M. G. Helander, T. K. Landauer, & P. V. Prabhu (Eds.), *Handbook of human-computer interaction* (pp. 1317-1348). Amsterdam: Elsevier Science.

Han, J. Y. (2005). Low-cost multi-touch sensing through frustrated total internal reflection. In *Proceedings of the 18th Annual ACM Symposium on User Interface Software and Technology* (pp. 115-118). New York: ACM Press.

Hawthorn, D. (1998). Psychophysical Aging and Human Computer Interface Design. In *Proceedings of the Australasian Computer Human Interaction Conference*.

Hinckley, K. (2008). Input technologies and techniques . In Sears, A., & Jacko, J. A. (Eds.), *The human-computer interaction handbook: fundamentals, evolving technologies, and emerging applications* (p. 161). Taylor & Francis CRC Press.

Hodges, S., Izadi, S., Butler, A., Rrustemi, A., & Buxton, B. (2007). ThinSight: versatile multi-touch sensing for thin form-factor displays. In *Proceedings of the 20th annual ACM symposium on User interface Software and Technology*. USA, Newport, Rhode Island.

Huckauf, A., & Urbina, M. (2007). Gazing with pEYE: new concepts in eye typing. In *Proceedings of the 4th symposium on Applied perception in graphics and visualization* (pp.141-141).

Hutchinson, T. E., White, K. P., Martin, W. N., Reichert, K. C. & Frey, L. A. (1989). Human-Computer Interaction Using Eye-Gaze Input. *IEEE Transactions on systems, man, and cybernetics*.

Iwase, H., & Murata, A. (2002). Empirical study on improvement of usability - for touch-panel for elderly - comparison of usability between touch-panel and mouse. *Systems, Man and Cybernetics, IEEE International Conference* (pp. 252-257).

Iwase, H., & Murata, A. (2003). Design proposals to assist older adults in using a computer mouse. *IEICE Transactions on Information and Systems . E (Norwalk, Conn.)*, *86-D*, 141–145.

Jacob, R. J. K. (1991). The use of eye movements in human computer interaction techniques: What you look at is what you get. *ACM Transactions on Information Systems*, *9*, 152–169. doi:10.1145/123078.128728

Jacob, R. J. K. (1993). Eye movement-based human-computer interaction techniques: Toward non-command interfaces. *Advances in Human-Computer Interaction*, *4*, 151–180.

Jordan, P. W. (2002). *An Introduction to Usability*. London: Taylor & Francis.

Kammerer, Y., Scheiter, K., & Beinhauer, W. (2008). Looking my way through the menu: The impact of menu design and multimodal input on gaze-based menu selection. In *Proceedings of the 2008 Symposium on Eye Tracking Research & Applications – ETRA* (pp. 213-220).

Kim, S.-G., Kim, J.-W., & Lee, C.-W. (2007). Implementation of multi-touch tabletop display for HCI . In Jacko, J. (Ed.), *Human-Computer Interaction, Part II* (pp. 854–863). Heidelberg, Deutschland: Springer-Verlag Berlin.

Liepmann, D., Beauducel, A., Brocke, B., & Amthauer, R. (1999, 2001). *Intelligenz-Struktur-Test 2000 R*, Göttingen, Deutschlang: Hogrefe Verlag.

Lin, H.-H., & Chang, T.-W. (2007). *A camera-based multi-touch interface builder for designers*. *Human-Computer Interaction*. HCI Applications and Services.

Luczak, H., & Frenz, M. (2008). Kompetenz - Erwerb, Erhalt, Ausbau, In Heinz Kowalski, CW Haarfeld (Hrsg), *Stärkung der persönlichen Gesundheitskompetenz im Betrieb - Bis 67 fit im Job* (pp. 19-59): Köln, Deutschland.

Luczak, H., & Stemann, M. (2008). Ergonomic Design and Intervention Strategies in Health Promotion for Ageing Workforces, In Conrad, H.; Heindorf, V.; Waldenberger, F., Palgrave Macmillan (Hrsg) (2008). *Human Resource Management in Ageing Societies* (pp. 144-156): Hampshire, UK: Palgrave.

Mehta, N. (1982). *A flexible machine interface*. M.A.Sc. Thesis, Department of Electrical Engineering, University of Toronto, Canada.

Micire, M., Drury, J. J., Keyes, B., & Yanco, H. A. (2009). Multi-touch interaction for robot control. *Submitted for Conference publication. IUI 2009 Workshop*, Florida.

Morris, C. (1946). *Signs, language und behaviour*. New York: Prentice-Hall.

Morris, M., Huang, A., Paepcke, A., & Winograd, T. (2006). Cooperative gestures: Multi-user gestural interactions for co-located groupware. *CHI 2006*, Montréal, Québec, Canada.

Murata, A. (2006). Eye-Gaze Input Versus Mouse: Cursor Control as a Function of Age. *International Journal of Human-Computer Interaction*, *21*, 1–14.

Naegele, G. (2004). *Zwischen Arbeit und Rente: Gesellschaftliche Chancen und Risiken älterer Arbeitnehmer*. Augsburg, Deutschland: Maro-Verlag.

Nair, S. N., Lee, C. C., & Czaja, S. J. (2005). Older adults attitudes toward computers: Have they changed with recent advances in technology? In *Proceedings of the 49th Annual Meeting of Human Factors and Ergonomics Society* (pp. 154–157).

Nakatani, L. H., & Rohrlich, J. A. (1983). Soft machines: A philosophy of user-computer interface design. In *Proceedings of the ACM Conference on Human Factors in Computing Systems* (pp. 12-15). New York: ACM Press.

Olwal, A., Feiner, S., & Heyman, S. (2008). Rubbing and tapping for precise and rapid selection on touch-screen displays. In *Proceedings of the 2008 SIGCHI conference on Human Factors in computing systems* (pp. 295-304), Italy.

Pak, R., McLaughlin, A. C., Lin, C. C., Rogers, W. A., & Fisk, A. D. (2002). An age-related comparison of a touch screen and a novel input device. In *Proceedings of the Human Factors and Ergonomics Society 45th Annual Meeting.*

Park, D. C., & Schwarz, N. (2000). *Cognitive Aging: A Primer.* London: Psychology Press.

Pickering, J. A. (1985). Touch-sensitive screens: the technologies and their application. *International Journal of Man-Machine Studies, 25,* 249–269. doi:10.1016/S0020-7373(86)80060-8

Pitrella, F. D., & Käppler, W.-D. (1988). *Identification and Evaluation of Scale Design Principles in the Development of the Sequential Judgment, Extended Range Scale. Forschungsinstitut für Anthropotechnik. FAT-Bericht Nr. 80.* Wachtberg.

Rau, P.-L. P., & Hsu, J.-W. (2005). Interaction devices and web design for novice older users. *Educational Gerontology, 31,* 19–40. doi:10.1080/03601270590522170

Rekimoto, J. (2002). Smartskin: An infrastructure for freehand manipulation on interactive surfaces. In *Proceedings of the 2002 SIGCHI Conference on Human Factors in Computing Systems,* USA.

Riviere, C. N., & Thakor, N. V. (1996). Effects of age and disability on tracking tasks with a computer mouse: Accuracy and linearity. *Journal of Rehabilitation Research and Development, 33*(1), 6–15.

Rogers, W. A., Cabera, E. F., Jamieson, B. A., & Rousseau, G. K. (1995). Automatic teller machines and older adults: Usage petterns and training needs. In *Proceedings of the 103 Annual Convention of the American Psychological Association.*

Sachs, L. (1999). *Angewandte Satistik, Anwendung statistischer Methoden.* Heidelberg, Deutschland: Springer Verlag.

Schneider, N., Vetter, S., Kausch, B., & Schlick, C. (2009). Age-differentiated Visualization of Network Plans for Project Management Software. *17th World Congress on Ergonomics,* Beijing.

Scott, S. D., & Carpendale, S. (2006). Investigating tabletop territoriality in digital tabletop work. *Technical Report 2006* (pp. 836-826). Department of Computer Science, University of Calgary, Canada.

Sengpiel, M., Struve, D., Dittberner, D. & Wandke, H. (2008). Entwicklung von Trainingsprogrammen für ältere Benutzer von IT- Systemen. *Wirtschaftspsychologie aktuell, 10,* 94-105.

Shneiderman, B. (1998). *Designing the User Interface* (Wesley, A., Ed.).

Sibert, L. E., & Jacob, R. J. K. (2000). Evaluation of eye gaze interaction. In *. Proceedings, CHI 2000,* 282–288.

Smith, M. W., Sharit, J., & Czaja, S. J. (1999). Aging, motor control, and the performance of computer mouse tasks. *Human Factors, 41*(3), 389–396. doi:10.1518/001872099779611102

Soukoreff, R. W., & MacKenzie, I. S. (2004). Towards a standard for pointing device evaluation, perspectives on 27 years of Fitts' law research in HCI. *International Journal of Human-Computer Studies, 61,* 751–789. doi:10.1016/j.ijhcs.2004.09.001

Tobias, C. L. (1987). Computers and the elderly: A review of the literature and directions for future research. In *Proceedings of the Human Factors Society 31st Annual Meeting* (pp. 866–870), USA.

Torres, D. A. (2006). Evaluating a pen-based computer interface for novice older users. *Conference on Computers & Accessibility ASSETS'06,* Portland, Oregon, USA. Association for Computing Machinery.

Umemuro, H. (2004). Lowering elderly Japanese users' resistence towards computers by using touchscreen technology. *Universal access in the information society*, 3, 276-288.

Vercruyssen, M. (1996). Movement control and speed of behavior . In Fisk, A. D., & Rogers, W. A. (Eds.), *Handbook of Human Factors and the Older Adult* (pp. 55–86). San Diego, CA: Academic Press.

Walker, N., Philbin, D. A., & Spruell, C. (1996). The use of signal detection theory in research on age-related differences in movement control . In Rogers, W. A., Fisk, A. D., & Walker, N. (Eds.), *Aging and skilled performance. Advances in theory and applications* (pp. 45–64). New Jersey: Lawrence Erlbaum Associates.

Ware, C., & Mikaelin, H. H. (1987). An evaluation of an eye tracker as a device for computer input. In *Proc. ACM CHI '87* (pp. 183-188).

Widgor, D., Penn, G., Ryall, K., Esenther, A., & Shen, C. (2007). Living with a tabletop: analysis and observations of long term office use of a multi-touch table. *Second Annual IEEE International Workshop on Horizontal Interactive Human-Computer System.*

Wobbrock, J. O., Rubinstein, J., Sawyer, M. W., & Duchowski, A. T. (2008). Longitudinal Evaluation of Discrete Consecutive Gaze Gestures for Text Entry. In *Proceedings of the Eye Tracking Research & Application Symposium* (pp. 11–18), ETRA.

Wu, M., & Balakrishnan, R. (2003). Multi-finger and whole hand gestural interaction techniques for multi-user tabletop displays. In *Proceedings of the UIST '03 Vancouver* (pp. 193-202). BC, Canada.

Wu, M., Shen, C., Ryall, K., Forlines, C., & Balakrishnan, R. (2006). Gesture registration, relaxation, and reuse for multi-point direct-touch surfaces. In *Proceedings of the First IEEE International Workshop on Horizontal Interactive Human-Computer Systems* (pp. 185-192), Washington, DC.

Xiao, M., Hyppolite, J. R., Pomplun, M., Sunkara, S., & Carbone, E. (2005). Compensating for the Eye-Hand Span Improves Gaze Control in Human-Computer Interfaces. In *Proceedings of the HCI 2005.*

Yarnold, P. R., Stewart, M. J., Stille, F. C., & Martin, G. J. (1996). Assessing functional status of elderly adults via microcomputer. *Perceptual and Motor Skills, 82,* 689–690.

Zhai, S., Morimoto, C., & Ihde, S. (1999). Manual and Gaze Input Cascaded (MAGIC) Pointing. *Proc. ACM CHI '99* (pp. 246-253).

Zöllner, M., Keil, J., Behr, J., Gillich, J., Gläser, S., & Schöls, E. (2008). Coperion 3D - A virtual factory on the tabletop. 5th Intuition 2008. *Proceedings: Virtual Reality in Industry and Society: From Research to Application*, Italy.

Chapter 12
Psychological and Social Problems of Automation and Computerization

Vladimir Munipov
MIREA University, Russia

ABSTRACT

This chapter discusses the ergonomic, psychological and social problems of operators of large complex systems. It is noted that the category of activity is the most important one in the Russian ergonomic and psychological knowledge. It is analyzed the relationship between information models and conceptual-image ones. It emphasizes that in the Soviet Union the notion of cognitive revolution makes not sense because cognitive processes were treated in the works of L. Vygotsky, S. Rubinstein and A. Leontiev as forms of activity. The article indicates the influence of works of G. Bradley on the development of social and psychological aspects of ergonomics in the former Soviet Union and Russia.

INTRODUCTION

In the former Soviet Union, as in the USA, ergonomics bore clearly psychological orientation because just psychologists in the country began to develop ergonomics. The solution of ergonomics problems is impossible without psychological competence. At the same time ergonomics formulates new problem before psychology and set requirements and criteria when solving these problems. The development of psychology is stimulated by the problems of ergonomics which

introduces into its context new kinds of human activity, means of its realization and means of studying it. The bringing ergonomics into psychology closer open possibilities for serving important theoretical problems and practical tasks of humanization of working life – development of standards of hazard prevention, development requirements regarding machines, workplaces and human working techniques. Basic goals were: reducing risk of accidents; environmental influences such as noise vibration, concussion, and hazardous substances; as well as physical and psychological stress and strain at work (Munipov, 1976). The first subject of ergonomic investigations was

DOI: 10.4018/978-1-60960-057-0.ch012

large complex systems, focusing on the human and social aspects of them. Many investigations are devoted to ergonomic problems of design, construction and utilization of automatic control systems. Ergonomists who take part in improving existing and designing new automatic systems of controlling complex production processes. Ergonomists participate in studying problems of man-computer interaction, including working out languages for their dialog. In VNIITE (All-Union research institute of industrial design) study of visual thinking was conducted. Visual thinking is defined as a kind of human activity, the product of which consists in the origin of new image, in the creation of new visual forms bearing a certain meaningful load and making the meaning be visual (Zinchenko et al., 1973). Also in VNIITE the investigations were conducted concerning the system of control of the computer user's safety and the method of estimating a visual fatigue when working with displays.

Ergonomic investigations become important in solving scientific and technological tasks in the field of space flight. Space ergonomics is also passing from special psychophysiological studies to the investigation of activity of cosmonauts on board the space ship. Ergonomists, together with other specialists, are solving tasks of effective organization of all aspects of space ship team's performance, paying special attention to studying motivation, physiology of the working organism, psychological climate, group interaction, and psychophysiological aspects of cosmonaut's leisure time organization. Keeping up all these aspects of cosmonaut's performance to a necessary level provides for a success of the entire flight.

Aviation ergonomics has much in common with space ergonomics. Aviation ergonomics is to provide good dynamic properties of aircraft and effectiveness of information presentation. The automation of aircraft control put forward the problem of effective pilot-equipment interaction under performance conditions. Flights at supersonic speeds and extremely low altitudes brought essential changes into the pilot's performance and required ergonomists' participation in solving a number of complex problems/ Ergonomic studies are considered very important for the design and operation of the ground control systems.

Human factors problems are of vital importance for the shipbuilding industry, as complex automation of control processes. In shipbuilding, as well as in aviation and some other fields, methodological principles of ergonomic design are being intensively worked out (Munipov, 1978, 1979).

Large complex systems are managed by controllers and operators, whose activity is being justly compared with the activity of commander tackling important strategic tasks. One need merely mention the operators of the Space Telecommunications Centre or the Integrated Power System of the USSR. In highly automated areas of production man's executive functions become functions of control. Here, man is the governor of the process as a whole, with the emphasis in his activities switching to the development, planning and prognosis of the process of human activity. There is the characteristic redistribution of the functions of human activity towards creative mental activity, having the decisive role to play. In the characteristic of the operator's qualification there is a corresponding shift of the accent from skill to knowledge.

The main function of the operator (a group of operators) in an automated control system is to take decisions, which usually implies the processing of information enabling man to work out a sequence of purposeful acts aimed at resolving a problem situation and achieving the necessary goal. Optimising decisions on the basis of automated data processing become the pivotal problem in automated control. Because of the complexity of the organizational and functional structures of control in any field of human activity this problem becomes ever more urgent and acute. It assimilates the approach to the tasks and methods of fulfilling them from various fields of knowledge: natural, technical and humanitarian sciences.

Research and development connected with the design of automated control systems have created the premises for integrating technical disciplines and the sciences of man and his/her activity, leading to the emergence a set of psychological problems. The practical tasks in the design, engineering and running of these systems constantly run up against the problem of the human factor. In order to prognosticate, evaluate and analyze the efficiency of control complexes and automated data processing systems it is important to know the quantitative characteristics of man's mental activity, without which such evaluations prove to be vulnerable. Unless the functional significance and the psychological mechanisms in man's processing of data and solution of problems are brought out, there may be serious errors in the distribution of functions between men and the means of automation. The professional training of the operators taking decisions at various levels of control systems cannot ignore the problem of correspondence between man's individual psychological properties and the requirements of rational organization of decision-making, which for their part are determined by the structure of control activity. The study of sensory, perceptive and mnemic functions is necessary for organizing the process of information back-up and preparation of decisions in control systems. We have deliberately left out the socio-psychological aspects of the problem of decision-making and categories like risk, responsibility and motivation, because, for the time being, they have been less adequately studied than the information back-up of decisions.

The solution of problems in automated control systems is a process oriented upon man, which assumes man's connection with man, implying introspection and self-evaluation, and reflexive elements of communication. This is frequently forgotten, because the link is obscured by intervening technical components of the system. But technique and its mathematical data back-up constitute an ancillary instrument for the solution of problems. Technique always operates on a lower level of problem solution than that of man's, and man always remains the vehicle of strategic thinking. In this context, it appears that the results of psychological research into decision-making in automated control systems acquire a more general significance as a possible means for enhancing the efficiency of control activity in general.

The activity of operators of automated systems is complex and mediated. As a rule, they are deprived of the possibility of directly observing the object of control and have to make use of the relevant data coming in along the information channel. The main type of activity of operators of automated control systems is work with information models which are reflections of the state of the object of human activity (the object of control), the system itself, the environment and modes of influencing them, organized in accordance with a definite system of rules. Physically, information models are realized with the aid of the means used to reflect information (indicators, displays, screens, etc.).

Information models are not always easily related to reality. The operator's work with them frequently fails to satisfy the requirements of speed and precision. The main reason here is that when devising information models engineers, as a rule, try to solve the problem of reflecting in it the system of interconnections of the object, while failing to take account of the specific features of the psychological structure of man's work with that object. This ignores the obvious fact that information models are produced for operational work in the process of which the operator transforms the information they contain. Moreover, definite types of information models must correspond to each other class of problems. The logic of problem solution defines the choice of principle on which the information model is structured.

The operator of a control system frequently has to carry out a great number of conversions of the information presented on the reflection devices, so as to move from model to the reality and to reduce the information to a form fit for decision-making.

Some intermediate results of these conversions are sometimes comprehended by the operator as images of reality, notions, schemes, models and behaviour programmes. Psychologists, physiologists and other specialists, who have turned to the long-forgotten study of image phenomena, have been looking closely at this world of the operator's images and notions.

Evaluation of information, its analysis and generalization is effected on the basis of a comparison between the accepted information model and the inner conceptual-image model of the situation (control system) which the operator has developed in the process of instruction and training. The conceptual image model is the product of the operator's comprehension of the existing situation with an eye to the problem before him. The content of this model includes images and models of the real and projected situation, and the significance of the aggregation (of programmes) of possible governing actions and executive reactions of the system. It also includes subjective (and frequently vaguely defined) elements like the notion of the purposes and criteria of the functioning of the system, motivations of activity, knowledge of the consequences of the decisions taken, etc.

In many control systems, the operators could have fulfilled their functions clearly, reliably and without special tension, being guided by the set of conceptual features and rules. But this does not happen because the information appears to the operator as a set of perceptive features which are not evidently linked with the conceptual features. These difficulties of moving from the perceptive to the conceptual features, on which the rules and instructions are based, pose the task of agreeing the conceptual and the information models which make full use of the operator's psychological possibilities in receiving and processing information and taking decisions.

The mediated perception of information creates a number of additional difficulties for the operator, who has to live in a real and simultaneously artificial world of signs, codes and symbols.

He becomes accustomed to manipulating them. However, every model, especially a laconic one, contains some uncertainty, which time and again creates the possibility either of habituation or a stronger emotional impact than that of the real world.

Sometimes the operator becomes accustomed to the model and ceases to relate it to the real situation. This may result in a substitution of ostensible for genuine motivation of actions and loss of vigilance. In such instances, the objective perception of the model needs to be revived (Zinchenko et al., 1976). The problem of interconnections of the information model and conceptual image model appears to have another aspect, which G. Bradley defines as "objective and subjective environments" (Bradley, 2006).

Technical systems are requiring strictly coordinated group control. Here, the stability and quality of activity are determined not so much by the individual contribution of each participant as by the character and degree of their interaction, which, besides, is mediated by technical means.

The study of the regularities operating in such groups has led to the creation of an experimental model of interconnected and interdependent activity in control, in which the whole regulation of the system is mediated. For this purpose the Soviet psychologist F. Gorbov has developed the idea of the homeostat, special device, which he designed, consisting of three or more control panels (depending on the number of examinees). The task of each of the members of the group being examined is to set the pointer on his panel at the zero mark. Each examinee receives information from his own indicator, acts on it, and simultaneously on the indicators of his partners. From his control panel, the experimenter can vary the difficulty of the tasks being set by changing the interconnection coefficient. The task is deemed to be fulfilled only when all the examinees manage to set their pointers at the zero mark. All the movements of the levers and of all the pointers are recorded on an oscillograph, which makes it possible to trace, not only the character of the action of the group as a whole but also the tactics of each of the members. The recording of a number of psychophysiological indicators helps to judge the emotional state of the examinees.

The simulation of group activity has helped to establish that successful fulfillment of experimental tasks is connected with the capability of the groups, as an integral system, to learn a process in the course of which conflict situations frequently arise. F. Gorbov and V. Lebedev say: "Similar situations tend to occur in teams servicing automated systems. In experiment and in life such conflict situations frequently arise due to inadequate training for understanding the intricate course the process of control tends to run within the group with the aid of the instrument readings or, in other words, the 'new language'. This means that man has yet to learn to 'see' the actions of his partners and the course of the process as a whole by means of the readings on the instruments on his control panel" (Gorbov et al., 1975).

Taking a firmly humanistic view, ergonomists, psychologists and designers look to the future as automation and computerization transform and impact on lives of people, and explore issues including stress, power, competence and psychosocial communication. Automation and computerization is frequently entering upon a stage of development making technically feasible projects based on systematized and coherent conceptions of human activity. The process of design starts from the assumed technical potentialities of the system, this is the basis for determining the place and functions of man, the operator (or group of operator); here, account is mainly taken of man's limitations (the relatively small volume of information which he can process in a unit of time, the slowness of his responses, his inadequate resistance to various disturbances, so on). There is need to consider another way. This is to start the elaboration of technical assignments from the idea of making machines cater for man's activity and, consequently, taking account above all of

man's positive potentialities as the operator and the user, that is, taking account not of his shortcomings, but of his advantages, as compared with the technical system.

The concept of human-centered design was formulated in 1970s in VNIITE. However, the idea could not make a reality of good design in the USSR in view of total domination of technics-centered design in the country. Only once, starting from the rule of contraries, i.e., meticulously analyzing how the neglect of human-centered design had led to the frightful consequences, I was able to test principles and methods of human-centered design on the real object bearing in mind the Chernobyl disaster. In this case, design, building, operation and detection of the causes of the accident had taken place without ergonomists' participation. In December 1989, I prepared a report named "Human engineering analysis of Chernobyl Accident.", but at that time there was no possibility of publishing it in the USSR. I learned for the first time that an operative group under the ruling of the Central Committee of the Communist Party of the Soviet Union had been established and that this group had undertaken severe scrutiny of all publications concerning the Chernobyl accident. According to the decision of this operative group secret instructions were given. They ordered: "to intensify the propaganda measures directed towards the exposure of false insinuations of the bourgeois mass media and special organs about the events that took place at the Chernobyl nuclear power plant".

I am very grateful to M. Kumashiro, a well-known Japan ergonomist, as organizers of the 1st UOEN International Symposium and 1st Pan-Pacific Conference on Occupational Ergonomics (Kitakyusu, Japan, 10-13 July 1990) invited me to present a report, the content of which was unpredictable because nobody had previously spoken on this matter (Munipov, 1991). During my report there was silence in the crowded room, because the Japanese are very sensitive regarding everything relating to nuclear power. After

I completed the presentation, there was total silence, which frightened me. For a moment an idea flashed in my head – perhaps the report had not been understood and had been poorly prepared. However, suddenly everyone rose in applause (Munipov, 1992).

Theoretical basis of ergonomics mainly relates to psychology, sociology, and industrial design. Since here we cannot be deep into the basis in general, let us give only an example.

Soviet psychology has evolved on the basis of historical approach to the development of human mental processes. L.S. Vygotsky played a considerable role in establishing this principle. In analyzing practical activity, psychologists emphasize the tool as the most important component of human activity. This component creates the qualitative uniqueness of human activity in comparison with animal behavior. The tool is not simply added on to human activity: rather, it transforms it. Action with a tool implies a combination of activation and human creative adaptation. Tools themselves appear as supplementary organs created by humans. The mediated nature of human activity clearly plays a leading role in the analysis of practical activity.

One of Vygotsky's central theses is that mental processes change in human beings as their processes of practical activity change (i.e., the mental processes become mediated). The sign (language, mathematical sign, mnemotechnic means, etc.) emerges as such a mediational link. Language is the most important form of the sign. In using auxiliary means and signs (for example, in making a notch in a stick in order to remember), humans produce changes in external things; but these changes subsequently have an effect on their internal mental processes. By changing the milieu, humans can master their behavior and direct their mental processes. Mediated mental processes initially emerge as functions distributed among members of social groups and only later become the internal psychological function of a single person. At the same time, mediated mental processes signify the development of new forms

of interfunctional relations. The emergence of: (1) logical thought as opposed to situational thought that is unmediated, (2) mediated memory as opposed to unmediated memory, and (3) voluntary attention as opposed to involuntary attention are all examples of the development of higher mental functions. Writing is mankind's artificial memory, which gives human memory an immense advantage over animal memory. With the help of speech, humans master thought, since the logical processing of their perception is conducted through a verbal formulation (Wertsch (ed), 1981).

The category of activity is the most important one in the Russian system of ergonomic and psychological knowledge (Zinchenko (ed), 1970-1986, Zinchenko et al, 1976). The original term in Russian is "dejatel'nost" which carries with it the idea of doing in order to transform, specifically the transformation of a material object. The most important aspect of activity theory is Leontiev's observation that activity is the smallest meaningful unit of analysis and the recognition that the definition of activity necessarily includes a definition of the context in which it is performed. Psychology has amassed a wealth of factual material on the structure of human activity, thus making it possible to describe such essential components as the need, motives, tasks, actions and operations (the task integrates the goal and the conditions for its attainment). Psychology knows of facts demonstrating mutual transitions of these components. This discipline has also accumulated extensive evidence on the specific features of the two principal forms of human activity, the "external" and the "internal" ones, and on their mutual transitions. The "external" or object-related, practical activity is primary in relation to the "internal" – cognitive, mental activity. The dynamics of human activity follows a complex pattern, and so does the dynamics of regulatory psychic images.

"The problem of meaning" is a term used by the activity theory. A.N. Leontiev explains it by the following example: "A day filled with many actions, successfully carried out by a person who in the course of their execution felt them to be adequate, can nonetheless leave that person with unpleasant, sometimes even oppressive, emotional "aftertaste". Against the background of ongoing life with its current tasks "aftertaste" is not clearly distinguishable. But the moment comes when the person looks back at himself and in thought goes over the events of the day, and then the emotional signal gathers strength and indicates unambiguously which of those events is responsible for the unpleasant feeling. And it may turn out that it is the *success* achieved by a friend, but prepared by himself, in reaching a common goal – a goal which was, he had thought, the only object his actions held in view. Now it is apparent that this was not so, that the main driving force for him had been personal success and advancement. This realization brings him face to face with "the problem of meaning", the task of recognizing his own motives or more precisely their real internal relationship to one another" (Leontiev, 1971).

This concept is not altogether monosemantic in Leontiev's conceptual usage. It is important to distinguish three uses, which may be indicated by the following three antitheses: (1) meaning-signification; (2) meaning-emotion; (3) presence of meaning (meaningfulness) – absence of meaning (meaninglessness). The first of these is derived from the fundamental opposition of *knowledge* and *attitude*: as signification is a unit of objective knowledge of reality, so meaning is a unit of subjective (partial) attitude to it. This first usage of the concept "meaning" is an abstraction from actual forms of its existence in consciousness. The second antithesis, meaning-emotion, in fact distinguishes between two basic forms of its existence in consciousness. Emotion is the immediate, direct expression of a person's attitude to one or another event or situation, while meaning is mediated by significations and knowledge in general, by the person's cognition of himself and his life: meaning is emotion plus thought, emotion enlightened by thought. The third antithesis,

meaningfulness-meaninglessness, has quite a different origin. Its source is in the concept of the "meaning-forming motive". Only when a subject's activity, and the course of events in general, is proceeding in a direction tending towards realization of his meaning-forming motives, will the situation have meaning (be meaningful). If things are proceeding otherwise the situation becomes meaningless (Vasilyuk, 1988).

Only the approach emanating from the point of view of the psychology of social interaction, A. A. Leontiev wrote, can give us the key to the correct treatment of the nature of meaning and its interrelationship with other philosophical and psychological categories (Wertsch, 1981).

Information science is often linked to a cognitive revolution; it is treated as a new cognitive discipline which has branched from many social, natural and technical sciences. Occasionally, the cognitive science is designated by the fairly polysemantic term "mind" which denotes reason, thinking, psyche and consciousness simultaneously. It is viewed as a sociological, psychological and natural science premise for the information science and for further development of computing engineering, including artificial intelligence. The revolutionary nature of the cognitive science is emphasized for the simple reason that it emerged by way of opposition to behaviorism and to the whole cycle of behavioral sciences that had held sway in the American humanities until the 1960s. In the Soviet Union, the notion of a cognitive revolution makes no sense because the opposition did not take on such acute forms (Zinchenko et al, 1989). In works of L. Vygotsky, S. Rubinstein, A. Leontiev and many other psychologists, cognitive processes were treated as forms of activity. It is on the works on the cultural-historical theory of psyche and consciousness developed by L. Vygotsky, on the psychological theory of activity expounded by A. Leontiev, A. Luria and A. Zaporozhets and on the theory of the physiology of activity advanced by N. Bernstein that ergonomics relies.

N. Bernstein demonstrated on the basis of sufficient and concrete evidence that movement must be analyzed as something goal-determined from within, "elucidated" by a psychic reflection, of a given situation and itself an essential factor in that reflection (Bernstein, 1966).

After many years of relative obscurity, English scientist P. Turner marked, interest on activity theory has experienced a renaissance with the publications in USA, Great Britain, Denmark, Finland. S. Bodker has applied activity theory to the analysis of applications for the Danish Labour Inspection Service. E. Christiansen studied computer use in police work using an activity theory framework (Turner, 2006).

VNIITE had much in common in its research with approaches to solving problems of G. Bradley. Y. Soloviev was creating VNIITE in 1962 so that it would gain an image as the most open Soviet institution behind the Iron Curtain. In 1975 Y. Soloviev was elected as ICSID President. VNIITE was created with the aim "that it is important to have a balance between pure technical research and development and the behavioral and social science disciplines" (Bradley, 2006). There is a balance to all related disciplines, and psychology is not represented only with some terms and contents but it is integrated with its basic pattern of thinking. VNIITE's management considered it was crucial for designer and ergonomist to understand clearly the social, economic and political background of what to do. Socially industrial design and ergonomic design include a description of human characteristics and activity, as well as environmental, cultural and development context in which an activity is performed; a description of the designed systems, cooperative task activities, organizational structure. Socially industrial design and ergonomic design integrate all these factors into development large complex systems. VNIITE's staff did its best that "cross-disciplinary research, in particular about interaction between technology, organization and humans, was recognized" (Bradley, 2006). In 1973, one of the more

meaningful of VNIITE's works was presented to the Italian Unita Company. It was an advanced lathe and it considered as the biggest achievement of industrial design and ergonomics. The significance of this project was the attraction of maximum attention to the person through the equipment design. At that time designers, ergonomists and other specialists worked together as an effective team (Munipov, 1978). VNIITE was "to integrate international, national and local research approaches". As with G. Bradley (Bradley, 2006), Y. Soloviev and V. Munipov served as project managers for interdisciplinary research.

The task was being solved in VNIITE's R&D – "a new type of engineer is being educated" (Bradley, 2006). There is a requirement for engineer in technical and computer sciences to have a broader humanistic and behavioral scientific orientation and knowledge (Munipov (ed.), 1983). Education programs were developed in VNIITE and other R&D organizations on the basis of scientific investigations. In 2001 V. Munipov and V. Zinchenko published the textbook " Ergonomics. The Human-Centered Ergonomic Design of Tool, Technology, Hardware, Software and Environment" (Munipov et al, 2001) that was recommended by the Ministry of Education of Russian Federation as a textbook for students of highest educational institutions. As a result of this a change is taking place in enrollment requirement for some technical universities in 2006. The author of this paper and five other scientists received a prize of Government of Russian Federation in the field of education for realization of a number of the R&D in practice.

One can continue the enumeration of the common themes of research and Bradley and VNIITE, however, I should indicate the main difference. It is that the task of creation of information society is the intention neither in the Soviet Union nor in Russia. Accordingly, nobody dealt with the psychological and social problems of this society. Russia, which has become almost raw power, thus today closed the path to the information society.

At the same time the nearest neighbor of Russia-the former poor and backward province of Czarist Russia - Finland- has become the information society with an information economy.

It was emphasized in proceedings of the meetings of World Summit on the Information Society (WSIS) held in the city of Geneva in 2003 and in Tunis in 2005: " At an early stage it was stated that the information society must be based on the Universal Declaration of Human Rights – including civil and political rights, as well as social, economic and cultural rights" (Bradley, 2006). The assertion, that democracy and human rights in the Western sense do not match to the country, is frequently justified and implemented in practice in Russia. G. Bradley ends his book with the phrase, which is logical and essentially completes the statement of World Summit: "We are in unique position in history where we should take on responsibility to use the technology to promote peace, and deepen democracy and the quality of life for all" (Bradley, 2006). Many Russian scientists are aware of "the responsibility to use the technology to promote peace, and deepen democracy and the quality of life for all". By studying the activities of people in large systems Russian ergonomists in theory turned to psychological, ergonomic and social problems of the Information Society. Hopefully, G. Bradley and her colleagues would find interesting and useful scientific solutions in the research of Russian ergonomists The author includes many Bradley's provisions in a series of his lectures in Moscow State University of Psychology and Education and in Moscow Institute of Radioengineering, Electronics and Automatics. Particular attention is devoted by him to the work "Humans on Net. Information and Communication Technology (ICT), Work Organisation and Human Being", published in 2001 and edited by G. Bradley, as well as her book "Social and community informatics: human on the net", published in 2006. The author tries to answer all questions on Education and Training of the European Commission (2001) and ones that G. Bradley poses in his book:

- A knowledge society, a cognitive society: What does it mean?
- How and why are these so-called historical revolutions happening?
- What kind of transformation in the nature of work and in the organization of production is induced by the information society?
- Increasing the level of qualifications to meet the globalization of the labour market: what exactly does it mean?
- What are the ethical rules of the information society?
- A broad base of knowledge: how and in which education structure?
- Flexibility, mobility: how, and at what price?
- To what degree can we accept the concept of employability? Where is it negotiated? Who will pay for it?
- What are the consequences for the workers of the so-called learning organization?
- What about the *customization* of education? Is it not a way of absolving the employers from their obligations?
- Lifelong learning: why not also lifelong training? A semantic slip of tongue? Who will be responsible? The individuals? The employers? The unions?
- Validation, certification, accreditation of programmes throughout life: By whom? How?
- How to restore a collective approach in the different processes of working, of training, of negotiating…? (Bradley, 2006).

Students lively and with a great interest perceive and discuss the content of these lectures. Young people understand that they will live and work in the information society.

It is important to note that the study of the book of G. Bradley "Psychosocial Work Environment", which had been read by me as the first book of the author, was, without exaggeration, a discovery for me and helped me to define the new frontiers of research. After that I began to closely monitor Bradley's publications. Engineers, who brought new technologies to the possible perfection, were the heroes of Silicon Valley. Being trained and working in Silicon Valley, G. Bradley grasped by some "animal" instinct that just psychologists, sociologists and researchers of organizational behavior would become the heroes of a future Swedish "Silicon Valley". This idea formed the meaning of her and her family's life, and thus she has made an enormous contribution to the development of information society.

In 1986 in Stockholm my personal acquaintance with this wise, charming, smart and friendly woman happened on the first Work with Displays Unit Conference. In 1994 I received an invitation to the Fourth International Symposium on Organizational Design and Management held in Stockholm. The Symposium was informative and interesting, with hot discussions on emerging issues of macroergonomics, and of social and psychological aspects of computerization. The impetus for this unique collective creativity came from G. Bradley and H.M. Hendrick. At the same time she found time and strength for the care and attention to almost every participant of the symposium. Works of G. Bradley had an impact on the development of ergonomics in the former Soviet Union. We compared our investigations of many psychological and social aspects of development of automation and computerization with the research that G. Bradley has done at the same time.

We often found the proximity of the positions, in other cases, saw the looming prospect of research, sometimes adjusted our scientific approaches.

I was strongly impressed by the three qualities of G. Bradley. If the woman conceived to do something in science, she will do; she will give up her life for something, but she will do that. The second quality expresses by the idea of one English philosopher: If you have knowledge, let others light their lamps from it. Bradley's lamp continues to attract scientists and specialists of many countries, including Russia. Also I admire the ability of Bradley to vary with time.

Especially I recall the meeting, when after my report she said: "Vladimir, do not report in such a serious style, you should be smiling." It seems to me that she has done many serious works and deeds with smiling all the time and so she has achieved such outstanding success.

ACKNOWLEDGMENT

The author is grateful to Michael Munipov for his participation in preparing the article.

REFERENCES

Bernstein, N. A. (1966). *Essays in the Physiology of Movement and Activity*. Moscow: Medicine Publishers. (in Russian)

Bradley, G. (2006). *Social and Community Informatics. Human on the Net*. London: Routledge.

Gorbov, F. D., & Lebedev, V. I. (1975). *Psycho-neurological Aspects of the Work of Operators*. Moscow: Medicine Publishers. (in Russian)

Leontiev, A. N. (1971). *Needs, Motivations, Emotions*. Moscow: Moscow University Press. (in Russian)

Munipov, V.M. (1976). Ergonomics and psychological science, (in Russian). *Questions of psychology*, 5, 3-17.

Munipov, V. M. (1978). Applied Ergonomics in the USSR. *Applied Ergonomics, 9*(4), 215–222. doi:10.1016/0003-6870(78)90082-0

Munipov, V. M. (1979). Ergonomics as a Factor in Social and Economic Development. *Ergonomics, 22*(6), 607–611. doi:10.1080/00140137908924645

Munipov, V. M. (Ed.). (1983). *Ergonomics: Principles and Recommendations. A Manual* (in Russian). Moscow, RU: VNIITE.

Munipov, V. M. (1991). Human engineering analysis of Chernobyl Accident . In Kumashiro, M., & Megan, E. D. (Eds.), *Towards human work: Solution to problems in Occupational Health and Safety*. London: Taylor and Francis.

Munipov, V. M. (1992). Chernobyl Operators: Criminals or Victims? *Applied Ergonomics, 23*(5), 337–342. doi:10.1016/0003-6870(92)90295-7

Munipov, V. M., & Zinchenko, V. P. (2001). *Human-Centered Ergonomic Design of Tool, Technology, Hardware, Software and Environment*. Moscow: Logos. (in Russian)

Turner, P. (2006). Critical Reappraisal of Activity Theory . In Karwowski, W. (Ed.), *International Encyclopedia of Ergonomics and Human Factors* (2nd ed., *Vol. 1*). London: Taylor and Francis.

Vasilyuk, F. (1988). *The psychology of experiencing*. Moscow: Progress Publishers.

Wertsch, J. (Ed.). (1981). *The Concept of Activity in Soviet Psychology*. New York: Sharpe Inc.

Zinchenko, V. P. (Ed.). (1970-1986). *Works of VNIITE* (in Russian). Series 1-32. Moscow: VNIITE.

Zinchenko, V.P., Gordon V.M. & Munipov, V.M. (1973). Study of Visual Thinking (in Russian). *Soviet Psychology*, XII(2).

Zinchenko, V. P., & Munipov, V. M. (1976). Man and Modern Production. [Moscow: USSR Academy of Sciences.]. *Social Sciences*, 4.

Zinchenko, V. P., & Munipov, V. M. (1989). *Fundamentals of Ergonomics*. Moscow: Progress.

Chapter 13

Cognitive and Organizational Complexity and Behavior:
Implications for Organizational Design and Leadership

Hal W. Hendrick
University of Southern California, USA

ABSTRACT

Historical findings concerning the nature of the higher-order structural personality dimension of cognitive complexity and related conceptual systems and the sociotechnical model of organizational complexity are summarized, including the relationship of the two. The author's own research findings on early trainer and traumatic event effects on one's complexity level are described. The relation of complexity level to creativity, leader behavior and influence, interpersonal and self-perception, group task performance, and matching individual and organizational position complexity, are reviewed. Implications of complexity level for organizational design and the design of information and training systems are noted.

INTRODUCTION

During the past five decades there has been a growing body of research that I believe is highly relevant to our understanding of individual differences in human performance, including values, attitudes, motives, creativity, and stylistic leadership and work behavior. This research concerns the higher-order structural personality dimension of *cognitive complexity*, or concreteness-abstractness of thinking. The fact that the high technology societies of the world appear to be undergoing significant, yet

understandable age-related demographic changes in this higher-order personality dimension further enhances its value to us in understanding human performance, including how it relates to organizational design, management, and the structure of information and training systems.

This area of structured personality research had its origins in the classical work of Piaget (1948) on child development. Among others, one group of researchers of particular relevance to this paper has extended the study of concreteness-abstractness into the adult range: Professors O.J. Harvey, D. E. Hunt, and H. Schroder (1961) in

DOI: 10.4018/978-1-60960-057-0.ch013

the area of conceptual functioning or *conceptual systems* and behavior.

Cognitive complexity, or concreteness-abstractness, is reported to have two major structural dimensions, *differentiation* and *integration* (Bariff & Lusk, 1971; Harvey, et al., 1961; King & Hicks, 2007). Operationally, differentiation can be defined as the number of dimensions extracted from a set of data, and integration as the number of interconnections between rules for combining structured data (Bariff and Lusk, 1971). A concrete cognitive style is one in which relatively little differentiation is used in structuring concepts. Experiential data are categorized by the individual into relatively few conceptual dimensions, and within concepts, there exists relatively few categories or shades of gray. In the extreme, a concept is divided into just two categories, characteristic of either/or, black/white, absolutist thinking. In addition, concrete thinkers are relatively poor at integrating conceptual data in assessing complex problems and developing unique or creative, insightful solutions. In contrast, cognitively complex persons tend to demonstrate high differentiation and effective integration in their conceptualizing (Harvey, 1966; Harvey, et al., 1961).

Although all persons tend to become more abstract over time, our development curve tends to flatten in early adulthood. At what degree of cognitive complexity this plateauing occurs, and to what extent, appears to depend primarily on two factors: How open one is to learning from one's experience, and how much exposure one has had to diversity. We all start out in life with very limited exposure to diversity, and thus have few conceptual categories in which to place experiential information, and few rules and combinations of rules to integrate our experiential information in problem solving and decision making. As we gain new experiences, and *if* we are open to learning from those experiences, we develop new conceptual categories and more rules and rule combinations for integrating our conceptual data (Harvey, 1966).

How open we are to learning from our experiences depends on the nature of one's early training environment at home and school (Blatt, 1971). In particular, the nature of the "trainer" role appears to be critical. In general, the more absolutist and authoritarian the parent, teacher or other trainer, the greater is the likelihood that *active* exposure was inhibited, and that the child will plateau at a relatively concrete level of conceptual functioning (Harvey, et al., 1961). The more relativistic and less authoritarian the training, the more the trainer encourages the child to think things through and draw personal conclusions, and the more the trainer instills a strong positive sense of self worth in the child, the more abstract or cognitively complex the child will become in his or her conceptual functioning as an adult.

COGNITIVE COMPLEXITY AND CONCEPTUAL SYSTEMS

During the mid 1900's Professors O.J. Harvey of the University of Colorado, David E. Hunt of Syracuse University, and Harold M. Schroder of Princeton University, who had been doing attitude research, noted that persons who had similar attitudes towards one thing tended to have similar attitudes towards many other things – that they had a similar *attitude pattern*. By the same token, they were able to identify others who had attitude patterns, but different from the first group's. These researchers wondered if these different attitude patterns really were reflections of basic underlying differences in how people perceive reality (i.e., if you and I conceptualize reality differently, then it makes sense that we would have different attitudes about issues in our world); and so they set about to determine if this was the case. (O. J. Harvey, personal communication, 1978).

Based on their original research, Harvey, et al. (1961) concluded that there appear to be at least four fundamentally different ways in which people organize or structure and integrate their experiences of reality. Further, these four ways appear to lie along an invariant developmental continuum, with the underlying dimension being concreteness-abstractness of thinking, or cognitive complexity. As individuals develop greater differentiation and integration in their conceptual functioning, they may move on to a new, more cognitively complex way of viewing reality. These four systematic ways or stages, in order of their developmental occurrence, are labeled simply as conceptual systems 1, 2, 3, and 4 (Harvey, et. al, 1961). While the four conceptual systems represent points along the cognitive complexity continuum, the specific location of those points can vary somewhat from person to person. As shown in Figure 1, imagine the cognitive complexity dimension as a 9-point scale, with 9 representing the highest level of complexity. Research, including my own, has shown that individuals with System 1 conceptual functioning can range from 1 to 5 on this concreteness-abstractness scale; with System 2 functioning from 3 to 7; System 3 from 6 to 8; and System4 functioning from 8 to 9.

In their initial research, Harvey, et al. (1961) identified the following sets of characteristics associated with each conceptual level of functioning. Subsequent research, including my own, consistently has confirmed these findings.

System 1 Functioning: Conventional (Conformist) Thinking and Behavior

Regardless of culture or nationality, all persons start out with a highly concrete System 1 orientation toward reality. As persons gain experience, they become more abstract in their conceptual functioning, but still may maintain a System 1 perspective. System1 persons tend to see their social world vertically – like a giant bureaucratic organizational chart. What is important is to know where one fits in heirarchally. In comparison with persons with other, more abstract, conceptual orientations, System 1 persons are characterized by conventional thinking and behavior, and they tend

Figure 1. Complexity level and conceptual systems

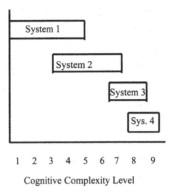

Cognitive Complexity Level

to rely on rules, regulations, tradition, and other *external* sources of "authority" as the basis for their decisions. In comparison with more abstract functioning individuals, the research consistently has shown System 1 persons to have a relatively high need for (a) structure and order and (b) simplicity and consistency, to be relatively (c) authoritarian, (d) absolutist, (e) closed in their belief systems, (f) ethnocentric, (g) paternalistic, (h) personally rigid, (i) have a low tolerance for ambiguity, (j) highly accepting of prevailing rules, norms, and social roles - and to see them as relatively static and unchanging, and (k) to have a high belief in external fate control.

Research, to date, suggests that approximately 5O% to 55% of the American adult population is operating primarily from a System 1 perspective; but that there are systematic differences by age group. Among those who are in their 80's or older, approximately 80% may be operating at the System 1 level. Among those adults in their 50's and younger, less than half are operating from a System 1 orientation. Those in their late 50's, 60's and 70's represent the national average. Limited research in other industrialized countries suggests a similar pattern.

Although age related, these differences are not age *caused*. Rather, other factors, such as generational differences in child rearing patterns, addressed later, and amount of childhood and adolescence exposure to diversity through such things as media, education, travel, etc. appear to be the most important factors. Of particular note, since World War II, there has been a tremendous increase in means that expose us to diversity, including TV, libraries, the commercial airplane, and especially, the internet. In addition, childrearing patterns in many instances have become less authoritarian.

System 2 Functioning: General Negativism

As individuals become more abstract, the System 1 conception of reality eventually may "break down". These individuals react by becoming focused on, and sensitized to what is "wrong" with the "system" - its institutions and persons who exercise authority and restraint over their lives. From a developmental standpoint, the individual appears to learn more about oneself as *distinct* from the generalized cultural standards that had been applied to both self and others during System 1 functioning (Hunt, 1966). In their moral decision-making, System 2 persons often seem in a kind of psychological vacuum. They tend to see the external norms, which heretofore they had relied upon, as having let them down and, thus, no longer reliable. As yet, they have not replaced this external basis for their decisions with an *internalized*, principled basis. About all System 2 persons can do is react in a distrustful, negative manner. Like System 1 individuals, but to a lesser extent, System 2 conceptualizers tend to have a high need for structure and order and simplicity and consistency, be absolutist, closed minded, not highly creative, and personally rigid. Unlike System 1 persons, they tend not to reject the prevailing rules, norms, and social order, and to advocate change. Often, movement into System 2 conceptualizing occurs during the latter high school and college age years. Behaviorally, persons may have either an "approach" or "avoidance" reaction: They may suddenly become campus left-wing activists or, alternately, simply "drop out" from the society

that has disappointed them. In either case, it is likely to be an indiscriminate "throw the baby out with the bathwater" reaction. If asked what they believe should replace the existing social order, they often will advocate some kind of anarchy - such as a simplistic belief of "let everyone do their own thing".

For most persons who enter the System 2 stage, it is a reactionary, transitory one - perhaps a few months to several years in duration. As they gain further experience and become more abstract, they move on to a System 3 orientation. Although as many as 20% of those in their teens may be in this stage at any given time, only several percent of adults plateau at this level. Those that do provide a source for radical left wing organizations - groups that have high sounding causes but inhumane means of accomplishing them, such as terrorism. I have seen intelligent, assertive, System 2 functioning adults literally tear an organization apart.

System 3 Functioning: The World is People

The System 2 breaking away from the norm, and learning about how one is distinctly *oneself*, provides the basis for eventually empathically understanding and accepting differences in others from *both* oneself and the norm (Hunt, 1966). With development of this more abstract and empathic realization about others, the individual moves into System 3 conceptualizing. As an overview, for System 3 functioning persons the world is *people*. Instead of seeing differences in values, religion, race, lifestyles, beliefs, etc. as deviant or "less than", as do more concrete functioning persons, System 3 individuals tend to value these differences as enriching their personal lives and the human condition. Instead of seeing their social world vertically, they tend to see it horizontally– people are valued not by their hierarchical position, but by their character.

In marked contrast to System 1 individuals, System 3 functioning persons tend to demonstrate a low need for structure and order, and for simplicity and consistency, and often will express a preference for complexity and change. They tend to have a high tolerance for ambiguity, low absolutism, low ethnocentrism, and an openness of beliefs - in fact, they *expect* their beliefs to change with increased experience. System 3 persons tend to be moderately authoritarian, but do not hold authority figures in awe, and expect to be questioned when they are in positions of authority. Rules, regulations, and procedures are accepted as useful, but also are seen as needing review and, sometimes, modification (or elimination) as things change to ensure that they remain functional. They tend to have both a high need for people and for helping others. They thus tend to be "joiners" and are empathically concerned with the human condition and factors that affect the quality of life.

In the United States, approximately 30% of the adult population operates from a System 3 orientation; but again, there is a systematic age relationship. Only 10% to 15% of those in their 80's and older appear to be operating from a true System 3 orientation. Among those in their mid 20's to mid 50's, close to half appear to be functioning at a System 3 level. Again, those in their late 50's, 60's and 70's represent the average. Based on very limited research, this same pattern appears to characterize other industrialized countries.

System 4 Functioning: Autonomous, Creative Behavior; Conceptual Maturity

The major developmental task at the fourth conceptual level is the *integration* of standards that apply to both self and others. This integration enables the individual to understand both self and others as occupying different positions on the *same transcendent dimension*, rather than seeing self and others simply as being on differ-

ent standards. In accomplishing this integrating task, the individual develops greater autonomy in thought and action (Hunt, 1966).

To an even greater extent than System 3 thinkers, System 4 conceptualizers have a low need for structure and order and simplicity and consistency, are relativistic rather than absolutist, open minded, creative, flexible, and have a high tolerance for ambiguity. Like System 3 persons, System 4 individuals are people-oriented, but are *not* highly people dependent - they thus tend *not* to be joiners; and will be very open and direct in expressing their views, even when they may be unpopular. Although others may have a high-perceived self-worth, it seems to be the norm among System 4 persons.

In terms of their empirically identified characteristics, System 4 individuals appear to be the same persons which, through very different research approaches and models, Maslow identified as true *self actualizers,* and the famous American psychologist, Carl Rogers, as *fully functioning persons.* All three approaches have identified approximately 8% to 10% of the adult population as falling into this group (Hendrick, 1981).

Characteristics Unrelated to Conceptual Systems

It should be noted that several important characteristics that might seem highly related to cognitive complexity and conceptual stage are not. First, when education level is held constant, only a weak correlation is found between abstractness of functioning and general intelligence (Harvey, et. al, 1961). Some of the most brilliant persons from all walks of life appear to have been, and are, System 1 functioning individuals. Secondly, conceptual functioning does not appear to be related to generosity, friendliness, or numerous other valued personality characteristics.

Other Characteristics Related to Abstractness and Conceptual Systems

More cognitively complex functioning has been found to be related to (a) completeness and effectiveness of cue utilization, (b) readiness and ability of persons to relinquish previous assumptions or approaches and change their set in order to complete tasks, (c) use of more novel, yet appropriate responses to problems, and (d) value differences (Harvey, et al, 1961; Hendrick, 1979). With respect to values, System 1 persons score higher than more abstract functioning individuals on Scott's Scale of Values for self-control, honesty, kindness, loyalty, religiousness, and the desire for power and influence; System 2 persons value self-control, honesty, kindness, loyalty and religiousness *less* than all others, and creativity and independence somewhat higher than System 1 persons; System 3 individuals score relatively low on their valuing of self-control and independence, and as high as System 1 persons on kindness, and intermediate on the other values; System 4 conceptualizers value creativity and independence highly, give low value to self-control and religiousness, and are intermediate on the other four dimensions. (Davis, 1966).

CONTRIBUTIONS TO OUR UNDERSTANDING BY THE AUTHOR

Cognitive Complexity Level and Childrearing Patterns

Harvey, et al. (1961) proposed that reaching a plateau at a particular stage of conceptual functioning is related to exposure to a particular dominant trainer pattern during one's childhood. The essential characteristics of the four trainer patterns identified are as follows.

System 1 Trainer Pattern

Trainers of System 1 adults were hypothesized to have been authoritarian, absolutist, ethnocentric, and closed minded; and to have relied on external sources in their moral reasoning. By the trainer's behavior, conformity rather than creativity of thought and action was emphasized, and the child was given little opportunity to explore values and power relationships.

System 2 Trainer Pattern

System 2 adults' trainers were hypothesized to have characteristics similar to those of System 1 trainers, but also to have been arbitrary and inconsistent. Consequently, the child learned not to trust authority figures or the institutions of social control that they represent.

System 3 Trainer Pattern

System 3 adults were hypothesized to have had trainers who were permissive, overprotective, indulgent, and somewhat socially dependent on the trainee. This enabled the child to take advantage of the dependency relationship to develop skill at manipulating others and, through this, to avoid facing the world alone. The permissive atmosphere allowed the child greater freedom than the System 1 and 2 trainer patterns to explore ideas, values, and relationships.

System 4 Trainer Pattern

System 4 adults were hypothesized to have had trainers who themselves functioned in a highly abstract manner. They tended to relate to the child as an older, experienced adult to a younger, developing adult. The child's behavior was shaped primarily by positive reinforcement, including being rewarded for exploring and trying the different rather than for overt responses matched to narrowly prescribed standards of the trainer. The child was intrinsically valued by the trainer as a person in his or her own right.

To test the above-hypothesized relationships, I had 198 practicing managers and engineers, enrolled in nine sections of my graduate organizational behavior classes between 1976 and 1979, write a one-page essay describing their childrearing. As part of their essay, these adults were specifically asked to (a) state the nature of their relationship with each parent, or surrogate parent, including the extent to which each parent was authoritarian or permissive, and (b) Indicate how each parent responded when they deviated from parental rules. 156 or 79% of the responses fell clearly into one of four trainer patterns, highly similar to those hypothesized by Harvey, et al. (1961). The others could not be classified into a distinct pattern. All 198 participants were administered Harvey's This I Believe Test (TIB), a measure of both cognitive complexity and conceptual systems (See Harvey, et. al 1961). For the 79% that could be categorized, the correlation between trainer pattern and Conceptual system was .62 (p. <. 001).

In general, the conceptual system level of the individuals matched the hypothesized corresponding trainer pattern, but with one exception: The System 4 adults (21 students) were fairly evenly split between having had either the System 3 or System 4 trainer pattern. Most frequently, those persons who had experienced the System 3 trainer pattern reported it for only one of the parents, usually the mother, with the father's role being either largely absent or less influential, and/or that of disciplinarian.

Cognitive Complexity and Traumatic Events

During the 1976-1995 period, I interviewed over 50 persons who experienced the System 1 trainer pattern while growing up, yet had made the transition to System 3 or 4 functioning. The one common

characteristic that these persons seem to possess, and to which they attribute their breaking away from the System 1 mold, is having undergone a traumatic event in their adult lives (e.g., near death, death of a loved one, divorce, combat in Viet Nam) which upset their lives and caused them to seriously question their views of reality.

While it appears traumatic events can lead to development of greater abstractness, it often is not the case. Harvey (1966) and Hunt (1966) have emphasized that exposure to diversity can be superoptimal as well as suboptimal, and thus not facilitate conceptual growth.

Cognitive Complexity and Creativity

In 1968, during a required undergraduate introductory psychology class at the U. S. Air Force Academy, over 600 students were asked to write down as many uses as they could think of for their uniform shoulder boards within a five minute period. All students also were administered the Abstract Orientation Scale (AOS)), a measure of cognitive complexity that has shown good correlation with Harvey's TIB and various measures of related dimensions (see Hendrick, 1979, 1990 for a brief summary of AOS validation studies). The cognitive complexity scores then were correlated with both numbers of uses and instructor ratings, including my own, of originality of the uses. For both number of uses and originality of uses, the cognitively complex students scored significantly higher (p<.001) than the more cognitively concrete students. Similar, but less striking results were found for uses of both a pencil and paper clip.

In a related study, the students were asked to write down how they would take their roommate's girl friend out on a date and have him appreciate it. The replies were rated for creativity by two instructors, with a third instructor rater being used to decide the issue when ever there was a disagreement between the first two. The abstract functioning students scored significantly higher on creativity than did the cognitively concrete group (p<.001). Using the students' Harvey TIB measures of conceptual system, we found no significant difference between System 3 and System 4 students' replies. The results of these studies are consistent with the cognitive complexity and conceptual systems literature, and lend construct validity to the model.

Cognitive Complexity and Interpersonal Perception

Fundamental to the interpersonal influence or leadership process appears to be the ability to perceive the behavioral cues of others (Harvey, 1966). Harvey (1966) has summarized a number of studies by himself and others demonstrating that abstract persons have a greater sensitivity to minimal cues and a greater ability to use them appropriately and completely. In order to determine if this ability also applies to interpersonal perception, I had 117 senior and junior male undergraduate students view the film, *Twelve Angry Men*, which frequently has been used in interpersonal perception research. The first 38 minutes of the film depicts the deliberations of the jury at the end of a murder trial. The film is rich in its portrayal of group dynamics phenomena. Issues of leadership, conformity, and deviation are highly visible in the emerging patterns of interpersonal relationships of the jurors. Each juror exemplifies a distinct personality and his arguments and nuances of behavior easily suggest a degree of attitudinal and behavioral flexibility. The initial vote of the jury is 11 to 1 "guilty". The film was stopped at the point where the jurors are about to take a second vote. The students were informed that during the remainder of the film, the jurors would change their vote, one by one, resulting in a final vote of 12 to 0 for not guilty. Each class member then was handed a form, depicting the jury seating arrangement, and asked to number the jurors in the order in which they would change their votes to "not guilty". Each student's ranking then was compared with the actual order in which

the jurors switched their vote, and a composite error score was computed. These error scores were correlated with their scores on the AOS measure of cognitive complexity. The resulting correlation was .44 (p<. 001), suggesting that the cognitively complex students indeed did make better use of the available cues. (Hendrick, 1990).

As part of a leadership influence study, described later, the students' own rankings of their effectiveness, as compared with that of the other class members, were compared with the composite group rankings and an error score for each student was determined. These error scores were correlated with the students' respective AOS scores. The resulting r was .39 (p<. 001), suggesting that the more abstract functioning students were somewhat more accurate in their self perceptions, as well as in their perceptions of their classmates. (Hendrick, 1990).

Cognitive Complexity and Group Task Performance

One of the most dramatic differences between abstract and concrete functioning persons that I have observed has been in two studies of group task behavior (Hendrick, 1979). In these two studies, the cognitive complexity levels of 100 cadets at the U. S. Air Force Academy and 100 experienced managers enrolled in a graduate management program at a large private university were assessed using the AOS. The five highest and five lowest scorers in each of 20 class sessions were assigned to *abstract* and *concrete* problem-solving groups, respectively. The group problem-solving task used was the Broken Squares exercise, described by Pfeiffer and Jones (1969) in their handbook. The exercise consists of five identically sized cardboard squares, consisting of three sections, thus forming a puzzle, with no two puzzles being alike. At the beginning of the task, each participant is given an envelope containing three puzzle pieces, each from a different square. The participants are instructed to complete all five squares as quickly as possible. They further are instructed that they are not to talk or gesture, can only pass pieces to the person to their right or left around the table, and must wait for pieces to be passed to them. The 20 concrete groups took almost twice as long as the 20 abstract groups to complete the task ($p<.001$). Compared to concrete groups, abstract group members interacted at a faster pace and demonstrated better cue utilization ($p<.001$). No differences were found between the undergraduate and graduate groups.

In addition to the systematic observations of group problem solving behavior, several other behavioral characteristics on which there were striking differences between the concrete and abstract groups were informally noted. These included (a) a tendency of abstract groups to demonstrate greater flexibility of set by a willingness to break up completed squares to try alternate combinations; (b) a tendency of abstract groups to test the rules to determine their real limits, whereas concrete groups did not; and (c) a tendency of concrete group members to focus primarily on their own individual task, whereas abstract team members tended also to focus on the work of the other team members.

Cognitive Complexity and Stratified Systems Theory

Stratified systems theory holds that hierarchical differentiation of jobs in organizations differ systematically in their cognitive complexity requirements and that managers perform most effectively and are happiest when their own cognitive complexity level matches that of their position (Stamp, 1981). Based on this hypothesis, I assessed the cognitive complexity levels of 22 hotel General and Resident Managers for a large hotel chain were assessed using both the AOS and a composite of four scales of the Guilford-Zimmerman Temperament Survey (Hendrick, 1986). All 22 managers were assessed by their superiors as being successful in their present

positions. The 22 managers each were evaluated by the Hotel Division's Vice President for Operations Support in terms of his potential for promotion to Area Manager – the next hierarchical level and one in which the manager exercises supervision indirectly over a group of hotels and their employees, thus making it more cognitively complex. Of the nine managers scoring as cognitively complex, seven were evaluated as having high potential for promotion to Area Manager. Of the thirteen managers scoring as cognitively concrete, only four were evaluated as having high potential for promotion (phi $=.57$, $p<.01$). These results appear to offer partial support for the stratified systems hypothesis.

Cognitive Complexity and Interpersonal Communication

Implicit in the cognitive complexity literature is a message concerning communicating with persons of differing levels of complexity which is consistent with my 40 years of experience as both an organizational consultant and teacher of practicing managers: Namely, express your message in terms of the *other* person's conceptual reality - to use a trite but true expression, from where he or she is "coming from". With concrete functioning persons, it is important to express ideas in specific, concrete terms. For example, if trying to persuade a concrete functioning manager to approve some organizational change intervention, it is important to describe the intervention in a clear, step-by-step fashion and, especially, the rationale for the intervention in terms of how it will improve the manager's "bottom line". In contrast, more abstract functioning managers are likely to respond positively to a description of the approach in terms of its underlying rationale and its less tangible benefits, such as improving employee job satisfaction and commitment, reducing stress, and being "the right thing to do" from a human consideration point of view.

Use of the Cognitive Complexity Dimension in Organizational Design

Organizational structures generally are acknowledged to have three major dimensions: *Complexity, formalization,* and *centralization* (Bedeian and Zammuto, 1991; Robbins, 1983; Stevenson, 1993). Like cognitive complexity, organizational complexity also has the two major components of *differentiation* and *integration*. Organizational differentiation refers to (a) the number of hierarchical levels or *vertical* differentiation, (b) the degree of departmentalization and specialization, or *horizontal* differentiation, and (c) the geographical dispersion of organizational units and employees, or *geographical differentiation*. Increasing any of these increases the organization's complexity. Organizational integration refers to the mechanisms that are used to coordinate and control the differentiated elements. These include such things as standard operating procedures, committees, task teams, information systems, integrating offices and vertical hierarchy (e.g., one boss supervises two or more subordinate units, thus serving as the integrator). Formalization refers to the extent to which operations rely on formalized procedures, standardized communications and detailed job descriptions, rather on employee expertise and decision-making. Centralization refers to the extent to which decisions are made by managers, higher up in the organization, versus being delegated to lower employee levels.

Among other factors, the optimal degrees of complexity, formalization and centralization to incorporate into an organization's design depend on the characteristics of the work force. In particular, the (a) degree of education and training or *professionalism,* and (b) the psychosocial characteristics of the employees (Robbins, 1983). With respect to the psychosocial characteristics, I have found one of the most useful factors to consider is that of cognitive complexity (Hendrick, 1981).

Given the characteristics, already described, it is not surprising that, in my 40 years of consulting,

I have found concrete functioning managers and employees alike to prefer the clear, unambiguous structure and formalization of bureaucratic organizational designs. In contrast, abstract functioning managers and employees usually prefer low formalization, decentralized decision-making; and are very comfortable in more complex or less structured, more ambiguous organizations (e.g., professionalized, matrix, and continuously changing or free-form designs).

In a study by me of a rapid prototyping, highly unstructured unit of a large telecommunications corporation, the manager was very concerned because three of his brightest software engineers were unhappy and wanted to transfer to a more traditional bureaucratic department. He was wondering if the problem was his organizational design or leadership style. I tested the cognitive complexity of the unit's engineers and found that all but the three that were unhappy were cognitively complex and very happy with the organization and it manager. The three cognitively concrete engineers were uncomfortable with the lack of structure and high ambiguity, so wanted to transfer to a more traditional, structured environment.

Cognitive Complexity and Leadership

Based on our coverage of cognitive complexity, it is not surprising that cognitively concrete leaders behave differently than cognitively complex ones. Let's take a look at the differences.

Cognitively Concrete (System 1) Functioning Leaders

In general, System 1 functioning managers tend to be authoritarian and task oriented. When not under stress, they also can sometimes appear to be people oriented, but will revert to low consideration behavior when they are under stress. Participative management does not fit with a hierarchically oriented, concrete, System 1, conception of reality. If forced to use participative management by their superiors, it has been my observation that they will let subordinates (and they do see them as subordinate) participate in decisions such as where to place the unit's coffee pot, but only minimally or not at all on important decisions – especially those in which the manager is ego involved. As characteristic of concrete functioning persons in general, they tend to see things in concrete, black-white ways; perceive persons as either for them or against them (i.e., there is no middle ground); and often communicate with subordinates and others perceived as having a lower status in a Parent to Child manner. They tend to have difficulty dealing with ambiguity and change, which can cause them considerable stress, and highly value structure and order. These characteristics are particularly noticeable in highly concrete functioning leaders, but also can be seen, at least to some extent, in those at intermediate levels of cognitive complexity who still are operating out of a System 1 conceptual orientation toward reality.

Cognitively Complex Functioning Leaders

In contrast to the above, cognitively complex (System 3 and 4) leaders tend to be very people oriented, empathic, and show high consideration behavior. Use of participative leadership comes easy for them. They tend *not* to see things simply as either-or, black-white; but rather as more complex, and in some cases, ambiguous. They handle both ambiguity and change more easily than their concrete functioning colleagues, and in fact, expect things to change. A major difference between System 3 and 4 functioning persons is that System 3 functioning leaders sometimes do not provide enough structure for their more concrete functioning subordinates, and are more dependent on their subordinates and peers liking them. System 4 leaders will provide structure as well as consideration, and can operate more

autonomously. In general, cognitively complex leaders are more creative than cognitively concrete ones (as one illustration of this, see the study of cognitive complexity and creativity by my colleagues and myself, described earlier).

In a leadership course at the USAF Academy, another instructor and I systematically observed cognitively concrete and abstract student behaviors during a series of class exercises throughout the course. Our observations generally were consistent with the findings noted above. Cognitively concrete students were more authoritarian, less open to opinions of others, more absolutist in their views, and took longer to change their opinions in light of new information. In contrast, the more abstract functioning students were more truly participative and empathic, open minded, relativistic in their views, and more flexible in their opinions. A few years later, I replicated the above study with 53 practicing managers and engineers in three of my graduate organizational behavior courses at the University of Southern California, and obtained similar results.

Cognitive Complexity and Leadership Behavior and Influence

117 male upper class undergraduate students, enrolled in eight sections of an advanced leadership class, were administered the Abstract Orientation Scale (AOS), a measure of cognitive complexity, noted earlier. During the course, the students participated in group discussions of case studies and reading materials and took part in various classroom exercises involving dimensions of leadership behavior. These discussions and exercises provided opportunity for each class section member to become aware of each other member, the resources he brought to the class section, and his method and pattern of participation. At the end of the course, each student ranked all of the students in his section, including himself, in terms of the degree of influence exercised in the classroom. These rankings were summed for each

student to determine his composite score. The product moment correlation between composite score and AOS score was .29 (p<. 01), suggesting that the more cognitively complex students tended to have somewhat greater influence on the group (Hendrick, 1990).

Observations by me and the other instructor of the cognitively concrete and cognitively abstract students' behaviors during the class exercises were generally consistent with previous findings for System 1 and Systems 3 & 4 functioning persons, cited earlier. Cognitively concrete persons were more authoritarian, less open to opinions of others, more absolutist in their views, and took longer to change their opinions in the light of new information. In contrast, the more abstract functioning students were more truly participative and empathic, open minded, relativistic in their views, and more flexible in their opinions.

A few years later, I replicated the above study with 53 practicing managers and engineers in three of my graduate organizational behavior courses at the University of Southern California and obtained similar results.

IMPLICATIONS FOR THE DESIGN OF INFORMATION AND TRAINING SYSTEMS

Based on the above, it should not be surprising to find that in designing management information systems, more cognitively concrete persons want their information presented in a clear, unambiguous, step-by-step approach, and are less concerned about the underlying rational, principles, or conceptual basis of the material. In contrast, cognitively complex persons prefer to have material presented in a manner that enables them to grasp the underlying concepts and principles (Bariff & Lusk, 1977). It also follows that the above also would likely hold true for the software design of information displays.

Similar to the findings for information systems, training systems designed for relatively concrete functioning persons should present material in a clear step-by-step manner. In contrast, cognitively complex persons will want material presented in a way that provides an understanding of the underlying concepts and general principles, or cognitive map, and are somewhat less concerned about a lock-step concrete presentation of the materials.

CONCLUSION

From the above historical review of cognitive complexity and its relation to conceptual systems and behavior, and my research contributions to our knowledge of cognitive complexity and performance, it should be apparent that the cognitive complexity dimension could be of considerable benefit to persons designing organizations and information and training systems. From my experience, I believe that many of the inconsistencies in human performance, often found between persons in the same or similar situations, can be explained by knowledge of the complexity levels of the individuals involved. Similarly, knowledge of the complexity levels of persons in a given environment can better enable us to design that work system to better enhance worker performance and satisfaction.

REFERENCES

Bariff, M. L., & Lusk, E. J. (1977). Cognitive and Personality Tests for the Design of Management Information Systems. *Management Science, 23*(4), 820–829. doi:10.1287/mnsc.23.8.820

Bedeian, A. G., & Zammuto, R. F. (1991). *Organizations: Theory and Design*. Chicago, IL: Dryden Press.

Blatt, M. (1971). The Effects of Classroom Discussion Upon Children's Moral Judgment . In Kohlberg, L., & Turiel, E. (Eds.), *Moral Research: The Cognitive-Developmental Approach*. New York: Holt, Rinehart and Winston.

Davis, K. (1966). Some Correlates of Responses to the "This I Believe Test" . In Harvey, O. J. (Ed.), *Experience, Structure, and Adaptability*. New York: Springer.

Harvey, O. J. (1966). Experience, Structure, Flexibility, and Creativity . In Harvey, O. J. (Ed.), *Experience, Structure, and Adaptability*. New York: Springer.

Harvey, O. J., Hunt, D. E., & Shroder, H. M. (1961). *Conceptual Systems and Personality Organization*. New York: Wiley.

Hendrick, H. W. (1979). Differences in Group Problem-Solving Behavior and Effectiveness as a Function of Abstractness. *The Journal of Applied Psychology, 64*(5), 518–525. doi:10.1037/0021-9010.64.5.518

Hendrick, H. W. (1981). Abstractness, Conceptual Systems, and the Functioning of Complex Organizations . In England, G., Negandhi, A., & Wilpert, B. (Eds.), *The Functioning of Complex Organizations* (pp. 25–50). Cambridge, MA: Oelgeschalger, Gunn & Hain.

Hendrick, H. W. (1986). Matching Individual and Job Complexity: Validation of Stratified Systems Theory. In *Proceedings of the Human Factors Society 30th Annual Meeting* (pp. 999-1001). Santa Monica, CA: Human Factors Society.

Hendrick, H. W. (1990). Perceptual Accuracy of Self and Others and Leadership Status as Functions of Cognitive Complexity . In Clark, K. E., & Clark, M. B. (Eds.), *Measures of leadership* (pp. 511–520). West Orange, NJ: Leadership Library of America.

Hunt, D. E. (1966). A Conceptual Systems Change Model and its Application to Education . In Harvey, O. J. (Ed.), *Experience, Structure and Adaptability*. New York: Springer.

King, L. A., & Hicks, J. A. (2007). What Ever Happened to "What Might Have Been" (section on "Happiness and Complexity: Two Sides of Maturity")? *The American Psychologist, 62*(7), 625–636. doi:10.1037/0003-066X.62.7.625

Pfeiffer, J. W., & Jones, J. E. (1969). *A Handbook of Structured Experiments for Human Relations Training (Vol. 1)*. Iowa City, IA: University Associates Press.

Piaget, J. (1948). *The Moral Judgment of the Child*. Glencoe, IL: Free Press.

Robbins, S. R. (1983). *Organization Theory: The Structure and Design of Organizations*. Englewood Cliffs, NJ: Prentice Hall.

Stamp, G. (1981). Levels and Types of Managerial Capability. *Journal of Management Studies, 18*(4), 277–297. doi:10.1111/j.1467-6486.1981.tb00103.x

Stevenson, W. B. (1993). Organizational Design . In Golembiewski, R. T. (Ed.), *Handbook of Organizational Behavior*. New York: Marcel Dekker.

Chapter 14

Individuation and Diversity:
The Need for Idiographic HCI

Sebastiano Bagnara
University of Sassari, Alghero, Italy & Deep Blue Research and Consulting, Italy

Simone Pozzi
University of Sassari, Alghero, Italy & Deep Blue Research and Consulting, Italy

ABSTRACT

Nowadays, our life is characterized by an increasing complexity and variety in the use of technology: highly idiosyncratic experiences in technology use have become rule rather than exceptions. Such "normal" variety has an impact on the field of Human-Computer Interaction by posing a new challenge, that of 'individuation', i.e. passing from research and design for the 'average user', to research and design for 'individuals'. We maintain that HCI is in the middle of such a transition and that it should actively develop proper means to address the complexity of idiosyncratic uses of technology. Such a transition will mark a shift from 'nomothetic' to 'idiographic' approaches.

INTRODUCTION

Some time ago, Alexander Luria posed the distinction between 'classical' and 'romantic' science in his autobiographic book "The Making of Mind: A Personal Account of Soviet Psychology" (Luria, 1979). According to him, the classical approach in psychology reduces phenomena to their elementary components and achieves understanding by means of abstract models, with the ultimate consequence of failing to appreciate the properties of the living whole. Romantic science should,

instead, be concerned with the understanding of "the way a thing or event relates to other things or events." The more perspectives we include in our analysis, the closer we get to a full understanding of the qualities, characteristics and rules of the subject under study.

Luria applied the romantic approach to two famous cases described in (Luria, 1968) and in (Luria, 1972). The former book "The Mind of a Mnemonist" is about a hypermnestic man, with a literally limitless memory. His memory capabilities were assessed and studied by Luria, who also renders a vivid portraiture of how the subject constructs the world, of the way he behaves. In the

DOI: 10.4018/978-1-60960-057-0.ch014

latter book, "The Man with a Shattered World", Luria describes a memory impairment, which affected the Soviet soldier Zasetsky after a bullet wound to the brain. The book is about Zasetsky's struggle to relearn even the simplest mental activities, to put together and make sense of the fragments of reality in his head. Again, the book is more about the personal drama of the Zasetsky, and his efforts to regain an orderly relationship with the world, rather than about the study of cognitive processes per se. In both books, Luria pursues the romantic science approach by seeking empathic identification with the patient's experience, by describing the case under study from both the external perspective of the psychologist and from the patients' perspective.

The challenge that Luria addresses in the two books is not new in psychology. It concerns the opposition between the nomothetic and the idiographic approaches. The nomothetic approach studies events and persons as examples of some general law. Its aim is to identify the general features of psychological processes, to describe the "average behaviour" across individuals, and to establish rules applicable to the largest possible number of persons. On the other hand, the idiographic approach studies events and persons as unique cases. Its aim is to understand specific instances of behaviour of one single individual.

In this contribution, we claim that the tension between the nomothetic and the idiographic approach is becoming increasingly central in HCI research, and that HCI should actively develop means to cope with the increased complexity and variety of our life, in which highly idiosyncratic uses of technology have become the norm rather than exceptions.

LONG TERM DYNAMICS IN TECNOLOGY USE AND HCI

Many changes are affecting the relationship between humans and technologies. We will briefly review some of them with the aim to outline some long-term dynamics and to show how research on diversity and individuation is increasingly becoming central in HCI.

The Dynamic Use of Technology in Work and Everyday Life

The use of technology could be considered as restricted to work and being relatively stable till the Eighties (technology was only used in certain specific workplaces in highly standardised situations), when the 'information revolution' has brought about some drastic changes, making technology widespread in many different contexts and situations of use (Malone, 2004). The relationship between the human and the machine could not be treated as a fixed one any longer. It started to depend on the social context, on the material used in the interaction, on the contents of it. Moreover, the relationship became increasingly shaped by the specific user and on her/his specific goals.

No one could have taken home her/his working tools from the Tayloristic factory, while working tools are now part of our houses and of our personal life. Nowadays, it is possible to work at home: technology is everywhere. At variance with the Tayloristic era, today's workplaces are very much similar to each other, and not very different from entertainment and leisure situations: all imply the use of computers. Those who lack computer skills are at risk of being cut off from work. However, the digital divide is not limited to work, but is also present in everyday life and affects people's social relations.

The supply side is no longer setting the pace of the market. The demand side is doing it. And demands are differentiated by nature and changing rapidly. In responding to demands, work has to cope with such variability. Work is aimed to deliver novelty and innovation, thus constantly requiring novel activities in uncertain conditions. It is made of often quite new activities to be performed in unfamiliar settings. In these days, when markets are characterised by uncertainty, work goals are never stable and well defined. The value of work depends by its originality. Communication and collaboration have become key means to cope with uncertainty.

Consequently, HCI no longer addresses work-related problems only, but it also studies leisure and entertainment (Bodker and Sundblad, 2008). People nowadays engage in interactions with the machines not only to work, but to fulfil personal goals and desires. HCI has to contribute to the creation of fulfilling experiences. HCI researches now go beyond 'human needs' and focus more on 'desires'. The Apple iPod does not solve any music-related problem. It instead leverages on the experience of listening to our favourite music. HCI is not anymore concerned with efficacy or efficiency (i.e. the 'functional characteristics' of a system) only, but should also address the subjective dimensions of user experience (like aesthetic pleasure, motivation, engagement, etc.) (Rullo, 2008).

Modern interfaces are better conceived as windows on complex activities, on social worlds. For instance, the interface of an online role playing game (*Multi User Dungeon/Domain - MUD*) is purely textual (see Figure 1), but still users are able to develop complex narrations, often with the joint participation of tens of players at the same time. Users use the interface to enter a different world.

The passage towards the changing nature of work and everyday experience is well captured by Himanen who describes the shift from "work as pain" to "work as self-realisation" in his book on the hacker's ethic (Himanen, 2001). Hackers engage in work for (i) enthusiasm and passion, (ii) wish to express their creativity and self-realisation, often in spontaneous aggregations, (iii) will to share their competencies and skills with a community of peers, in order to make the community advance and to gain a more prominent status in the community itself. Hackers work because they are driven uniquely by internal motivations, because they want to fulfil their expectations. They rate their success only by the metric of their own zeal.

Gaming is another case of such a general change of approach. Game interfaces are windows on complex set of activities. Users enter game world through the interface. The interface is the access door to an ongoing narration, which is nowadays often a collective one, both in work and in leisure.

Changes in the Market Structure: The Long Tail

A market driven by desires is by its very nature more dynamic and diverse than traditional markets. Chris Anderson (Anderson, 2006) described how this market can also follow different economic rules than traditional markets. In old-fashioned markets, 80% of the revenues are generated by 20% of the products, resulting in the 80-20 rule

Figure 1. The textual interface of a MUD

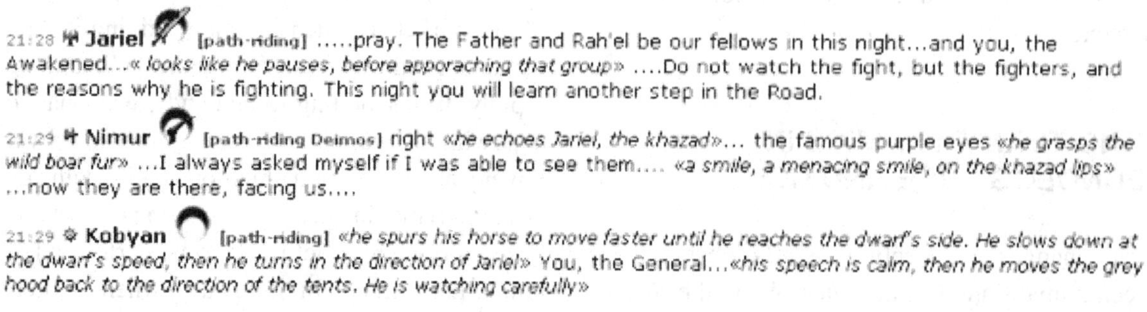

21:28 ⚕ **Jariel** 🏹 [path-riding] .....pray. The Father and Rah'el be our fellows in this night...and you, the Awakened...« *looks like he pauses, before apporaching that group*» ....Do not watch the fight, but the fighters, and the reasons why he is fighting. This night you will learn another step in the Road.

21:29 ⚕ **Nimur** 🎣 [path-riding Deimos] right «*he echoes Jariel, the khazad*»... the famous purple eyes «*he grasps the wild boar fur*» ...I always asked myself if I was able to see them.... «*a smile, a menacing smile, on the khazad lips*» ...now they are there, facing us....

21:29 ⚘ **Kobyan** 🌙 [path-riding] «*he spurs his horse to move faster until he reaches the dwarf's side. He slows down at the dwarf's speed, then he turns in the direction of Jariel*» You, the General...«*his speech is calm, then he moves the grey hood back to the direction of the tents. He is watching carefully*» (also known as the Pareto rule). The Pareto rule has been found valid for many formats (e.g., it applies to books, TV shows, videogames, etc.), but it does not remain true for digital markets.

Anderson surveyed different online stores and found that approximately 98% of the products sells at least one copy every three months. Anderson mentions the case of Rhapsody (an online music service that streams music for subscribed users): Compared to a traditional record store, Rhapsody makes available more than what would be a standard figure of 40 thousand songs, as its users can browse and select among 750 thousand songs. What is more noticeable, around 400 thousand songs sell at least one copy every month. For a traditional store, the cost of keeping an archive as large as that would exceed the potential income, while for online stores the additional cost is totally negligible. The long tail (depicted in Figure 2) is made of these songs which would not be available in a traditional store.

The key point from an economic perspective is that the aggregate income derived from the long tail can be as important as the income from the top-sellers. When Anderson wrote the initial article in 2004, Rhapsody was making 22% of its income from the long tail, Amazon 57% and Netflix 20%.

Getting back to our main line of reasoning, a 'long tail market' is more diverse than a traditional market. While in traditional markets, users group around few options, a long tail market makes it possible for them to pursue highly idiosyncratic preferences. And it is also economically viable for providers to satisfy their requests.

HCI is following this transition, from an applied science of ease of interaction to the science of supporting rewarding human-machine interaction experiences. However, while the design side of HCI seems to be well advanced in supporting idiosyncratic uses, the analysis side is still focused on the average user. HCI would need to bridge this gap and develop methods and techniques to identify, analyse and design for small niches of specific users, be they experts and trained professionals, or just groups of people with the same desires and preferences.

Figure 2. The long tail – image adapted from Anderson's newspaper article

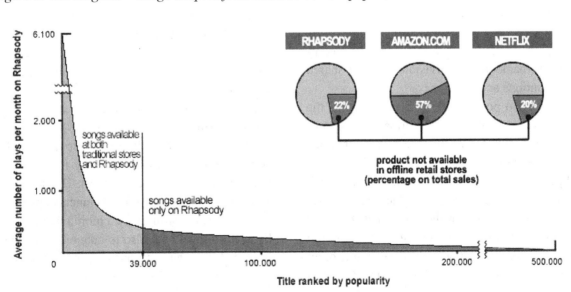

The End of Tool Stability

In a recent paper, Scott (Scott, 2009) questions the validity of "old-fashioned" usability methods in the current technological scenario. Scott focuses the discussion mostly on usability, and she reviews five factors that make traditional usability not effective. These five factors well summarise some of major changes in the technological scenario.

The key one of these factors is the pace of technological change. The life cycle of traditional software-based products and services could last years, even one decade for very complex pieces of software. It took huge investments for big firms to design a new piece of software, to develop and implement it, to market it. So long periods of time had to pass from one major release to the following one. Nowadays, the life cycle has been shortened dramatically. The design and development phases can now be iterative, thus making the deployment phase almost immediate. Once the product has been developed, it can be marketed immediately, then revised (i.e. re-enter into the design phase) and deployed again as a matter of weeks. Some web applications are refined continuously in their first days of life and producers keep delivering new releases every month. New features may be introduced incrementally, without having to re-purpose the whole software, on the basis of users' live feedback. Scott also mentions how this pace is even faster in the open source community, thanks to the 'invisible hand' of shared contributions and revisions.

A second point made by Scott concerns the increasing complexity of Information Communication Technologies (ICT). Software products used to be stand-alone applications, whose quality of performance was entirely based on "internal" factors. Current software products are instead networked systems, in the sense that they rely on an array of other services to function in the proper manner. Scott presents the example of an application for the Apple iPhone named "Urban Spoon". It is a restaurant recommendation sys-

tem that tracks the user's location and provides recommendations based on proximity and on users' ratings. For this application to work at least five different software components need to be in place and interact together: the web store interface for purchasing and downloading the application, the application interface on the iPhone, the web interface to rate restaurants, the restaurant database, the resolution of the Global Positioning System (GPS) coverage in a given area. The user experience with this application is shaped by all these components. For instance, if the restaurant database is not frequently updated by an active user community, or if it provides only limited choices in certain areas, the overall quality of interaction gets diminished. On the contrary, the database quality may be perfect, but that would irrelevant if the GPS tracking system could not resolve the location in less than a mile. Most web applications are nowadays 'mash-ups', a name used for applications created by merging one kind of data with another. The heightened complexity of such applications makes it difficult to define their boundaries, to trace where they start and where they finish. It also contributes to dramatically increase their pace of change: whenever any of the main components gets upgraded or refined, the interaction experience changes.

A third point relates to the stability of contexts of use. As computing devices get more pervasive and get to move around with their users, we may expect users to interact with them in markedly different contexts. As Scott says "they live in a variety of different environments, scenarios, and contexts of the users' choosing […] Most contexts of use today, however, live in the 'long tail'. The context of use varies significantly from user to user, or day to day" (Scott, 2009). The same device may be used in different manners depending on the context, for instance a mobile phone may be used to speak, but also to take notes, to shed light, to text friends, to track your position, etc. All these uses entail different modalities of interaction, either context-dependent or personalised ones, which make of the application a different one each time it gets used in a different manner.

The last characteristic mentioned by Scott is the ever-expanding base of users and the active role they are playing in reshaping the ICT tools. Active repurposing of software applications used to be carried out only by a small community of hackers, while it is now becoming feasible for a larger and larger user community. Ten or twenty years ago, publishing information (either digitally or on paper) required a certain level of expertise, not to mention the prohibitive costs of dedicated machinery and software. Today, easily available, cheap online tools allow users with limited computer literacy to publish, share, modify, and enrich contents. At the same time, the Internet is making all this content available to everyone. Everyone can read the contents we post, but they can also creatively re-use it, by cut and paste, by linking to it, by enriching it with personal comments or tags. This phenomenon is known as 'user-generated content' (UGC), that is the capability of users to easily produce data and publish them on the web. The extent of such a shift cannot be downplayed.

This week approximately 600.000 blogs will be opened, adding up to the more than 70 millions listed by Technorati in 2007. It is most likely that even these figures will be far from reality, since blog number doubled in 2007. In 1996, the web was composed on around 250 thousand sites, nearly all of which could be defined as 'online publications', i.e. they were similar to read-only archives of information. Nearly 45 millions of users used to browse and search through those sites. Nowadays, web sites are close to 100 millions and users have topped one billion.

What is more important, one third of published contents is enriched or created by users. It is not only about publishing online your own photos, it is also about the decentralisation of software development. The distinction among producers, publishers, distributors and consumers is getting blurred, both as far as roles are concerned and in terms of time (all phases dissolve in a unique

phase). Users are all becoming content producers, publishers and developers as much as they are consumers. This does not only concern blogs or personal sites, it can also affect professional domains like journalism. For instance, citizen journalism can now count hundreds of web sites, while other services let users collaboratively set the agenda (digg.com is one good example). The web used to deliver a type of service similar to the power grid, where users simply have to connect to the grid with their appliances to enjoy the service, but it has now become more similar to the telephone network, whose value comes from the number of users aggregated around it.

Again, this has an impact on the pace of technological change, as user-driven innovation goes by quicker than the traditional industrial process. It also increases variability, as each individual is now able to repurpose the tool for her/his own idiosyncratic use, for a unique set of preferred interaction modalities.

HCI AS A SCIENCE OF DIVERSITY: THE NEED FOR PERSONALISED TECHNOLOGIES

The variety of users and contexts of use is unlikely to be understood by traditional HCI methods, which mostly rely on the similarity between users and on highly shared usage patterns. HCI should instead shift its focus from designing for the intermediate user (i.e. the average user) to designing for diversity (i.e. designing for individuals).

A way by which HCI is currently addressing diversity is that of personalization. Personalization supports the diversity of users by means of malleable tools, that can shaped as preferred by each user, for instance by changing the interface layout, activating special features, providing automation for frequently performed actions. Some computer applications do not even require the user intervention to adapt, as they self-modify themselves by tracking the user's frequent behaviours.

For instance, Microsoft Office cascade menus automatically "shorten" themselves, displaying only those options that have been frequently chosen by the user.

The key concept to understand personalization is that of 'preferred interaction modalities'. The interaction with a tool is shaped both by its physical characteristics and also by the way we interact with it. The same tool can be used to achieve two markedly different purposes if the user employs two different set of interaction modalities (e.g. a book can be read, or thrown against someone, or used to hold papers in place, etc.). Interaction modalities tell the user how to use that specific tool, they represent 'knowledge in use', knowing 'how to do something with that tool'.

As discussed in the previous section, different interaction modalities are elicited depending on both the preferences of each user and the context of use. For instance, a mobile phone can be used on the move (e.g. while driving a car, on a plane, walking, cycling, etc.), in different places (e.g. in a cinema, at a conference, outside in direct sunlight, in a restaurant, in a meeting, etc.), by a different user. Each of these situations is likely to rely on a different set of interaction modalities, as users interact with the phone differently when trying to send a text message, while placing a phone call, shedding light in a dark room, or writing a personal note or reminder.

In summary, interaction modalities may change depending on different users, on situations of use, on more long-term dynamics like changes of users' needs, desires, preferences, physical characteristics (ageing and disability being the most notable ones). Personalised technologies should address the variability of interaction modalities by ensuring that each user can rely on her/his favourite set in each different situation, or that users can customise the tool to best suit personal preferences.

A specific HCI research field on personalization relates to 'multimodal interaction'. This field covers research on input methods different than those based on keyboard and mouse, the application of which spans from mass market product to assistive devices. To name but the principal research areas, interfaces based on speech recognition, pointing, gaze direction or gesture recognition can be exploited to ease human-computer interaction for people with reduced dexterity or motor impairments, but can also be implemented to support hands-free tasks, for instance to reduce risk of infections in pre-operatory debriefs for surgeons, during operations to cut operation time, to have a military aircraft pilot fly the aircraft while gaze-pointing at a target. Another particular case is that of Brain-Computer Interfaces, where the user may self-regulate brain activity (detected by the EEG - electroencephalogram - electrical activity of the brain) in order to move a cursor on the computer screen.

Under the same category, we may also mention 'sonification', i.e. the use of non-speech audio to convey information. 'Sonification' is typically used in situations where the user's eyes are busy elsewhere, such as in a laboratory or production line; where extracting temporal information is important; or where the data presentation requirements exceed the bandwidth of visual means" (Walker and Kramer, 2006). Successful applications can be found in the healthcare domain (for instance the hearth rate sound during surgery), or to convey additional information in Geographic Information Systems (e.g. abrupt changes in height or depth). The same technique is also exploited in assistive devices, typically for visually impaired users, for instance to support the exploration and construction of graphs and diagrams, or the interaction with scroll bars and other navigation items.

The last example we would like to briefly mention for multimodal interaction is that of gesture-based interaction. On the one hand, gesture research is a natural province of research on technology accessibility, because, compared to point and touch interfaces, gesture-based interfaces are easier to use by people with diminished visual acuity. On the other hand, the iPhone interaction modality (based on gestures, rather than on touch) has brought gesture-based interfaces to the mass public.

It is not by a fortuitous case that we observe concurrent research efforts on multimodal interfaces for specific uses (e.g. doctors and pilots) and for assistive technologies. The need is the same: to design personalised technologies that take into account the diversity of different users/activities.

To summarise the line of argument in few words: each user has some preferred ways of interacting with her/his computer, which may change driven by needs, desires or everyday contingencies. Personalization addresses such differences and changes.

IDIOGRAPHIC RESEARCH

The need for personalised technologies bears a deep impact on the HCI field. Personalization means that all users should be treated as equally important, that the idiosyncratic use of one specific user should be considered as relevant as the standard use of the mass of "average users". Outliers are as important as the users 'in the middle of the distribution'. This stands true from the economic point of view, as outliers form the long tail and may be a remarkable source of revenue. Furthermore, outliers also affect HCI methodological aspects. To understand specific users, we need methods that delve into the complexities and intricacies of single users' interactions with the system, into the minute details that differentiate one user from the others.

A similar issue is not new. As briefly mentioned in the introduction, psychology has been dealing for long with the opposition between the nomothetic approach and the idiographic approach. Nomothetic approaches are concerned with the identification of general and universal mechanisms of human behaviour. The (often implicit) assumption is that common universal mechanisms should be identified by studying the average person,

while within group variability is treated either as error or as differences in ability/skill/experience (Karwowski and Cuevas 2003 in Hancock et al., 2009). On the other hand, idiographic approaches study each individual as a unique personality, and refuses the idea that individual differences be "an annoyance rather than a challenge to the experimenter. His goal is to control behaviour, and variation within treatments is proof that he has not succeeded. Individual variation is cast into that outer darkness known as 'error variance'" (Cronbach, 1957).

Idiographic research gathers instead data on single individuals, not considering them necessarily as a representative part of any group, sample or population. Idiographic studies are the typical province of medicine. Similar to the two Luria's books mentioned in the introduction, other famous examples include the studies of Oliver Sacks (Sacks, 1970) and Antonio Damasio (Damasio, 1995). These studies share the idea that brain disorders (and damages) may be studied as revealing moments of the way the brain works.

In a similar manner, idiographic HCI should study individuals because knowledge gained through these researches can be revealing for the design of new technologies and applications. The design of new technologies should not only take advantage of regularities in the users' general characteristics, but should also target person-specific interactions. The methodological challenge is a revolutionary one and is going to impact on all the aspects of HCI as a discipline.

First of all, a different unit of analysis would be needed to perform 'individualised user studies'. Individual characteristics would be better understood by enlarging the scope to include aspects traditionally outside of "mainstream cognitive" HCI, like for instance motivation, personality, emotions, socio-cultural aspects (Szalma, 2009). These factors have profound effects on individual performance and need to be considered when studying human-computer interaction. For instance, Baldwin (Baldwin, 2009) demonstrates how individual characteristics (such as age, or sense of direction) should be considered when designing in-vehicle navigation systems. Drury and colleagues (Drury et al., 2009) review different measures that can be applied to differentiate among individual performances in inspection tasks. Research on individuals questions our very conception of the user, so the unit of analysis should also be extended in time (and not only in scope). Individuals exhibit vast changes over a lifetime, due to aging and intervening disabilities, but also due to extensive training, or to the development and practice of specialised competencies. There is also large variation in shorter intervals of time, like for in-session fatigue or in particular contextual conditions. Individuality concerns not just inter-individual differences, but just as much intra-individual differences.

New methods and techniques should also be developed to gather data and to represent results of HCI studies. For instance, current user experience or usability methods have a very limited access to users, typically in a laboratory setting for a very short period, while it is indeed the case that personalised technologies usability (or user experience) unfolds and change over a longer time period, often affected by spontaneous users' adaptations, or by the variability of contexts in which the user moves. Individualised user research would need to gather data on technology use over longer periods and across different contexts, ideally understanding how human-computer interaction changes with continuous use. Some HCI practitioners have, for instance, turned personal mobile devices into data gathering devices (with the user's consent) to support studies with the experience sampling method, which aims to examine user experience where it occurs, 'in situ'. Users are thus always connected to the researcher, feeding data on a variety of experiences, in different contexts and over a long time frame (Lew, 2009).

Once extensive user data have been gathered, HCI would still be confronted with the issue of how to analyse them. At the present moment,

HCI still lacks structured methods that can help make sense of such complex data sets, inherently dynamic, noisy and multi-level. Specific events are currently analysed case by case, but HCI has no disciplined method of analysing larger sets of 'individualised data'. Statistical analyses to plot variability and distribution are well suited for a nomothetic approach, while there is still no comparable method for idiographic research. This is also a major concern for the presentation of results. As well put by Hancock: "Quite simply, how does one illustrate individual differences that are truly unique to each individual? This means, how does one plot and communicate the findings from studies of true individuation?" (Hancock et al., 2009).

In the same work just cited, Hancock suggests that inspiration should be sought in visual and media arts, because of their mastery in telling individual stories. Regardless of the form of analysis and results presentation adopted, the major point discussed here refers to how knowledge produced by idiographic research can be encoded and transmitted. Without a shared consensus on such a matter, it is really unlikely for idiographic research to progress beyond "impressionistic research", with too many methods of analysis and presentation formats.

The last point we would like to touch relates to the design part of HCI, that is how to intervene after analysis. In traditional HCI, regularities in users' characteristics have been the basis to develop and design new technologies. The individuation approach should instead understand how to gain useful knowledge for design out of person-specific interactions. This should take HCI a step even further than ethnographic approaches.

Ethnography addresses the need for user studies not to limit themselves to user requirement elicitation, but to understand also the rich fabric of complex, socially-organized settings. Some HCI authors have focused on the issue of the 'implications for design' to question the naïve assumption that we can move from user studies to design in a straightforward manner (Dourish, 2006). This passage is always a critical one, where a "translation" of the knowledge produced in the data gathering phase is required to make it of some use for the following design phase. The same 'thick data' should be gathered on individuals and the same translation issue should be addressed. Some HCI fields (e.g. assistive technologies, applications for highly specialised fields, etc.) have been addressing such an issue for nearly twenty years now, so it may be worthwhile moving our attention to their methods and techniques for this challenge.

The opposition between nomothetic and idiographic approaches is currently reflected in a variety of domains and HCI applications. The radically different approaches brought forward by Google and Facebook is probably the most noticeable case that can be described here. Google provides search results by aggregating the browsing behaviour of thousands of anonymous users, in order to identify high relevance web sites and to provide browsing recommendations. In such an approach, specific individual users are not important at all, what mainly matters is the central part of the curve, where the majority of users is clustered. In other words, Google is providing recommendations on the basis of the "average user" behaviour. If you search for a restaurant recommendation, you get as a result what the average user thinks, and not what a specific individual thinks.

Facebook is instead based on a smaller network of users (even though it has currently more than 200 millions users, approximately one fifth of the internet users) and is currently trying to develop individualised recommendations. For instance, Facebook has recently introduced two software tools (named Connect and Open Stream) that let users access their Facebook profile even when navigating on other web sites. The practical consequence is that when an user accesses a restaurant recommendation site, the web site gets to know her/his Facebook contacts and delivers recommendations primarily based on those specific users' preferences. It is as if the Facebook user is navigating the Facebook web (populated by individuals, i.e. her/his friends), instead of accessing the aggregated data of many anonymous users.

In conclusion, if you are primarily concerned with the average user, no one can beat the amount of data stored by Google, but if you had rather find out what specific individuals think, then the Facebook web is the place to be. The individuation trend does not only concern the academic HCI field, but it also bears a relevance for big players, such as Google (who flourished at the end of the Nineties-beginning of Two Thousand) and Facebook (whose success became manifest in the last three years).

CONCLUSION: INDIVIDUAL-CENTRED HCI

The study of individuals implies that users be considered in their wholeness and uniqueness, and not only for some specific characteristics (e.g. physical, or cognitive, or practice-based, etc.). This means including human values in HCI leading principles. Technologies are not neutral, they have an impact on social and cultural values. Such an impact is probably the only sensible criterion to steer design. This is similar to the shift from a technology-driven approach to a user-centred one, provided that we complement the old-fashioned criteria (e.g. efficacy, efficiency, usefulness) with social ones. HCI should be able to analyse the multi-faceted issues brought by technological innovation, be those of a cultural, social, political, or even ethical nature. HCI has to move further, from a technology-driven approach, and a user-centred approach, towards individual-centred approach.

To address this change, Harper et al. (Harper et al., 2008) suggested that HCI should focus on two immediate challenges. Firstly, user-centred design should explicitly include the analysis of social issues in the development process, in order to design individual-centred innovation. Secondly, HCI should develop methods and techniques to foster dialogue with the humanities. Design trade-offs are likely to increasingly concern socio-cultural aspects, with their large variation across different contexts, communities, and individuals. The concept of privacy means something different in our workplace or in our family, in a small town or in big cities.

HCI should no longer study the interaction between technology and an undifferentiated user, that has to be defined as broadly as possible to fit anybody, rather it needs tools to address each user's needs and diversities. Even very peculiar ones. To have a truly 'individual-centred' design approach, the characteristics of individuals certainly deserve the same level of detailed attention that HCI has devoted to displays and devices.

A potential pitfall for the individuation trend is that of designing overly specific solutions. While it is true that every user is different, it is not feasible to have a different design solution for each one. For this reason, HCI should work on disciplined ways of overcoming the gap between individual users and design. There is a need to identify disciplined ways of considering the individual's characteristics, using them as design leverages, and at the same time being able to separate unnecessary peculiarities. HCI should go beyond user-friendly tool customisation as the preferred solution to the problem of individual differences to fully address and take care of the complexities of individual interactions.

REFERENCES

Anderson, C. (2006). *The long tail: why the future of business is selling less of more*. New York: Hyperion.

Baldwin, C. L. (2009). Individual differences in navigational strategy: implications for display design. *Theoretical Issues in Ergonomics Science, 10*(5), 443–458. doi:10.1080/14639220903106379

Bodker, S., & Sundblad, Y. (2008). Usability and interaction design-new challenges for the Scandinavian tradition. *Behaviour & Information Technology, 27*(4), 293–300. doi:10.1080/01449290701760682

Cronbach, L. J. (1957). The two disciplines of scientific psychology. *The American Psychologist, 12*(11), 671–684. doi:10.1037/h0043943

Damasio, A. R. (1995). *Descartes' error: emotion, reason, and the human brain*. New York: Harper Collins.

Dourish, P. (2006). *Implications for Design. CHI: Conference on Human Factors in Computing Systems*. Montréal, Québec, Canada.

Drury, C. G., Holness, K., Ghylin, K. M., & Green, B. D. (2009). Using individual differences to build a common core dataset for aviation security studies. *Theoretical Issues in Ergonomics Science, 10*(5), 459–479. doi:10.1080/14639220802609887

Hancock, P. A., Hancock, G. M., & Warm, J. S. (2009). Individuation: the $N = 1$ revolution. *Theoretical Issues in Ergonomics Science, 10*(5), 481–488. doi:10.1080/14639220903106387

Harper, R., Rodden, T., Rogers, Y., & Sellen, A. (Eds.). (2008). *Being Human: Human-Computer Interaction in the year 2020*. Cambridge, UK: Microsoft Research Ltd.

Himanen, P. (2001). *The Hacker Ethic and the Spirit of the Information Age*. New York: Random House.

Lew, G. S. (2009). What Do Users Really Do? Experience Sampling in the 21st Century. *HCI International 2009*. San Diego, USA.

Luria, A. R. (1968). *The mind of a mnemonist; a little book about a vast memory*. New York: Basic Books.

Luria, A. R. (1972). *The man with a shattered world; the history of a brain wound*. New York: Basic Books.

Luria, A. R. (1979). *The Making of Mind*. Cambridge, MA: Harvard University Press.

Malone, T. W. (2004). *The Future of Work: How the New Order of Business Will Shape Your Organization, Your Management Style, and Your Life*. Cambridge, MA: Harvard Business School Press.

Rullo, A. (2008). The soft qualities of interaction. *ACM Transactions on Computer-Human Interaction, 15*(4), 17. doi:10.1145/1460355.1460359

Sacks, O. (1970). *The Man Who Mistook His Wife For A Hat: And Other Clinical Tales*. New York: Touchstone.

Scott, K. M. (2009). Is Usability Obsolete? *Interaction, 16*(3), 6–11. doi:10.1145/1516016.1516018

Szalma, J. L. (2009). Individual differences in human-technology interaction: incorporating variation in human characteristics into human factors and ergonomics research and design. *Theoretical Issues in Ergonomics Science, 10*(5), 381–397. doi:10.1080/14639220902893613

Walker, B. N., & Kramer, G. (2006). Sonification . In Karwowski, W. (Ed.), *International Encyclopedia of Ergonomics and Human Factors*. Boca Raton, FL: Taylor & Francis. doi:10.1201/9780849375477.ch195

Chapter 15
Usable Privacy–Enhancing Identity Management:
Challenges and Approaches

Simone Fischer-Hübner
Karlstad University, Sweden

John Sören Pettersson
Karlstad University, Sweden

ABSTRACT

A critical success factor for Privacy-Enhancing Technologies (PETs), and for Privacy-Enhancing Identity Management in particular, will be user-friendly and intelligible user interfaces that are legally compliant and convey trust. Such user interfaces have to meet challenges such as the user-friendly representation of complex PET concepts (such as "pseudonyms", "unlinkabilty" or "anonymous credentials") that are unfamiliar to many users, the provision of security, the enforcement of legal privacy principles, such as informed consent or transparency, as well as the mediation of reliable trust to the end users. In this paper, we will discuss such challenges for usable privacy-enhancing identity management and will provide some HCI guidelines for addressing those challenges.

INTRODUCTION

In today's network society, users have lost effective control over their personal spheres. When communicating via the Internet, users are leaving many personal data traces at various sites, which can be easily compiled to extensive personal profiles. These processes of personal data collection and processing are often not transparent for the individuals concerned. It is however critical to our society and to democracy to retain and maintain the individual's autonomy and thus to protect privacy and particularly the individual's right to informational self-determination. Powerful tools for technically enforcing user control and informational self-determination as well as the privacy principle of data minimisation can be provided by privacy-enhancing Identity Management systems, as those which have been developed within the EU FP6 integrated project PRIME ("Privacy and Identity Management for Europe"[1]) and its follow-up EU FP7 integrated project PrimeLife ("Privacy and Identity Management for Life"[2]).

DOI: 10.4018/978-1-60960-057-0.ch015

Identity Management (IDM) can be defined to subsume all functionality that supports the use of multiple identities, by the identity owners (user-side IDM) and by those parties with whom the owners interact (services-side IDM). According to Pfitzmann and Hansen (2008), identity management means managing various partial identities (i.e. set of attributes, usually denoted by pseudonyms) of a person, i.e. the administration of identity attributes including the development and choice of the partial identity and pseudonym to be (re-)used in a specific context or role. Privacy-enhancing IDM is also sufficiently preserving unlinkability (as seen by an attacker) between the partial identities of an individual person required by the applications.

With privacy-enhancing identity management such as with PRIME, all interactions are a priori anonymous, and individuals can choose to act under different pseudonyms with respect to communication partners or activities, and furthermore have control over whether or not interactions and pseudonyms can be linked with each other or not. Moreover, PRIME provides tools that help individuals to define who has the right to do what under which conditions with their personal data, as well as tools providing transparency about who has received what personal data related to them and possibilities to trace personal data being passed on.

Privacy-enhancing identity management implies that users can make informed choices about the releases of personal data, the selections of credentials for proving personal properties, and about their privacy and trust policy settings. For enabling users to make well-informed decisions, user interfaces (UIs) are needed that inform them about the trustworthiness and the privacy policies of their communication partners as well as the implications of personal data releases. These user interfaces should be informative while not being perceived as intrusive, intuitive, legally compliant and trustworthy. Privacy-enhancing identity

management technologies will only be successful if they are accepted and applied by the end users.

Therefore, several challenges have to be addressed regarding the user interfaces such as how to represent complex Privacy-Enhancing Technology (PET) concepts that are unfamiliar to most users in a user-friendly way, how to provide security against phishing and spoofing attacks, how to enforce legal privacy principles and how to mediate reliable trust.

In this chapter, we will discuss these challenges and problems for meeting them in more detail. Then, we will propose a list of recommendations for designers of privacy and identity management systems to address these challenges. These recommendations also include concrete suggestions of possible approaches to meet those challenges that we have elaborated within the PRIME and PrimeLife projects or that have been suggested by others.

RELATED WORK

This chapter is based on results from the HCI activities of the PRIME and PrimeLife projects. Earlier results from the HCI work within the PRIME project have also been reported, e.g. in (Fischer-Hübner et al. 2008) and (Pettersson 2008). However, this paper contains substantial updates of PRIME project results and includes also some first results from the PrimeLife project's HCI work.

There has been some previous related work discussing HCI challenges and HCI Guidance for secure system (e.g., Herzog 2007, Johnston et al. 2004, Yee 2002, Garfinkel 2005) and for privacy-enhancing technologies (e.g., Patrick et al. 2003, Patrick and Kenny 2003). Also very recently Dhamija and Dusseault discuss flaws of identity management posing HCI and security challenges and provide some recommendations how to address them (Dhamija and Dusseault 2008). However, in contrast to our work presented in this chapter, none of those related publications has had a specific focus on HCI of privacy-enhancing identity management. Consequently, as our work addresses HCI challenges and recommendations specific for privacy-enhancing identity management, it partly overlaps with the previous work mentioned above, but also covers many other aspects.

CHALLENGES

Privacy-enhancing identity management systems will only be successful if they are accepted and will be applied by the end users, which requires the development of user interfaces that are user-friendly, intelligible and which mediate trust. Another important task of the user interface developers is to map legal privacy principles, mainly postulated by the EU Data Protection Directive 95/46/EC (EU Directive 1995) and the EU E-Communications Privacy Directive 2002/58/EC (EU Directive 2002), into HCI requirements and subsequently into user interface design solutions, so that the user interfaces are actively enforcing privacy legislation. For achieving these goals, several challenges need to be met, in particular the ones that we discuss in the following subsequent sections.

User-Friendly Representation of Complex PET Concepts

Privacy-enhancing Identity Management and other privacy-enhancing technologies are based on technical concepts such as pseudonyms, unlinkability, anonymous credentials as well as privacy policy negotiation and management that are unfamiliar to many end users and often do not fit to their mental pictures of what is technically feasible. Often no direct or obvious real-world analogies exist for these concepts.

Our HCI work in PRIME and PrimeLife revealed for instance the difficulty for users to understand the concept of anonymous credentials. Traditional credentials require that all attributes are disclosed together if the holder wants to prove certain properties and have the drawback that different uses of the same certificate can be linked to each other. In contrast to traditional credentials, anonymous credentials as proposed by Camenisch and Lysyanskaya (2001) make it possible for a user to prove to a web site that she has a certificate with specific properties, without actually revealing the certificate itself or any extra information. For example, if a user named Jane has an anonymous passport credential from her state, she can prove that she is older than 18 in case that she wants to shop a video online which is only permitted for adults. Anonymous credentials also have the property that different shows of a credential cannot be linked with each other. If for instance Jane later wants to purchase another video for adults online at the same video shop, she can again prove that she is over 18 with her anonymous credential without that the video shop is able to recognise that the two proofs are based on the same credential. This means that the two purchases by Jane cannot be linked as purchases done by the same person. Hence, the metaphor of real-world credentials does not fit for anonymous credentials.

In mockup-based user tests conducted within PRIME, we have noticed that people easily mistake that with proofs of "age > 18" based on anonymous credentials as much data as contained in the source credential is revealed (and not only the fact that the holder is over 18). Short pre-test information on anonymous credentials does not seem to influence this perception. For instance, in a post-test interview, one participant mentioned explicitly that his personal number found in his passport will be sent to the service provider, even though the window asking for data release stated the request as: *Proof of "age > 18" (built on "Swedish Passport")*. In the PrimeLife project, first usability tests were performed for mockups based on the paradigm of derived virtual cards containing only a selection of attributes or characteristics of attributes to illustrate the fact that only those data of the virtual card are revealed. However, first pilot usability tests for these mockups showed as well that most users did not understand the data minimisation property of anonymous credentials.

Other examples of complex PET concepts are privacy policy management and negotiation, which are part of privacy-enhanced identity management systems. In PRIME, the user's release policy (or her so-called "privacy preferences") defines the user's preferences regarding the release/disclosure of her personal data. At the services side, a so-called data handling policy (or simply "privacy policy") specifies how and what data are processed by the service in question. If personal data are requested from a user by a service provider, the PRIME user-side system can compare ("match") the services side's privacy policy with the user's release policy (privacy preferences) and warn the user in case of a mis-match. For ordinary users defining and adapting a privacy-friendly data release policies is a complex and error-prone task which usually requires some expertise about basic legal privacy concepts and principles. In the non-electronic world no equivalent task exists, which means that ordinary users have no experiences with how to define and manage their release polices. Without assistance, most users would not define and use release policies at all or could accidentally define or choose release policies, which are not as privacy-friendly as the users would like them to be.

Informational self-determination means that users are able to decide how their personal data are used. This should not necessarily have to involve determining how technicalities such as anonymous credential proofs or pseudonymisation are carried out. From a usability perspective such technicalities should on the contrary rather be invisible to the users. However, when it comes to understanding the risk of being identified across different interactions with one or several service providers, some sort of notion about digital identity must be understood by the user.

Mapping Legal Principles

Another important task of the user interfaces is to enforce and promote legal principles such as informed consent or transparency, so that the user interfaces are not only privacy-compliant, but also enhance the users' understanding, awareness, and control.

For enforcing the privacy principle of 'transparency' as a prerequisite of user control, a special challenge is to design user interfaces that are informative while user-friendly: Users must be well informed about the consequences when releasing data, and consequently there are legal requirements for providing information to the users (e.g. Art. 10, 11 EU Directive 95/46/EC) that need to be met by the user interfaces. However, users should not be confronted with excessive or badly structured information – such information is usually perceived as bothersome and ignored by the users. Providing transparency also requires that PET concepts are made understandable. Hence, the challenges to represent complex PET concepts in an understandable way and of providing security are also a part of the challenge to map legal privacy principles to UI solutions.

A special challenge is also the development of UI constructs for obtaining really informed and unambiguous user consent for the disclosure of personal data, which is usually often a prerequisite for the lawful data processing (see for instance Art. 7.a EU Directive 95/46/C or Art. 9 EU Directive 2002/58/EC). Ordinary click-through dialog windows, which are often used also in combination with long legal statements, may cause users to click the "I Accept" button too easily if the preference settings have filled in all the requested data for them. Putting up "Are you really sure?" boxes does not resolve the problem as people may often click the "I Accept" or "OK" button even more automatically if they have to go through an extra dialogue box every time (Raskin 2000). Also Dhamija et al. conclude that when confronted with dialog boxes such as for end-user license agreements, users tend to quickly skim the text and efficiently swat away the dialog boxes without having read or understood what they consented to (Dhamija and Dusseault 2008).

In the PISA project ("Privacy Incorporated Software Agent", an EU FP5 project), it was studied how privacy principles derived from the EU Data Protection Directive 95/46/EC can be translated into HCI requirements and what are possible design solutions to meet those requirements (Patrick et al. 2003). The derived HCI requirements were grouped into the four categories of comprehension (to understand, or know), consciousness (be aware or informed), control (to manipulate, or be empowered) and consent (to agree). In the PRIME project, we have extended these privacy principles and HCI requirements from the PISA project with a special focus on improved HCI constructs for enhancing transparency and for obtaining informed consent (see also Fischer-Hübner et al. 2008 and below).

Mapping Social Requirements

While legal concepts are often based on generally held notions of what fair actions include and do not include, there are aspects of PETs that are outside legal requirements and also outside usability requirements strictly defined. Such aspects include for instance adoption and trust.

"Trust is important because if a person is to use a system to its full potential, be it an e-commerce site or a computer program, it is essential for her to trust the system" (Johnston et al. 2004). Usability tests of early PRIME prototypes have shown that there are problems to make people trust the claims about the privacy enhancing features of the systems (see Fischer-Hübner and Pettersson 2004, Andersson et al. 2005). Although test users were first introduced into the aims and scope of privacy-enhancing identity management, the tests revealed that many of the test users did not trust the claim that the tested system would really protect their data and their privacy. Some participants voiced doubts over the whole idea of attempting to stay private on the Net. "Internet is insecure anyway" because people must get information even if it is not traceable by the identity management application, explained one test participant in a post-test interview. Another test subject stated: "It did not agree with my mental picture that I could buy a book anonymously". Another factor contributing to the lack of trust that was revealed by our usability tests was that test subjects generally had difficulties to mentally differentiate between user side and services side identity management. In post-test interviews the test subjects sometimes referred to functionalities from both the web site and the user side identity management system as if these were one. Consequently, they also had difficulties to understand that the user side identity management console, where the user can manage her electronic identities, can be trusted by the user because it is within the user's control, whereas the web site is under the service provider's control.

Similar findings of a lack of trust in privacy enhancing technologies were also reported by Günther and Spiekermann in a study on the perception of user control with privacy-enhancing identity management solutions for RFID environments, even though the test users considered the PETs in this study fairly easy to use (Günther and Spiekermann 2005).

Trust plays a major role in privacy-enhancing identity management, because users do not only need to trust their own platforms to manage their data accordingly but also need to trust communication partners and their remote set of platforms that receives personal data to process their data in a privacy-friendly manner.

Provision of Security

Besides fulfilling normal application security requirements, the user interfaces also need to be "secure" in the sense that they should have reasonable countermeasures against common types of Internet fraud attacks, such as phishing (an attempt to fraudulently acquire sensitive information, such as user names, PINs and credit card details, by masquerading as a trustworthy web site).

Only in recent years, research has been done on how to inform users of when to trust web sites – there are indeed problems of mediating trustworthy information because the user must understand which indicator to look at. Unscrupulous web site owners naturally will use all means available to fool innocent visitors. For instance, they will use trust signs they have not been awarded or simply copy the appearance of other sites.

Most users cannot distinguish a legitimate web site from an illegimate phishing one that is designed to capture identity data and credentials (Dhamija and Dusseault 2008). In an illuminating study on this topic in which 22 participants were shown 20 web sites and asked to determine which ones were fraudulent, the researchers "found that 23% of the participants did not look at browser-based cues such as the address bar, status bar and the security indicators, leading to incorrect choices 40% of the time. We also found that some visual deception attacks can fool even the most sophisticated users" (Dhamija et al. 2006). Another study concludes: *"We confirm prior findings that users ignore HTTPS indicators: no participants withheld their passwords when these indicators were removed. We present the first empirical investigation of site-authentication images, and we find them to be ineffective: even when we removed them, 92% participants who used their own accounts entered their passwords"* (Schechter et al. 2007).

HCI GUIDANCE FOR PRIVACY & IDENTITY MANAGEMENT DEVELOPERS

In this section, we will provide a list of recommendations that developers of privacy-enhancing identity management systems should follow in order to address the challenges discussed above. We also provide approaches how those recommendations can be implemented, which were elaborated by our HCI research activities within PRIME and PrimeLife projects or by others. These recommendations and approaches are summarising some of the from our perspective most important HCI guidelines for privacy and identity management. For a more detailed and extensive document of HCI Guidelines for privacy-enhancing identity management, please refer to Pettersson (2008). In addition to those guidelines specific for privacy and identity management, general design principle such as the ten usability principles by Nielsen (1994) should be followed as well.

Do Research on Mental Models and Derive Good Metaphors

For developing intelligible user interfaces for privacy-enhancing identity management, it will be of key importance to do research on the users' mental models of privacy-enhancing technology concepts such as the concepts of unlinkability or anonymous credentials, which are usually poorly understood by end users. The human tendency to create mental models can be used by HCI specialists to guide users to develop appropriate modes, or to examine what models already exist and account on them (Patrick et al. 2003).

Also, user interfaces based on real-world metaphors are easier to comprehend. However, as stated above, often no direct or obvious real-world analogies exist for the concepts in question. Within PRIME, research on alternative UI paradigms for privacy-enhancing identity management based on the metaphor of a town map has been conducted, which should make the process of selecting the right privacy preferences fitting the users' demands when contacting a services side more simple and comprehensible (see also Bergmann et al. 2005, Pettersson et al. 2005). Different areas on the map represent different default privacy preference settings. Icons for services put into the "Public Area" of the town map will for instance be accessed anonymously by default, whereas icons put in the "Neighborhood" of where the user's house is located represent web sites where the user is 'recognisable'. The approach to use different default privacy preference settings for different areas within a town should make it easier for a novice user to see and select the options available once she has grasped the town map metaphor.

A special case of metaphors are icons that can increase learnability if they are carefully chosen. For instance, with the data track icon used for PRIME prototypes most users correctly associated the feature that behind this icon they are able to see the data traces that they have left online, as various usability tests showed (See Figure 1).

A caveat is in place: icons, especially if used in the area of security and privacy, need to be self-explaining and have to clearly suggest the concept that they are representing so that non-intended actions are not performed by the user.

Provide a Selection of Pre-Defined Settings with the Possibility of "On the Fly" Customisation

As security and privacy protection are often secondary goals of ordinary computer users (Herzog 2007), it is not realistic to assume that users will spend much time and efforts on privacy configurations. Moreover, as mentioned above, the task of defining a user's privacy preferences is a complex and error-prone task.

Therefore, the user-side IDM system should provide options of pre-defined privacy configurations. These should include predefined "standard" privacy preferences, from which a user can

Figure 1. Data track icon used in PRIME

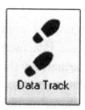

choose from. For a simplified handling of privacy preferences, it should be possible to choose and customise the privacy preferences "on the fly" (i.e. when a services side is requesting data) rather than demanding that the user selects them by hand before she can use them. The set of predefined privacy preferences should represent the users' privacy interests and thus should also include the most privacy-friendly options for acting anonymously or for releasing as little information as needed for a certain service.

In the PRIME and PrimeLife projects, we have defined a set of three predefined privacy preferences (so-called "PrivPrefs"). The first PrivPref defines the preference of releasing no personally-identifiable data at all, i.e. the preference of remaining anonymous. The second PrivPref defines the preference of releasing only the minimal data needed for a certain purpose while the third PrivPref allows revealing more data than needed (usually in return for certain benefits, e.g. to release an email address for receiving special offers as a bonus customer). For each combination of communication partner (services side) and purpose, one of these privacy preference (PrivPref) types can be assigned, meaning that this type of privacy preference will be applied if personal data is requested by that services side for that specific purpose. If for a combination of a services side and purpose, no PrivPref type has been assigned, the preference (PrivPref) of "no personally-identifiable data" is taken by default. Furthermore, as suggested above, these preference settings can be adapted "on the fly". If for example a user agrees to release data needed for a service (e.g., to reveal her address to a delivery service for the delivery of purchased items), the user will at the same time be asked whether she wants to change the PrivPref type for the respective services side and purpose from "No personally-identifiable data" to "only minimal data". This approach of offering pre-defined preferences, from which a user can choose "on-the fly"', should simplify privacy policy management for the users. Users can also be warned about excessive data requests if the PrivPref type "only minimal data" has been chosen. For this, a table of types of data needed for certain purposes is used, which could be provided by trustworthy organisations such a data protection commissioners (see (Bergmann 2009) for more details).

Choose the Most Privacy-Friendly Setting as a Default

For users that do not bother or are unsure about settings, it is reasonable to have "maximum privacy" switched on from start as a default and at every new visit of a services side, so as to deflect e.g. phishing attacks. As mentioned above, we have in the PRIME and PrimeLife projects proposed a set of pre-defined privacy preferences (PrivPrefs), where the 'anonymous' one (*"no personally-identifiable data"*) should be activated by default if no other privacy preference has been chosen by the user, which is for example useful for anonymous browsing. With this privacy preference, no personally identifiable data should actively be released by default. Transaction pseudonyms are used, i.e. user actions should not be linkable beyond the transaction so long as no specific data are released.

Use HCI Constructs for Obtaining Really Informed Consent for Personal Data Disclosures

The Article 29 Data Protection Working Party has also investigated what information should be provided in what form to users in order to fulfill all legal provisions of the EU Data Protection Directive 95/46/EC for ensuring that individuals are informed of their rights to data protection (Art. 29 WP 2004). The Art. 29 Working Party recommends providing information in a "multi-layered format under which each layer should offer individuals the information needed to understand their position and make decisions". They suggest three layers of information provided to individuals: The short notice (layer 1) must offer individuals the core information required under Article 10 of the Directive 95/46/EC, which includes at least the identity of the controller and the purpose of processing. In addition, a clear indication must be given as to how the individual can access additional information. The condensed notice (layer 2) includes in addition all other relevant information required by Art. 10 of the Directive such as the recipients or categories of recipients, whether replies to questions are obligatory or voluntary and information about the individual's rights. The full notice (layer 3) includes in addition to layers 1 and 2 also "national legal requirements and specificities." The Art. 29 Working Party sees short privacy notices as legally acceptable within a multi-layered structure that, in its totality, offers compliance. The "Send Personal data?"- window developed in PRIME for obtaining informed consent as illustrated in Figure 6 corresponds to such a short privacy notice, which in turn corresponds concept-wise to a JITCTA ("Just-In-Time Click-through Agreement") as proposed by Patrick et al. (2003).

As discussed above, click-through dialogs have the disadvantage that users tend to click the *OK* button too easily without having read the text. Presenting data items in cascading menus to select data or credentials, as shown in Figure 2, has the effect that the user must read the text for making the menu choices, which means that in this case she should make more conscious selections. Naturally, such cascading context menus would then need to also include the other information

Figure 2. Menu-based approach for selecting credentials (Camenisch et al. 2006)

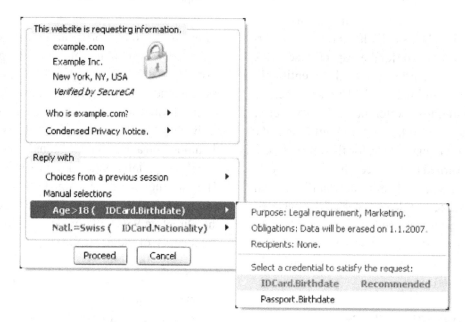

that is relevant for data disclosures, and therefore the cascading context menus depicted in Figure 2 are also following the Art. 29 WP recommendation for a multilayered structuring of privacy policies. However, this user interface design is not suitable if many data fields have to be filled; the design is intended as a special feature for very simple data requests where the user might have to select among a few credentials asserting a specific data claim.

"Drag-and-Drop Agreements" (DADAs) were also elaborated in PRIME in the context of the town map based user interface paradigm as a method for raising the consciousness about the nature of data disclosure (Figure 3). Symbols were used to represent personal data of a user (placed in his house on the town map)– this allowed users to visibly drag-and-drop data icons from his house to icons representing the receivers. Here, the user not only has to pick a set of predefined data (corresponding to clicking "I Accept" or "I Agree" in a pop-up window), but choose the right personal data symbol(s) and drop them on the right receiver symbol. These explicit actions to some

extent offer a guarantee for more conscious user consent.

Provide Means for Making Data Processing Transparent for End Users

This guideline concerns at least two different contexts of user actions. One is the context where the user transfers data to some services sides, and the other is when the user wants to know how data already sent has been processed.

For the first case, as discussed above, it is hard to request from any user to read lots of information. Presumably, the users' main focus is on other things than reading privacy statements from the service provider in question. As suggested by the Art. 29 Working Party, the information (i.e. the privacy notices) should thus be structured to display only the most important information leaving the rest to deeper levels to be called upon by the user if she is interested.

For the second case, it cannot be left to the user to remember all the sides where she has

Figure 3. Drag and drop agreement

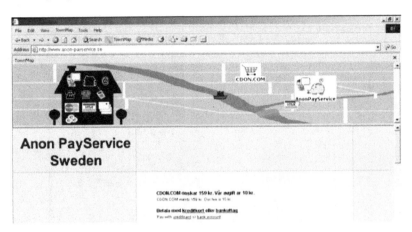

left some information. Rather a history function, such as Data Track in the PRIME prototype must keep track of her data releases. Such a data track function should store at the user's side all transaction records comprising personal data sent, pseudonyms used for transactions, credentials that were disclosed, date of transmission, purposes of data collection, recipient (i.e., the data controller) and all further details of the privacy policy that the user and recipient have agreed upon. Easy tools for finding relevant records about past data disclosures must be part of such a data track.

A simple search box was found unsatisfactory in early usability tests because the general user is unaware of what the system does and is not sure of what to search for. In Figure 4, which shows a recent implementation of the Data Track, the simple search box is supplemented by a few template sentences putting search boxes within meaningful frames: "Who has received my [dropdown list with data or data types]?". In addition, a slider provides the possibility to highlight an individual transaction record as a small page and the whole data track is depicted as a stack of cards. It is possible to browse the Data Track by scrolling the record slider.

During the final phase of the PRIME project we run a small test comparing the (still prototypical) PRIME Data Track with Microsoft's CardSpace. The focus in CardSpace on visual although virtual "identity cards" is also reflected in its history functions; users had to search data "per card", while our prototype Data Track allowed for searches across the templates used for data releases. The latter is more of a traditional database design which, admittedly, can be more demanding but this solution was definitively more liked by the test participants although they managed to solve tasks more easily with CardSpace. Further usability laboratory tests of the final PRIME integrated prototype also showed that the test users really appreciated the idea and possibilities of the data track (Köffel et al. 2008).

As has been proposed in the PRIME project from early user test data, such a history function should preferably also support the user in contacting the data recipients (i.e., the data controllers) and, if these organisations do not respond, support the user in contacting data protection authorities and/or other benevolent organisations (see also next section).

Provide Online Functions for Enabling Users to Exercise Their Rights

Pursuant to Art. 12 EU Directive 95/46/EC, every individual has the right to access her data as

Figure 4. Data track

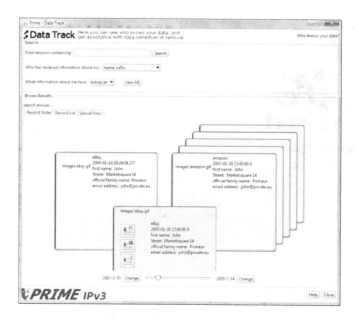

well as the right to ask for rectification, erasure, or blocking of data concerning her as far as the processing does not comply with the requirements of the Directive, in particular when the data are incomplete or inaccurate. As surveys have shown (e.g. Eurobarometer 2008), individuals are usually not aware of all their privacy rights. And even if they are, they rarely exercise them because it means too much effort to find out whom to address, to compile a letter, often to be personally signed on paper, to send it, wait for an answer, write reminders etc. When using pseudonyms (e.g., from an identity management system), this may even be more complicated because the data controller needs a proof that it communicates with the specific pseudonym holder.

We recommend that the interface should provide obvious tools for exercising the individual's rights on-line (as well as at the physical address as a fall back). These tools at the user side identity management system should preferably provide the individual with direct access to her data stored at the data controller's side or at least help her in finding out about the address of the data controller (from the privacy policy), generating requests,

giving the needed authentication (even if a pseudonym is used), monitoring the complaint status, compiling reminders, and – in case of problems – addressing the supervisory authority in charge (see also (Fischer-Hübner et al. 2008)). Tools for exercising rights could be integrated with the data track function presented above. Once the user has "tracked" specific transaction records, the data track user interface provides buttons that the user can click for activating such online functions.

Such online functions will not only improve the individual's possibilities to exercise their privacy rights. It can also enhance trust in the services sides that allow users to exercise their rights online, as the research on social trust factors in PRIME suggest that trust in a service provider can be increased if procedures are transparent and reversible (Andersson et al. 2005).

Provide a Trust Evaluation Function

A trust evaluation function can communicate reliable information about trustworthiness and assurance (of providing the stated functionality) of communication partners. For allowing the user to do well-informed decisions, trust and assurance information needs to be presented to the user at least at the moment when she is requested to release personal data to a communication partner. The user interfaces for giving consent should therefore be augmented with a trust evaluation function to check the trustworthiness of service providers that are not familiar to the user. Trust information can also be displayed when a website is contacted

A trust evaluation function should be based on suitable parameters for measuring the trustworthiness of communication partners and for establishing reliable trust. It should display both information about the communication partner's trustworthiness in terms of privacy practices and of the reliability as a business partner. Both will be important aspects for influencing the user's trust.

A model of social trust factors, which was developed by social science researchers in the PRIME project and which was summarised in (Andersson et al. 2005), states that trust in a service provider can be established by monitoring and enforcing institutions, such as data protection commissioners, consumer organisations and certification bodies. Turner (2001) showed that for ordinary users to feel secure when transacting with a web site depended on factors as, 1. the company's reputation, 2. their experiences with the web site, and 3. recommendations from independent third parties.

Privacy seals certified by data protection commissioners or independent certifiers (e.g., the EuroPrise seal[3], the TRUSTe seal[4] or the ULD Gütesiegel[5]) provide therefore especially suitable information for establishing user trust.

Such static seals can be complemented by dynamic (in real-time generated) seals conveying assurance information about the current security state of the services side's system and its implemented privacy and security functions. Such dynamic seals can be generated in real-time by an "Assurance Evaluation" component that has been implemented within the PRIME framework

(Pearson 2006). Dynamic seals that are generated by tamper-resistant hardware can be regarded as third-party endorsed assurances, as the tamper-resistant hardware device can be modeled as a third party that is not under full control of the services side.

Further information sources by independent trustworthy monitoring organisations that can measure the trustworthiness of services sides can be blacklists maintained by consumer organisations (such a blacklist exists for example in Sweden) or privacy and security alert lists, such as list of alerts raised by data protection commissioners or Google's anti-phishing blacklist. The mockup shown in Figure 5 that we developed within the PrimeLife project is based on such parameters.

The selection of parameters used for trust evaluation should depend on the user's trust policy settings. Further evaluation parameters are possible: The European Consumer Centres have launched a web-based solution, Howard the owl, for checking trust marks and other signs of trust-

Figure 5. Mockup for trust evaluation results (3rd layer)

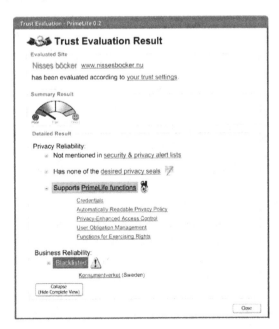

worthiness that could be used as well when evaluating a web shop[6].

As mentioned above, also reputation metrics based on other users' rating can influence user trust. Reputation systems, such for instance the one in eBay, can however often be manipulated by reputation forging or poisoning. Besides, the calculated reputation values are often based on subjective ratings by non-experts, for whom it might for instance be difficult to judge the privacy-friendliness of communication partners.

For the design of our trust evaluation function mock-ups, we followed the following design principles comprising general HCI principles as well as design principles, which should in particular address challenges and usability problems that we have encountered in pervious usability tests:

- Use a Multi-layered structure for displaying evaluation results, i.e. trust evaluation results should be displayed in increasing details on multiple layers in order to prevent an information overload for users not interested in the details or the evaluation. Our mockups have been structured into three layers displaying a short status view with the overall evaluations for inclusion in status bars and in the "Send Personal Data?" window (1st layer, see Figure 6) displaying also the services side's short privacy policy and data request, a compressed view displaying the overall results within the categories privacy seals, privacy & security alert lists, support of PRIME functions and blacklisting (2nd layer), and a complete view showing the results of sub categories (3rd layer, see Figure 5).
- Use a selection of meaningful overall evaluation results. For example, in our mock-ups, we use a trust meter with a range of three possible overall evaluation results that provide a semantic by their names (which should be more meaningful than for instance percentages as used by some

reputation metrics). The three overall results that we are using are (see trust meter in Figure 2):
  ○ "Poor" symbolised with a sad-looking emoticon and red background colour (if there are negative evaluation results, i.e. the side is blacklisted or appears on alert lists);
  ○ "Good" symbolised with a happy looking smiley and green background colour (if there is no negative, but some positive results, i.e. the side has a seal or supports PrimeLife functions and is not appearing on black/alert lists);
  ○ "Fair" symbolised with a white background colour (for all other cases, i.e. the side has no seal, is not supporting PrimeLife functions, and is not appearing on black/alert lists).

- Make clear who is evaluated - this is especially important, because as we mentioned above our previous usability tests have revealed that users have often difficulties to differentiate between user and services side (Pettersson et al. 2005). Hence, the user interface should make clear by its structure (e.g., by surrounding all information referring to a requesting services side, as illustrated in the "Send Personal Data?" window Figure 6), and by wording that the services side and not the user side is evaluated. If this is not made clear, a bad trust evaluation result for a services side might also lead to reduced trust in the user side IDM system.
- Structure the trust parameters visible on the second and third layers into the categories "Business reliability" (comprising the parameter "blacklisted") and "privacy (comprising the parameters of security & privacy alert lists, privacy seals and PrimeLife function support). This structure should illustrate that the trust parameter used have

different semantics and that scenarios with companies that are "blacklisted" for bad business practices, even though they have a privacy seal and/or support PrimeLife functions do not have to be contradictory, as they refer to different aspects of trustworthiness.

- Inform the user without unnecessary warnings - our previous usability tests showed that extensive warnings can be misleading and can even result in users loosing their trust in the PrimeLife system. It is a very difficult task for the systems designer to find a good way of showing an appropriate level of alerting (see also below).

First usability tests for three iterations of our PrimeLife trust evaluation function mockups were performed in the Ozlab testing environment of Karlstad University in two rounds with ten test persons each and one round with 12 tests persons. The tests clearly showed that such a function is much appreciated by end users. The presentation of overall evaluation results on top level, especially the green and red emoticons as well as the fact that the services side was evaluated were well understood. Some users had problems though to understand the "neutral" evaluation result (in case a side has no seal, is not supporting PrimeLife functions, is not blacklisted and does not appear on alert lists), which we first phrased with "ok", and then "fair". However, in the post-test interviews, there were no clear preferences for other names (such as "Not bad", "No alert"). Hence, the illustration of "neutral" results is one of the most difficult issues and still needs to be investigated further (see also (Fischer-Hübner et al. 2009)).

Help Users Detect Phishing Attacks

As suggested by Dhamija and Dusseault (2008), identity management systems should support mutual authentication rather than only focusing on user authentication. This means that also the

services sides need to authenticate themselves for the users.

In particular, users should be provided with help to detect spoofing attacks. If, for example, the identity management system detects that this web service has never been visited by the user before, it can as Microsoft's CardSpace does notify the user about this. Such a feedback alerting the user of a suspected attempt of fraud should be visibly displayed by the user interface.

In our mockups presented in Figure 6, the system could not show the company's logo if it does not recognise the web address as an address that the user has visited before. In the same figure, the trust evaluation result will alert if the web address is found on a phishing blacklist. Compare also the study of the effectiveness of web browser warnings by Egelman et al. (2008) referred below.

Pay Special Attention to the Design and Phrasing of Security & Privacy Alerts

For traditional web browsing, the browser itself is nowadays trying to inform the user about potential risks and definitive risks. However, as reported by Egelman et al. (2008), the implementation of

Figure 6. "Send Personal Data?" window displaying the overall trust evaluation result (1st layer)

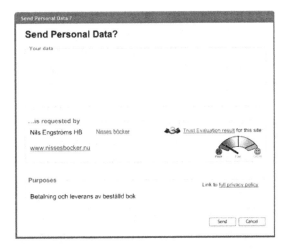

these warning is crucial. Non-obstructive warnings are often not noticed at all, while warnings that the user has to deal with before continuing on a dangerous or potentially dangerous website can be dismissed by users who have seen them so many times before. Egelman et al. suggest: *"Altering the phishing website* – Phishing indicators need to distort the look and feel of the website such that the user does not place trust in it."* This would make people not to habitually trust (what seems to be) a familiar web site or familiar brand name.

Besides this risk that users might not notice the seriousness of warnings, from our experiences from usability tests performed in PRIME and PrimeLife (Köffel et al. 2008), we see at least two more problems that privacy alerts must address:

- Users may try to get rid of intrusive privacy warnings by changing to less privacy-friendly settings. In usability tests of early privacy policy management mockups, we experienced that very prominent warnings, informing test users about a mismatch between her privacy preferences and the services side's privacy policy, led to some test users panic and reacting by changing to more "generous" privacy preference settings in order to eliminate the warning.
- As mentioned above, our previous usability tests also showed that extensive warnings can be misleading and can even result in users loosing their trust in the identity management system. Therefore, alerts should only be displayed in serious cases. In cases where for instance the trust evaluation of a side reveals that the side has no privacy seal and is not implementing PrimeLife functions, rather a "neutral" result than an alerting "poor" evaluation result should be displayed, as the majority of services sides today, including even the ones of privacy-friendly organisations, actually wont fulfill those requirements yet. Also, the yellow colour should be avoided for illustrating

such "neutral" evaluation results (besides green for "good" results and red for "poor" results), as yellow is symbolising a state right before an alarming red (i.e. the traffic light metaphor should not be used in this context).

Hence, a careful phrasing and design of alerts, which should be carefully tested, is of key importance.

CONCLUSION

In this paper we have discussed usability challenges for privacy-enhancing identity management. Moreover, we provided a list of recommendations that developers of privacy-enhancing Identity Management Systems should follow in order to address the above challenges. Some approaches of how those recommendations can be implemented were discussed, which were partly developed within the EU FP6 project PRIME. However, many of these approaches did not offer an ultimate solution and still left open questions. Further research is needed for developing improved or novel innovative approaches for addressing these and other challenges. This will also be a task within the EU FP7 project PrimeLife ("Privacy and Identity Management for Life"), which started in March 2008 and which conducts further research on mental models and metaphors, trust and assurance HCI as well as simplified policy administration. A special focus of PrimeLife is on privacy-enhancing identity management solutions for social communities, which will require novel HCI solutions (in addition to the HCI solutions that we have for client-server applications), as they have to take the specific legal, social and technical aspects of social communities into account.

ACKNOWLEDGMENT

We acknowledge the EU FP 6 project PRIME for financial support. Moreover, parts of the research leading to these results has received funding from the EU 7th Framework programme (FP7/2007-2013) for the project PrimeLife. The information in this document is provided "as is", and no guarantee or warranty is given that the information is fit for any particular purpose. The PrimeLife consortium members shall have no liability for damages of any kind including without limitation direct, special, indirect, or consequential damages that may result from the use of these materials subject to any liability which is mandatory due to applicable law.

REFERENCES

Andersson, C., Camenisch, J., & Crane, S. Fischer-Hübner, S., Leenes, R., Pearson,S., Pettersson, J.S., & Sommer, D. (2005). Trust in PRIME. In *Proceedings of the 5th IEEE Int. Symposium on Signal Processing and IT*, December 18-21, 2005, Athens, Greece.

Article 29 Data Protection Working Party. (2004). Opinion on More Harmonised Information provisions. 11987/04/EN WP 100, November 25 2004.

Bergmann, M. (2009). User Friendly Policy Management and Presentation. In Fischer-Hübner et al.

Bergmann, M., Rost, M., & Pettersson, J. S. (2006). Exploring the Feasibility of a Spatial User Interface Paradigm for Privacy-Enhancing Technology. In *Proceedings of the Fourteenth International Conference on Information Systems Development (ISD'2005)* (pp. 437-448), Karlstad, August 2005. Published in Advances in Information Systems Development, Springer-Verlag, Germany.

Camenisch, J., & Lysyanskaya, A. (2001). Efficient non-transferable anonymous multi-show credential system with optional anonymity revocation. In *Advances in Cryptology - Eurocrypt 2001* (pp. 92-118), 2045.

Camenisch, J., Shelat, A., Sommer, D., & Zimmermann, R. (2006). Securing user inputs for the web. In *Proceedings of the Second ACM Workshop on Digital Identity Management* (pp. 33-44). Alexandria, Virginia, USA, November 03 - 03, 2006. DIM '06. New York: ACM.

Data Protection in the European Union. Citizens' perceptions (2008, February). *Flash Eurobarometer*. Retrieved from http://ec.europa.eu/public_opinion/flash/fl_225_en.pdf

Dhamija, R., & Dusseault, L. (2008). The Seven Flaws of Identity Management: Usability and Security Challenges. *IEEE Security and Privacy*, *6*(2), 24–29. doi:10.1109/MSP.2008.49

Dhamija, R., Tygar, J. D., & Hearst, M. (2006). Why Phishing Works. *CHI 2006 Proceedings*. *ACM Conference Proceedings Series*. ACM Press.

Directive 2002/58/EC of the European Parliament and of the Council of 12 July 2002 concerning the processing of personal data and the protection of privacy in the electronic communications sector, Official Journal L No. 201, 31.07.2002.

Directive 95/46/EC of the European Parliament and of the Council of 24 October 1995 on the protection of individuals with regard to the processing of personal data and on the free movement of such data, Official Journal L No. 281, 23.11.1995.

Egelman, S., Cranor, L., & Hong, J. (2008). You've Been Warned: An Empirical Study of the Effectiveness of Web browser Phishing Warnings. *CH 2008 Proceedings*, Florence/Italy, April 5-10.

Fischer-Hübner, S., Köffel, Ch., Wästlund, E., & Wolkerstorfer, P., (2009). PrimeLife HCI Research Report, Version V1. PrimeLife EU FP7 Project Deliverable D4.1.1.

Fischer-Hübner, S., & Pettersson, J. S. (Eds.). (2004). Evaluation of early prototypes. PRIME deliverable D6.1.b.

Fischer-Hübner, S., Pettersson, J. S., Bergmann, M., Hansen, M., Pearson, S., & Casassa-Mont, M. (2008). *Digital Privacy – Theory, Technologies, and Practices* (Aquisti, , Eds.). Auerbach Publications.

Garfinkel, S. L. (2005). *Design Principles and Patterns for Computer Systems That Are Simultaneously Secure and Usable*. PhD Dissertation, Massachusetts Institute of Technology, May 2005.

Günther, O., & Spiekermann, S. (2005). RFID and the perception of control: The consumer's view, in *Communications of the ACM, 48*(9), 73-76.

Herzog, A. (2007). *Usable Security Policies in Runtime Environments*. Linköping Studies in Science and Technology, Dissertation No. 1075. Linköping University.

Johnston, J., Eloff, J. H. P., & Labuschagne, L. (2003). Security and human computer interfaces. *Computers & Security, 22*(8), 675–684. doi:10.1016/S0167-4048(03)00006-3

Köffel, Ch., Wästlund, E., & Wolkerstorfer, P. (2008). PRIME IPv3 Usability Test Report V1.2.

Nielsen, J. (1994). Heuristic evaluation. In Nielsen & Mack (Eds.), *Usability Inspection Methods*. New York: John Wiley & Sons. Retrieved from http://www.useit.com/papers/heuristic/heuristic_list.html

Nielsen, J. (2004). Jacob Nielsen's Alertbox, User Education Is Not the Answer to Security Problems. Retrieved from http://www.useit.com

Patrick, A. S., & Kenny, S. (2003). *From Privacy Legislation to Interface Design: Implementing Information Privacy in Human-Computer Interaction*. Privacy Enhancing Technologies Workshop (PET2003), Dresden/Germany.

Patrick, A. S., Kenny, S., Holmes, C., & van Breukelen, M. (2003). Human Computer Interaction. In van Blarkom, G.W., Borking, J.J., & Olk, J.G.E. (Eds.), *Handbook for Privacy and Privacy-Enhancing Technologies* (pp. 249-290). PISA project.

Pearson, S. (2006). Towards Automated Evaluation of Trust Constraints. In *Trust Management* (LNCS 3986, pp. 252-266).

Pettersson, J. S. (Ed.). (2008). HCI Guidelines. PRIME deliverable D6.1.f.

Pettersson, J. S., Fischer-Hübner, S., & Bergmann, M. (2006). Outlining Data Track: Privacy-friendly Data Maintenance for End-users. In *Proceedings of the 15th International Conference on Information Systems Development (ISD 2006)*, Budapest, 31st August - 2nd September 2006. Springer Scientific Publishers.

Pettersson, J. S., Fischer-Hübner, S., Danielsson, N., Nilsson, J., Bergmann, M., Clauß, S., et al. (2005). Making PRIME usable. *SOUPS 2005 Symposium on Usable Privacy and Security*, Carnegie Mellon University, July 6-8 July, 2005, Pittsburgh. Available in ACM Digital Library.

Pfitzmann, A., & Hansen, M. (2008, February 15). Anonymity. Unlinkability, Undetectability, Unobservability, Pseudonymity, and Identity Management – A Consolidated Proposal for Terminology, Version v0.31. Retrieved from http://dud.inf.tu-dresden.de/literatur/Anon_Terminology_v0.31.doc#_Toc64643839

Raskin, J. (2000). *The Humane Interface – New Directions for Designing Interactive Systems*. New York: ACM Press.

Schechter, S. E., Dhamija, R., Ozment, A., & Fischer, I. (2007). The Emperor's New Security Indicators: An evaluation of web site authentication and the effect of role playing on usability studies. *IEEE Symposium on Security and Privacy*, May 20-27, 2007, Oakland, California.

Turner, C. W., Zavod, M., & Yurcik, W. (2001). Factors that Affect the Perception of Security and Privacy of E-commerce Web Sites. In *Proceedings of the Fourth International Conference on Electronic Commerce Research*, Dallas, TX.

Yee, K.-P. (2002). User interaction design for secure systems. In [Springer-Verlag.]. *Proceedings of the International Conference on Information and Communications Security, ICIC, 02,* 278–290.

ENDNOTES

[1] https://www.prime-project.eu/
[2] http://www.primelife.eu/
[3] https://www.european-privacy-seal.eu/
[4] http://www.truste.org/
[5] https://www.datenschutzzentrum.de/guete-siegel/index.htm
[6] ready21.dev.visionteam.dk

Chapter 16
Living Lab:
An Open and User-Centric Design Approach[1]

Birgitta Bergvall-Kåreborn
Luleå University of Technology, Sweden

Anna Ståhlbröst
Luleå University of Technology, Sweden

ABSTRACT

In this chapter we focus on a new research area, Living Lab that introduces new ways of managing innovation processes. A Living Lab can be viewed as both an innovation milieu and an innovation approach, and the aim of this chapter is to clarify these two perspectives, as well as to illustrate how they can enrich each other. This is done by presenting one Living Lab milieu, Botnia Living Lab, and its key components; and one Living Lab approach, FormIT, and its key principles. The presentation is done on two levels, one general level and one case specific level. The case focuses on involving citizens in the design of an e-service aimed to increase their influence in a municipality and its development. Through this we learnt that the key components of a Living Lab constitutes important structures that enhance the process and as such the principles.

INTRODUCTION

Living Lab has become an umbrella concept for a diverse set of innovation milieus emerging all over Europe. Even though they differ in many ways, both in focus and approach, there also are a few common denominators pulling them together (Shami, 2008).

In order to join forces, coordinate activities, and share learning experiences, a European Network of Living Labs has developed. The aim of the network is to offer a gradually growing set of networked services to support the "Innovation Lifecycle" for all actors in the system: end-users, SMEs, corporations, the public sector, and academia. Today, the network consists of 129 Living Labs, after the third recruitment wave have finished.

Our definition of Living Lab The definition of Living Lab given by the network is that "a Living Lab is an open innovation environment in real-life settings in which user-driven innovation is the co-creation process for new services, products, and

DOI: 10.4018/978-1-60960-057-0.ch016

societal infrastructures. Living Labs encompass societal and technological dimensions simultaneously in a business-citizens-government-academia partnership."

The rationale behind these new milieus, to open company boundaries toward their environment and to harvest creative ideas and work capabilities existing among different stakeholder, is similar in its approach to other open methodologies, e.g., open innovation (Chesbrough 2003; Chesbrough and Appleyard, 2007), crowdsourcing (Brandel 2008; Hempel 2007), and involving lead users (Von Hippel, 1986; Von Hippel & Katz 2002). Living Labs also share many characteristics with user-centred approaches such as "participatory design" and "socio-technical design" (Bekker & Long, 2000).

In this chapter, we will focus on Living Labs aimed to create a shared arena in which digital services, processes, and new ways of working can be developed and tested with user representatives and researchers.

Since Living Labs is a rather new research area, the amount of supporting theories for understanding the concept is limited (Feurstein et al. 2008). The same is true when it comes to methodologies, methods, and tools. Here, there is a lack of systematic analyses and reflection on available methods and tools and their suitability to the Living Lab context (Følstad 2008). Thus, Feurstein et al. (2008) argue for a structuring of the approaches used in Living Labs in order to gain an overview of what is used and to what extent.

In this chapter, we take a different approach by focusing on one Living Lab milieu, Botnia Living Lab, and one Living Lab approach, FormIT (Bergvall-Kåreborn et al. 2008; Ståhlbröst & Bergvall-Kåreborn 2008) and reflecting on their strengths and weaknesses in relation to given Living Lab components and principles. The aim of the chapter is to clarify these two perspectives, and to illustrate how they can enrich each other. By this, we participate in the building of a common knowledge base of existing practice that later can be accessed.

In the following, we present the concept of Living Lab and its key components and principles. Subsequently, we introduce Botnia Living Lab, followed by FormIT. Thereafter, a description of our research method and a case that illustrates the milieu and the approach is given. After this we reflect on the key principles and key components, as well as the relation between. Finally, the chapter ends with some final remarks.

LIVING LABS

Living Lab started to emerge in the beginning of 2000 (Markopoulos and Rauterberg, 2000), with an initial focus on testing new technologies in home-like constructed environments. Since then, the concept has grown; today, one precondition in Living Lab activities is that they are situated in a real-world context.

During the design of the concept, Living Labs has been defined as an environment (Ballon et al. 2005; Schaffers et al. 2007), as a methodology (Eriksson et al., 2005) and as a system (CoreLabs. 2007). We do not see these three definitions as contradictory but rather as complementary perspectives. Depending on which perspective one takes, certain themes come into focus. With the environment perspective, objects such as technological platforms and user communities come to the forefront. With the methodology perspective, it is processes such as data transfers and methods for user involvement that are highlighted. Based on this we define Living Lab as follows.

A Living Lab is a user-centric innovation milieu built on every-day practice and research, with an approach that facilitates user influence in open and distributed innovation processes engaging all relevant partners in real-life contexts, aiming to create sustainable values.

In this chapter, we present Living Lab as a system for design and innovation consisting of both a milieu and an approach. One way of illustrating a Living Lab milieu can be seen in Figure 1. The *technology and infrastructure* component outlines the role that new and existing ICT technology can play to facilitate new ways of cooperating and co-creating new innovations among the partners and stakeholders. *Management* represent the ownership, organisation, and policy aspects of a Living Lab. The Living Labs *partners and users* bring their own specific wealth of knowledge and expertise to the collective, helping to achieve higher standards of excellence of every area. *Research* symbolizes the collective learning and reflection that take place in the Living Lab, and should result in contributions to both theory and practice. Finally, *approach* stand for proposed standards and methods that emerge as best practice within the Living Labs environment.

In relation to the Living Lab methodology five key principles have been suggested as a result of the CoreLabs project (CoreLabs. 2007). However, based on our experiences from the Swedish Living Lab Network (OLLSE) we have redefined these concepts (Bergvall-Kåreborn et al. 2009a). In this work we have worked very close with colleagues from Halmstad Living Lab (Bergvall-Kåreborn et al. 2009b). Below we describe these five new key principles: Openness, Influence, Realism, Value and Sustainability. As the Living Lab concept is multi-disciplinary, we will discuss these principles with reference to literature from related areas such as economy, innovation, organization, information systems, participatory design and human-computer interaction.

Openness

In open innovation literature (Chesbrough, 2006) the perspective of openness is of concerns firms driving innovation processes to reach for example new products, services or new markets. However,

Figure 1. Key components of a living lab (Bergvall-Kåreborn et al. 2009b)

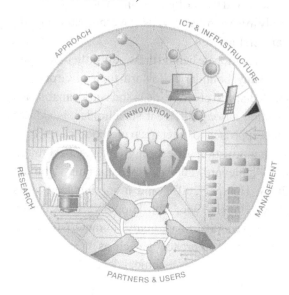

Figure 2. Living lab key principles (Bergvall-Kåreborn et al. 2009b)

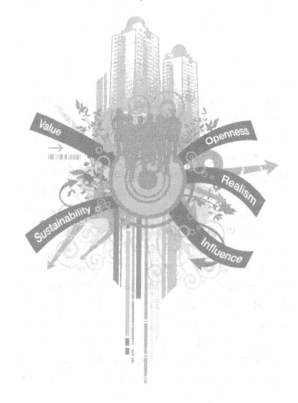

openness can also be discussed based on e.g. an individual, team or firm level. In these cases openness concern how to support open mindsets on an individual or team level or openness and knowledge transfer between different levels in an organization. Openness can also be seen as an overarching philosophy that is being used as the basis of how various groups and organizations operate.

In a Living Lab, digital innovations are created and validated in collaborative multi-contextual empirical real-world environments. Openness is crucial for the innovation process in a Living Lab, where it is essential to gather a multitude of perspectives that might lead to faster and more successful development, new ideas and unexpected business openings in markets. However, to be able to co-operate and share in a multistakeholder milieu, different levels of openness between the stakeholders seems to be a requirement. To stimulate creativity and create new ideas that can be turned into applications and bring value through use, Eriksson et al. (2005) suggest open collaboration between people of different backgrounds, with different perspectives that have different knowledge and experiences. More people, including consumers, need to be involved in the innovation process. This is argued by Thomke & von Hippel (2002) who claim that users are often the source of innovations. The concept of user driven innovation (von Hippel, 1988) suggests that users are capable innovators. Thereby it can be argued that involvement of end users or consumers in the innovation process is important, hence they should be vital part of an innovation system.

It could be expected from a business and innovation perspective that smaller enterprises might have strong incentives to be involved in Living Lab processes. Small and micro enterprises often lack the resources and knowledge that larger organizations have. One way to strengthen smaller enterprises' innovation capacity is by collaborating with other actors such as academia, the public sector and other enterprises (Eriksson et al. 2005). Living Lab and similar innovation milieus might thereby strengthen the innovation capacity due to cross-fertilization and open collaboration between different actors. The Living Lab may also provide an arena where different stakeholders are needed to in order to commercialize and bring products and services to market, either support existing relations between business stakeholders or as a milieu where new partners get the chance to meet and collaborate.

In our projects we have experienced openness on different levels, but we have also experienced when processes close up due to e.g. IPR issues. The challenge is to create a milieu where stakeholders are motivated to and have incitement to share knowledge. Specifically business stakeholders might need economically tangible incitement whereas user groups often are driven by other motives. These motives need to be identified and acted upon. Furthermore, the motives for engagement might also differ quite radically depending on the specific Living Lab context.

Influence

A key aspect of the influence principle is to view "users" as active and competent partners and domain experts. As such their involvement and influence in innovation and development processes shaping society is essential. Equally important is to base these innovations on the needs and desires of potential users, and to realize that these users often represent a heterogeneous group. This means utilizing the creative power of Living Lab partners, whilst facilitating their right to influence these innovations. By stressing the decision making power of potential users and domain experts the principle differs from related concepts such as participation, involvement, and engagement which instead focus on the activities carried out by users and users' psychological state (Barki & Hartwick, 1989; Baroudi et al. 1986).

In order to reduce the diversity and ambiguity related to the principle of influence, and to increase its positive impact in practical studies, it is prudent to define and explain the concept as clearly as possible. To manage this we propose three dimensions linked to influence: why, who, and how. When it comes to the why of influence, two motivations can be identified in the literature: a political and a technical perspective. The political perspective is based on the central tenet that users have a moral right to influence technological decisions affecting their private and professional life. The technical perspective is founded on the notion that the effective participation of skilled users can contribute to high quality products as well as system acceptance. The who of influence is related to making reflective choices on who to involve in a particular study while the how refers to the process of participation and on different degrees of participation and influence linked to different partners.

Based on our experience the meaning assigned to the principle of influence differs quite a lot among different partners and users. However, to take the step from participation or involvement to influence, domain experts' and users' needs and ideas should be clearly traceable in concepts, prototypes, and the finished product. In all our projects users have exercised influence over the design of the final systems; their needs and suggestions have influenced the design and been implemented as functions and features in the prototypes and final systems. However, in most projects they have been given this influence because the partners kept open minds and wanted to base the solution on user needs rather than on their own predetermined view on what users like. However, there is a reoccurring difference between how users and domain experts are portrayed and the actual roles, activities and responsibilities assigned to them (Beath & Orlikowski, 1994). While users often are described as drivers and shapers of technology they still very often are treated as a homogeneous and passive group that carry out activities assigned to them. Hence, one important issue that Living Labs need to manage is how to assure that participation, influence and responsibility among different partners harmonizes with each other and with the ideology of the user influence of the project.

Realism

One of the cornerstones for the Living Lab approach is that innovation activities should be carried out in a realistic, natural, real life setting. Orchestrating realistic use situation and user behavior is seen as one way to generate results that are valid for real markets in Living Lab operations (CoreLabs, 2007). However, the aim to create and facilitate realism is an endeavor that needs to be grappled with on different levels and in correlation to different elements such as contexts, users, use situations, technologies, and partners. The principle does not separate between the physical and the online world. Instead we argue that activities carried out in both worlds are as real and realistic to its actors. Being inspired by the online reality we argue that IT based tools and methodologies can function as twin-world mediators (Attasiriluk, et al. 2009) which facilitate the interconnection between real-world devices and their virtual counterparts. Following Mingers & Willcocks (2004) we also argue that ideas, concepts, meanings, and categories are equally real as physical objects. These are emergent from, but irreducible to, the physical world and have causal effects both on the physical world and the social world. This means that to understand roles, behavior, and relationships related to the innovation process we need to go beneath the surface and not only focus on what is observable.

Relating realism to Checkland's real-world concept (Checkland, 1999), means that the "real-world" situation reflects people's interpretation of their current situation. People's interpretations and how they perceive the situation is related to people's worldview, or what they view as important for them; hence, what is viewed as the reality for one person does not necessarily mean the same for another person. This means that what is important and motivating for one partner, is not necessarily important to another partner, which is a rationale for why it is crucial to involve a diversity of perspectives in the innovation process.

When it comes to facilitating as realistic use situations as possible two different approaches can be observed in relation to Living Labs. In the first approach, environments for test and evaluation of products or services are created in ways that are similar to the real world (Markopoulos & Rauterberg, 2000), while in the second approach products and services are tested and evaluated in users' real world environments (Schumacher & Niitamo, 2008).

Another important aspect related to the principle of realism, but not specifically addressed by the principle, is the fact that different stakeholders face different realities. This means that what is important and motivating for one stakeholder, is not necessarily important to another stakeholder. For example, as a researcher, the reality can be focused on producing scientific results, while SMEs' reality can be to earn money by developing a new IT system. Different perspectives and views on the reality are also often mentioned reasons for why it is crucial to involve users as well as many different stakeholders in the development process. The reality aspect is also considered by focusing on involving real users, not using personas or other user representative theories.

Value

The notion of value and value creation in a Living Lab concerns several different aspects such as economical value, business value and consumer/ user value. Economical value is highly tangible and can be viewed from different stakeholder perspectives. Living Lab activities or outcomes in the shape of innovations can often be transformed into economical value. Therefore these activities or outcomes can be assessed and evaluated from an economical value perspective.

Business value is a somewhat more intangible term that includes all forms of value that determine the health and well-being of a firm in the long-run. Business value expands the concept of economical value to include other forms of value such as e.g. employee value, customer value, supplier value, managerial value and societal value. Business value also often embraces intangible assets not necessarily attributable to any stakeholder group such as intellectual capital and a firm's business model.

There is a growing recognition that providing superior value for users is a key aspect for business success (Boztepe, 2007). One way to mitigate competition and open up entirely new markets is by focusing on creating advances in customer value (Kim & Mauborgne 2005). One key attribute that distinguishes breakthrough products from their closest followers, is according to Cagan & Vogel (2002), the significant value they provide for users.

According to Kuusisto (2008) the concept of value adding services or products imply that value is contained in the product or the service. The value is created and offered by the producer. Another perspective is the value-in use concept that focuses on the experience perceived by a user interacting with products or services in use situations. This concept implies that the customer is always a co-creator of the value. According to this concept, the customers experience and perception are essential to be able to determinate user value (Kuusisto, 2008).

Consumer value can also be defined in terms of the monetary sacrifice people are willing to make for a product. The primary focus here is on the point of exchange where money is seen as an index of value. According to this perspective, the assumption is that at the moment of purchase, the consumer makes a calculation and evaluation of what is given (value) in respect to what is taken in terms of money (Boztepe, 2007). Consumer value and consumer needs are also important aspects of adoption and diffusion theory. Based on our experience, a Living Lab has the opportunity to create value based on all aspects of the value term. However, a Living Lab might also provide insights about how users perceive value. These insights can guide the innovation process to be able to deliver innovations that are perceived as valuable from both an economical, business, and a consumer perspective.

Sustainability

Sustainability refers both to the viability of a Living Lab and to its responsibility to the wider community in which it operates. Focusing on the viability of the Living Lab highlights aspects such as continuous learning and development over time. Here, the research component of each Lab plays a vital role in transforming the everyday knowledge generation into models, methods and theories. Other important aspects related to the sustainability of a Living Lab is the partnership and its related networks since good cross-border collaboration, which strengthens creativity and innovation, builds on trust, and this takes time to build up. In order to succeed with new innovations, it is important to inspire usage, meet personal desires, and fit and contribute to societal and social needs. However, in line with the general sustainability and environmental trends in society it is of equal importance that Living Labs also take responsibility of its environmental, social, and economic effects.

Among these five principles, three stands out, as they represent the core of Living Labs. The first is influence, since the main role of Living Labs is "to engage and empower users to participate in the generation of valuable and sustainable assets toward objectives set up by its partners and customers" (CoreLabs. 2007, p. 9). This relates strongly to user-centric approaches of different types, such as "participatory design" and "socio-technical design" (Bekker & Long 2000).

The second is openness, which can be related to open innovation (Chesbrough, 2003; Chesbrough & Appleyard, 2007), crowdsourcing (Brandel, 2008; Hempel, 2007), and involving lead users (Von Hippel, 1986; Von Hippel & Katz, 2002). The third is realism and focus on real-world settings. This principle also is the most distinguishing characteristic of a Living Labs compared to both open approaches and user-centric approaches. Due to this, we will focus on these three principles in this chapter.

BOTNIA LIVING LABS

The Living Lab described in this chapter is called Botnia; it focuses on developing innovative IT services or products, with real users, from the basis of user needs, in a real-world context. This Living Lab is open for all kinds of IT stakeholders and aims to facilitate the collaboration process between all relevant stakeholders in the value-chain, and to help these stakeholders manage their innovation processes with users. During its life cycle, the aim of Botnia has altered. In the beginning, the main objective was to facilitate user tests of innovations for SMEs and researchers. This focus has matured and increased, and today Botnia not only performs user tests, but also aims to support processes in which users are involved as equal co-creators of innovations in close cooperation with companies, users, academia, and authorities.

In this cooperation, a few stable partners have been crucial for the sustainability of the Living Lab, especially in the start-up phase. Two very important contributors to the environment are Ericsson and TeliaSonera. Besides these large telecommunication companies, there also are a number of small and medium-sized companies that have followed and contributed to the development of Botnia. On the public side, there is a close relationship between Botnia and researchers in diverse sciences. Each science, as well as each partner, contributes in its specific knowledge area. Besides these more stable partners, there are many companies and public authorities that are more loosely coupled to the Lab. They might participate in a project and then cease the relation to Botnia when the project ends.

Over the years, Botnia has built up a community of end-users with which they easily can communicate; hence, they are the centre of the organisation. This community includes 5,800 test pilots who have, as private persons, voluntarily chosen to be part of the Living Lab community. One unifying factor among these test pilots is their curiosity to try new technical artefacts and to get the opportunity to influence them. What separates them are demographical and psychosocial factors (Ståhlbröst, 2004). The blend of people available through this community makes it possible to select and tailor a test target group in relation to the needs and wants of the test initiator. Here, the test initiator can be represented by customers buying a user test or the test initiator can come from within the Living Lab organization. The only requirement test pilots must meet is to have access to a mobile phone.

Since Botnia aims to involve real-world users in real-world use situations throughout the innovation process, each study becomes customised in accordance with the unique requirements for that particular study. The contexts for each individual study can differ substantially, from reindeer herders in rural areas to city residents in traffic jams, even though the focus of Botnia always is to develop innovative IT services or products.

The technology and infrastructure platforms are available through the Living Lab collaboration partners. This platform, with its Living Lab portal, constitutes the focal point of the Living Lab since this is where projects are presented to the end-users and where end-users are recruited. The portal also is where the interaction between end-users and other partners takes place. In order to extend the number of users a Living Lab can access there are a number of EU-funded research projects that aim to connect different platforms together in order to widen the scope of the activities that can be carried out.

As with the technological platform and infrastructure, there is a need to learn more about the methodologies, methods, and tools that are used in Living Lab situations, and also to reflect on their suitability. There is no lack of existing methodologies, methods, and tools used in individual Living Labs, but there are few studies that reflect on the methods used in relation to the unique character of Living Labs. There also is a need to develop new methodologies, methods, and tools specific to the aim and context of Living Lab, especially new distributed methods for user involvement, since users are involved in the development process independent of their location. One such methodology, developed based on the practice within Botnia, will be presented in the next chapter.

Another important aspect of Botnia's methodological and organisational structure is the "living" aspect. This means that the people involved in any development project "live" with the process and constantly check how the process proceeds, thus being prepared for any necessary adjustments to ensure, for example, that users are stimulated to participate, or that the development process proceeds as planned. If the process does not proceed as planned, the aim is to gather data about what has happened and how the plans can be adjusted accordingly. The Living Lab organisation in which we are involved is based on the development project that currently is running; hence, the project's aim and process highly influence the Living Labs activities, participants, and structure. This can mean, for example, that if a certain competence is missing in the organisation, SMEs can be involved to fill that spot. Finally, the Living Lab setting also enables sharing experiences across partners as well as for research. Botnia aims to harmonise the development process and the innovations, among four main stakeholders; companies, users, authorities, and researchers. The close relationship between research and development is one important characteristic.

FORMIT: AN ILLUSTRATION OF A LIVING LAB METHODOLOGY

In this section, we present the framework of ideas and characteristics of FormIT before we introduce the general shape of FormIT, in order to give a holistic view of the methodology. The kernel of this chapter is concept design, and this part of FormIT therefore will be presented in more detail through an illustration of a case later in this chapter.

Framework of Ideas

FormIT is inspired by three theoretical streams: Soft Systems Thinking (SST), Appreciative Inquiry (AI), and NeedFinding (NF). From the first stream, Soft Systems Thinking (Checkland, 1981; Checkland et al. 1990; Checkland & Holwell, 1998), the assumption that changes can occur only through changes in mental models is utilised. This implies that we need to understand both our own as well as other stakeholders' worldviews, and we need to be clear about our interpretations and the base on which they are made. The second stream, Appreciative Inquiry (Cooperrider & Avital, 2004; Cooperrider & Whitney, 2005; Cooperrider et al. 2005; Norum, 2001), has encouraged us to start the development cycle by identifying different stakeholders' dreams and visions of how IT can improve and support the lives of people. This includes a focus on opportunities, related to specific trends, contexts, or user groups, and on the positive and life-generating experiences of people (Holst & Ståhlbröst, 2006; Ståhlbröst & Holst, 2006).

This way of thinking is closely aligned with the philosophy behind SST, since it also highlights the importance of people's thoughts about themselves and the world around them in a design situation. Hence, instead of starting the process by searching for problems to solve in a situation, we identify what works well and use this as a basis for design.

The third stream, NeedFinding, has two different inspirational sources. The NeedFinding concept, as such, and its motivation finds its origin in a paper by Patnaik and Becker (1999). Patnaik and Becker argue that the main motivators for the NeedFinding approach are that needs are not influenced highly by trends; hence, they are more long lasting. The needs generation process, on the other hand, is inspired by Kankainen and Oulasvirta (2003) and Tiitta (2003). These authors inspire us to focus on user needs throughout the development process, and to use these as a foundation for the requirement specification (See Figure 3).

Characteristics of FormIT

Grounded in these three theoretical streams, FormIT enables a focus on possibilities and strengths in the situation under study; this is fundamentally different from traditional problem-solving approaches. In our perspective, identifying opportunities is the basis for appreciating needs since needs are opportunities waiting to be exploited (Holst & Ståhlbröst, 2006; Ståhlbröst & Holst, 2006). Hence, FormIT strongly stresses the importance of the first phase in the concept design cycle, usually referred to as analyses or requirements engineering. Since this phase creates the foundation for the rest of the process, errors here becomes very hard and expensive to correct in later stages. This also is the phase in which users can make the strongest contributions, by actually setting the direction for the design rather than mainly responding to (half finished) prototypes. Since users' needs and requirements can change as users gain more knowledge and insights into possible solutions, it is important to continually reexamine their needs and make sure they correlate to given requirements.

In accordance, the FormIT method is iterative, and interaction with users is an understood

Figure 3. The FormIT process (Ståhlbröst, 2008)

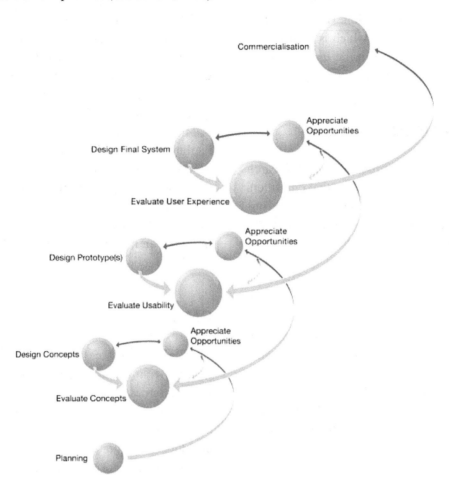

prerequisite. The idea is that knowledge increases through iterative interactions between phases and people with diverse competences and perspectives (Holst & Mirijamdotter, 2006; Mirijamdotter et al. 2006). In this way, knowledge increases through dialogue among participants. The idea is that the cross-functional interaction enables the processes of taking knowledge from one field to another to gain fresh insights, which then facilitates innovative ideas. The shared understanding of the situation informs and enriches the learning processes and thus facilitates changes in perspective and leads toward innovative design-processes. This, in turn, increases our qualifications to design IT systems that answer to user needs (Ståhlbröst & Holst, 2006).

General shape of FormIT

The FormIT process can be seen as a spiral in which the focus and shape of the design becomes clearer, while the attention of the evaluation broadens from a focus on concepts and usability aspects to a holistic view on the use of the system; see Figure 2.

In this process three phases – Generate Needs, Design, and Evaluate – are repeated in three iterative cycles. The first cycle is called Concept Design, the second Prototype Design, and the third Final System Design. The name of the cycle indicates the expected output of each cycle. Besides these three cycles, two additional phases are included in the figure. The first is planning, seen in the upper right hand corner of the figure, and the second is commercialisation. The focus of this chapter is concept design, which is managed in the first cycle, illustrated in the upper level of figure 2.

RESEARCH METHOD

In this study, we have chosen an action research approach. Action research means that one enters a real-world situation with the aim of both improving it and creating knowledge (Baskerville & Wood-Harper, 1998; Checkland & Holwell, 1998). It is an established method within social sciences, including information systems (Baskerville and Wood-Harper 1996; Jönsson, 1991), and is thought to produce highly relevant results because it is grounded in practical action and aims to solve immediate problem situations while informing theory. Baskerville and Wood-Harper (1996) even argue that "action research is one of the few valid research approaches that researchers can legitimately employ to study the effects of specific alterations in systems development methodologies" (p. 240).

Action research also is a methodology well suited for Living Lab since both approaches emphasise interaction between theory and practice, involve many different stakeholders with distinct roles relevant in the situation, and highlight the importance of constant reflection in order to follow wherever the situation leads.

Focusing on both the practical and the theoretical in a situation, and how they enrich each other, fits well with the dual role we have had in this study. Our project role and responsibility were to appreciate technological opportunities that could improve citizens' possibilities and willingness to participate in municipality development. Our research aim was to develop FormIT further through reflection on our experiences of applying the methodology in this particular situation. This also meant that we gained knowledge on how a

Living Lab milieu and a Living Lab approach can enrich each other.

The key components of a Living Lab can be found on two different levels. One describes the general framework of a Living Lab, while the other describes separate projects carried out within the general framework. While the first level brings stability and continuity to the lab, the second facilitates spontaneity and represents the living aspect of a lab. To illustrate this, we have separated the two levels into the Botnia Living Lab and the SMART case. Since the data gathering in the case is mainly a part of the aim of improving the situation it will be integrated and reported in the Case section.

CASE

The background to the SMART case was a general feeling that citizens lack opportunities to communicate easily with public authorities. This results in few citizen-driven suggestions and opinions for how the municipality should develop. To facilitate active participation among citizens, the project aimed to develop IT services that increased citizens' abilities to influence and improve the society.

The SMART project had three different but intertwined purposes:

- to give product and service developers the opportunity to engage citizens and user groups in their change, quality, and innovation processes
- to give citizens and individuals the opportunity to engage in these innovation processes
- to create opportunities for a dynamic region where boundary-crossing cooperation becomes usual in the change processes on all levels from product development to community building.

The project was carried out in an interactive manner in cooperation among citizens, companies, and authorities. Here, this meant local universities, municipalities, and private SME companies, as well as citizens. All of these partners brought valuable knowledge and expertise into the project. The universities brought knowledge about user-centric methods for design; the municipalities contributed with the situation as such, and with visions on how they would like the interaction with citizens to be; the SMEs brought the technical know-how to the project; and the citizens contributed their stories about how they interacted with public authorities today and how they would like to interact.

The citizens' participating in the project was heterogeneous in character, with a blend of ages, gender, civil status, and occupation. The citizens were between 18–50 years old, and there were 11 men and 13 women. The participants were selected from the Living Lab community based on where they lived, their age, gender, and occupation. The aim of the heterogeneous group was that, to some extent, they should represent a broad range of citizens. Diverse groups also have the benefit of generating mixed perspectives that challenge the statue quo and presents alternative ways of viewing situations.

The technology should facilitate the possibility for citizens to interact and communicate with public authorities when a need occurred, independent of time or space. Based on this, it was decided to explore and develop the concept of "reaction media." It also was decided that the service should be able to run on both mobile and stationary devices.

To gain understanding of the potential users and their situations, focus group interviews were used as the main data-collection method. In this study, five focus group interviews, each with four to six citizens, were carried out, as well as one individual interview. These focus group interviews lasted between one to two hours. The focus of the interviews was to discuss citizen's experiences and thoughts related to communication with municipalities and governments.

The stimulus material we used in these focus groups was scenarios related to communication with authorities, alarm, and suggestions for improvement of society. Whenever the focus group discussion stopped, we introduced a new theme or question.

From the user stories, needs were generated and translated into requirements for designing the prototype. It is the design team's role to develop concepts, mock-ups, or prototypes that incorporate the needs of the users. This does not mean that users cannot participate in this work; it is meant as a clarification of the different knowledge assets held by different roles and where their responsibilities lie (Bergvall-Kåreborn et al. 2008).

In this project, no evaluation of the prototype took place, since we were unable to recruit the necessary number of users to conduct a relevant test; this was despite a number of recruitment activities. We decided not to recruit citizens from the Living Lab community since these people have a bias toward technology-interested people, early adopters, and a willingness to influence situations. They also had participated in questionnaires and focus group interviews in the beginning of the project, and we wanted people who were new to the project and its ideas. Therefore, we advertised for test people in the local newspapers three times, but despite this repeated effort we only managed to recruit about ten people. Therefore, we decided not to have a regular evaluation; instead, we did an internal test within the project.

The result of the project was a well functioning prototype for a system in which citizens could enter a Web portal and give suggestions for improvements or alert hazardous situations. The portal could be entered either via mobile phones or PCs. However, it never was implemented at the municipalities. The reasons for this never were investigated. But, a simpler version of the concept was developed and implemented about a year later. Even though this might not be seen as a success story, it is our experience that it represents quite a standard illustration of many development projects. Studies indicate that only 15 percent of companies' development time is invested in products that reach the market (Feurstein et al. 2008).

REFLECTING ON KEY PRINCIPLES

In this section, we discuss and reflect on how the Living Lab principles relates to key components in the SMART case.

Openness

The principle of openness emphasises that the innovation process should be as open as possible. The idea is that multiple perspectives bring power to the development process and achieve rapid progress. The openness supports the process of user-driven innovation.

In the SMART project, many different stakeholders participated and each had an agenda and perspective. The weakest link in the partnership was the municipalities. Though they were positive about the project and its endeavour, they did not participate operationally in the project. This can be one important reason why the system never was implemented into their organisation. Hence, the SMART project points to the importance to have both strategic and operational commitment among key stakeholders.

In relation to the last part of the principle, that inclusion of many different stakeholder perspectives supports the process of user-driven innovation, we want to offer a world of warning. It is important to recognise that inclusion of multiple stakeholders does not guarantee a user-driven innovation process.

A lesson learnt from the SMART project, as well as from earlier projects, is that openness is easier said than done. This is true on many different levels. Firstly, the evaluation phase in our project clearly illustrated that citizens do not join automatically just because we want them to or ask them to do so. This always has been the case, but in voluntary use situations it becomes even more noticeable. In work settings, participating in development projects often is part of the work role, but no such driving force exists in relation to systems developed for private use.

When it comes to actually listening to the citizens and taking their ideas into consideration, the project managed very well, and most of the generated needs were included in the final design of the system. This can be related both to an openness in the design team for this way of working and to the nature of FormIT. FormIT's framework of ideas strengthens this way of working—AI, through its appreciative nature, SST though its focus on diverse perspectives as a way to challenge present frames of thought, and needfinding, with its focus on understanding users and their needs. The openness principle therefore is related closely to the empowerment principle, as we will indicate when we discuss this principle.

Realism

Realism is one of the principles that clearly separates Living Lab from traditional systems development as well as other kinds of open co-creation environments, such as Second Life. The principle highlights the necessity to facilitate realistic use situations and behaviour as much as possible in order to generate results that are valid for real markets.

Understanding the citizens and their interaction with public authorities was difficult, since there was no clear and limited application environment. It would have been possible to observe them in their real-world environment but, considering the limited amount of interaction that most people have with public authorities, this would have required long observation cycles and very patient citizens. An alternative would have been to focus on people visiting public authorities, but this would generate understanding only of single and isolated encounters, and we wanted a systemic view of people's relationship with these authorities. Hence, we carried out our appreciative user study in traditional ways: meeting for focus group interviews in easily accessible locations.

To set them in a real-world mode, we presented a number of scenarios and asked the focus groups to relate to these and reflect on how they thought they would behave in similar situations.

Another important aspects related to realism, but not specifically addressed by the principle is the fact that different stakeholders view reality different. This also is one often mentioned reason why it is crucial to involve users as well as many different stakeholders in the development process. Instead of trying to understand someone, we should let people participate and tell their own stories, and learn form this.

Influence

The key element of the influence principle is to base innovations on humans' needs and desires, and to utilise the creative power of user communities. Influence and empowerment of users is also a key characteristic in FormIT, and it is visible in many different ways. Firstly, users and other stakeholders are seen as partners in the innovation process, not just as co-designers, which is common in most systems development projects. Inherent in being a partner, from an end-user perspective, is the power of choice. People can choose if, when, and to what extent they want to participate.

Secondly, including potential end-users guarantees participation and facilitates involvement. However, in our view, influence is the key element and this is assess based on the exten to which user needs and ideas can be traceable in the concepts, prototype, and finished product. Not the extent to which users have participated in meetings. FormIT's iterative process between phases and between cycles makes it possible for users to judge whether their participation and involvement contributed to and influenced key deliverables.

As was said in relation to openness, the citizens had influence over the final system. Their needs and suggestions were taken seriously and implemented as functions and features in the prototypes and final system. However, as is often the case, they had influence because the partners kept open minds and wanted to base the solution on real user needs rather than on their own predetermined views of what citizens like.

The technical system as such also aimed to empower citizens by giving them the possibility to influence their municipality. But, when we look at the system that actually was implemented, this system was less empowering. Here, the citizens were not able to give suggestions about what they prioritised as important; instead, the system only allowed input on issues that the municipality selected as important to get feedback on. Hence, it is important to have an open discussion with all stakeholders on what empowerment represents. Is it the freedom to set a boundary or to give comments within an already defined boundary. Our view is that empowerment requires the possibility to set boundaries.

REFLECTING ON KEY COMPONENTS

In this section we alter the perspective and reflect on how the key components express themselves in practice. Starting with the partners and users, we found that the user community is one crucial asset and that it is important that these communities represent the mixture that reflects the surrounding society. However, these user communities have a tendency to be biased toward technically mature and curious people who like to have influence on societal changes. In the SMART study, we acknowledged the biased population and aimed to recruit users who were not involved actively in the community. However, we found it difficult to recruit users who did not have biases, since these are personal characteristics that make them eager to contribute to these processes. Looking at the partnership in a Living Lab we have found that it is important to have a mixture of large, medium, and small organisations as well as long and short term partnerships. As with the user community, diversity in the kind of partners that contribute to the Living Lab is positive from a development and innovation perspective since they can bring different opportunities, resources, and, experiences to the collaboration.

When it comes to research it was rather difficult to carry out appreciative user studies in a real-world setting since the situation we aimed to study was a relatively small and seldom occurring part of the citizens everyday life. In the project we were, therefore, not able to carry out the need generation phase in the real-world situation of the citizens. Instead, we facilitated discussions focused on their interaction and reflection on their real world experience related to the SMART-application. This indicates the need for mobile tools that empower the citizens and give them the opportunity to express their thoughts, experiences, and ideas regardless of where and when they arise.

In relation to technology and infrastructure we have found that technological support constitutes one focal point for user interaction in Living Labs. In Botnia, the user community is one important place where potential users can be accessed easily. However, having a large user community also includes the necessity to create enough activities to keep the users active and motivated to participate, yet at the same time not overload them. From an empowerment perspective, the user community is more geared toward information to users. Further, communication and interaction is initiated from Botnia and its needs rather than from the user community and its needs. Hence, to facilitate empowerment for the users, a more balanced relationship needs to be established. To make this community even more heterogeneous, it is important to create cooperation between

individual Living Labs in the European Network of Living Labs (ENOLL).

The approach of Living Lab can differ quite a lot depending on the nature of the other Living Lab components. For example, influence of users or openness is always important but they can take many different forms. In our study we used the FormIT methodology and found that it harmonized well with the basic idea of Living Labs. It is open and facilitates empowerment of users. However, its week point is in relation to realism. Here we find that there still is much work to be done before the process actually meets the vision of truly taking place in the users' real-world contexts throughout the whole innovation process, as well as being truly user-driven.

Management of a Living Lab involves all the traditional management aspects of any organisation but also adds some specific challenges. The question of ownership is one such issue. Because, even though a Living Lab is a network of organisations there is usually one organisation that hosts the Living Lab and this organisation becomes something of a front figure for the Lab. For Botnia Living Lab it is Centrum for Distance-Spanning Technology at Luleå University of Technology that hosts the Living Lab. This means that they provide the technical infrastructure, manages the partnerships, and is responsible for tactical planning and daily operations while a board of directors with industrial majority sets the strategic direction for the Living Lab. The constellation of the Living Lab partnership, intellectual property rights, and long term financial support are other important issues belonging to the management of a Living Lab.

FINAL REMARKS

In this chapter, we have presented a Living Lab environment called Botnia and a methodology called FormIT. We have reflected on how they correspond to key components and principles of Living Labs and how these components and principles can enrich each other.

Among the three principles, we find that it is within realism that we often lack the knowledge and experience to truly interact in the user's real-world environment throughout the whole development process. Considering that this principle also is the principle that distinguishes Living Labs from other open and user-centred approaches, it is important to gather more knowledge in this area. It also is important to gain deeper understanding of the relationship between the three principles of openness, influence, and realism in order to understand how they can strengthen each other in future development projects.

In relation to the key components we found that it is difficult to recruit representative user groups. Participating in the development of new technology attracts people with certain personal characteristics. In relation to the three components research, technology and infrastructure, and, approach we observe that it is the principle of realism that is hardest to achieve. One reason for this can be the shift in design context that is taking place, which, result in a lack of methods and tools that can support these new design contexts. When it comes to the management of a Living Lab it is important to have a mixture of stable and flexible partnerships, since the stable give continuity to the Lab while the more flexible partners contribute new perspectives and ideas.

Finally, based on the above discussion and final remarks we conclude that the key components of a Living Lab constitutes important structures that enhance the process and as such the key principles.

ACKNOWLEDGMENT

We thank the Swedish Foundation for Strategic Research and Vinnova - Research and Innovation for Sustainable Growth for supporting our work.

REFERENCES

Ballon, P., Pierson, J., & Delaere, S. (2005). Open Innovation Platforms for Broadband Services: Benchmarking European Practices. In *16th European Regional Conference, Porto, Portugal.*

Baskerville, R. L., & Wood-Harper, A. T. (1998). Diversity in Information Systems Action Research Methods. *European Journal of Information Systems, 7,* 90–107. doi:10.1057/palgrave.ejis.3000298

Baskerville, R. L., & Wood-Harper, T. A. T. (1996). A Critical Perspective on Action Research as a Method for Information Systems Research. *Journal of Information Technology, 11,* 235–246. doi:10.1080/026839696345289

Bekker, M., & Long, J. (2000). User Involvement in the Design of Human-Computer Interactions: Some Similarities and Differences between Design Approaches. In McDonald, S. & Cockton, G. (Eds.), *People and Computers XiV: Proceedings of the HCI 2000* (pp. 135-147). New York: Springer.

Bergvall-Kåreborn, B., Holst, M., & Ståhlbröst, A. (2008). Creating a New Leverage Point for Information Systems Development. In Avital, M., Boland, R., & Cooperrider, D. (Eds.), *Designing Information and Organizations with a Positive Lens* (pp. 75–95). Oxford, UK: Elsevier Science /JAI Press.

Bergvall-Kåreborn, B., Ihlström Eriksson, C., Rudström, Å., Svensson, J., Ståhlbröst, A., & Åkesson, M. (2009a). *Clarifying the Living Lab Concept.* Luleå, Sweden: Luleå University of Technology.

Bergvall-Kåreborn, B., Ihlström Eriksson, C., Ståhlbröst, A., & Svensson, J. (2009b). A Milieu for Open Innovation - Defining Living Lab. In Huizingh, Conn, K. R. E., Torkkeli, S., & Bitran, M (Eds.). *Proceedings of the 2nd ISPIM Innovation Symposium,* New York.

Brandel, M. (2008). CROWD SOURCING: Are You Ready to Ask the World for Answers? *Computerworld, 42*(10), 24–26.

Checkland, P. B. (1981). *Systems Thinking, Systems Practice.* Chichester, UK: John Wiley & Sons.

Checkland, P. B., Forbes, P., & Martin, S. (1990). Techniques in Soft Systems Practice Part 3: Monitoring and Control in Conceptual Models and in Evaluation Studies. *Journal of Applied Systems Analysis, 17*, 29–37.

Checkland, P. B., & Holwell, S. (1998). Action Research: Its Nature and Validity. *Systemic Practice and Action Research, 11*(1), 9–21. doi:10.1023/A:1022908820784

Chesbrough, H. (2003). *Open Innovation: The New Imperative for Creating and Profiting from Technology.* Cambridge, MA: Harvard Business School Press.

Chesbrough, H., & Appleyard, M. (2007). Open Innovation and Strategy. *California Management Review, 50*(1), 57–76.

Cooperrider, D. L., & Avital, M. (Eds.). (2004). *Advances in Appreciative Inquiry, Constructive Discourse and Human Organisation.* Oxford, UK: Elsevier.

Cooperrider, D. L., & Whitney, D. (2005). *Appreciative Inquiry - A Positive Revolution in Change.* San Francisco: Berrett-Koehler Publishers.

Cooperrider, D. L., Whitney, D., & Stavros, J. M. (2005). *Appreciative Inquiry Handbook,* San Francisco, SF: Berrett-Koehler Publishers.

CoreLabs. (2007). *Living Labs Roadmap 2007-2010: Recommendations on Networked Systems for Open User-Driven Research, Development and Innovation* (pp. 1–61). Open Document. Luleå, Luleå University of Technology, Centrum for Distance Spanning Technology.

Eriksson, M., Niitamo, V. P., & Kulkki, S. (2005). *State-of-the-art in Utilizing Living Labs Approach to User-centric ICT innovation - a European approach.* Finland: Centre of Distance Spanning Technology at Luleå University of Technology, Sweden, Nokia Oy, Centre for Knowledge and Innovation Research at Helsinki School of Economics.

Feurstein, K., Hesmer, A., Hribernik, K. A., Thoben, K. D., & Schumacher, J. (2008). Living Labs: A New Development Strategy . In Schumacher, J., & Niitamo, V. P. (Eds.), *European Living Labs - A New Approach for Human Centric Regional Innovation* (pp. 1–14). Berlin, DE: Wissenschaftlicher Verlag.

Følstad, A. (2008). Living Labs for Innovation and Development of Information and Communication Technology: A Literature Review. *The Electronic Journal for Virtual Organisations and Networks, 10*, 100–131.

Hempel, J. (2007). Tapping the Wisdom of the Crowd. *Business Week Online, 27.*

Holst, M., & Mirijamdotter, A. (2006). Framing Multi-Disciplinary Teams: Sense Making Through the POM-model. In A. Basden, A. Mirijamdotter, & S. Strijbos (Eds.), *12th Annual CPTS Working Conference - Integrating Visions of Technology* (pp. 111-131). Maarssen, The Netherlands.

Holst, M., & Ståhlbröst, A. (2006). Enriching the Process of Appreciating Needs with Storytelling. *International Journal of Technology . Knowledge and Society, 2*(4), 61–68.

Jönsson, S. (1991). Action Research. In H.-E. Nissen, H. K. Klein, & R. Hirschheim (Eds.) *Information Systems Research: Contemporary Approaches and Emergent Traditions* (pp. 371-396). Amsterdam, NL: North-Holland.

Kankainen, A., & Oulasvirta, A. (2003). Design Ideas for Everyday Mobile and Ubiquitous Computing Based on Qualitative User Data. In N. Carbonell, & Stephanidis (Eds.), *User Interface for All* (LNCS 2615, pp. 458-464).

Markopoulos, P., & Rauterberg, G. W. M. (2000). Living Lab: A White Paper. IPO Annual Progress Report (pp. 53-65).

Mirijamdotter, A., Somerville, M. M., & Holst, M. (2006). An Interactive and Iterative Evaluation Approach for Creating Collaborative Learning Environments. [EJISE]. *The Electronic Journal of Information Systems Evaluation, 9*(2), 83–92.

Norum, K. E. (2001). Appreciative Design. *Systems Research and Behavioral Science, 18*(4), 323–333. doi:10.1002/sres.427

Patnaik, D., & Becker, R. (1999). Needfinding: The Why and How of Uncovering People's Needs. *Design Management Journal, 10*(2), 37–43.

Schaffers, H., Cordoba, M., Hongistro, P., Kallai, T., Merz, C., & Rensburg, J. (2007). Exploring Business Models for Open Innovation in Rural Living Labs. In *Proceedings of the 13th International Conference on Concurrent Enterprising* (pp. 49-56). Sophia-Antipolis, France.

Shami, T. A. (2008). Living Labs: Good Practices in Europe . In Schumacher, J., & Niitamo, V. P. (Eds.), *European Living Labs - A New Approach for Human Centric Regional Innovation* (pp. 15–30). Berlin, DE: Wissenschaftlicher Verlag.

Ståhlbröst, A. (2004). Exploring the Testbed Field. In *27th Information Systems Research Seminars in Scandinavia, IRIS 27*, Falkenberg, Sweden.

Ståhlbröst, A. (2008). *Forming Future IT - The Living Lab Way of User Involvement*. Department of Business Administration and Social Sciences. PhD Thesis. Luleå, Luleå University of Technology, Sweden.

Ståhlbröst, A., & Bergvall-Kåreborn, B. (2008). FormIT - An Approach to User Involvement . In Schumacher, J., & Niitamo, V. P. (Eds.), *European Living Labs - A New Approach for Human Centric Regional Innovation* (pp. 63–76). Berlin, DE: Wissenschaftlicher Verlag.

Ståhlbröst, A., & Holst, M. (2006). Appreciating Needs for Innovative IT Design. *International Journal of Knowledge . Culture and Change Management, 6*(4), 37–46.

Tiitta, S. (2003). Identifying elderly people's needs for communication and mobility. *Include 2003*.

Von Hippel, E. (1986). Lead User: A Source of Novel Product Concepts. *Management Science, 32*(7), 791–805. doi:10.1287/mnsc.32.7.791

Von Hippel, E., & Katz, R. (2002). Shifting Innovation to Users via Toolkits. *Management Science, 48*(7), 821–833. doi:10.1287/mnsc.48.7.821.2817

NOTE

This chapter is a modified version of a previously published paper. Bergvall-Kåreborn, B. and Ståhlbröst, A. 2009. "Living Lab: An Open and Citizen-Centric Approach for Innovation," *International Journal of Innovation and Regional Development* (1:4), pp. 356-370.

Section 4
ICT in Work Life
and Private Life:
Organisational and Psychosocial Aspects

Chapter 17
ICT Tools and Transform in Work:
From Computer Supported Work to Knowledge Work

Eila Järvenpää
Aalto University School of Science and Technology[1], Finland

Stina Immonen
Aalto University School of Science and Technology[2], Finland

ABSTRACT

In this chapter, we consider ICT (information and communication technologies) as a tool that has significantly changed our work. We deal with the relationship between work and ICT, and changes in work due to the development of ICT, and their relationship with worker well-being and stress. Our aim is to consider major trends in research starting from studies about office work and computers and ending up to the use of ICT in knowledge work. We cover mainly a period from 1970's to the end of 2000's. Our main interest is on various types of information and knowledge processing work where implementation of new tools has clearly followed the general development of ICT solutions. The scope of the chapter is in the transition from traditional office work towards knowledge work from the viewpoint of worker well-being. Our research questions are 1) what connections and research trends can be identified between ICT supported work and stress and well-being at work and 2) what is the role and connection of ICT on knowledge work. Based on our literature study from electronic databases surprisingly few research articles focussing on ICT's role on knowledge worker wellbeing or knowledge work as such were found. Only a surprisingly small fraction of the research concerning ICT or tools seems to integrate relations between technology, work and worker well-being. However, we know much about the physiological or psychological reactions of the use of VDT (visual display units) applications. This relatively narrow, even if important focus is not enough for workplace and job designers' knowledge accumulation and exploitation. There is a risk that new researcher generations are maturing without being aware of the rich Northern European and German research tradition in developing the quality of work life. Thus, the existing body of knowledge is not fully exploited anymore. This also challenges our university teaching.

DOI: 10.4018/978-1-60960-057-0.ch017

INTRODUCTION

From the early stages of mankind people have used tools to conduct their tasks whether concerning their immediate survival in the environment or preparing tools for the forecasted needs. Designing, producing and utilising these primitive, simple tools took most likely place within relatively closed, small communities. At the same time, the designer, manufacturer and user of the tool was the same person or a member of her/his family. In other words, the connection between the tool designer, maker, and user was seamless, and the purpose and requirements of the tool were well understood. The key concept of the design, even if not explicated, must have been functionality, and the best available know-how was taken in use both during the design and production process and in the final use of the ready made tool. Learning by imitating and doing, repeating successful processing methods, and later on using language and visuals to pass on traditions e.g. about most value-adding and usable tools, have been powerful means of sharing existing and creating new knowledge.

The Legacy of Industrialism

Most of these archaic fundaments we can still relate to our current and future working life but at the same time something has also dramatically changed. Western industrial history shows how planning and designing, manufacturing and usage of products were in the name of efficiency separated from each other. Grounds for this industrial philosophy were set in Taylorism, and the mass production concept together with standardization of work, tools and methods by Fordism only reinforced 'the one fits all thinking' in designing working tools and methods, managing work, leading organisations, and even in fulfilling customers' needs. Since early 1900 on, the Western working life has been influenced by the legacy of Taylor and Ford, only the modern applications

of their management and production philosophies may appear slightly modified from the original ones. However, even if the need for standardised, physical human labour has significantly decreased, and the demand of non-routine, highly skilled knowledge work has increased, our management systems and leadership paradigms still overly rely on the world view of tangible, measurable work performance and controllable workers. Technological advancements from mechanisation to automation and information digitalization have emancipated us from repetitive, routine-based, often also from physical labour. We argue though, that most of the design of modern tools, methods and processes takes place too far from the actual workers. Only recently open source software development and crowd sourcing have brought the end-users closer or even into the core of ICT (information and communication technology) tool design and programming. We can still question, if we have really taken into account the nature of current work in designing and implementing the numerous amount of various ICT solutions and information systems. Often users become frustrated when ICT doesn't support their work flow, disrupts working and thinking processes, and in some cases even destroys output of several hours' work due to "computer crash" or errors in computer programs. However, already in studies conducted in 1970s working with computers was shown to cause stress to users.

The Ambiguous Nature of Knowledge Work

In knowledge work, the relationship between knowledge workers, their context-specific work content and ICT tools and methods used to complete the tasks can be argued to be especially complex and complicated. Skill requirements are usually high, and learning of new skills is continuous. For example, Järvenpää and Immonen (2002) have differentiated knowledge work from information work based on the level of processing knowledge and information in the work. Knowledge work involves with high expertise with creative problem solving, ability to abstract thinking and analytical skills. Knowledge work processes and refines information and knowledge into more value adding form of knowledge. Information work rely more on routines of editing, manipulating and transferring the content.

In general, knowledge work, as one dimension of work, means working from and with predominantly abstract, even theoretic knowledge. We need to understand the job content of knowledge work to be able to design and implement proper ICT tools for knowledge workers. However, in reality, ICT tools are usually designed for general use, not for a specific knowledge work. In addition, there are different kinds of knowledge works, and thus different kinds of ICT tools are needed for communication and knowledge sharing both on individual, team and organizational levels.

Our Aim and Research Questions

In this chapter, we deal with changes in work in relation to ICT development, and especially the relationships between ICT and recognition of knowledge work, taking into account worker well-being and stress. Our aim is to consider major trends in research starting from studies about office work and working with computers and ending up to the use of ICT in knowledge work. We cover mainly a period from 1970's to the end of 2000's. Our main interest is on information processing work where implementation of new tools has clearly followed the general development of ICT solutions from large computer systems to micro computers (work stations and personal computers (PC) with video or visual display units (VDT) and to current mobile technologies (portable wireless devices, local area networks, the Internet etc.).

The focus of our chapter is in the transition of research from office work towards knowledge work in relation to ICT application, taking into account research on worker well-being and stress.

We will discuss how research on computer supported information processing work has developed as such and especially related to worker stress and well-being (and job satisfaction) at work. Thus, our research questions are

- What connections and research trends can be identified between ICT related work and well-being and stress at work in different periods of time?
- What is the role and connection of ICT on knowledge work?

We will concentrate on the major trends in research on relationship between different work types and ICT applications especially from well-being and stress point of view. We are interested in the development and change in research focus related to ICT and its connections to changes in work, from information processing work to knowledge work.

Accordingly, we are interested in how much and in what ways researchers have dealt with these issues. Finally, we shall draw conclusions on what still seem to be "the blind spots" in our understanding about the nature of knowledge work and work-related wellbeing of knowledge workers.

INFORMATION AND COMMUNICATION TECHNOLOGY AND KNOWLEDGE WORK

Fritz Machlup is recognised to be the first who identified knowledge industry and information work in his 1962 published book 'The Production and Distribution of Knowledge in the United States' (Martin 1999). Machlup's book is dated to the rise of the information society concept emphasising a shift in the economy from the production of goods to the production and distribution of information. Martin (ibid.) shows a growth of 100 milliards of dollars (measured in 1992 dollars) in ICT investment during two decades' period, from

25 milliards in 1970 to 125 milliards in 1992 in the United States. From the mid 1990s, the expenditure on ICT products - namely on information technology equipment such as computers and related hardware, communication equipment as well software - has on average varied between 15 to 20 percent of each OECD country's gross fixed capital formation (excluding residential construction). OECD Factbook 2009 states that software has been the fastest growing component of ICT investment.

"...In many countries, its [software] share in non-residential investment multiplied several times between 1980s and 2006. In 2007, software's share in total investment is highest in the United States, the United Kingdom, Sweden, Finland, Denmark and France." (OECD 2009, p.174)

ICT Applications and Information Processing

According to Martin (1999), there are at least three explanations why investment in ICT has grown since 1970's. First, Martin (1999) refers to Beniger's[3] (1986) argument of 'crisis of control', where the ability to move goods exceeded the ability to track the movement of those goods. Complex information streams about products and markets demanded better information processing technologies. Second, the low productivity of the information processing sector focussed the interest in improving the efficiency of electronic information technologies. Referring to Jonscher (1983), the rate of efficiency improvement in information processing (essentially white-collar) work was historically much slower than in production work. Introducing new data processing, communication and storage technologies changed this pattern. Finally, Martin refers to Garnham[4] (1990) arguing that information has become the latest commodity goods in the need to find new

markets and thereby information is now gathered, quantified and priced.

Modern ICT is a versatile mixture of hardware and software equipment and services (Andriessen 2003). It includes telecommunication infrastructures, e.g. networks of cable or mobile systems, satellites, etc., data-transport services, e.g. telephone net, data net, telematic services, i.e. value adding services such as WWW, videotext, more or less intelligent terminals: telephone, computer, applications, both for stand-alone and for interactive purposes, such as word processors, e-mail applications and video-conferencing. In this chapter, we are especially interested in ICT applications that are used in demanding information processing work. These applications usually are such as VDT (visual display units), office automation/word processing, calculation systems, CAD systems, intranet, internet, data mining, collaboration technologies, and social media. Collaboration technology refers to ICT applications that support communication, co-ordination, co-operation, learning and/or social encounters through facilities such as information exchange, shared repositories, discussion forums and messaging (Andriessen 2003). New media or social media refers to web-based services, e.g. blogging, Wikis, social networking sites (Hearn et al., 2008).

ICT applications especially for managing knowledge include a variety of different kinds of tools and systems for knowledge acquisition, knowledge processing, knowledge/idea creation, sharing of tacit and explicit knowledge, knowledge storing (databases, intranet), and communication. These applications can be divided into systems and tools reflecting their functions in human knowledge processes such as supporting knowledge dissemination, knowledge acquisition, or knowledge storing (Mäki et al., 2001, Toivonen et al. 2007). Knowledge dissemination refers to active transferring of knowledge to defined target groups using selected dissemination on point-to-point or point-to-many basis. Technologies like computer networks, real-time video conferencing, online data bases, and internet etc. distribute information both point-to-point and point-to-many.

Knowledge acquisition includes locating of knowledge, access to knowledge needed, as well as tools for processing acquired knowledge. Again, applications are many e.g. from office tools, search engines and management information systems to social media. In knowledge storing existing information is organized and stored in e.g. electronic databases and interlinked Web pages. Naturally, many of above mentioned applications are used for more than just one function in knowledge processes.

Definitions of Different ICT Related Work Types

Office work, often referred as white-collar work, is a general term for clerical work covering both professional and semi-professional personnel e.g. from engineers to journalists, judges and scientists or from bookkeepers to travel agents. Typically, it is or at least to its major part, non manual desk work requiring special education and updated skills in using computerized technology. Office work can be both mentally and physically demanding consisting not only of VDT work such as data entry, data control, word processing, data searching and reading documents (Vink and Kompier, 1997) but also interaction with internal and external customers of the work. According to Seppälä (2001) many studies on VDT work have shown that physical and mental wellbeing in computer-based office work is related to ergonomic features of the workstation, illumination and glare, job content and task variety, hours and intensity of working with video display unit, time pressure and workload, computer skills, age, gender and educational level.

Computer or computer-based work refers to jobs involving mentally demanding tasks, usually using complex routines with high demands on working memory and problem solving (e.g. Sharit et al. 1998). Cook and Salvendy (1999, p.

14) describe computer-based work with following characteristics:

• conceptual work tasks are modelled in computer software,
• core work tasks are contained in computer memory, interface designs allow "physical realisation" of work tasks and job organisation,
• task organisation is not constrained by physical attributes of work tasks,
• task demands are primarily cognitive and physical demands are limited to data entry and manipulation of devices.

These characteristics fit for computer tasks both in industry and office environment. Typically, these are jobs with tasks of data entry, information retrieval or use of graphical user interface with no other accessory materials (Sharit ibid.).

Information Work

Information work is historically connected to library and information science meaning those services librarians have provided to their customers in their information needs. However, as already discussed, the rapidly grown investment in ICT has also meant increase of information processing occupations which can be named as information work. Martin (1999) describes this, referring to Susan Zuboff, development where tasks have been 'carved out' of higher, more skilled positions creating occupations where more routine and less body of knowledge are required to perform them. Following Fritz Machlup's conceptual scheme about information work from 1962, Martin (ibid.) categorises the following as routine information occupations consisting of highly codified and rule-bound activities:

• transporter (delivers exactly what is received),

- transformer (changes the form but not the content of the information) and
- processor (changes both form and content of the information by routine procedures)

Knowledge Work

Knowledge work as a concept was popularized and legitimized already in the late 1960s (Bell 1968, Drucker 1969). Nevertheless, Kelloway and Barling (2000, p. 5-8) argue that there is still little consensus to what constitutes knowledge work. They find at least three thematic definitions of knowledge workers. First, knowledge work has been defined as a profession. Second, knowledge work has been described as an individual characteristic. Finally, knowledge work has been defined as an individual activity.

Knowledge work as a profession follows the scheme of Martin's (1999) and Machlup's categorisations. Here, three types of higher level information work, the non-routine information occupations involve non-codified or non-rule bound activities like creativity, synthesis, and meaning making. These work types Martin (1999) describes as

- interpreter (changes form and contents of information and uses imagination to create in the new form effects equivalent to those he feels were intended by the original message),
- analyser (uses own judgement and intuition in addition to accepted procedures so that the original information can barely be recognised) and
- original creator (draws on a rich store of information, adds his own inventive genius and creative imagination so that only relatively weak and indirect connections to the original can be found).

Knowledge work as an individual characteristic refers to the creation of value, or being innovative

rather than incumbency in a particular position. This sets up two 'classes' of workers: those who display creativity and those who don't. Knowledge work as an individual activity defines knowledge work in terms of the balance between "thinking" and "doing" activities. This approach sets focus on behavior, on what employees do on their day-to-day activities.

The currently dominant view on knowledge work conceptualizes it as involving the intensive and exclusive use of predominantly abstract, theoretical knowledge (Hislop 2008). Kelloway and Barling (2000) suggest that knowledge work should be viewed as one dimension of work. While all work to some extent involves the use of knowledge, knowledge work can be defined as work which is characterized primarily by the application of knowledge rather than physical effort. Thus, knowledge workers work from knowledge and with knowledge (Scarbrough 1999), transforming the objects of their work into symbolic form while maintaining the systems and tools which they employ (e.g. Pyöriä 2005).

MATERIAL AND METHODS

To answer our research questions about 1) the connections and research trends between different types of ICT related work types and well-being and stress at work in different periods of time, and 2) what is the role and connection of ICT in knowledge work we conducted a systematic literature study as follows. First, we used Google Scholar search engine to illustrate the general research interest in different types of office and knowledge work in different time periods (see Table 1). We used article titles as the search criteria with exact phrases such as "office work", "knowledge work", "computer work", "information work", "virtual work", "telework", "mobile work" and "digital work" as search words in business and social sciences related data. The phrases used were selected as they indicate different types and

Table 1. Amount of Google Scholar results with different types of information processing work (search done 30 June 2009). Google Scholar covers peer-reviewed articles, theses, books, abstracts, and other scholarly literature of research including also multiple versions of them published in English. The search was conducted using the exact phrases.

Work types as	Amount of results						
exact search phrases*	-1979	1980-1984	1985-1989	1990-1994	1995-1999	2000-2004	2005-2009
Office work	4490	840	1250	1660	2560	4360	5460
Computer work	511	314	523	669	1240	1880	1610
Information work	687	402	572	651	1210	1770	1480
Telework	2	2	48	81	311	350	116
Knowledge work	169	92	170	381	1420	4030	4750
Virtual work	99	20	24	47	320	940	847
Mobile work	76	31	61	125	208	478	505
Digital work	2	3	8	18	133	489	813
TOTAL	6036	1704	2656	3632	7402	14297	15581

*Search in business, administration, finance, economics, social sciences, arts and humanities in Google Scholar.

Table 2. Number of search results from different scientific data bases (search done 30.6-7.7. 2009). The search was focused on only article/content item title with the search phrase office work, knowledge work, computer work, information work or information and communication technology (ICT) combined with one of the following: wellbeing/well-being, stress or stressors, job content/demand/characteristic/ satisfaction and tools. Period of search was limited from 1986 to 2009. Search was not limited to any specific sciences within the data bases.

Search result from ABI Inform, Emerald, JSTOR, and ISI Web of Knowledge	Total* amount of found items	Stress or stressors in item title	Wellbeing or well-being in item title	Job content/ demand/ character-istic/ satisfaction in item title	Tools or technology in item title
Office work	110	3	0	2	1
Computer work	58	12	1	0	0
Information work	139	1	1	0	13
Knowledge work	171	0	0	0	5
IT or ICT**	7970	5	1	8	19

*The total amount equals to the number of items having one of the following work types in the title: office work, knowledge work, computer work, or information work.

**Both abbreviations IT and ICT as written versions such as information technology, information and communication technology were used.

nature of office work and knowledge work. Each search dealt with a five years' period.

Thereafter we conducted systematic literature searches in the following scientific literature data bases: ABI Informs, Emerald, JSTOR and ISI Web of Knowledge (see Table 2). We selected "office work", "knowledge work", "computer work", and "information work" as keywords of the content-related search based on the findings of the frequency of these work types in Google Scholar. The focus of the search was to find research articles discussing about the well-being of the workers and the role of ICT in the work. Again, as key words in the article title we used the following: stress, stressors, well-being or wellbeing, job satisfaction, technology and tools. All search results are dated from 30 June to 7 July 2009.

RESEARCH TRENDS ON RELATIONSHIP BETWEEN WORK AND ICT

Computerisation or office automation has unquestionable affected working environment, skill demands and job characteristics of (so called industrial blue-collar work as well as) office and expert white-collar work. Rapid technological advancements have also kept researchers interested in following the change in ICT related work. Table 1 shows some clear trends in the breakthrough points in prevalence of certain ICT related work types within academic community/or in research activities.

Office work has naturally been acknowledged already long before "computer time" as one of the ways of differentiating mainly mental work without significant physical labour from pure physical work. Interestingly, the phrase "office work" seems to have maintained its relevance throughout the decades, and maybe only in the most recent years it has been losing its dominating position to knowledge work.

Entering the new millennium shows a clear growth in scientific publications about knowledge work measured by Google Scholar. It is notable, though that the breakthrough (from 380 hits to 1400 hits) of the concept of knowledge work took place already in the mid 90's, it was surprisingly late considering the origins of the concept many decades earlier. Interest towards computer work started to grow already in mid 80's but only in the mid 90's both computer work and information work clearly doubled their publication amounts. Conceptualising and studying information work is one manifestation of a commonly accepted phenomenon reflecting information society. Later in 2000, the usage of computer and information work has consolidated on the equal amounts being still clearly smaller in volume than office or knowledge work but more than virtual, mobile or digital work. To conclude, it seems that the mobile, digital as well as virtual work have established themselves to academic writing, but maybe the real rise of these is still to come. Meanwhile, the concept of telework has clearly lost its attractiveness as a description of ICT related work type.

Research Connecting Work Types, Well-Being and Tools

For determining the focus of a research article we used the item's title as the most concentrated form of the content of the publication. In other words, if one hand, none of the computer aided work types was mentioned in the title, the articles were interpreted to have their focus on something else than identifying or understanding more about information processing work types as such. On the other hand, if information or communication technology or both were mentioned in the title, this technology could be also related to the work as such or to workers' wellbeing. Table 2 shows that according to selected scientific data bases information and communication technology indeed has drawn much attention in scientific research and writing (about 8000 items since 1986) but examples of having both the work type and technology in the same title are surprisingly few (about 20 articles since 1986).

Office Work

The only article title combining office work and tools (Table 2) was from the subject area of geriatrics and gerontology dealing with screening tools for streamlining initial assessment of the geriatric patient. These screens can quickly identify signs of delirium, dementia, depression, and adverse drug effects; vision and hearing deficits; risk for future impairments in activities of daily living; incontinence, and malnutrition (Sherman 2001) and thus facilitate the reporting work of the nursing personnel.

The articles about office work in relation to worker wellbeing dealt with factors of work environment such as heat and noise, or work with VDTs concentrating mainly on musculoskeletal discomfort and eyestrain (Seppälä 2001, Witterseh et al. 2004). As Table 2 shows, office work is not that much used in relation with stress or wellbeing neither with job satisfaction. The research has dealt office work mainly from viewpoints of ergonomics, human-computer interaction or worker experiences about implementing new technologies (Seppälä 2001).

Computer Work

Computer work or computer-based work has mainly been dealt with in connection to experienced stress or measured stress outcomes (Table 2). These articles relate either to physiology, psychology or ergonomics. Based on the article titles found from the selected data bases, two thirds of them concentrated on musculoskeletal or other bodily problems mainly due to visual or postural stressors. For example, all very recently conducted research by Hjortskov et al. (2004), Larsman et al. (2009), Mork (2007), Schleifer et al. (2008) or Treaster et al. (2006) suggest that the solutions

to stress related challenges in computer work are to be found from organising the work differently e.g. having sufficiently long rest periods during the working day. These authors did not question the content of the computer work, whether the job contents as such would be rich enough to provide sufficient variation in work activities during the work hours. The only article found about computer work and wellbeing (Henning et al. 1997) dealt the issue similarly, namely providing evidence that frequent short breaks from continuous computer-mediated work can benefit worker productivity and wellbeing.

Information Work

Information work has most often been related either to tools or technology (Table 2). As expected, majority of the found items relates to information science, library science or information systems. These articles deal with tools such as wikis to be used in librarian work. The few exceptions from this line of research were from subject areas of management or applied psychology. For example, Hempel (2004) discusses the direct and indirect effects of technology on human resource management work pointing out that HR professions shift away from past administrative orientation towards more strategic development of the organisation. This transition requires from HR personnel new skills of mastering new technologies of human resource information systems and understanding of business and associated work processes of the organisation. Finally, only one article dealing with wellbeing and stress in information work was found. Van den Berg and Schalk (1997) studied how the concepts of Type A behaviour (e.g. having more negative emotional reactions during frustrating situations, reporting heavier subjective workloads than Type Bs), emotional wellbeing, work overload, and role-related stress are related. They studied office workers of a large insurance company, library and staffing organisation. Their results showed that role-related stress and work overload are important stress factors in information work. However, in their study, Type As are not more vulnerable to work overload than others. Thus, the researchers conclude that more studies should be directed at the causes of work overload and role ambiguity. They recommend that communication should be improved to solve the problems of role-related stress and experienced work overload.

Knowledge Work

We found no articles about knowledge work related to stress or wellbeing or any of the following: job content, job demand, job characteristics or job satisfaction (Table 2). It seems that the long tradition of job design and quality of working life has been ignored when dealing with more complex information processing work. However, knowledge work and tools or technology seems to be a more popular subject for research. Those articles we found discuss how to support knowledge work teams (e.g. Shani et al. 2000, Pyöriä 2005) or knowledge work (e.g. Schultze and Boland Jr. 2000, Linger 2006) with ICT. All these authors emphasise that in order to support the work practices they should be identified – both the content and context - and understood first.

As Pyöriä (2005) states, the role that technology can take is automation of routine work and if used properly it can indirectly contribute to creating more space for interpersonal interaction by eliminating routine communication. The article by Quinn (2005) deals with flow in knowledge work where technology was now the content of the work. He (ibid. p. 632) concludes that flow experience is connected to high-performance experience which is real and relevant phenomenon in knowledge work. Moreover, the degree to which people experience flow depends on the types of jobs and tasks as well as on the clarity and difficulty of their goals. He also continues that when people experience high performance,

they also tend to derive more joy from their work, feel like they have more control over their work.

Information and Communication Technology In Work

In our study, the number of those articles discussing information and communication technology in relation with stress or wellbeing, or even job satisfaction was higher than those trying to connect the technology to information processing activities in work (Table 2). Actually, in majority of the articles, IT or ICT were used as an attribute of work or occupational group, e.g. information technology project managers (Richmond and Skitmore 2006), information technology personnel (Kuo and Chen 2004), information technology workers (Lim 2008, McMurtrey et al. 2002), information technology employees (Reid et al. 2008), information technology professionals (Aziz 2004, Loh et al. 1995, Lounsbury et al. 2007, Raghavan et al. 2008) or consultants (Wallgren and Hanse 2007). In other words, the focus in this type of research is on particular ICT-related occupational groups and on their experienced stress or well-being. The research treats either ICT or the work as a "black box". How the technology is supporting or hindering workers in their work is a theme that is often excluded from the research setting.

Few of the found articles dealt with implementation of information technology (Korunka and Vitouch 1999, Salanova et al. 2004) and in few articles the authors discussed the implications of working with information technology (Arnetz, 1997, Engstrom et al. 2005). Korunka and Vitouch (1999) emphasise the importance of user interface design, user training, and user participation in the implementation process when new ICT tools are developed and applied for the work processes. Salanova et al. (2004) state that the technology implementation style in a company is more related to workers' subjective cognitive well-being (e.g. job satisfaction and role ambiguity) than to affective well-being (e.g. job related enthusiasm, job related comfort). Arnetz (1997) raises the issue of the risks of bodily, mental and psychophysiological reactions of employees using VDTs especially when the two-way interaction between ICT environment and the users has been ignored in the design. In Engstrom's et al. (2005) study ICT support was used in health care helping the nursing staff in monitoring the dementia patients. Here, the technology in use did not only increase the personnel's job satisfaction but also the quality of care.

Table 2 shows also articles that combine both ICT and tools in the article title. These articles deal with a wide variety of research themes of which at least three different categories were easily found. One category is articles presenting use of ICT tools in specific industry branches such as construction, health care, or aviation industry etc. Typically, the articles study the effectiveness and efficiency of ICT tools in some core processes of the production. The second type of articles deal with ICT tools in relation to training and education having the emphasis on facilitated learning. The third type is clearly an emerging category of articles that deal with ICT tools enhancing or facilitating communication in communities and participation to social media. Even if all these themes are highly relevant and interesting in our work life, they are not in the focus of our research interest in this article.

DISCUSSION

We conclude our main findings of this study as follows:

- ICT connected to information processing work is a research area attracting numerous researchers and producing a lot of publications. The amount of scientific items recognised by Google Scholar and published between 2000 and 2009 is larger than the amount of the publications of all the previous decades together.

- Knowledge work as a type of information processing work has matured its position as an identified work type while other work types such as computer work, information work, virtual work, mobile work and digital work are either loosing their attractiveness or still waiting for their breakthrough. Through out the decades, office work has remained in its stable, high positioning in the research agendas.

- Only a surprisingly small fraction of the research concerning information and communication technology or tools seems to deal with the relations between technology, work and worker well-being. Most commonly, these studies have concentrated on the physiological or psychological reactions of the use of VDT applications.

- ICT's role in the design and content of knowledge work and in the productivity and well-being of a knowledge worker seems still be undervalued or at least not much studied in work life related research and development.

The role of technology in information processing work seems to be very instrumental. Occupations and professions where large amounts of data need to be processed, complex information and knowledge from different sources need to be collected, combined and utilised, or new knowledge need to be created can without question benefit from advanced ICT. However, this notion has maybe led us to adopt a too technology-driven approach towards knowledge work. Even if we know much about, for example user-centered design and implementing technologies in work in general, we still seem to miss a clear focus on how knowledge work could be facilitated (not prohibited) with the technologies. This will need more context and content sensitive research in knowledge work practices, especially in how knowledge is acquired, shared, exploited and created. Only based on this kind of research knowledge we can design and develop tools that really help us in our information and knowledge processing work.

Traditionally researchers and developers from e.g. human factors and organisational behaviour disciplines have been interested to improve workers' performance, well-being and motivation by providing recommendations on how to design jobs, work environments and tools, or organisational support. When dealing with knowledge work, there is a risk that we "forget" to ask the same fundamental questions about individuals' work conditions and tools, task and role clarity, feedback and communication demands, autonomy or dependency on others, support from control and reward systems as we have done in job design of blue-collar work. The principles of healthy job contents and organisations are still very relevant and valid, of course. In the light of our study though, it is alarming that so few article items from electronic data bases were retrieved that would have raised the questions of knowledge workers' well-being and the role of ICT in their work. For new researcher and developer generations this might form a challenge to build a firm bridge between the existing context-sensitive knowledge of work and industrial psychology, and the emerging new work types and ways of working triggered by for example evolving IC-technology. In other words, there is a risk that new researcher generations are maturing without being aware of the rich Northern European and German research tradition in developing the quality of work life. Thus, the existing body of knowledge is not fully exploited anymore. This also challenges our university teaching.

While stating this we also acknowledge the several limitations of our study. First, our findings are strictly connected to our methodological choices. Using only a selection of scientific data bases and Google Scholar inherently restricts the outcome. We recognise that using only English words as key words and most importantly using only electronic data bases biases our results. The scientific journal based data bases used in this study do not include books, conference papers and conference publications, dissertations, or research reports published by research institutes and university departments. Thus, a lot of relevant studies are excluded in our analysis. Since we used only English key words, a lot of studies published in other languages are excluded. However, research on work life is published e.g. in Swedish, German, French or Finnish.

The publishing policy of the journals included in the data bases may affect our findings in terms of the number of articles found in data bases. The criteria for data and data analysis required in scientific journals may not fit with the research paradigms applied in work life research. In work life research, data is often collected in one or some organizations concentrating on certain office or knowledge work (and ICT tools used in work). Even if research in the research area may be comprehensive, the research findings are published in publications that are not included in the data bases we used.

Still, we emphasise that even if the absolute number of items we found might not be totally correct, our results illustrate the main stream trends in the research. And as knowledge workers, we also acknowledge the challenge of collating and compiling all the relevant information from the information oversupplied world. In this respect, this chapter may also serve as an example of an outcome of information technology driven study about knowledge work.

REFERENCES

Andriessen, J. (2003). *Working with Groupware: understanding and evaluating collaboration technology*. New York: Springer.

Arnetz, B. B. (1997). Technological stress: psychophysiological aspects of working with modern information technology. *Scandinavian Journal of Work, Environment & Health, 23*(3), 97–103.

Aziz, M. (2004). Role stress among women in the Indian information technology sector. *Women in Management Review, 19*(7), 356–363. doi:10.1108/09649420410563412

Bell, D. (1968). *The coming of post-industrial society: A venture in social forecasting.* New York: Basic Books Inc. Publishers.

Christensen, H., & Lundberg, U. (2002). Musculoskeletal problems as a result of work organization, work tasks and stress during computer work. *Work and Stress, 16*(2), 89–90. doi:10.1080/02678370213265

Cook, J. R., & Salvendy, G. (1999). Job enrichment and mental workload in computer-based work: Implications for adaptive job design. *International Journal of Industrial Ergonomics, 24,* 13–23. doi:10.1016/S0169-8141(98)00084-5

Drucker, P. F. (1969). *The age of discontinuity: Guidelines to our changing society.* New York: HarperCollins Publishers.

Engstrom, M., Ljunggren, B., Lindqvist, R., & Carlsson, M. (2005). Staff perceptions of job satisfaction and life situation before and 6 and 12 months after increased information technology support in dementia care. *Journal of Telemedicine and Telecare, 11*(6), 304–309. doi:10.1258/1357633054893292

Ezoe, S., Araki, S., Ono, Y., Kawakami, N., & Murata, K. (1993). Work stress in Japanese computer engineers: Effects of computer work or bioeducational factors? *Environmental Research, 63*(1), 148–156. doi:10.1006/enrs.1993.1136

Hearn, G., Foth, M., & Gray, H. (2008). Applications and implementations of new media in corporate communications. An action research approach. *Corporate Communications: An International Journal, 14*(1), 49–61. doi:10.1108/13563280910931072

Hempel, P. S. (2004). Preparing the HR profession for technology and information work. *Human Resource Management, 43*(2-3), 163–177. doi:10.1002/hrm.20013

Henning, R. A., Jacques, P., & Kissel, G. V. (1997). Frequent short rest breaks from computer work: Effects on productivity and well-being at two field sites. *Ergonomics, 40*(1), 78–91. doi:10.1080/001401397188396

Hislop, D. (2008). Conceptualizing knowledge work utilizing skill and knowledge-based concepts. *Management Learning, 39*(5), 579–596. doi:10.1177/1350507608098116

Hjortskov, N., Rissen, D., Blangsted, A. K., Fallentin, N., Lundberg, U., & Sogaard, K. (2004). The effect of mental stress on heart rate and blood pressure during computer work. *European Journal of Applied Physiology, 92*(1-2), 84–89. doi:10.1007/s00421-004-1055-z

Järvenpää, E., & Immonen, S. (2002). Tietointensiivisten organisaatioiden dynamiikka: Tietotyö, johtaminen ja organisaatioiden verkostot. Working paper no. 28/Work and organisational psychology. Helsinki University of Technology.

Jonscher, C. (1983). Information resources and economic productivity. *Information Economics and Policy, 1*(1), 13–35. doi:10.1016/0167-6245(83)90016-1

Kawakami, N., Roberts, C.R., & Haratani, T. (1995). Job stress characteristics of computer work in Japan. *Advances in Human Factors/Ergonomics, 20*(2), 705-710.

Kelloway, E. K., & Barling, J. (2000). Knowledge work as organizational behaviour. *International Journal of Management Reviews, 2*(3), 287–304. doi:10.1111/1468-2370.00042

Korunka, C., & Vitouch, O. (1999). Effects of the implementation of information technology on employees' strain and job satisfaction: a context-depemdent approach. *Work and Stress, 34*(4), 341–363.

Kuo, Y.-F., & Chen, L.-S. (2004). Individual demographic differences and job satisfaction among information technology personnel: an empirical study in Taiwan. *International Journal of Management, 21*(2), 221–231.

Larsman, P., Thorn, S., Sogaard, K., Sandsjo, L., Sjogaard, G., & Kadefors, R. (2009). Work related perceived stress and muscle activity during standardized computer work among female computer users. *Work – A Journal of Prevention Assessment and Rehabilitation, 32*(2), 189-199.

Lim, S. (2008). Job ssatisfaction of information technology workers in academic libraries. *Library & Information Science Research, 30*, 115–121. doi:10.1016/j.lisr.2007.10.002

Linger, H. (2006). Supporting collaborative knowledge work: A methodology for developing ICT tools for biomedical research. *Neural Networks, 3931*, 261–271.

Loh, L., Sankar, C. S., & Yeong, W. Y. (1995). Job orientation, perceptions, and satisfaction: a study of information technology professionals in Singapore. *Information & Management, 29*, 239–250. doi:10.1016/0378-7206(95)00022-X

Lounsbury, J. W., Moffitt, L., Gibson, L. W., Drost, A. W., & Stevens, M. (2007). An investigation of personality traits in relation to job and career satisfaction of information technology professionals. *Journal of Information Technology, 22*, 174–183. doi:10.1057/palgrave.jit.2000094

Mäki, E., Järvenpää, E., & Hämäläinen, L. (2001). Managing knowledge processes in knowledge intensive work. In *Proceedings of the 2nd ECKM 2001 - CA The 2nd European Conference on Knowledge Management*. Bled School of Management, Slovenia, November 8-9, 2001.

Martin, S. B. (1999). Employment in the information age. Information technology and information work. *The Journal of Policy . Regulation and Strategy for Telecommunications and Media, 2*(3), 271–283.

McMurtrey, M. E., Grover, V., Teng, J., & Lightner, N. (2002). Job satisfaction on information technology workers: the impact of career orientation and task automation in a case environment. *Journal of Management Information Systems, 9*(2), 273–302.

Mork, P. J., & Westgaard, R. H. (2007). The influence of body posture, arm movement, and work stress on trapezius activity during computer work. *European Journal of Applied Physiology, 101*(4), 445–456. doi:10.1007/s00421-007-0518-4

OECD. (2009). Investment in ICT. Science and technology. OECD Factbook. Retrieved March 5, 2010 from http://puck.sourceoecd.org/pdf/factbook2009/302009011e-07-02-02.pdf

Pyöriä, P. (2005). Information technology, human relations and knowledge work teams. *Team Performance Management, 11*(3/4), 104–112. doi:10.1108/13527590510606307

Quinn, R. (2005). Flow in knowledge work: high performance experience in the design of national security technology. *Administrative Science Quarterly, 50*(4), 610–641.

Raghavan, V. V., Sakaguchi, T., & Mahaney, R. (2008). An empirical investigation of stress factors in information technology professionals. *Information Resources Management Journal, 21*(2), 38–62.

Reid, M. F., Riemenschneider, C. K., Allen, M. W., & Armstrong, D. (2008). Information technology employees in state government – A study of affective organizational commitment, job involvement and job satisfaction. *American Review of Public Administration*, *38*(1), 41–61. doi:10.1177/0275074007303136

Richmond, A., & Skitmore, M. (2006). Stress and coping; a study of project managers in a large ICT organization. *Project Management Journal*, *37*(5), 5–16.

Salanova, M., Cifre, E., & Martin, P. (2004). Information technology implementation styles and their relation with workers' subjective well-being. *International Journal of Occupations and Production Management*, *24*(1), 42–54. doi:10.1108/01443570410510988

Scarbrough, H. (1999). Knowledge as Work: Conflicts in the Management of Knowledge Workers. *Technology Analysis and Strategic Management*, *11*(1), 5–16. doi:10.1080/095373299107546

Schleifer, L. M., Spalding, T. W., Kerick, S. E., Cram, J. R., Ley, R., & Hatfield, B. D. (2008). Mental stress and trapezius muscle activation under psychomotor challenge: A focus on EMG gaps during computer work. *Psychophysiology*, *45*(3), 356–365. doi:10.1111/j.1469-8986.2008.00645.x

Schultze, U., & Boland, R. J. Jr. (2000). Knowledge management technology and the reproduction of knowledge work practices. *The Journal of Strategic Information Systems*, *9*, 193–212. doi:10.1016/S0963-8687(00)00043-3

Seppälä, P. (2001). Experience of stress, musculoskeletal discomfort, and eyestrain in computer-based office work: A study in municipal workplaces. *International Journal of Human-Computer Interaction*, *13*(3), 279–304. doi:10.1207/S15327590IJHC1303_1

Shani, A. B., Sena, J., & Stebbing, M. W. (2000). Knowledge work teams and groupware technology: learning from Seagate's experience. *Journal of Knowledge Management*, *4*(2), 111–124. doi:10.1108/13673270010336602

Sharit, J., Czaja, S. J., & Nair, S. N. (1998). Subjective experiences of stress, workload, and bodily discomfort as a function of age and type of computer work. *Work and Stress*, *12*(2), 125–144. doi:10.1080/02678379808256855

Sherman, F. T. (2001). Functional assessment – Easy-to-use screening tools speed initial office work-up. *Geriatrics*, *56*(8), 36–40.

Toivonen, M., Smedlund, A., & Järvenpää, E. (2007). *The impacts of information technology on the stock of and flow of a firm's intellectual capital.* In L.A. Joia (Ed.), *Strategies for Information Technology and Intellectual Capital: Challenges and Opportunities* (pp. 111-126). Hershey: Information science reference.

Treaster, D., Marras, W. S., Burr, D., Sheedy, J. E., & Hart, D. (2006). Myofascial trigger point development from visual and postural stressors during computer work. *Journal of Electromyography and Kinesiology*, *16*(2), 115–124. doi:10.1016/j.jelekin.2005.06.016

Van den Berg, P. T., & Schalk, R. (1997). Type A behavior, well-being, work overload and role-related stress in information work. *Journal of Social Behavior and Personality*, *12*(1), 175–187.

Vink, P., & Kompier, M. A. J. (1997). Improving office work: a participatory ergonomic experiment in a naturalistic setting. *Ergonomics*, *40*(4), 435–449. doi:10.1080/001401397188071

Wallgren, L. G., & Johansson Hanse, J. (2007). Job characteristics, motivators and stress among information technology consultants: A structural equation modelling approach. *International Journal of Industrial Ergonomics*, *37*, 51–59. doi:10.1016/j.ergon.2006.10.005

Witterseh, T., Wyon, D. P., & Clausen, G. (2004). The effects of moderate heat stress and open-plan office noise distraction on SBS symptoms and on the performance of office work. *Indoor Air*, *14*(8), 30–40. doi:10.1111/j.1600-0668.2004.00305.x

ENDNOTES

[1] Former Helsinki University of Technology

[2] Former Helsinki University of Technology

[3] Beniger, J. (1986) The Control Revolution: Technological and Economic Origins of the Information Society. Harvard University Press. Cambridge, MA.

[4] Garnham, N. (1990) Capitalism and Communication: Global Culture and the Economics of Information. Sage, London.

Chapter 18
Sociotechnical Issues of Tele-ICU Technology

Peter Hoonakker
University of Wisconsin-Madison, USA

Kerry McGuire
University of Wisconsin-Madison, USA

Pascale Carayon
University of Wisconsin-Madison, USA

ABSTRACT

Intensive care units (ICUs) are highly complex organizations where lives are hanging by a thread. Approximately 400,000 to 500,000 people die each year in American ICUs. The highly complex environment and large responsibilities put a burden on ICU staff including physicians and nurses. Research has shown that ICU physicians and nurses report high levels of workload and burnout that are related to lower quality of care provided to ICU patients and patient safety problems. Furthermore, there is a shortage of ICU personnel. In the past decades, the number of critical care beds has increased while the number of hospitals offering critical care services has decreased. Telemedicine may be one solution to deal with the shortage of ICU personnel. The tele-ICU technology represents the application of telemedicine in ICUs: ICU patients are monitored remotely by physicians and nurses trained in critical care. Recent estimates show that a nurse in the tele-ICU environment can monitor as many as 50 ICU patients in different ICUs, using the most recent telemedicine technology that provides access to patient information as well as video and audio links to patient rooms. The physicians and nurses in the tele-ICU collaborate with the physicians and nurses in the ICUs in what can be considered virtual teams. We know little about how the virtual team characteristics affect communication and trust between the participating members of the team. Furthermore, we know little about how the technological environment of the tele-ICU may affect the physicians and nurses' workload and possibly burnout, and how this may affect quality of care and patient safety. In this chapter we describe the ICU and tele-ICU from a sociotechnical perspective, and examine how organizational factors may affect the jobs of nurses in the tele-ICU, and possible consequences for quality of work life, quality of care and patient safety.

DOI: 10.4018/978-1-60960-057-0.ch018

INTRODUCTION

The delivery of health care is going through major changes, including reduction of hospital stays and increasing severity of hospitalized patients. The provision of critical care provided to patients spread over large geographical regions such as the US or Australia has become increasingly difficult because of shortage of critical care staff (in particular, physicians and nurses) and lack of access to critical care expertise. Telemedicine is seen as an answer to providing care remotely (Field 1996; Norris 2002); the tele-ICU technology is the application of telemedicine to support critical care. In this chapter, we review sociotechnical issues related to the implementation of tele-ICU technology. We first explain the challenges related to critical care and then describe the tele-ICU technology. We discuss the major sociotechnical issues related to the tele-ICU technology, i.e. communication, trust, conflict management and performance of tele-ICU nurses and physicians.

GENERAL CONTEXT OF ICUS

People are living longer than ever before. The number of older Americans, people age 65 and older, is expected to double from 36 millions in 2009 to 72 million by 2030 (Administration on Aging, 2009). A study comparing the number of adverse events between patients under age of 65, and patients 65 and older, demonstrated that adverse events are more prevalent among the older patients (Thomas and Brennan 2000). Care of the older patient is frequently more complex because of the high number of drug orders and procedures performed, and the fact that older patients frequently do not present typical signs and symptoms of diseases (Thomas and Brennan 2000; Breslow, Rosenfeld et al. 2004). Between 1985 and 2000, the number of critical care beds has increased by 26.2% in the US, while the total number of hospitals offering critical care services has decreased

by 13.7% (Halpern, Pastores et al. 2004). Due to the current shortage of ICU qualified staff, only 10 - 12% of US ICUs offer 24-hour coverage by intensivists (Pronovost, Angus et al. 2002). This statistic is worrisome as numerous studies have shown that the presence of intensivists can reduce mortality, morbidity, length of stay, resource utilization, and ICU charges (Pronovost, Angus et al. 2002; Breslow, Rosenfeld et al. 2004) as well as reduce the risk of death by 40% (Pronovost, Angus et al. 2002).

Approximately 400,000 to 500,000 people die each year in ICUs (Angus, Linde-Zwirble et al. 1996). The ICU is a fast-paced, complex, high-risk, and team-oriented environment. Patients in ICUs are critically ill and receive roughly twice as many medications as non-ICU patients (Wu, Pronovost et al. 2002). A study conducted by Donchin et al. (1995) estimated that 1.7 errors occurred per patient per day in ICUs. Many of these errors appear to be system-related and therefore patient safety researchers suggest system approaches to reduce errors and improve the quality of care in ICUs (Carayon, Hundt et al. 2006).

ICU: Organizational Characteristics

From an organizational theory perspective, ICUs can be considered complex organizations providing services (Hoonakker, Carayon et al. 2008). The complexity of ICU patients requires clinicians from multiple disciplines (e.g. internal medicine, surgery, anesthesiology, radiology, nursing, pharmacy, respiratory therapy) to coordinate care. There are several causes for the complexity, including great uncertainty in the process of care, the diversity of the processes involved, and the need for quick decision-making required by urgent situations (Lamothe 1999). The team model of care and the multidisciplinary team approach to ICU care have been emphasized by the Society of Critical Care Medicine (Parillo 1995; Rainey and Shapiro 2001) and the American Association of Critical Care Nurses (Evans and Carlson 1992).

Studies in the US and in Europe have described the organization of ICUs (Groeger, Strosberg et al. 1992; Vincent, Suter et al. 1997), and show large diversity of organizational arrangements of ICUs, in particular in the US (Groeger, Strosberg et al. 1992).

Some studies have identified the organizational characteristics that contribute to improved ICU patient care outcomes; very few studies have examined the relationship between patient care outcomes and working conditions and work organization. Carlson et al. (1996) argue that the use of an ICU team, admission and discharge criteria, protocols and guidelines, and the principles of evidence-based medicine can improve ICU outcomes, performance and cost effectiveness. A large observational study was conducted to examine the relationship between ICU organizational characteristics and outcomes of abdominal aortic surgery (Pronovost, Jenekes et al. 1999). The absence of daily rounds by an ICU physician was correlated with a 3-fold increase in in-hospital mortality and a range of complications (i.e. cardiac arrest, septicemia, acute renal failure, and re-intubation). A study by Rapoport et al. (2000) examined the relationship between ICU organizational factors and pulmonary artery catheter use. Using data from a retrospective study of 10,217 non-operative patients, they found that the presence of a full-time ICU physician was correlated with a two-thirds reduction in the probability of catheter use. Other studies have confirmed the patient care benefits of daily rounds by an ICU physician (Dimick, Pronovost et al. 2001), the presence of full-time critical care specialists (Brown and Sullivan 1989; Miranda 1992; Hanson, Deutschman et al. 1999), the presence of physicians trained in critical care medicine (Reynolds, Haupt et al. 1988), and intermediate care units (Dhond, Ridley et al. 1998).

Knaus, Rousseau, Shortell, Zimmerman, and colleagues (Knaus, Draper et al. 1986; Shortell and Rousseau 1989; Shortell, Rousseau et al. 1991; Shortell, Zimmerman et al. 1994) have extensively studied organizational characteristics

and performance of ICUs. In a study of ICUs in 13 tertiary care hospitals, Knaus et al. (1986) used a severity of disease classification system (Apache II) to identify organizational characteristics associated with better care. Coordination of care and involvement and interactions of nurses and physicians were associated with improved patient care. The methodology used in the National ICU study is described in detail in several articles (Draper, Wagner et al. 1989; Shortell and Rousseau 1989; Shortell, Rousseau et al. 1991; Shortell, Zimmerman et al. 1994). Their conceptual framework was based on the structure-process-outcome model of Donabedian (1966). Shortell et al. (1991) hypothesized that "a team-oriented, achievement oriented culture and leaders who set high standards and provide necessary support provide more open, accurate, and timely communication, effective coordination with other units, and more open collaborative problems solving approaches". The study by Shortell et al. (1991) showed that communication and coordination in the ICU are positively associated with quality of care and negatively related with turnover intention of nurses.

The literature shows that direct communication (face-to-face communication or real time communication) is the preferred mode of communication in ICUs (Moss, Xiao et al. 2002). However, due to the interruptive nature of ICUs, direct communication may contribute to communication breakdown and medical errors (Coiera, Jayasuriya et al. 2002). According to the Joint Commission (Joint Commission on Accreditation of Healthcare Organizations (JCAHO) 2007), two-thirds of the root causes of sentinel events between 1995-2005 were communication-related.

ICU: Job Demands and Stress

The heavy workload of hospital nurses is a major problem for the American health care system. Nurses are experiencing high workload due to four main reasons (Carayon and Gurses 2008):

(1) increased demand for nurses, (2) inadequate supply of nurses, (3) reduced staffing and increased overtime, and (4) reduction in patient length of stay. The demand for nurses is increasing as a result of population aging, and the supply of nurses is not adequate to meet the current demand: the nursing shortage is projected to grow more severe as future demand increases and nursing schools are not able to keep up with the increasing educational demand (US DHHS HRSA 2006; Kuehn 2007). When a nursing shortage occurs, the workload increases for nurses who remain on the job (Baumann, Giovannetti et al. 2001). In response to increasing health care costs since the 1990s, hospitals have reduced their nursing staff and implemented mandatory overtime policies to meet unexpectedly high demands, which significantly increased nursing workload. Increasing cost pressure forced healthcare organizations to reduce patient length of stay. As a result, hospital nurses today take care of patients who are sicker than in the past, and their work is more intensive (Aiken, Sochalski et al. 1996). A recent development in the US healthcare, i.e. the implementation of healthcare information technology (HIT), can produce numerous changes in the organization of work in health care and may cause additional stress.

Workload and stress are high in ICUs (Hay and Oken 1977; Cross and Fallon 1985; Boumans and Landeweerd 1994; Goodfellow, Varnam et al. 1997; Le Blanc, de Jonge et al. 2001; White and Dorman 2001; Gurses, Carayon et al. 2009). The reasons are mainly the same as the reasons for the increased workload of nurses in general. In recent years, ICUs have had to deal with rapidly expanding medical technology and, subsequently, increasing job complexity; cost containment because of the rapid increase in health care costs, which has reduced the resources available to nurses in the ICU (Le Blanc, de Jonge et al. 2001). In a large cross-sectional study (N=2090) in 13 different European countries, Le Blanc et al (2001) examined the relationship between tasks

of ICU nurses and their well-being as measured by burnout and job satisfaction. The different task categories were defined as: operational tasks (medical care/technical nursing activities, psychological support of patients, physical care); organizing tasks (contacts with the nurse manager, with physicians, and with colleagues from their own team); preparatory tasks (replenishing work supplies, collecting equipment); and supportive tasks (training and coaching, coordinating care). Two scoring dimensions were used: for each task ICU nurses had to indicate (1) how demanding the task was and (2) how satisfying the performance of such a task was. Results of the study show that ICU nurses experience operational tasks as most demanding, but also as most satisfying, and that organizing tasks were perceived as least demanding, but also least satisfying. The demanding aspects of operational tasks were related to burnout (Le Blanc, de Jonge et al. 2001).

In summary, from an organizational perspective, ICUs are very complex organizations where coordination and communication play an important role. What happens when a technology such as the tele-ICU technology is implemented in this complex work system? The tele-ICU will have a major impact on the ICU work system; but it is also important to examine the work system of the tele-ICU. Will tele-ICUs reduce some of the coordination and communication problems, or only add to them? How are communication patterns between the ICU and the tele-ICU established? Do tele-ICUs help to improve quality of care and patient safety? Some of the high workload in ICUs may be reduced by using tele-ICU nurses to monitor patients in the ICU. However, what about the workload of the tele-ICU nurses? Some estimates show that tele-ICU nurses should be able to monitor as many as 50 patients in 5 ICUs at the same time. How do they handle that high cognitive workload? Do nurses in the tele-ICU suffer as much from burnout as ICU nurses?

Table 1. Examples of telemedicine over time

Examples of telemedicine	Data
Telegraphy	1830s-1920s
Telephone	1870s-now
Radio	1920s-now
Television	1950s-now
Space technologies, e.g. satellite based communications	1960s-now
Digital technologies	1990s-now

TELEMEDICINE AND VIRTUAL TEAMS

Telemedicine utilizes information and telecommunication technologies to transfer medical information for diagnosis, therapy and education (Norris 2002). Although most applications of telemedicine such as tele-surgery and tele-radiology are relatively new, earlier examples of telemedicine have existed for more than 100 years.

There are four different applications of tele-medicine:

1. Tele-consultation
2. Tele-education
3. Tele-monitoring
4. Tele-surgery

Tele-consultation is used to support clinical decision-making and is the most frequent example of telemedicine. Tele-consultation can take place between two (or more) Health Care Providers (HCPs), or between the patient and one (or more) caregivers, Data can be transferred in real time, for example in video-streaming, or in "store-and-forward". The best example of the latter is tele-radiology, i.e. the transmission of large X-ray files (Norris 2002).

Tele-education occurs when learning over a distance takes place, for example during the exchange between a care provider and a medical expert. There are different forms of medical

tele-education (Norris 2002): clinical education from tele-consultation; clinical education via the Internet; tele-medical courses via the Internet; and public education via the Internet.

Tele-monitoring is the use of telecommunications links to gather routine or repeated data on a patient's condition (Norris 2002). The purpose of monitoring is to decide if and when an adjustment is needed in the patient's treatment.

Tele-surgery means using tele-communication systems to guide robotic arms to carry out remote surgical procedures. Tele-surgery is still in its infancy, but significant progress has recently been made (Melvin, Needleman et al. 2002; Rawlings, Woodland et al. 2007; Müller-Stich, Reiter et al. 2009).

Description of the Tele ICU Technology

In the tele-ICU, the following three applications of telemedicine are combined: tele-consultation, tele-education, and tele-monitoring. Tele-consultation is used to give instructions to the ICU nurses and physicians about patient care. Tele-education is a result of the tele-consultation. Personnel in tele-ICUs are highly qualified: physicians who work in the tele-ICU are generally trained as intensivists and can provide supplementary care support to multiple ICUs from a remote location in real time. The remote team can be comprised of multiple clinicians: board-certified intensivists, critical care nurses, clerical personnel and, in some instances, a pharmacist. Personnel in the ICU (including residents on duty in the ICU) receive instructions or guidance from the tele-ICU and may have the opportunity to learn new skills and knowledge. Evidently, tele-monitoring is critical to the tele-ICU model. Personnel in the tele-ICU receive patient data in real time; one of the advantages of the tele-ICU technology is that personnel in the tele-ICU, using the continuous, real-time data may be able to *detect trends in*

Table 2. Tele- ICU category of care responsibilities

Category of Care	Responsibilities
1	Remote team is only allowed to intervene in emergencies.
2	Remote team executes daily care plan (set by on-site team) and implements all best practices.
3	Remote team provides all ICU services when there is no physician in the ICU and communicates with the attending physician for major issues.

patient status and can alert personnel in the ICU (Anders, Patterson et al. 2008).

The Leapfrog Group for Patient Safety is a voluntary program that aims to improve the quality and safety of health care (Eikel and Delbanco 2003; Jha, Orav et al. 2008). One practiced endorsed by Leapfrog is about physician staffing in ICUs, or the use of 'intensivists', which has been shown to reduce the risk of patients dying in the ICU by 40% (http://www.leapfroggroup.org/home). Because of significant shortages in intensivists, this practice has led to the emergence and expansion of tele-ICUs.

It is recommended that both the tele-ICU physician and tele-ICU nurse have at least five years of ICU experience. Some tele-ICU HCPs split their time between the ICU and the tele-ICU. The ICU determines the involvement of the tele-ICU by appointing each patient a category of care. Categories of care range from 1 to 3 and are additive. For example the tasks carried in category 1 also occur in categories 2 and 3. Table 2 provides a detailed description of the different categories of tele-ICU care.

Typically, tele-ICU HCPs use a color system for rounding on patients: each patient is assigned a color of red, yellow or green. Tele-ICU HCPs round on "red" patients every hour, on "yellow" patients every two hours and "green" patients about every four hours. Patients who are labeled green are stable and may have a discharge or transfer pending. Each tele-ICU HCP works at a workstation that is commonly composed of multiple monitors, a two-way camera, microphone, and a hot phone. Clinical data captured about the

ICU patient are directly streamed to the tele-ICU. Tele-ICU HCPs are dependent on information communicated over the phone or entered into the computer from the bedside to inform them on the current state of the patient. They monitor numerous clinical indicators, such as blood pressure, heart rate, ventilator settings, and oxygen saturation. Other data such as patient care plans, lab results, and X-rays are electronically sent or faxed to the tele-ICU. Most tele-ICU software uses "smart alarms" to alert the clinicians to possible significant changes in patient status.

Review of the Research on Tele-ICU Technology

To date, relatively few studies have examined the impact of tele-ICUs and most of the studies have focused on clinical and financial outcomes (Rosenfeld, Dorman et al. 2000; Breslow, Rosenfeld et al. 2004; Thomas, Chu-Weininger et al. 2007; Ries 2009; Zawada, Herr et al. 2009). Few studies have focused on the health care providers (HCPs) working in the tele-ICU. The study by Tang et al. (2007) examined the work of tele-ICU nurses and physicians, the study by Anders et al (2007) has explored interactions between the tele-ICU and the ICUs, the study by Ries (2009) examined clinical and financial outcomes of tele-ICU implementation as well as the effect on tele-ICU personnel, and the study by Thomas et al (2007) examined teamwork and patient safety.

Several studies have shown that the implementation of an ICU telemedicine program can improve clinical care outcomes (e.g., reduced length of stay, reduced mortality, reduced complications) and reduce healthcare costs (Rosenfeld, Dorman et al. 2000; Breslow, Rosenfeld et al. 2004; Zawada, Herr et al. 2009).

Tang et al. (2007) conducted an observational study of tele-ICU nurses and physicians in one tele-ICU. A task analysis tool was developed and implemented on a Tablet PC; the tool allowed the collection of time data on 'primary tasks' (e.g., doing rounds, handling specific patients), 'activities' (e.g., monitoring, communicating, looking for information), information sources, interruptions and people (i.e. staff in the tele-ICU and staff in the ICU). Results show that tele-ICU physicians and nurses interact with ICU staff about 7 and 6 times per hour respectively. This study also highlighted the importance of capturing data on interruptions and sources of interruptions, as well as data on the use of various information sources; this is particularly important in the information-intensive environment of ICUs.

Anders and colleagues (2007) performed 40 hours of observation of eight tele-ICU nurses and one tele-ICU physician in one tele-ICU. During periods of low workload, questions were asked to clarify specific activities. Results showed that the tele-ICU fulfills three functions: (1) anomaly response: tele-ICU nurses processed information related to alerts and alarms and contacted other staff in the tele-ICU or the ICU if they perceived the need for follow-up or action; (2) access to specialized expertise: experienced tele-ICU nurses were observed to mentor junior ICU nurses, ICU nurses had access to expertise and experience of the tele-ICU nurses therefore augmenting their knowledge base; and (3) sense-making: tele-ICU nurses can make sense of what is happening with patients because they have access to many sources of data and have the resources (time, expertise) to synthesize the data.

The research on tele-ICUs is extremely limited; in particular *nursing issues* related to tele-ICU have been overlooked (Cummings, Krsek et al. 2007). Only two of the published studies on tele-ICUs

are relevant to these issues; both studies examined nurses in single tele-ICUs (Anders, Patterson et al. 2007; Tang, Weavind et al. 2007). Therefore, the generalizability of the studies is limited. In addition, the studies had a limited scope: one study captured data on how tele-ICU nurses and physicians spend their time; the other study described the functions of the tele-ICU. No study has explored how tele-ICU HCPs deal with multiple interactions across varied ICUs, and their quality of working life and performance.

Virtual Teams

Research on virtual teams has significantly evolved in the past 10 years. Several reviews of the literature (Martins, Gilson et al. 2004; Powell, Piccoli et al. 2004; Hertel, Geister et al. 2005; Pinsonneault and Caya 2005; Cohen 2008) emphasize the *various types of configuration and structure* of virtual teams. Therefore, there has been a call for in-depth research on specific types of virtual team and for the need to clearly define the type of virtual team under study (Driskell, Radtke et al. 2003; Priest, Stagl et al. 2006). Virtual teams are defined as having the following characteristics: geographically dispersed, electronically dependent, dynamic, and comprising diverse members working remotely (Gibson and Cohen 2003; Gibson and Gibbs 2006; O'Leary and Cummings 2007). O'Leary and Cummings (2007) have proposed that geographic dispersion actually includes 3 dimensions: (1) spatial dispersion or the geographic distance among team members, (2) temporal dispersion or the time difference between team members, and (3) configurational dispersion or the various locations where team members are located. Table 3 lists characteristics of virtual teams and their definition for the tele-ICU. A virtual team consists of the interaction between tele-HCPs and ICU HCPs; therefore, the tele-HCPs have to deal with multiple virtual teams, i.e. multiple ICUs.

Table 3. Characteristics of virtual teams and tele-ICUs

Characteristics of virtual teams	Characteristics of tele-ICUs
Geographic dispersion (spatial dispersion)	YES. The tele-ICU HCPs are located in a central hub, which is at a distance from the ICUs.
Temporal boundary	NO. HCPs in the tele-ICU and the ICUs work at the same time.
Relational boundary	YES. The tele-ICU and the ICUs connected to the tele-ICU may or may not belong to the same organization.
Information and communication technologies	YES. Tele-ICU HCPs use various synchronous and asynchronous information and communication technologies.
Configurational dispersion	YES. Each tele-ICU HCP works with several ICUs in different locations.
Cultural diversity	YES. Various ICUs and hospitals have different work organizations and cultures. Cultural diversity is related to configurational dispersion.

PSYCHOSOCIAL AND ORGANIZATIONAL IMPACT OF TELE-ICU

Trust

There are multiple ways to define trust (Bigley and Pearce 1998; Rousseau, Sitkin et al. 1998). One of the most commonly cited definitions comes from Mayer et al. (1995):

... the willingness of a party to be vulnerable to the actions of another party based on the expectation that the other will perform a particular action important to the trustor, irrespective of the ability to monitor or control that other party (p. 712).

Trust is the foundation of teams. Characteristics of virtual teams affect the traditional ways in which team members create trust (Handy 1995; Aubert and Kelsey 2003) (Bradley, 2001). Due to the lack of social history, context (e.g., social similarity, shared values, and expectations) and co-location, a virtual setting may impede the development of trust between virtual team members (Lewicki and Bunker 1996; Kramer 1999). Virtual teams are composed of culturally diverse members who perform interdependent tasks with a common goal. They use electronic communication technologies as a link between their geographically dispersed locations to coordinate care. Frequent face-to-face

interaction between team members enables trust to be built by the sharing of norms, values, and experiences (Handy 1995; Jarvenpaa and Leidner 1999). Team relationships mature with frequency, duration, and diversity of experiences that help to confirm expectations. Trust transforms as a relationship develops (Mayer, Davis et al. 1995; Lewicki and Bunker 1996). Trust between individuals permits open communication and challenging ideas without the fear of repercussion, and also values diversity of opinions (Jarvenpaa, Knoll et al. 1998; Holton 2001; Conchie, Donald et al. 2006). Communication, group cohesion, collaboration, and conflict management are factors that may affect ICU patient care (Knaus, Draper et al. 1986; Conchie, Donald et al. 2006). A team that practices good teamwork can contribute to desirable patient and staff outcomes.

Tele-ICU nurses continuously alternate between ICUs and need to adapt to different team members (i.e. healthcare providers in the ICUs). The virtual team literature shows that communication, and establishing trust between the virtual team members is crucial for the performance of virtual teams (Iacono and Weisband 1997; Jarvenpaa, Knoll et al. 1998; King and Majchrzak 2003; Paul and McDaniel 2004). Good communication between the tele-ICU and the ICU is extremely important to make the tele-ICU model work. The tele-ICU nurses receive real time data on the status of the patients in the ICU. However, because they are operating from a remote location they are helpless in a crisis situation when they are not able to communicate their concerns, treatment suggestions, etc., to the nurses and doctors in the ICU. In other words: the nurses and physicians in the tele-ICU have to trust the nurses and physicians in the ICU to follow their instructions. Vice versa, the physicians and nurses in the ICU have to trust the physicians and nurses in the tele-ICU to provide them with timely, precise information and instructions on what to do. However, how is trust between the ICU and the tele-ICU established? The physicians and nurses in the ICU may have never met the physicians and nurses in the tele-ICU. How is trust in these virtual teams established? Research is needed to characterize communication and trust between ICUs and tele-ICUs.

Conflicts and Performance

Several studies show that virtual teams experience high levels of conflict as a result of two factors: the distance that separates them and their reliance on technology to communicate and work with one another (Hinds and Weisband 2003). Both distance and technology dependence can enhance conflicts and reduce performance in virtual teams. There are methods that can mitigate the negative effects of distance and use of mediating technologies (Hinds and Weisband 2003). For example, by increasing the frequency and length of contacts between virtual team members, and by actually meeting the other team members in person, teams seem to be able to overcome some of the negative effects (Kraut, Fish et al. 1992). Providing more information about the context, in order for their team members to better understand the context of a specific demand, can lead to better understanding among team members (Atkins, Boyer et al. 2002). The way technologies used by virtual teams are designed and implemented has a major impact on teamwork and performance; in addition, the level of training provided to the virtual team members

is also important for team effectiveness (Walther and Burgoon 1992; Hinds and Kiesler 1995; Hinds and Weisband 2003). The literature shows that the combination of working at a distance and the use information and communication technology (ICT) can have significant impact on team performance and conflict management. More research is needed to examine how the distance between the tele-ICU and the ICUs they monitor, as well as possible communication problems, caused by the technology used, may impact performance and cause possible conflicts.

CONCLUSION

ICUs are highly complex organizations where lives are literally at stake. Decisions often have to be made quickly, while at the same time there may be many parties involved in the decision making process. This puts a large burden on ICU staff. Furthermore, partly due to population aging, but also because of tremendous increase in medical knowledge, techniques and technology, there has been a large increase in ICU patients in the last decades. This is occurring in an environment of shortage of ICU personnel, in particular highly trained and skilled ICU nurses and physicians (i.e. intensivists). Between 1985 and 2000, the number of critical care beds has increased by more than 25%, while the total number of hospitals offering critical care services has decreased by 14% (Halpern, Pastores et al. 2004). Probably as a result of the shortage in ICU personnel and increased patient demands, ICU physicians and nurses report high workload and burnout, which can lead to lower levels of quality of care and patient safety problems. The literature also shows that communication and coordination in hospitals, and in particular in ICUs, is of great importance (Shortell and Rousseau 1989; Shortell, Rousseau et al. 1991; Hoonakker, Carayon et al. 2008; Hoonakker, Carayon et al. 2008). A possible solution for dealing with the shortage of ICU personnel is telemedicine. Telemedicine uses information and communication technologies (ICT) to transfer medical information for diagnosis, therapy and education. With telemedicine, in this case the tele-ICU, patients in ICUs can be monitored remotely, and when help is needed, the physician and/or nurse in the tele-ICU can provide information, support and recommendations to personnel in the ICU. One of the advantages of telemedicine is the ability to detect trends in patient status that personnel in the actual might have missed: these trends may be captured by the tele-ICU staff who monitor a continuous stream of information and the software to analyze it. However, there is little literature on the impact of telemedicine, and even less literature on tele-ICUs.

Personnel in a tele-ICU work in an environment that is similar to a traffic control or process control environment. We know little about the impact of ICT on physicians and nurses in the tele-ICU. Furthermore, personnel in the ICUs and the tele-ICU have to collaborate to provide the best care for ICU patients; therefore, they form virtual teams. The literature on virtual teams shows that interactions in virtual teams can be very complex (Jarvenpaa and Leidner 1998). The communication technologies used by the virtual teams speed up interaction. In a virtual organization, a person may interact with different teams frequently and rapidly because of electronic communication technologies. The HCPs in the tele-ICU continuously alternate between ICUs and need to adapt to different team members (i.e. healthcare providers in the ICUs) and different structures of different ICUs. As mentioned before, a tele-ICU nurse can monitor as many as 50 intensive care patients in five different ICUs and therefore belong to as many as 50 virtual teams. However, little is known about how these nurses manage their interactions with 50 virtual teams at the same time, establish adequate communication patterns, and establish and maintain trust with physicians and nurses in the ICUs and in the tele-ICU.

The literature from these three domains (medical settings, and in particular ICUs and tele-ICUs; telemedicine; and virtual teams) shows that we know very little about the sociotechnical environment, work organization and quality of working life of tele-ICU nurses, and its impact on the quality and safety of care provided to ICU patients. By combining the literature of these three domains, it becomes clear that we need to learn more about the following factors: the impact of the tele-ICU technology on the work of physicians and nurses in the tele-ICU and in the ICUs, the possible high workload in tele-ICUs, communication between the tele-ICU and ICUs, and trust between the tele-ICU and the ICUs.

In the past decades, we have made tremendous progress in the development of ICT and our understanding of sociotechnical and psychosocial issues of ICT (Bradley, 2006). ICT developments in health care have resulted in life saving technologies that can be operated from a distance. However, this chapter has also shown that we are still very dependent on human beings, and the interactions between human beings to take advantage of these developments. Psychosocial issues, such as establishing good communication patterns and developing trust between members of virtual teams, are key factors both in the health care domain and in virtual teams. Lack of communication and trust can result in lower quality of care provided to ICU patients and patient safety problems.

We recently initiated a research project (http://cqpi.engr.wisc.edu/vicu_home) to examine the sociotechnical issues of tele-ICU, in particular from the viewpoint of nurses in the tele-ICU. This study will shed light on the psychosocial issues of tele-ICU.

ACKNOWLEDGMENT

This research has been made possible with a grant from the National Science Foundation (NSF

08-550: Virtual Organizations as Sociotechnical Systems (VOSS), PI: Pascale Carayon).

REFERENCES

Administration on Aging. (2009). Aging statistics. Retrieved April 24, 2009, from http://www.aoa.gov/AoARoot/Aging_Statistics/index.aspx

Aiken, L. H., Sochalski, J., & Anderson, G. F. (1996). Downsizing the hospital nursing workforce. *Health Affairs*, *15*(4), 88–92. doi:10.1377/hlthaff.15.4.88

Anders, S., Patterson, E. S., Woods, D. D., & Ebright, P. (2007). Projecting Trajectories for a New Technology Based on Cognitive Task Analysis and Archetypal Patterns: The Electronic ICU. *8th Annual Naturalist Decision Making Conference*. Asilomar, CA.

Anders, S., Patterson, E. S., Woods, D. D., & Schweikhart, S. (2008). Shifts in Functions of a New Technology Over Time: An Analysis of Logged Electronic Intensive Care Unit Interventions. *Human Factors and Ergonomics Society 52nd Annual Meeting*. New York, Human Factors and Ergonomics Society.

Angus, D. C., Linde-Zwirble, W. T., Sirio, C. A., Rotondi, A. J., Chelluri, L., & Newbold, R. C. III (1996). The effect of managed care on ICU length of stay: implications for medicare. *Journal of the American Medical Association*, *276*(13), 1075–1082. doi:10.1001/jama.276.13.1075

Atkins, D., Boyer, D., Handel, M., Herbsleb, J., Mockus, A., & Wills, G. (2002). *Achieving speed in globally distributed project work*. Winterpark, CO: Human Computer Interaction Consortium.

Aubert, B. A., & Kelsey, B. L. (2003). Further understanding of trust and performance in virtual teams. *Small Group Research*, *34*(5), 575–618. doi:10.1177/1046496403256011

Baumann, A., Giovannetti, P., O'Brien-Pallas, L., Mallette, C., Deber, R., & Blythe, J. (2001). Healthcare restructuring: the impact of job change. *Canadian Journal of Nursing Leadership*, *14*(1), 14–20.

Bigley, G. A., & Pearce, J. L. (1998). Straining for shared meaning in organization science: Problems of trust and distrust. *Academy of Management Review*, *23*(3), 16. doi:10.2307/259286

Boumans, N. P. G., & Landeweerd, J. A. (1994). Working in an intensive or non-intensive care unit: does it make any difference? *Heart & Lung*, *23*, 71–79.

Bradley, G. (2001). Information and Communication Technology (ICT) and Humans - How we will live, learn and work . In Bradley, G. (Ed.), *Humans on the Net: Information and Communication Technology (ICT), Work Organization and Human Beings* (pp. 22–44). Stockholm: Prevent.

Bradley, G. (2006). *Social and Community Informatics - Humans on the Net*. London/New York, UK/NY: Routledge.

Breslow, M. J., Rosenfeld, B. A., Doerfler, M., Burke, G., Yates, G., & Stone, D. J. (2004). Effect of a multiple-site intensive care unit telemedicine program on clinical and economic outcomes: An alternative paradigm for intensivist staffing. *Critical Care Medicine*, *32*(1), 31–38. doi:10.1097/01.CCM.0000104204.61296.41

Brown, J. J., & Sullivan, G. (1989). Effect on ICU mortality of a full-time critical care specialist. *Chest*, *96*(1), 127–129. doi:10.1378/chest.96.1.127

Carayon, P., & Gurses, A. P. (2008). *Nursing workload and patient safety - A human factors engineering perspective. Patient safety and quality: An evidence-based handbook for nurses*. Rockville: Agency for Healthcare Research and Quality.

Carayon, P., Hundt, A. S., Karsh, B.-T., Gurses, A. P., Alvarado, C. J., Smith, M., & Flatley, B. P. (2006). Work system design for patient safety: The SEIPS model. *Quality & Safety in Health Care, 15*(Suppl I), i50–i58. doi:10.1136/qshc.2005.015842

Carlson, R. W., Weiland, D. E., & Srivthsan, K. (1996). Does a full-time, 24-hour intensivist improve care and efficiency? *Critical Care Clinics, 12*(3), 525–552. doi:10.1016/S0749-0704(05)70260-8

Cohen, M. H. (2008). Professional communication and teamwork. *Creative Nursing, 14*(1), 17–23. doi:10.1891/1078-4535.14.1.17

Coiera, E. W., Jayasuriya, R. A., Hardy, J., Bannan, A., & Thorpe, M. E. C. (2002). Communication loads on clinical staff in the emergency department. *MJA, 176*, 415–418.

Conchie, S. M., Donald, I. J., & Taylor, P. J. (2006). Trust: Missing piece(s) in the safety puzzle. *Risk Analysis, 26*(5), 1097–1104. doi:10.1111/j.1539-6924.2006.00818.x

Cross, D. G., & Fallon, A. (1985). A stressor comparison of four speciality areas. *The Australian Journal of Advanced Nursing, 2*, 24–36.

Cummings, J., Krsek, C., Vermoch, K., & Matuszewski, K. (2007). Intensive care unit telemedicine: Review and consensus recommendations. *American Journal of Medical Quality, 22*(4), 239–250. doi:10.1177/1062860607302777

Dhond, G., Ridley, S., & Palmer, M. (1998). The impact of a high-dependency unit on the workload of an intensive care unit. *Anaesthesia, 53*, 841–847. doi:10.1046/j.1365-2044.1998.00522.x

Dimick, J. B., Pronovost, P. J., Heitmiller, R. F., & Lipsett, P. A. (2001). Intensive care unit physician staffing is associated with decreased length of stay, hospital cost, and complication after esophagal resection. *Critical Care Medicine, 29*(4), 753–758. doi:10.1097/00003246-200104000-00012

Donabedian, A. (1966). Evaluating the quality of medical care. *The Milbank Memorial Fund Quarterly, 40*, 166–206. doi:10.2307/3348969

Donchin, Y., Gopher, D., Olin, M., Badihi, Y., Biesky, M., & Sprung, C. L. (1995). A look into the nature and causes of human errors in the intensive care unit. *Critical Care Medicine, 23*, 294–300. doi:10.1097/00003246-199502000-00015

Draper, E., Wagner, D., Russo, M., Bergner, M., Shortell, S., & Rousseau, D. (1989). Study design - data collection. *Critical Care Medicine, 17*(12), S186–S193. doi:10.1097/00003246-198912000-00007

Driskell, J. E., Radtke, P. H., & Salas, E. (2003). Virtual teams: Effects of technological mediation on team performance. *Group Dynamics, 7*(4), 297–323. doi:10.1037/1089-2699.7.4.297

Eikel, C., & Delbanco, S. (2003). John M. Eisenberg Patient Safety Awards. The Leapfrog Group for Patient Safety: rewarding higher standards. *Joint Commission Journal on Quality and Safety, 29*(12), 634–639.

Evans, S. A., & Carlson, R. (1992). Nurse-physician collaboration: Solving the nursing shortage crisis. *Journal of the American College of Cardiology, 20*(7), 1669–1673. doi:10.1016/0735-1097(92)90464-X

Field, M. J. (Ed.). (1996). *Telemedicine: A Guide to Assessing Telecommunications in Health Care*. Washington, DC: National Academy Press.

Gibson, C. B., & Cohen, S. G. (Eds.). (2003). *The last work - conclusions and implications. Virtual Teams That Work - Creating Conditions for Virtual Team Effectiveness*. San Francisco, CA: Jossey Bass.

Gibson, C. B., & Gibbs, J. L. (2006). Unpacking the concept of virtuality: The effects of geographic dispersion, electronic dependence, dynamice structure and national diversity on team diversity. *Administrative Science Quarterly, 51*(3), 451–495.

Goodfellow, A., Varnam, R., Rees, D., & Shelly, M. P. (1997). Staff stress on the intensive care unit: a comparison of doctors and nurses. *Anaesthesia, 52,* 1037–1041. doi:10.1111/j.1365-2044.1997.213-az0348.x

Groeger, J. S., Strosberg, M. A., Halpern, N. A., Raphaely, R. C., Kaye, W. E., & Guntupalli, K. K. (1992). Descriptive analysis of critical care units in the United States. *Critical Care Medicine, 20*(6), 846–863. doi:10.1097/00003246-199206000-00024

Gurses, A. P., Carayon, P., & Wall, M. (2009). Impact of performance obstacles on intensive care nurses' workload, perceived quality and safety of care, and quality of working life. *Health Services Research, 44*(2), 422–443. doi:10.1111/j.1475-6773.2008.00934.x

Halpern, N. A., Pastores, S. M., & Greenstein, R. J. (2004). Critical care medicine in the United States 1985-2000: An analysis of bed numbers, use, and costs. *Critical Care Medicine, 32*(6), 1254–1259. doi:10.1097/01.CCM.0000128577.31689.4C

Handy, C. (1995). Trust and the Virtual Organization. *Harvard Business Review, 73*(3), 40–50.

Hanson, C. W., Deutschman, C. S., Anderson, H. L., Reilly, P. M., Behringer, E. C., Schwab, C. W., & Price, J. (1999). Effects of an organized critical care service on outcomes and resource utilization: A cohort study. *Critical Care Medicine, 27*(2), 270–274. doi:10.1097/00003246-199902000-00030

Hay, D., & Oken, D. (1977). The pscyhological stresses of intensive care unit nursing . In Moos, R. H. (Ed.), *Coping with physical illness* (pp. 381–396). New York: McGraw Hill.

Hertel, G., Geister, S., & Konradt, U. (2005). Managing virtual teams: A review of current empirical research. *Human Resource Management Review, 15,* 69–95. doi:10.1016/j.hrmr.2005.01.002

Hinds, P. J., & Kiesler, S. (1995). Communication across boundaries: Work, structure, and the use of communication technologies in a large organization. *Organization Science, 6,* 373–393. doi:10.1287/orsc.6.4.373

Hinds, P. J., & Weisband, S. P. (2003). Knowledge sharing and shared understanding in virtual teams . In Gibson, C. B., & Cohen, S. G. (Eds.), *Virtual Teams That Work* (pp. 21–36). San Francisco, CA: Jossey-Bass.

Holton, J. (2001). Building trust and collaboration in a virtual team. *Team Performance Management: An International Journal, 7*(3/4), 36–47. doi:10.1108/13527590110395621

Hoonakker, P. L. T., Carayon, P., Douglas, S., Schultz, K., Walker, J., & Wetterneck, B. T. (2008). Communication in Intensive Care Units and the Relation with Quality of Care and Patient Safety . In Snelwar, L. I., Mascia, F. L., & Montedo, U. B. (Eds.), *Human Factors in Organizational Design and Management, IX* (pp. 715–721). Santa Monica, CA: IEA Press.

Hoonakker, P. L. T., Carayon, P., Walker, J., & Wetterneck, B. T. (2008). *Coordination in the ICU and the Relation with Quality of Care and Patient Safety.* Healthcare systems Ergonomics and Patient Safety (HEPS 2008) conference, Strasbourg, France.

Iacono, C. S., & Weisband, S. (1997). Developing trust in virtual teams. *Thirtieth Hawaii International Conference on System Sciences.* Wailea, HI.

Jarvenpaa, S. L., Knoll, K., & Leidner, D. E. (1998). Is anybody out there? Antecedents of trust in global virtual teams. *Journal of Management Information Systems, 14*(4), 29–64.

Jarvenpaa, S. L., & Leidner, D. E. (1998). Communication and Trust in Global Virtual Teams. *Journal of Computer-Mediated Communication, 3*(4).

Jarvenpaa, S. L., & Leidner, D. E. (1999). Communication and trust in global virtual teams. *Organization Science, 10*(6), 791–815. doi:10.1287/orsc.10.6.791

Jha, A. K., Orav, E. J., Ridgway, A. B., Zheng, J., & Epstein, A. M. (2008). Does the Leapfrog program help identify high-quality hospitals? *Joint Commission Journal on Quality and Patient Safety, 34*(6), 318–325.

Joint Commission on Accreditation of Healthcare Organizations (JCAHO). (2007). Sentinel events statistics, March 31, 2007. Retrieved August 7, 2007, from http://www.jointcommission.org/SentinelEvents/Statistics/

King, M., & Majchrzak, A. (2003). Technology Alignment and Adaptation for Virtual Teams Involved in Unstructured Work . In Gibson, C. B., & Cohen, S. G. (Eds.), *Virual Teams That Work* (pp. 265–291). San Francisco, CA: Jossey-Bass.

Knaus, W. A., Draper, E. A., Wagner, D. P., & Zimmerman, J. E. (1986). An evaluation of outcome from intensive care in major medical centers. *Annals of Internal Medicine, 104*, 410–418.

Kramer, R. M. (1999). Trust and distrust in organizations: Emerging perspectives, enduring questions. *Annual Review of Psychology, 50*, 569–598. doi:10.1146/annurev.psych.50.1.569

Kraut, R. E., Galegher, J., Fish, R. S., & Chalfonte, B. (1992). Task requirements and media choice in collaborative writing. *Human-Computer Interaction, 7*(4), 375–407. doi:10.1207/s15327051hci0704_2

Kuehn, B. M. (2007). No end insight to nursing shortage: Bottleneck at nursing schools a key factor. *Journal of the American Medical Association, 298*(14), 1623–1625. doi:10.1001/jama.298.14.1623

Lamothe, L. (1999). Hospital reconfiguration: A professinal challenge. *Ruptures, 6*, 132–149.

Le Blanc, P. M., de Jonge, J., de Rijk, A. E., & Schaufeli, W. B. (2001). Well-being of intensive care nurses (WEBIC): a job analytic approach. *Journal of Advanced Nursing, 36*(3), 460–470. doi:10.1046/j.1365-2648.2001.01994.x

Lewicki, R. J., & Bunker, B. B. (Eds.). (1996). *Developing an maintaing trust in work relationships. Trust in organizations: Frontiers of theory and research.* Thousand Oaks, CA: Sage.

Martins, L. L., Gilson, L. L., & Maynard, T. (2004). Virtual teams: What do we know and where do we go from here? *Journal of Management, 30*(6), 805–835. doi:10.1016/j.jm.2004.05.002

Mayer, R. C., Davis, J. H., & Schoorman, E. F. (1995). An integrative model of organizational trust. *Academy of Management Review, 20*(3), 709–734. doi:10.2307/258792

Melvin, W. S., Needleman, B. J., Krause, K. R., Schneider, C., Wolf, R. K., Michler, R. E., & Ellison, E. C. (2002). Computer-enhanced robotic telesurgery. *Surgical Endoscopy, 16*(12), 1790–1792. doi:10.1007/s00464-001-8192-9

Miranda, D. R. (1992). Critically examining intensive care. *International Journal of Technology Assessment in Health Care, 8*(3), 444–456. doi:10.1017/S0266462300013738

Moss, J., Xiao, Y., & Zubaidah, S. (2002). The operating room charge nurse: Coordinator and communicator. *J Am Med Inform Assoc, 9*(Nov - Dec Suppl), S70-74.

Müller-Stich, B., Reiter, M., Mehrabi, A., Wente, M. N., Fischer, L., Köninger, J., & Gutt, C. N. (2009). No relevant difference in quality of life and functional outcome at 12 months' follow-up—a randomised controlled trial comparing robot-assisted versus conventional laparoscopic Nissen fundoplication. *Langenbeck's Archives of Surgery, 394*(3), 441–446. doi:10.1007/s00423-008-0446-8

Norris, A. C. (2002). *Essentials of Telemedicine and Telecare*. New York: John Wiley & Sons.

O'Leary, M. B., & Cummings, J. N. (2007). The spatial, temporal, and configurational characteristics of geographic dispersion in teams. *Management Information Systems Quarterly*, *31*(3), 433–452.

Parillo, J. (1995). A silver anniversary for the Society of Critical Care Medicine - Visions of the past and future: The presidential address from the 24th Educational and Scientific Symposium of the Society of Critical Care Medicine. *Critical Care Medicine*, *23*(4), 607–612.

Paul, D. L., & McDaniel, R. R. (2004). A field study of the effect of interpersonal trust on virtual collaborative relationship performance. *Management Information Systems Quarterly*, *28*(2), 183–227.

Pinsonneault, A., & Caya, O. (2005). Virtual teams: What we know, what we don't know. *International Journal of e-Collaboration*, *1*(3), 1–16.

Powell, A., Piccoli, G., & Ives, B. (2004). Virtual teams: A review of current literature and directions for future research. *The Data Base for Advances in Information Systems*, *35*(1), 6–36.

Priest, H. A., Stagl, K. C., Klein, C., & Salas, E. (2006). Virtual teams: Creating context for distruibuted teamwork. In Bowers, C., Salas, E., & Jentsch, F. (Eds.), *Creating high-tech teams - Practical guidance on work performance and technology* (pp. 185–212). Washington, DC: American Psychological Association. doi:10.1037/11263-009

Pronovost, P. J., Angus, D. C., Dorman, T., Robinson, K. A., Dremsizov, T. T., & Young, T. L. (2002). Physician staffing patterns and clinical outcomes in critically ill patients - A systematic review. *Journal of the American Medical Association*, *288*(17), 2151–2162. doi:10.1001/jama.288.17.2151

Pronovost, P. J., Jenekes, M. W., Dormant, T., Garrett, E., Breslow, M., & Rosenfeld, B. A. (1999). Organizational characterisitcs of intensive care units related to outcomes of abdominal aortic surgery. *Journal of the American Medical Association*, *281*(14), 1310–1317. doi:10.1001/jama.281.14.1310

Rainey, T. G., & Shapiro, M. J. (2001). Critical care medicine for the 21st century. *Critical Care Medicine*, *29*(2), 436–437. doi:10.1097/00003246-200102000-00040

Rapoport, J., Teres, D., Steingrub, J., Higgings, T., McGee, W., & Lemeshow, S. (2000). Patient characteristics and ICU organizational factors that influence frequency of pulmonary artery catheterization. *Journal of the American Medical Association*, *283*(3), 259–2567.

Rawlings, A., Woodland, J. H., Vegunta, R. K., & Crawford, D. L. (2007). Robotic versus laparoscopic colectomy. *Surgical Endoscopy*, *21*(10), 1701–1708. doi:10.1007/s00464-007-9231-y

Reynolds, H. N., Haupt, M. T., Thill-Baharozian, M. C., & Carlson, R. W. (1988). Impact of critical care pysician staffing on patients with septic shock in a university hospital medical intensive care unit. *Journal of the American Medical Association*, *260*(23), 3446–3450. doi:10.1001/jama.260.23.3446

Ries, M. (2009). Tele-ICU: A new paradigm in critical care. *International Anesthesiology Clinics*, *47*(1), 153–170. doi:10.1097/AIA.0b013e3181950078

Rosenfeld, B. A., Dorman, T., Breslow, M. J., Pronovost, P., Jenckes, M., & Zhang, N. (2000). Intensive care unit telemedicine: Alternate paradigm for providing continuous intensivist care. *Critical Care Medicine*, *28*(12), 3925–3931. doi:10.1097/00003246-200012000-00034

Rousseau, D. M., Sitkin, S. B., Burt, R. S., & Camerer, C. (1998). Not so different after all: A cross-discipline view of trust. *Academy of Management Review, 23*(3), 393–404.

Shortell, S. M., & Rousseau, D. M. (1989). *The Organization and Management of Intensive Care Units*. University of California-Berkeley.

Shortell, S. M., Rousseau, D. M., Gillies, R. R., Devers, K. J., & Simons, T. L. (1991). Organizational assessment in intensive care units (ICUs): construct development, reliability, and validity of the ICU nurse-physician questionnaire. *Medical Care, 29*(8), 709–726. doi:10.1097/00005650-199108000-00004

Shortell, S. M., Zimmerman, J. E., Rousseau, D. M., Gillies, R. R., Wagner, D. P., & Draper, E. A. (1994). The performance of intensive care units - does good management make a difference. *Medical Care, 32*(5), 508–525. doi:10.1097/00005650-199405000-00009

Tang, Z., Weavind, L., Mazabob, J., Thomas, E. J., Chu-Weininger, M. Y. L., & Johnson, T. R. (2007). Workflow in intensive care unit remote monitoring: A time-and-motion study. *Critical Care Medicine, 35*(9), 2057–2063. doi:10.1097/01.CCM.0000281516.84767.96

Thomas, E. J., & Brennan, T. A. (2000). Incidence and types of preventable adverse events in elderly patients: population based review of medical records. *BMJ (Clinical Research Ed.), 320*(7237), 741–744. doi:10.1136/bmj.320.7237.741

Thomas, E. J., Chu-Weininger, M. Y. L., Wueste, L., Lucke, J. F., Weavind, L., & Mazabob, J. (2007). The impact of a tele-ICU provider attitudes about teamwork and safety climate. *Critical Care Medicine, 35*, A145.

US DHHS HRSA. (2006). *Report to congress the critical care workforce: a study of the supply and demand for critical care physicians*. Washington, D. C.: US Department of HHS HRSA.

Vincent, J. L., Suter, P., Bihari, D., & Bruining, H. (1997). Organization of intensive care units in Europe: lessons from the EPIC study. *Intensive Care Medicine, 23*, 1181–1184. doi:10.1007/s001340050479

Walther, J. B., & Burgoon, J. (1992). Relational communication in computer mediated interaction. *Human Communication Research, 19*, 50–88. doi:10.1111/j.1468-2958.1992.tb00295.x

White, M., & Dorman, S. M. (2001). Receiving social support online: implications for health education. *Health Education Research, 16*(6), 693–707. doi:10.1093/her/16.6.693

Wu, A. W., Pronovost, P. J., & Morlock, L. (2002). ICU incident reporting systems. *Journal of Critical Care, 17*(2), 86–94. doi:10.1053/jcrc.2002.35100

Zawada, E. T. J., Herr, P., Larson, D., Fromm, R., Kapaska, D., & Erickson, D. (2009). Impact of an intensive care unit telemedicine program on a rural health care system. *Postgraduate Medicine, 121*(3), 160–170. doi:10.3810/pgm.2009.05.2016

Chapter 19
The Interplay between Humans and Technology:
A Techno–Utilitarian Approach

Jacques Steyn
Monash University, South Africa

ABSTRACT

A brief overview of how computers, more specifically ICT, have changed over the past half a century is presented. Decades ago, when Gunilla Bradley began investigating the use of computer systems from a psychosocial perspective, ICT was used predominantly in the work environment, particularly for data capturing. Systems were designed for the workplace. Since then computer technology has changed significantly expanding to private and social use as well as for entertainment and communication. This chapter is about the history and development of ICT of which Bradley was a part. Now, at the end of her career, ICT will move beyond social aspects. The question is: what is next? - especially as work-place metaphors are still used for interface design. I propose that the human aspect should be the next dominant focus of attention, which implies a redesign of systems in order to reduce task load, effort and stress. This proposal is founded on a techno-utilitarian philosophy.

INTRODUCTION

When Gunilla Bradley began investigating the use of computer systems from a psychosocial perspective in the late 1960s, computers were used only in large organisations such as the military, government and corporations. The "market" covered was a small proportion of possible populations. Computers at that stage were number crunching machines, predominantly used for calculations and basic record keeping. Bradley's work naturally could only focus on the work environment, as computers were initially not used for other purposes yet.

Her interest was not so much on the computer engineering or technician side -- i.e. the whitecoats who managed computers in "secret" locations inaccessible except for the initiates -- but on the end-users: the data capturing clerks in typing pools. She considered their reactions to the work

DOI: 10.4018/978-1-60960-057-0.ch019

environment, and later defined psychosocial as "the process involving the interaction between the objective environment and the subjective one." (2006:51).

Computer technology has changed significantly since the 1960s, not only technically, but also regarding their use by humans. In her summary (chapter 3 in 2006) of developments in computing the focus is more on technological changes, such as miniaturization and chip innovations, but she does not neglect interface improvements and home entertainment technology (e.g. chapter 5 in 2006). My own summary presented here of the relatively short history of computers does not focus so much on the technological history than on the human and social aspects.

The first generations of devices were computers used for military and business purposes. Some later generations were networked. In large organisations there was a server with workstations on individuals' desks. All the computing power was on the server, and the terminals basically dumb display and input units. When the computing power was transferred to the terminal, which could now operate by itself, even without network connection, it was called a "personal computer" (the PC), which is a misnomer, as there was nothing personal about it - its main function was still office work, as demonstrated by the metaphors used for the interface: files, directories, and the name of the first general application "word processing", on which I will elaborate below.

With reference to computing power, the PC was actually a down-scaled computer, but it could operate on its own, independent of the server or network. The first PC's were, to put it crudely, just powerful typewriters, and the purpose of typing was creating documents for business and organisational purposes. Academics began writing books and articles on PCs, just as they previously did with typewriters. Later generations of PCs would have the added advantage of re-use of such documents, when copying sections of text

became easier, but that was not possible with the early generation of PCs.

Only from the 1990s did the PC became more "personal", as more application software products came on the market that were not primarily work-related. Entertainment products, particularly games, grew phenomenally, so that by the turn of the century the gaming industry surpassed the movie industry in financial turnover. The internet moved into the public domain, and especially the World Wide Web brought an immense digital library into middle-class homes, as well as facilitating communication by means of email. Just after the turn of the century, social networking tools were introduced that made networked communication even easier, as well as including multimedia functionality. At the time of writing some of the most popular online applications are tools focusing on the social aspects of human nature - Facebook, blogs, and twitter.

The brief history of computing, stretching over just half a century, thus saw extending its range of relevance from the workplace to homes, from formal office administration to entertainment and informal social activities, from restricted in-house network connectivity to informal global networks. Castells (2004a) and Giddens (1983) have somewhat different takes on technology and society, but they agree that ICT are social enablers. Despite these changes that penetrated society at large, and extended use to include many more and diverse social groups, human interaction models with the virtual world of information are still held hostage by workplace metaphors, by convoluted applications, and in short, by immature interfacing with the machinery of computers.

HISTORIES

The histories of different human endeavours are not the same, but similar patterns may be observed. This should not be read as a statement supporting technological determinism and progressivism, which assume that all kinds of developments follow the same paths. Technological development always has two sides: economical and personal. Mass uptake of technology with no financial benefit is unknown, at least to me. And technology that does not have personal and social (which in this context includes business as one type of social and cultural endeavour) benefit does not make much sense. The motor car has tremendous personal benefit: it offers freedom of movement, and each generation of cars has more features to make life easier. For example, the self-starter no longer requires turning a handle to crank the engine; when darkness approaches lights switch on automatically; navigation systems assist drivers not getting lost, and a very long list of functions that make driving quite a different experience than even half a century ago. This is not to say that modern cars are easier to use cognitively. Our physical stresses have been reduced manifold. But the cognitive load using a car has increased with a plethora of available buttons to push. The approach in this chapter is techno-utilitarian: the use of technology to make life easier by extending the power of our constrained physiological and cognitive abilities with the least possible effort.

HISTORY OF TECHNOLOGY

The great revolutions in the history of technology made things easier for human endeavours. We as humans are able to spend less energy on the tasks which technology can perform better. In general terms, the history of technology is briefly this. Our ancestors first extended muscle power by using stick and stones to dig, cut and throw. Ancient stone age mines at European locations such as Spiennes in Belgium, Grimes Graves in England, Krzemionki in Poland and many more suggest an extensive industry for making stone tools. Renfrew and Bahn (2004) noted that the Rijckholt mine in the Netherlands contains about 2.5 million axeheads. Dating of stone tools sug-

gest that our ancestors began to make use of them at least 2 million years ago. Later innovations were about newer materials (copper, iron) used for the same functions. An immense stone tool industry existed, manufacturing devices to make life easier. The tools were hand-operated, and served to mediate manipulation from the hand to the object that required manipulation. Such tools extended muscle-power.

The next revolution came when the extension of muscle power was mechanised. Some machines driven by various forms of energy (water, wind, fire, steam, fuel, electricity, nuclear energy) now directly worked on the material, while humans manipulated the machines. Operators were now one system removed from the materials on which the work is performed, and humans only indirectly in touch with the materials.

Using animals for transport extended bodily carrying power as well as mobility. Animals are of course not a technology, but technologies were attached to animals - the cart, the harness, stirrups, and so forth. Our ancestors extended our ability to move first to animals, and later to mechanised vehicles, both transport methods manipulated by controls. Controlling functions for transport have not changed much functionally since its inception, but the controlling technologies have changed dramatically. A control technology could be used to command a transport mechanism (whether animal-driven, wind-driven, fuel-powered, and others) to start or stop movement, the direction of movement (forward, backward, or degree left or right). Steering the direction of an animal with bridle technology involves pulling a string either left or right. Steering a car left or right fifty years ago was a mechanical process. Now it is possible to steer a car by wire, meaning that the driver manipulates an ICT layer that triggers the mechanics of steering. Large aeroplanes are no longer directly steered by pilots using mechanics. They now fly by wire. An additional layer, a computer layer was inserted.

As recent as only 100'000 years ago, as per available evidence, we began to extend our brain power by making symbolic marks. The oldest known *homo sapiens* "writing" (dated 77'000 years ago) is on a piece of ochre found in Blombos Cave in South Africa. There is a deliberate pattern of diagonal lines along the length of the piece, which indicates that by that time we had advanced cognitive abilities. Older art work was found at Berekhat Ram in Israel, probably done by *homo erectus* around 230'000 years ago, but it is debatable whether artistic patterns require the same cognitive skills than geometric patterns (Renfrew & Bahn, 2004). The dating of the origin of cognitive abilities is immaterial for this discussion, but it points to a very long history of extending cognitive power to external objects, although not as long as the use of stone tools.

The oldest known writing system is the cuneiform script of Sumer on clay tablets and dated to about 4000 years ago. A stylus was used to directly write the symbols on the clay. Archaeological finds of early artwork indicate the use of technology first for aesthetic purposes, and later for communicative purposes. Writing with pens, pencils and similar utensils all involved humans directly manipulating the material with technology. Later computers would, as with transport, become an intermediary layer. Our writing became digital in a virtual world that requires devices to render them in more real output forms, such as printing. Again we no longer manipulate the world directly, but indirect through virtual worlds.

Machines have become the dominant interfacers with the world, while humans became the controllers of machines, involved only indirectly with the world. Yet most of our control systems were designed in different eras, many of them in a mechanical era, and the interfaces following mechanical metaphors, based on levers and buttons. These were merely digitised without much thought and energy spent on more appropriate design of digital controlling interfaces. One reason for this was the limited available computing

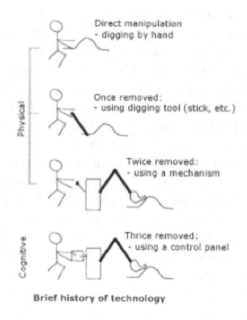

Figure 1. Brief history of technology

power and memory restrictions in the early days of computers. There just was not enough power and capacity to spend on interface design.

The history of designing controlling interfaces for mechanical technology extending muscle power is very long compared to the short history of extending cognitive power. The first comprehensive interfaces for extending cognitive power with computers were introduced about half a century ago, and the metaphors used came from the context of office administration. Functionally, these metaphors are very poor descriptors for what computers are used for today (Figure 1)

BRIEF HISTORY OF THE AUTOMOBILE

Viewing a forest from a hilltop results in quite a different perspective than when viewing it from a path within the forest. Reframing the mind's biases is often difficult, but when prompted by a different conceptual framework from a different domain, the trees often appear different too. This brief history of the automobile serves as a tool for reframing how we view the history of computing. This brief expose should not be seen as some form of historical determinism, an attempt to force the histories of two different technologies into a single mould of technological progressivism. The attempt is more heuristic, and to stimulate discussion from a different perspective.

Historians generally define the automobile as a device of transport that is self-propelled. Given this definition, wind-driven water-borne vehicles would of course also be automobiles. Bottorff (no date) reports that in 1335 the Italian, Guido da Vigevano, designed a wind-propelled terrestrial vehicle. The first vehicle that carried its own power source was designed by Nicholas Joseph Cugnot and constructed by a certain Brezin in 1769 (Wikipedia 2009b). It was steam-driven, and designed to move cannon around in Paris, France.

The first fuel-propelled vehicle was developed by Siegfried Marcus around 1870 in Vienna. The structure of the vehicle was still basically a wagon, except with no horses pulling it. Karl Benz built the first vehicle that did not mimic the cart or wagon. Drivers would have experienced an enormous amount of stress to change their cognitive schema from a vehicle similar to a horse-cart to a vehicle with no horse in front. Over the next half a century there was a proliferation of small car manufacturers, but output was relatively slow and low.

Perhaps stating the obvious, this all changed when Henry Ford introduced a production assembly line and making the car affordable to the middle class. The Model T Ford was first launched in 1908 and production of the model only stopped in 1927. Almost no changes were made to the car's design over the almost two decades of production, as Henry Ford was of the opinion that users do not need features other than those already offered. History proved him wrong. The Model T Ford, or Tin Lizzie, could be regarded as a personal transport mechanism, as opposed to public transport mechanisms. Attempts at self-propelled transport

had a history of several centuries, but became only widely used after several technological innovations (e.g. the internal combustion engine) and mass-production. There is a parallel here with the history of computers: the mass-produced PC originally was an office computer that later also became available for private use. There were of course several products available from other car manufacturers, but Ford set the tone for mass production, just as Microsoft set the tone for the PC among several other contenders. Neither Ford nor Microsoft offered the best quality products, but enough features that more or less satisfy most people, which is how technology is usually adopted (Garbarino & Edell, 1997).

The cars of today may share features with the first generation of cars, including the Model T Ford. Cars generally have four wheels, a chassis, a body, seats, and controls for the driver to manipulate the mechanic beast. These functions have not changed over the past century, and if animal drawn vehicles are included, they have not changed functionally since the first carts were drawn by animals. Technologically, however, every single component has undergone a very wide range of innovations, from the materials used to the mechanical engineering and design. And finally, the modern car has on-board computers that assist drivers to make their driving easier. Light sensors trigger headlights to automatically turn on and off; other sensors trigger both the on/off status as well as the speed of windscreen wipers; climate control ensures a constant temperature in the cabin, and in some cars even humidity is controlled. Dashboard displays inform drivers when the next service is due. All kinds of technologies were introduced for breaking, ranging from controlled traction, to alternating and pulsating breaking (all performed by the mechanics and electronics), while the driver only needs to activate these functions with the break pedal. Operations are relatively simple. Cognitive overload is mainly due to the wide range of functionality offered, and the fact that there is no global standard for matters such as the pattern for manual gear changing, or for the position of levers such as for indicators.

The point of this discussion is that the car has changed over the past century to became more user friendly (except for cognitive load), to address the human aspect more and more. I propose that contemporary PC technology and applications are still stuck in the same phase of development than the Model T Ford and the next phase of development in ICT would imply redesigning systems from a more user-friendly perspective. Computer technology has matured; interfaces have not.

This brief exploration of the history of the automobile and of computing should not be seen as an attempt to interpret history deterministically. There may be observable repeating patterns in human history, but the paths of change are not predetermined, and because of human agency, can take any direction. I also do not wish to fall into the trap of progressivism, so I deliberately made a statement about "paths of change", rather than the Victorian "paths of progress" language, which seems to be very prevalent within the ICT industry.

BRIEF HISTORY OF COMPUTING

Agar (1998) points out that literature on the history of computing is typically technical, and do not much reflect on ICT usage - i.e. not functional histories. He suggests the term *informatic history* for a history of computing that focuses on the overall information ecology, rather than just the history of technological items, e.g. chip development or application development. Here I offer an informatic history. The word "computer" was introduced for a device used for calculations that could be performed manifold faster than the human brain. The first applications all focused on calculations. Today, however, a small percentage of use, from a user's perspective, involves calculations.

Historians of computing often claim that computer technology began centuries ago, exemplified

with tools used for calculations, such as tally marks on objects, dating as far back as 30'000 years ago. The abacus, the first of which were probably invented in Babylon around 2400 BCE also features, and so does the more recent Difference Engine of Charles Babbage (1791-1871) -- see e.g. Frauenfelder (2005). Such trivialities may be as interesting as Guido da Vigevano's 1335 wind-propelled vehicle, but functionally irrelevant, as few contemporary users would regard their PCs as advanced calculators.

In the 1950s and 1960s physicists used computers at atomic energy laboratories for calculations, and the military extensively sponsored research in computing. There was a need to calculate the flight of a shell fired from a weapon to its target, and to do this very quickly and accurately. This is just arithmetic, and the human brain not particularly built for this, so errors were common. The computer was the ideal tool for such quick calculations.

Modern computers may essentially be calculators, but this definition is methodological, not functional. After all, all writing is scratching on a surface (the method), but it does not follow that the alphabet (a function) began as scratches. Developmentally perhaps the ability to make scratches is a prerequisite for writing, but writing does not necessarily flow from scratches. A significant breakthrough is required to turn informal random scratches into a formal, highly structured writing system.

Functional computing only really began in the 1950s when Grace Murray Hopper, who worked for the US Navy, developed a compiler for the UNIVAC which translated human language commands into machine code. Later she also worked on the FORTRAN and COBOL programming languages. Human language commands made programming much easier for programmers, but had no impact on end-users, except for programmers as "end-users", having the benefit that programs could be developed somewhat quicker. Technically, many such innovations were prerequisites for the development of ICT, but it was not until the 1970s that it would be possible to turn computers into devices that would be more friendly towards ordinary users, although the consumer market was still some time in the future.

The non-technical history of ICT, in a very brief statement, can be viewed as the expansion of the user base from a few closed social groups (the military, government and large corporations), to open and informal networks of social groupings, based on similar interests. Simultaneously, the communication media expanded from numbers to text, and eventually to multiple media channels -- i.e. full colour, audio, still pictures, and eventually moving pictures. This entire range is today available to all the computer user groups (including the closed groups).

Initially motor cars were used by a small proportion of the population who had access to such vehicles – they were just too expensive for the middle-class. Henry Ford changed that. With his production line approach, cars could now be mass produced, and that changed the history of transport. Today, in highly developed economies, the typical middle-class household owns a motor car, if not several. Transport was "personalized" as a commuter now did not depend on public transport networks to be mobile. This was of course also possible with the horse, but non-animate self-propelled vehicles had advantages such as less fatigue on long distances, and more riding comfort.

Similarly, the advent of the personal computer did much to contribute to the widespread use of computers. Initially PCs were only networked within large organisations. The advent of the World Wide Web in the 1990s changed that, as it put being networked within the reach of the middle-class too. In the beginning PCs were not powerful enough to handle colour, graphics, sound, or video, but since around the turn of the century standard PCs came equipped with such functionality. Whereas in the early days of the Web only nerds were able to fully use many different

media, channels and functionality for social networking, after the turn of the century tools became available to make it easy enough for the masses to participate in a media-rich network of social relationship. These developments have changed the nature of network communities forever, now being able to rise above the constraints of time and of geographical space. "Computing" was personalised and became available to the masses.

HISTORY OF WORD PROCESSING

The history of computing is briefly about a change from the use of computers in formal settings, particularly office administration, to informal social networks. One application in particular put the PC on the map. The ability to type documents digitally, and manipulate them in the virtual world, benefited the growth of computer usage, and benefited all societies in which writing is important. In the beginning of the twentieth century, the function of typing pools was to capture hand-written paper documents that other clerks created. Initially typing pools used typewriters to produce more readable documents than hand-written documents. The first generation of computer data capturers were essentially also working in typing pools, except that the document data was now captured electronically. Data capturing was a specialised activity, and done in a special venue, typically separated from other office workers, who completed the forms with the data that needed to be captured. The advent of the desktop computer and word processing changed this. Today office workers themselves do the data capturing. In fact, with online systems and home access to networks, consumers and clients may perform the data capturing tasks. The typing pool is no longer required.

This history is like an inverted pyramid: originally few people (data capturing clerks) did capturing; then more people captured data (the general office workers) and we are now moving into an era where everyone with access can do data capturing. The burden on typing pool kind of jobs is now spread over whole populations. It entered the social domain.

But none of this would have been possible without the PC and word processing applications. In the early 1970s IBM introduced word processing centres, which contained word processing machines, basically automatic typewriters and dictating machines, that were operated by word processing operators rather than secretaries or stenographers (Haigh 2006). By the late 1970s office automation became the fad in business computing, which implied that office workers could now, independently of typing pools, write their own documents on computerized devices. However, the vision to deploy these specialized work stations did not materialize, due to costs, as well as due to the human factor that managers did not take a liking to this new technology. The 1970s also saw the introduction of a range of computerized word processing typewriters (such as produced by IBM, Wang Laboratories, and Vydec) replacing automatic typewriters (Haigh 2006). The first word processors were stand-alone devices.

Around 1975 Xerox at PARC developed novel office automation concepts, including a Bravo text editor which was based on the notion of WYSIWYG (*What You See Is What You Get*).

In 1980 IBM released the Displaywriter word processing system, which included a screen which showed documents, hence the name indicating that what one writes is displayed. This Displaywriter is not to be confused with the product later released for the PC. DisplayWrite 1 software application for the IBM PC was released only in 1984, although it was based on the 1980 "computer typewriter" product.

In the 1970s and early 1980s marketing of the use of corporate computing emphasised office automation, rather than the personal computer. I recall how in the early 1980s we as academics were frustrated by our university computer services who still believed there was no future for the PC, and

the networked work station was to be the only method considered by IT Services. We bypassed university red tape by making a case for research to buy PCs that could handle character sets other than ASCII, which was just too cumbersome for the mainframers to develop.

In 1968 Doug Engelbart demonstrated a word processor at a Joint Computer Conference to demonstrate his vision of a system to augment human intelligence. This system had more useful features than any of our contemporary dominant word processor today, more than 40 years later. For example, his system allowed for creating highly structured documents of which parts could be expanded or hidden, depending on where the user wants to work (similar to contemporary Ajax-driven web pages that hide some information until instructed by a user to be exposed), collaborative editing (present systems, in my view, still have a long way to go in this regard), and sending messages from the system (Haigh, 2006). Despite this ground-breaking work that included the use of a mouse, scrolling, cutting and pasting between documents, his system did not get off the ground because of a difficult interface design and limited computer power. About a decade later Xerox took these concepts further in their personal workstation concept. Haigh highlights that Xerox' efforts were to "reinvent the office, rather than a philanthropic desire to advance knowledge" (2006: 21), and focused on the paperless office, with emphasis on office work. Until that time, computer output was predominantly text files. Xerox' Bravo text editor could produce documents with graphics and print in laser quality, similar to printing press quality, which was a move toward multimedia documents.

Another development, introduced by Wang Labs in 1982, was an attempt to offer an integrated multimedia office work station. This Office Information System was called Alliance and claimed to offer "data processing, word processing, audio processing, image processing and networking". It never took off as the system was too slow. There was not enough processing power in those days for such a complex system. Users are only prepared to wait when their degree of desperation matches frustration levels of having to wait for slow processing time. In 1984 Wang Labs introduced their Office system, which integrated word processing, telephony, and email (Haigh, 2006). Alliance was very far ahead of its time as this concept is along the lines of what I suggest with the multimedia "workspace" I will discuss further on. At that stage ICT systems were just not powerful enough to handle all this functionality. Today they are.

WordStar (produced by MicroPro) was launched in 1978 on the CP/M operating system. WordStar 3.0 was released in 1983. Despite a cumbersome user interface, this word processor put control in the hands of the user, and did indeed save time to correct mistakes. Prior to this, to correct a spelling mistake on a printed page, one had to place the page back into the typewriter, align it very carefully, and retype the character. With the PC word processor, rough editing could be done on the screen, and mistakes corrected, while a page with a mistake could be reprinted after corrected. In practice, this lead to waste of paper, especially when corrections covered syntax or additional words, which messed up the layout of the following pages as well. We have now become accustomed to reprint entire documents, at great expense to forests, and making a mockery of the original vision to create a paperless office. I have not come across a study comparing paper waste, but having observed printing habits over the past few decades, I am convinced we waste much more paper per person today than twenty to thirty years ago when we used typewriters.

In 1981 IBM launched its Personal Computer, which became the business standard. WordStar was ported to this operating system, and remained the dominant word processor for several years. IBM's DisplayWrite for PCs was a duplication of its word processing system DisplayWriter, a very cumbersome program to use, but forced down by business computer support services onto

office users. WordPerfect, originally designed in 1979-1980 for the city of Orem's Data General minicomputers was ported to the IBM PC operating system in 1982, and dominated the word processing market in the later 1980s. It surpassed WordStar, which stopped improving the software, and when they woke up in 1987 to introduce major changes with WordStar 4 and WordStar 2000, it was too late to recapture the market. WordStar continued to exist until the release of Version 7 in 1998-1999 after which it disappeared. In 1983 Microsoft released its word processor software, called Multi-Tool Word, but it was not a success, while the first attempt at Windows was released in 1985, but took off only after the release of Windows 3 in 1990.

In 1988 Amí, the first fully-functional Windows word processor, was released by Samna, but could not handle tables. The upgrade that could handle tables was called Amí Pro, released with Adobe Type Manager for Windows. In 1990 Lotus bought out Samna, and the product was renamed Lotus Ami Pro, later to be renamed again as Lotus Word Pro. After IBM bought out Lotus in 1995 the product was again renamed as IBM Lotus Word Pro. The table layout handling of this program is still the best ever of all word processing programs I have used, and I include the most recent versions of the most popular word processing applications. Its layout features in general has also not yet been surpassed by any other product on the market. It allowed for an object, including a character, to be placed anywhere on a page. The entire page frame acted as a surface, while all other word processors still regarded the end of the workable page as the last character entered. And of course, its selection panels were floatable, non-interruptive of workflow, while even today panels in word processors interrupt workflow.

What does the history of the word processor demonstrate? It originated as a typewriter aimed at typing pools in the context of large organizations - office work. Some op the functionality that was added was the move from black and white output to colour output, the addition of spell checkers, the inclusion of images, some collaboration abilities and communication abilities. But as a tool contemporary word processors are comparatively still primitive - like the Model-T Ford. Many of the great ideas that would have put the word processor on a different plane were ignored or squashed. Engelbart's collapsible structure, and proper collaboration functions are still absent; AmiPro's use of the workspace as a scratch pad, allowing the placement of objects by a mouse click is still ignored or difficult to control, and the worse of all, except for AmiPro, all word processors rudely interrupt workflow with modal panels, or require convoluted or unnecessary steps to complete tasks - especially system steps that were designed when computer power was still very limited, and introduced to prevent system crashes.

Functionally there have been no breakthroughs in word processing applications for decades. Except for cosmetic changes, and some changes under the hood (for example the move toward XML), very few improvements have been introduced in word processing application programs. Yet the consumer market is duped into forking out unnecessary money for each supposedly "new" version and upgrade. This immoral approach would not be tolerated by consumers in other product markets. Upgrading car models implies much more driving comfort and safety, but we are not forced to upgrade our cars every year. Consumers do not really get any benefit from upgrading application software. Some upgrades, in fact, are backward steps into the dark ages of computing. Let me give an example outside the domain of word processing. In my view the interfaces of the latest upgrades to both Adobe Photoshop CS4 and Adobe Dreamweaver CS4 are steps backwards. For example, in previous versions of Dreamweaver open documents could be floated anywhere on the screen estate. Now they can only be moved inside the application frame. In previous versions the HTML <title> content

showed in the top document bar along with the filename and path. This information has now been dropped for no usability reason at all. There is a host of other backward steps, but beyond the scope of this chapter.

Two decades ago Tognazzini (1992) stated that control panels should be modeless. With today's computer power it is an embarrassing shame that interfaces of application programs are still caught up in programming requirements of 40 years ago! It is also surprising that with the amazing processing power and memory capacity available today, we still require different applications to perform some task that could technologically speaking, easily be performed by a single program.

THE TECHNICAL, SOCIAL, AND THE HUMAN ASPECTS

The history of technical development involves three aspects: the technical, social, and the human aspects. With the human aspect I imply technology designed around human needs. Despite the evangelism of those in the field of HCI that computer systems should be user friendly, it is surprising that the present form of design of ICT applications is taken for granted, and that HCI research focuses so much on improving the status quo, rather than on designing functionally friendly systems from scratch.

Initially developments of a new technology are technical in nature. the basic generic design of cars is now stable, while technological innovations refine the existing functional modalities - e.g. energy efficiency, steering mechanisim refinement, gearbox refinement. The basic architectural design problems have been solved. For more than half a century the dominant innovations in ICT were technical. Once the basic technologies in ICT - the handling of colour, images, sound and video - became more widespread, ICT reached a mature enough stage that the social aspect could materialize. Social computing is a relatively new development, and tools facilitating social computing are still rudimentary, and require both architectural systems design and modality refinement. The basics of colour, image formats and so forth have more or less been sorted, but still requires architectural integration.

Contemporary ICT systems meet a whole range of human needs which were not possible in the early days. Bradley alludes to some of these needs in her chapter 5 (2006), such as the feeling of social belonging. The importance of such a need is evidenced by applications such as Facebook. The popularity of social media is due to the introduction of a single front-end that allows several features previously handled by different application tools.

Google Wave (2009) is an application designed from the social aspect, and encompasses novel approaches to "old" functions, such as email. Some new interface components were also introduced in Google Wave, which means that the human aspect is now considered. Google Wave (2009) illustrates what I mean with designing an application from a functional point of view. The development team took a few steps back, and asked what users really want to do. Human needs drove the design process.

Technical, social, and the human aspects do not follow linearly or chronologically one after the other. I propose it is the degree of dominance that would distinguish between the different aspects - I deliberately do not call them phases. Initially innovations are technical, then products become more socially consumable, and finally designs begin to consider human comfort and characteristics. These aspects are not progressively related. Even high technology incorporates the human aspect, although on a very basic level. After all, humans use technology. When driven technologically, the human aspect is typically added as an after thought.

The human aspect contains more than just the notion of being user friendly. It refers to designing for the human touch, and develop technologies

around that. It promotes designing to reduce stress by making effort seamless an non-demanding.

STRESS

Bradley traces the study of "psychological stress" back to Hans Seyle's work in 1926, which is defined in relation to over-stimulation and under-stimulation.

"Medically speaking, stress is our reaction to various kinds of irritation. Stress is a combination of defence and adjustment measures that is the organism's response to frustrations and other sources of irritation in its surroundings. In many cases this is a positive and appropriate reaction, while in other cases it is inappropriate or misdirected." (Bradley 1989, p. 146).

In typing pools, or batch-operators, the dominant stressors were physiological . Bradley lists stressors such as headaches and bodily pain (neck, back, shoulders). "Current research shows that prolonged continuous work at a VDT [computer screen] can cause problems in the neck, shoulders, and back. These are caused by poor seating posture and the fact that people spend far too long sitting and working at a VDT. (1989, p. 147).

There were also psychological stressors such as hectic work pace and work load that cause anxiety (2006, chapter 8). Today the dominant techno-stress is psychological due to information overload. Bradley mentions stressors such as: contact overload, lack of organizational filters, difficulty of separating noise from essentials, and so on (2006, p. 189). It is of course not only the workplace surroundings that cause irritation. Complex on-screen processes, especially unnecessary steps (such as long strings of mouse clicks), also cause irritation. My focus is on such on-screen irritations, as they could be avoided with better flowing interface designs.

Ergonomically designed workspaces may perhaps reduce physiological stresses, but systems should also be designed to reduce psychological stress. Despite some amazing developments and innovations, the computer industry is still in its infancy, as applications are not designed to reduce stress. It seems that innovation is primarily technological, while little attention is paid to the psychosocial aspects. Technological innovation seems to be driven by economic models. Developments are typically driven by administrative efficiency rather than reducing psychosocial effort. Where humans are indeed considered, it seems that interest in making their lives easier views them a just another cog in the wheels of industry rather than true compassion. Alexander (2006) relates that the Elmo workstool, developed between the world wars in the Elmowerk (Germany), was developed to increase worker efficiency and lessen fatigue, not because of compassion for workers, but to increase productivity. The word processor was introduced to increase the productivity of office paperwork. Humans are reduced to one of the components in the business process (the insulting "human capital"), reducing us to *homo economicus*.

This display did more than demonstrate specific ways to enhance physical comfort and support, however. It also illustrated an industrial need for regularity and uniformity in human motions and signalled the creation of a pathology of movements that did not fit industrial patterns. To combat this new pathology, the exhibition offered a solution: workers would be rendered efficient through a mechanical form of discipline in which their individual movements would be constrained, much as were those of a machine (Alexander 2006, p. 286).

Alexander also quotes a 1929 journal on labour health stating that the aim was "to eliminate 'all motion not directly necessary for work.' " (2006, p. 287). The emphasis is thus not primarily on worker comfort, but on streamlining the production process. The worker is merely a gear in the process. To make it run smoother, add more grease.

From a humane, psychosocial perspective, worker needs need to be considered, rather than the profit margin of the company. Bradley alluded that the psychological attitude of workers would indicate whether ICT reduces stress:

From a psychology-of-work viewpoint, it is desirable that a computer system contributes to the creation of work tasks and a work situation that implies as few employees as possible being subjected to the woes of either over- or understimulation. It is the individuals themselves that make this assessment (Bradley 1989, p. 11).

Surely if workers complain about physiological pains because of their bodily positions in front of computers, and of irritation with software, while the ICT industry does not introduce solutions to these complaints, it must be concluded that the assessment of their tools by the workers themselves is ignored.

ICT systems should be design so as to reduce stress. In this respect Csikszentmihalyi's "flow" is a useful concept. With flow he meant that when one is absorbed in an activity one likes, it is like being in the zone. One's entire being is involved. He mentions playing jazz, where the musicians are totally absorbed in the activity. I would add that if this flow is disrupted when a guitar string breaks, or if one of the musicians messes up a rift, results in stress. PC systems are often presently designed to interrupt such flow, and it causes unnecessary stress. Yet not much attention is paid to consider reducing stress in the design of ICT systems.

No technology could ever be designed to reduce human stress completely. After all, our human bodies have not evolved over the past few hundred thousand years to sit on a chair, bent over a desk and interface with a computer for hours at a time. The stresses Bradley investigated will most likely never go away, but systems could nevertheless be designed to reduce any stresses as far as possible. Perhaps it may be impossible to design away the causes of physical stress, but

I suspect it would be easier to design to reduce psychological stress.

PLACES: THE WORKPLACE AND THE THIRD PLACE

The history of ICT can also be constructed in terms of the "place" where ICT is used. In the beginning it was business systems that dominated, and developments focused on streamlining office work for efficiency. The workplace dominated ICT. Today ICT functions mainly in a virtual space, called *the third place* by Oldenburg (1989, 2001) - no longer only at the workplace, or at home, but in virtual worlds. In the section on the history of technology I suggested that through the course of time we moved further and further away from manipulating the real world directly. First we used tools directly on the objects we wished to manipulate. Then we mechanised the process, controlling the mechanics with levers and buttons. Today we have an additional layer, a digital layer with which we interface, and that layer operates the execution of the controls. We thus manipulate objects only indirectly, and operate in the third place, even if that place is about work.

Interface metaphors are often still stuck in the world of direct manipulation, which by itself is not necessarily a bad thing. We press virtual "buttons" on computer screens with "mouse" clicks. But the virtual world does not of necessity require the mechanical metaphors of the formal workplace, especially if the historical process has changed so much it no longer makes sense. We no longer use a stylus to make cuneiform marks on clay, so stylus would not be a good metaphor for writing. We no longer process words, and neither do we work with office files when we create a multimedia document, or participate in online social activities. Why are we stuck with such workplace metaphors? Metaphors should be relevant to the third place, which includes informal social chat-

ting, doodling, creating information parcels that contain a variety of media, and so forth.

The present generation of base software (i.e. windows-based operating system interfaces) is based on workplace metaphors. Applying ICT began in large organisations, such as the military, government and corporations, where files and directories are commonly used for office administration. Note that the dominant application suite of Microsoft is called "Office", not "Home"(the suite with this name is merely a scaled-down versions in terms of features, using the same office metaphors as the mother suite) or "Entertainment" or "Chatting". After the advent of the PC, particularly its multimedia abilities, and then joining of the PC to global networks, other social dimensions could be addressed by ICT: entertainment, private hobbies, and extending social networks into the virtual domain. If a suite were called "Chat Tools", it would mimic the social setting of conversation, mediated by technology. The medium does not have to be audio. But as in ordinary chatting, we may share information in other media, e.g. showing a magazine article (i.e. text) or photos from a vacation to a participant in the virtual conversation. Any of these media objects should be handled seamlessly and effortlessly. In such a suite metaphors such as "send" and "file" would not be used, but to "share" (for send) a "photo" (instead of having to select a photo file), while the system would handle technicalities to make the photo available to the addressee.

The workplace was the first domain of ICT, and systems were designed for the requirements of the workplace. The tools and metaphors used in ICT applications show this bias. The third place may indeed also serve as a workplace, but it is much more than that. It is a social place, and a place for personal gratification (such as entertainment). ICT tools of the third place require much more than the limited set of workplace tools, and it is unsuitable to use office metaphors for such a broad set of interests. The third place mimics the real 3D world we live in, addressing the complete set of human senses. This requires a different kind of interface.

HABITS, CUSTOMS

The office metaphor is deeply entrenched in ICT design. Changing this to a new set of metaphors would require a great deal of effort. Some habits die hard. In the history of the automobile new technologies have been introduced that demanded learning new ways for performing tasks, and to unlearn some habits.

The Model T Ford's transmission was controlled not with a gear lever, but with three foot pedals that had different results depending on their settings. What served as the modern accelerator pedal (the throttle) was a lever on the steering wheel. Imagine having driven this car for a long time, and then switching over to a car with different settings where one now had to use a hand-lever for gear changing, and a foot-lever for the throttle. The switch to such a new system would require immense cognitive effort to override the habit.

For many decades gear levers were mounted on the steering column, while the levers of sports cars were mounted on the floor. Today few cars have steering column mounted gear levers; most are on the floor. Now, once again, the trend, especially in luxury cars, is to let electronics handle switching gears, and have the control as a relatively small lever on the steering column . Drivers continuously have to adapt to new interfaces.

Different gear lever positions is not as confusing as the different patterns for changing gears. In manual cars, first gear could be anything from left front or back, while reverse could be in any corner. In some cars the lever has to be pushed in, and in others pulled out to engage reverse gear. Driving different cars with different configurations can be hazardous, especially when one's schema for gear changing was established driving one type, and then having to drive another type.

The same kind of confusion arises regarding indicator levers and windscreen wiper levers, which are in opposite positions in European and in American and Asian cars. It is disturbing that an established schema, developed through driving one particular setup, can be life-threatening when switching to another configuration and having to react to a threatening event by reflex, which would trigger reactions based on a schema.

Using ICT is not life-threatening (yet...?), so changing customs would not have such an effect. The common argument against changing the present set of office metaphors and interface customs assume that establishing new schema would be too costly in training workers to adapt to a new set. But this is a financial response, not a humane one. It is a response that assumes humans are mechanisms in the gears of corporate life.

The book publishing industry has been around for half a millennium, and we have grown accustomed to books, newspapers, magazines and such printed material in predominantly portrait orientation. The film and broadcast media, on the other hand, adopted a landscape orientation.

Unfortunately, despite its focus on documents and print in the early days of PCs, the landscape orientation was chosen for PC screens, resulting in the need for excessive scrolling. To see a whole portrait page on a landscape screen results in text too small to be of any use without scrolling, even on today's extra large screens. Ideally a screen should be in portrait orientation for the most efficient flow of text, as some early DTP programs indeed used, but landscape for video.

The convergence of the media results in a peculiar problem. The same computer screen is used for both documents and movies. To consider the needs of users, screens should thus be capable to be switched to any orientation. Such a design would put the user in control, even if it would require effort to change.

There is a very good reason why video is in landscape format. The world around us consists of a 360 degree horizontal view that contains an immense amount of predominantly visual information. The vertical view, by comparison, provides relatively little information -- only clouds and weather, and the moon, planets and stars, including perhaps flying birds, mountains and tree tops. Without visual enhancing technologies, such as telescopes, there is not much to see in the skies above us. So our typical 3D orientation is locked into the landscape format around us.

The portrait format for text also has a good reason. Early book makers realised this even without the assistance of scientific research, which only really began in-depth studies in the twentieth century (Nanavati & Bias, 2005; Rayner 1998). It seems that for on-screen reading text should not exceed a medium of about 55 character per line for ease of reading, comprehension and reading rates (Nanavati & Bias, 2005). This implies that the portrait orientation is better suitable for reading text.

Despite established habits and customs in ICT, particularly with reference to the office interface used for multimedia documents, it is time to revisit the metaphors in interface designs.

HUMAN PERCEPTION AND MULTIMEDIA

Stated crudely, humans are information processing "machines". Our perceptual system processes incoming information, and our information productive system outputs information. Modern neurobiology distinguishes nine perception systems (sight, hearing, touch, smell, taste, thermoception, proprioception, nociception, equilibrioception), several more than the five identified by the ancients, such as Aristotle. We experience these systems as an integrated whole. Not even the most advanced computer technology can mimic this. Although amazing developments in mimicking human senses have occurred in robotics and intelligent computing, the systems are not fully integrated and ready yet for mass-production. In

the domain of the PC, specialised systems (multimedia PCs) are still required, and very far from getting even remotely close to offer an integrated experience of all the sensory inputs. How can interfaces designed for an office, using office metaphors, offer adequate interface metaphors for such a multiple sensory world? They can not. Even if a computer extends the power of the brain, it still is a relatively primitive device in the present historical instance of time.

Humans have a complex set of perception (or input) systems, and several expressive (or output) systems that are used for messages in multiple media. Referring to the message, information media may be classified as follows:

- Atemporal visual information: such as text, photos
- Temporal information: such as music, narration
- Temporal visual information: such as video, animation

The temporal information classes require a timeline onto which the flow of information is mapped.

The above classification does not state anything about the production or interpreting processes, which both require time, but only about the message content. Scanning with the eyes through a photo requires time. But the information package, a text document, or a photo, does not contain a time property. Sound only addresses the auditory senses, while video may be watched without sound. All these facets need to be considered when designing an interface that should provide message producers with easy to use tools to create messages and the selection of media, and tools for message receivers to access information parcels in formats of their preference (without having to know the formats - i.e. the device should handle formats without the user having to pay attention to such technicalities).

THE MULTIMEDIA "DOCUMENT"

In the early days of ICT, computers had limited memory capacity, and processing power was weak compared to today's processing power. It was necessary to build small applications that were not too slow, nor consumed too much memory. Wang Laboratories' *Alliance* failed mainly because it was too slow and tried to do too many things with the then restricted available technology. This Office Information System was released in 1982, but by 1990 the company faced bankruptcy.

Only by the late 1990s could PC's handle multimedia objects, and only after year 2000 were networks capable to handle multimedia more or less adequately, although still primitively. Fullscreen on-demand online video is still a dream on networks, and given the present state of development, globally still several decades away, if ever achievable.

Given that ICT attempts to mimic the human senses and experiences, from an application point of view, what is required is a "workspace" on which a user can create multimedia objects: atemporal, temporal and temporal visual, while seamlessly and effortlessly switching between and integrating different media.

EFFORT AND LOAD

The physics law of entropy applies to human behaviour as well. Assume doing nothing is a state of rest - except of course for our physiological processes required to keep us alive. By implication then, any action we take requires effort and energy. Technological devices may reduce the basic effort involved in performing a task, but the technology itself should also require the least possible effort to use.

This is not always obvious in the domain of devices that extend the power of our brains. If a task is physical, it is quite obvious that a lever that needs to be pulled with a lot of effort requires redesign. It is not so obvious that in the domain of ICT that interfaces that require a lot of cognitive effort could be redesigned resulting in less effort.

Effort is measurable. Both physiological and psychological stress are measurable. For example, stress may result in an increase in the flow of blood, which could be measured, or the amount of energy spent may be measured. The amount of energy spent by an individual will depend on his interest, drive, or fear. For example, the motivation to perform a boring task on the job may be due to the fear of losing the job. In such a case the worker may be prepared to spend hours in front of a computer screen. Effort moving a mouse across a screen, or performing a long string of steps, are also measurable.

For the purposes of this chapter qualitative effort will refer to the amount of energy spent above the resting threshold, while task load will refer to the discernible discrete quantifiable "steps" to perform a task. I distinguish between three types of load that influence interface design: cognitive load, motor load, and time load.

Cognitive Load

Cognitive Load Theory was introduced in the early 1980s by among others, John Sweller (see e.g. 1988, 1994 and 2005), to analyse instructional techniques, particularly solving mathematical problems. The goal of solving a problem can be reached by many possible routes, many which are dead-ends, or which may lead in totally different directions, preventing reaching the goal, or at reaching the goal following a tiring route. During the process of problem solving there are decision points (which Sweller calls choice points) where a user needs to make a decision of which route to follow. The decision may not necessarily lead to the solution (reaching the goal). The best methods for problem solving depend on using schema, which are constructed through experience and include domain specific knowledge. If the solving path is complex, little learning takes place, and schema are not constructed, which means that next time the problem solver approaches the problem, he basically starts again as novice. According to Sweller, experts depend on cognitive schema that have been formed through experience, and direct the problem solver in choosing between possible routes. As schema are still under-developed in the brains of novices, they take longer to solve problems, and would also take more wrong choices.

A schema is a cognitive construct that organizes the elements of information according to the manner with which they will be dealt. An early discussion of schemas was presented by Bartlett (1932), who worked on the role of the sensory cortex in bodily postures, but who disliked the term. Later Miller's (1956) concept of a *chunk* addressed the same notion, and later still, Schank and Abelson's (1977) introduced the notion of scripts (also Schank 1982). Whatever label is used, a schema incorporates "standard" routines that are constructed through experience, which Bartlett called "active, developing patterns".

Schemas are not binary on-off constructs. A schema is constructed over time and thus becomes more informative through experience. One illustration to explain this is to visualise the history of a schema as an interlaced image that loads onto a networked computer canvas. Initially only some pixels are visible. As more information becomes available, more pixels are coloured and the picture becomes clearer. Schema construction starts at the beginning of the learning process, but becomes more refined as more information is added through experience. The more information a schema contains, the easier processing becomes. Perhaps in the starting phase the brain needs to spend more effort on concentrating, while once the schema reaches maturity, handling schema-based processes becomes effortless and "automatic".

Performing tasks using technologies such as ICT could be viewed as problem solving tasks. For example, if someone using a word processor wants to reduce the font-size of a particular word,

there are several steps required by the user interface that need to be followed. For a novice this is a problem that needs to be solved, while for an expert user, the steps could be followed automatically without much conscious thought (if he has a schema for it). There are nevertheless a certain number of steps that are required, and each one induces cognitive load (as well as motor load).

Cognitive load, as used in the context of interfacing with ICT, is defined as the number of discrete steps to be taken to reach the goal. This only applies to goal-directed tasks. When performing leisurely driven tasks, such as browsing, the goal is not so much completion of a task as the enjoyment of exploring, in which case the number of steps does not really matter to the user.

The number of steps that need to be calculated would also include the number of sub-routines that need to be performed. Sub-routines would be necessary deviations from the main path. For example, the main goal might be to write a one page document. Changing some text into bold font in this case would involve a sub-routine.

Users draw on memory to remember the paths (based on acquired schema) taken to reach the goal. Recalling such paths depend on at least two aspects:

- Frequency of use
- Complexity of the task

Tasks performed less frequently are remembered more poorly. There is no universal rule here. Remembering such steps will depend on a variety of idiosyncratic characteristics of the user - varying from interest, to degree of desperation and unique individual memory capacity.

Using applications for work, or a specific task, leads to stress if the path is not obvious or clear, or convoluted and confusing. The design goal should be to reduce stress levels in the interface, and to minimize the number of steps required to perform a task.

Motor Load

Motor load refers to the number of muscles used in order to perform a task. Some muscles are directly involved in the action -- such as moving a mouse -- while others would be indirectly involved -- such as keeping one's body in a seating posture in a chair while working. Fatigue from having to sit in the same position for long periods of time has been documented for a very long time. Bradley's work refers not only to emotional (or psychological) stress, but also to physical stress, such as pains in the neck, shoulders and back (see e.g. 2006).

In 1954 Paul Fitts proposed that when using technological interfaces, the time required to rapidly move to a target area is a function of the distance and the size of the target. This came to be known as Fitts' Law. Not only the number of muscles involved in an action should be considered, but also the order in which the muscles are operated. In this respect a corollary to Fitts' Law would be relevant: Effort increases exponentially when multiple targets need to be hit in order to reach the goal. To explain this, mark the four corners of a work surface as A (top left), B (top right), C (bottom left) and D (bottom right). Consider having to move a mouse with one's hand diagonally across the work surface from bottom right (D) to top left (A), then having to move back to the bottom right (D), and then to the top right (B), the order D-A-D-B. Moving the mouse left-right uses one set of muscles, while using the mouse forward-backward, another set, and diagonally, some combination of the two sets. It should be logically evident that energy would be conserved if the two separate D events could be collapsed into a single step, or if the triggers for such as an event sequence are at least located closely together to prevent having to move the mouse not only over long distances, but also in several different directions to complete the task.

Mouse movements, number clicks, typing keys, and other tasks that require the user's physiological motor system to be performed, all add to the task load. Present application interfaces are not particularly designed to reduce keystrokes or mouse movement, resulting in unnecessary user stress.

Time Load

Time load (more formally temporal mode) refers to the elapsed time to complete each step in the task-completion process. Humans are constrained spatio-temporally, and thus time load is important. Every action we take is performed through time. Time wasted when the work flow is interrupted would have a negative effect, and cause stress, no matter how minuscule. This is a logical statement, as in practice users may be so used to wasting time using present generation PCs (e.g. being habitually used to having to wait for applications to load), that they accept that it is necessary baggage for using technology. Interruptive tasks should be avoided - such as unnecessary pop-ups that the user is forced to close down before being able to continue. They take up unnecessary time, require motor input, and are disruptive to the main task at hand. However, not all interruptive tasks may be disruptive. In some cases supportive tasks need to be completed before the device can continue with the main task. In my view the majority of pop-up windows in present applications are unnecessary.

The number of perceptual channels involved in a task also play a role. Some channels may be dominant, which would be the fundamental channels for a particular task. For example, when reading, the visual channel is dominant, but there are nevertheless other channels involved. When turning a page, motor and touch may be the dominant channels, even if this is on a sub-routine level. Expert readers do not have to concentrate on turning a page, but do so unconsciously, based on their reading schemas. Such tasks are important for task completion. After all, without turning a page one cannot finish reading the document. Turning pages requires spending energy (this would be motor load, but also take time). Turning pages have nothing to do with understanding the message, but nevertheless need to be done in order to access the message - hence called a subsidiary task, which also needs to be considered when calculating the task load. Subsidiary tasks should be reduced as far as possible.

Some subsidiary tasks using ICT would be switching on a computer, moving a mouse, opening a window, starting a program, and in all these actions, having to wait (i.e. time load) for technology to complete the requested tasks. It should be self-evident that a device that makes programs available immediately when switched on would require much less task load than one for which one has to wait. The immaturity of the ICT industry shows by not having basic programming application procedures burnt into chips to be available immediately when switched on. There is no technical reason why this cannot be done - only business reasons. The ICT industry is unfortunately driven not by manufacturing user friendly devices, but by business models that in effect hamper the development of good and user-friendly products. It could be argued that historically large ICT corporations stifled the implementation of good technological concepts by worrying more about the continuation of their products than making life easier for users.

It might be possible to measure the stress levels of the different types of load, either by means of a cognitive model, and, or with tools such as fMRI. As there are constraints on the contexts within which fMRI scans can be performed, cognitive models may be useful until such time as measuring technologies can be implemented in a variety of contexts.

Garbarino and Edell (1997) point out that humans typically spend effort to reach a satisfactory goal, rather than the optimal goal. When decision making is complex, the effect is negative affect. People seem to be willing to forgo benefits to conserve cognitive effort. In the web design courses I have taught I alluded to this notion - what I call the Principle of the Degree of Desperation. When

searching the web, or wanting to download a file on low bandwidth, the time and effort a user is prepared to spend on the activity would depend on how desperate he wants that information or file. When searching for some specific information, and not finding it within the timeframe allowed by the degree of desperation, the user will give up quickly if desperation is low - not even reaching a satisfactory goal. However, if the information is regarded as important, the user might spend a great deal of time and effort trying to find that information. Web surfers, in particular, do not typically have a high degree of desperation and would quickly go elsewhere if they have to spend too much energy trying to find something on a particular website.

THE ULTIMATE "WORKSPACE" - A CREATIVE SPACE

The fact that humans are typically satisfied with less than the optimal goal illustrates that we wish to avoid effort. Reaching optimal goals require more effort. The design of technology should be such that optimal goals could be reached with the least possible effort, which can only be achieved by reducing the task load.

Gunilla Bradley's interests have changed along with technological developments. Later in her career she acknowledged the importance of social networks, and alluded to multimedia systems (2006, chapter 5). We are in the beginning of the explosion of social computing, while multimedia is still in an infant stage. This discussion of the ultimate workspace is based on ICT concepts that have been touted as the next big thing for more than a decade: multimedia platforms, convergence of media, ubiquitous access, etc. I suspect that if Bradley continued to be active in ICT, this might have been her next topic of interest - the socio-psychology of the human aspect of multimedia ICT.

Here follows some initial notes on an ultimate multimedia application program that collapses the functionality of entire present application suites into a single program. With a multimedia application I certainly do not have in mind the presently available tools for multimedia applications, which are extremely rudimentary. There is presently no easy to use application that can handle all the different media adequately in a single package. The text handling abilities of high-powered graphic tools is not suitable at all to create text documents. Some word processors appear to be able to handle multimedia. For example, in a text document one could add an image, and even sound. But such documents are merely containers of objects that have to be created using other applications to create high quality objects. What I propose here is a single application with the power to incorporate all the other functionality. This is technically possible.

In addition to the aspects of media (atemporal visual information, temporal information, and temporal visual information), there are two modes in the production of messages: creating the message, and sharing the message. When creating a message the information producer decides on which senses to address, and composes the message accordingly. It is possible that one medium may dominate, but most likely several media might be used in the same "document". A better formal metaphor for a multimedia "document" would be "information parcel" (or package). The tools to make this production possible should allow seamless switching between media -- in fact, the producer should not even be aware that medium switching is happening.

An application used for creating an information parcel should include functionality that today is handled by different applications. A multimedia application should be able to handle: text (word processing), images (both still and moving), structured data (database), calculations in tabular format (spreadsheet), presentation of information in chunks (presentation tools), sound (with differ-ent approaches ranging from MIDI to soundwaves, and include sound mixing), communication (such as done with Google Wave), and so on.

The mode of sharing the message would include the intention of the producer: is the message to be read, listened to, watched, a combination of these? Must the addressee respond? An information parcel may consist of a combination of media. Each would constitute a chunk within the message, and each might address a different set of senses. The technical aspects of message delivery should be immaterial. The addressee must be able to use any device at her disposal to access the message. This implies that the producer "sends" the message to a virtual repository, and technically this should be done in a device neutral medium such as a markup approach, e.g. XML. The producer should not even have to worry whether this message must be sent, to use contemporary technical jargon, in email format, SMS, web page, or whatever protocol. From a user point of view, file formats should become obsolete as they are system properties that should not concern users, just as the technicalities of the chemistry of fuel used in cars does not concern drivers.

The area in which information is created is traditionally called the "workspace", a metaphor which implies labour, but such information production spaces can be used for many other functions, such as conversation, entertainment and fun, and other human activities that have nothing to do with work. Such a virtual space, or arena, is an "area" in which information is created, compiled and packaged. It is a three dimensional space. Perhaps we should rather drop "work" from "workspace" and just use "space", even though this space would also include time, for temporal classes. The metaphor "space-time" would perhaps hint too much at high science to be user-friendly.

Two spaces are required: the creative space, and the information presentation space. Except when collaborating, producers of messages would not like their message to be altered by addressees. The presentation space would prevent editing. Ownership rights and similar issues would be protected within the presentation space. Note that this only concerns editing rights, not access rights (e.g. DRM), which is an issue I will not address here.

Only a single space (or creative space) on the computer screen, which in today's parlance would be a single window, needs to be opened to work on. There is no technical need to open multiple application programs. A non-interruptive (i.e. modeless) floating toolbox panel would contain user-defined actions (i.e. programming commands). A user should be able to drag and drop items into the floating toolbox. According to Harris (2006), user feedback on Microsoft Word 2003 indicated that the top most used commands were: 1. Paste, 2. Save, 3. Copy, 4. Undo, and 5. Bold. These actions could be included by developers as default commands in the active floating toolbox - and users could of course remove them from the box. But, the Save command is totally unnecessary. Saving could be done programmatically, and with today's processing power and memory capacity, changes could be saved character by character and pixel by pixel, without the user ever having to explicitly tell the computer to save data. Processing speed is today so fast, and memory so large, that a user should never be required to explicitly save a document or file. The system is capable of saving each keystroke, and can save endless previous versions of the document which can be retrieved if the user so wishes. But apart from data entry applications, this very basic method of reducing effort is not applied in any application programs

In such a "space" *Undo* would mean reverting to a previous version. In order to accommodate random reversion, data deleted could show in a different pane (i.e. window). For example, while writing, an author may realise that some reversion is required, but only the sentence four steps previously, while the last three sentences need to be kept. Such a reversion window may facilitate this kind of action.

The "work" space should act as a scratch pad - on whatever coordinate a user places a pointing

device, it should be the starting point of work. In this context "work" means creating data in any of the media: text, images, moving images, sound.

A modal process interrupts the present mode and route taken to reach the goal. It requires entering into another mode that requires attention from the user before one can proceed - e.g. a dialogue box that pops up and needs to be closed before one can continue. A modeless process does not stop any processes but is part of flow. It is quite possible to design systems that have modal process only by rare exception.

Here is one very simple example. In most word processors, including the most recent versions of OpenOffice or Microsoft Word, when selecting text formatting options, the action window must first be closed before one can continue working in the document – i. e. a modal approach. A much better design would be to make that window a floating panel that is non-interruptive, as was done by a word processor originally known as Ami Pro (Figure 2), then bought out by Lotus, and then by IBM, and renamed Word Pro. Selected text would immediately display the formatting features selected within the panel, without having to leave the panel. It is thus possible to toggle between different fonts and font styles until one is satisfied with the result. One could also continue to work in the document without having to close the floating panel, which can be placed anywhere on the screen. As far as usability is concerned, this is by

Figure 2. A modeless floating panel used to add features to text in IBM Lotus WordPro

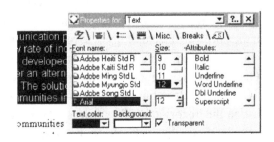

far the best ever word processor released on the market. Its table handling was absolutely brilliant.

Modal windows are invasive of work flow, especially if they are just information or notification windows, and even worse so when they take up large screen estate.

The above suggested "space" and guidelines for interfacing are self-evident if applications are built around user needs, and not so much driven by software corporations who are more concerned with dominating the market than providing human-centred applications. The concepts presented are very simple, but require a radical design approach to application development. There is nothing technically impossible preventing such an approach. Some of the suggestions are in fact quite old. As long as about two decades ago Bruce Tognazzini (1992) recommended that the Save command should become obsolete, and that modal panels should be avoided. Unfortunately developers are not adequately trained in the human side of ICT, so for the past almost twenty years this advice seems to be unknown in the domain of software developers.

CONCLUSION

The above serves as a very brief glimpse of what is technically possible for the design of ICT devices that would reduce effort, and thus stress. In this respect I do not refer to alternative input devices, such as Jeff Han's Multi-Touch Interaction (2006), but focus only on digital on-screen interfacing. It is by no means intended to be comprehensive, as this chapter is about considering how ICT has developed thus far in its short history, and where it might be going, given the underlying assumption that the purpose of technology is to reduce effort.

In very broad strokes, I gave some pointers to Gunilla Bradley's contributions to the journey of ICT history. It is time to move into the next phase in the history of ICT, which would be not so much about the technology, but about the socio-psychological aspects of ICT usage, which Bradley did indeed consider, and the basis of which I propose should be a techno-utilitarian approach.

Since the late 1960 when Gunilla Bradley began studying ICT and humans, the ICT landscape has changed significantly. Computers that were originally used only in large organisation for office administration and other formal tasks are now consumer products, used for private purposes and social networking. Yet ICT, particularly the PC and its applications, are still in the Model T Ford phase of development.

The question is, what next? This "next" should not be defined technologically, but how technology could be utilised by humans to perform tasks with less effort. Such a techno-utilitarian approach demands a fresh look at the design of ICT systems. It was suggested that perhaps we need to implement new metaphors, and to explain that, I gave a handful of examples of how application software could make much more sense, and be used with much less effort, addressing the human aspect.

The techno-utilitarian position I propose is a type of consequentialism which holds that the moral worth of an action is determined by its outcome, in this case less effort. The principle of least effort would be the measure to determine the value of a technological product, not only the product as a whole, but each of its components. Reducing effort reduces stress. Unnecessary cognitive load, motor load, or time spent on actions cause stress. ICT systems should be designed to reduce this.

The techno-utilitarian approach allows for a balance between the extremes of technological and cultural deterministic approaches. The utility of technology is to make life easier. By doing so, human behaviour, and possibly customs and habits may change. There is thus a continuous interplay between technological development and human adoption of new technologies.

Such a proposal is idealistic, as corporations dominating markets are not particularly threatened or interested in reconceptualising mass produced applications. But we could dream...

REFERENCES

Agar, J. (1998). Introduction: History of computing: Approaches, new directions and the possibility of informatic history. *History and Technology, 15*(2), 1–5. doi:10.1080/07341519808581938

Alexander, J. K. (2006). Efficiency and Pathology Mechanical Discipline and Efficient Worker Seating in Germany, 1929–1932. *Technology and Culture, 47*, 286–310. doi:10.1353/tech.2006.0109

Alty, J. L. (2003). Cognitive workload and adaptive systems. In Hollnagel, E. (Ed.), *Handbook of cognitive task design* (pp. 129–146). New Jersey: Lawrence Erlbaum Associates.

Annett, J. (2003). Hierarchical Task Analysis. In Hollnagel, E. (Ed.), *Handbook of cognitive task design* (pp. 17–35). New Jersey: Lawrence Erlbaum Associates.

Bartlett, F. (1932). Remembering: A Study in Experimental and Social Psychology. Cambridge University Press. Retrieved December 2009 from http://www.ppsis.cam.ac.uk/bartlett/RememberingBook.htm

Bauer, W., & Kern, P. (1994). Human Factors in office design - employee expectations and future trends. In G.E. Bradley & H. W. Hendrick (Eds.), *Human Factors in organizational design and management* (pp.67-72). Amsterdam, NL: North-Holland

Bottorff, W. W. (n.d.). What Was The First Car? A Quick History of the Automobile for Young People. Retrieved December 2009 from http://www.ausbcomp.com/~bbott/cars/carhist.htm

Bradley, G. E. (1989). *Computers and the psychosocial work environment*. London: Taylor and Francis.

Bradley, G. E. (2006). *Social and Community Informatics: Humans on the Net*. London: Routledge.

Bradley, G. E., & Hendrick, H. W. (Eds.). (1994). Human Factors in organizational design and management - IV. Development, introduction and use of new technology - challenges for human organization and human resource development in a changing world. In *Proceedings of the 4th International symposium on Human Factors in Organizational Design and Management*. Amsterdam, NL: North-Holland

Castells, M. (Ed.). (2004). *The network society*. Northampton, MA: Edward Elgar.

Castells, M. (2004a). Informationalism, networks, and the network society: a theoretical blueprint. In Castells, M. (Ed.), *The network society* (pp. 3–45). Northampton, MA: Edward Elgar.

Ceruzzi, P. E. (2005). Moore's Law and Technological Determinism. Reflections on the History of Technology. *Technology and Culture, 46*, 584–593. doi:10.1353/tech.2005.0116

Csikszentmihalyi, M. (1990). *Flow: The Psychology of Optimal Experience*. New York: Harper and Row.

Fitts, P. M. (1954). The information capacity of the human motor system in controlling the amplitude of movement. *Journal of Experimental Psychology, 47*(6), 381–391. doi:10.1037/h0055392

Frauenfelder, M. (2005). *The computer*. London: Carlton Books.

Garbarino, E. C., & Edell, J. A. (1997). Cognitive effort, affect, and choice. *The Journal of Consumer Research, 24*(2), 147–158. doi:10.1086/209500

Garson, B. (1988). *The Electronic Sweatshop: How Computers are Transforming the Office of the Future into the Factory of the Past*. New York: Simon and Schuster.

Giddens, A. (1984). *The Constitution of Society*. Los Angeles: Univ California Press.

Google Wave. (2009). Retrieved December 2009 from http://wave.google.com/

Haigh, T. (2006). Remembering the Office of the Future: The Origins of Word Processing and Office Automation. *IEEE Annals of the History of Computing, 4*(5), 6–31. doi:10.1109/MAHC.2006.70

Han, J. (2006). Multi-Touch Interaction Research. Retrieved December 2009 form http://cs.nyu.edu/~jhan/ftirtouch/

Harris, J. (2006). No distaste for paste (Why the UI, Part 7). Retrieved December 2009 from http://blogs.msdn.com/jensenh/archiove/2006/04/07/570798.aspx

Hollnagel, E. (Ed.). (2003). *Handbook of cognitive task design*. London: Lawrence Erlbaum Ass.

Hollnagel, E. (2003a). Prolegomenon to cognitive task design . In Hollnagel, E. (Ed.), *Handbook of cognitive task design* (pp. 3–15). London: Lawrence Erlbaum Ass.

Latour, B. (1993). *We have never been modern.* Cambridge, MA: Harvard University Press.

Lewis, R. (2001). Redesigning the Workplace. The North American Factory in the Interwar Period. *Technology and Culture, 42*(3), 665–684. doi:10.1353/tech.2001.0172

Mayer, R. E. (Ed.). (2005). *The Cambridge handbook of multimedia learning.* Cambridge, UK: Cambridge University Press.

Miller, G. (1956). The magical number seven, plus or minus two: Some limits on our capacity for processing information. *Psychological Review, 63*(1), 81–97. doi:10.1037/h0043158

Nanavati, A. A., & Bias, R. G. (2005). Optimal Line Length in Reading--A Literature Review. *Visible Language, 39*(2), 121–145.

Neerincx, M. A. (2003). Cognitive Task Load analysis: allocating tasks and designing support . In Hollnagel, E. (Ed.), *Handbook of cognitive task design* (pp. 283–305). London: Lawrence Erlbaum Ass.

Oldenburg, R. (1997). *The Great Good Place.* New York: Paragon House. (Original work published 1989)

Paas, F., Renkl, A., & Sweller, J. (2003). Cognitive Load Theory and Instructional Design: Recent Developments. *Educational Psychologist, 38*(1), 1–4. doi:10.1207/S15326985EP3801_1

Rayner, K. (1998). Eye Movements in Reading and Information Processing: 20 Years of Research. *Psychological Bulletin, 124*(3), 372–422. doi:10.1037/0033-2909.124.3.372

Renfrew, C., & Bahn, P. (2004). *Archaeology: theories, methods and practice.* London: Thames and Hudson.

Schank, R. C. (1982). *Dynamic memory.* Cambridge, UK: Cambridge University Press.

Schank, R. C., & Abelson, R. P. (1977). *Scripts, plans, goals, and understanding: An inquiry into human knowledge structures.* Hillsdale, NJ: Lawrence Erlbaum Associates.

Sweller, J. (1988). Cognitive Load During Problem Solving: Effects on Learning. *Cognitive Science, 12*(6), 257–285. doi:10.1207/s15516709cog1202_4

Sweller, J. (1994). Cognitive load theory, learning difficulty, and instructional design. *Learning and Instruction, 4*, 293–312. doi:10.1016/0959-4752(94)90003-5

Sweller, J. (2005). Implications of cognitive load theory for multimedia learning . In Mayer, R. E. (Ed.), *The Cambridge handbook of multimedia learning.* Cambridge, UK: Cambridge University Press.

Sweller, J., & Levine, M. (1982). Effects of goal specificity on means-ends analysis and learning. *Journal of Experimental Psychology. Learning, Memory, and Cognition, 8*(5), 463–474. doi:10.1037/0278-7393.8.5.463

Swierstra, T., & Jelsma, J. (2006). Responsibility without Moralism in Technoscientific Design Practice. *Science, Technology & Human Values, 31*(2), 309–332. doi:10.1177/0162243905285844

Tognazzini, B. (1992). *Tog on design*. Reading, MA: Addison-Wesley.

Wikipedia. (2009a). Fax. Retrieved December 2009 from http://en.wikipedia.org/wiki/Fax

Wikipedia (2009b). History of the automobile. Retrieved December 2009 from http://en.wikipedia.org/wiki/History_of_the_automobile

Wissner, A. (1994). Organization anthropotechnological contingencies an analytical approach. In G.E. Bradley & H. W. Hendrick (Eds.), *Human Factors in organizational design and management* (pp.613-617). Amsterdam, NL: North-Holland.

Chapter 20
Psychosocial Life Environment and Life Roles in Interaction with Daily Use of Information Communication Technology:
Boundaries between Work and Leisure

Ulrika Danielsson
Mid Sweden University, Sweden

Karin Danielsson Öberg
Umeå University, Sweden

ABSTRACT

The presence of ICT (Information Communication Technology) in our psychosocial work environment and in our personal lives, has increased rapidly during the past 40 years. This way of interacting with ICT is often characterized in terms of access to information and social networks with the possibility of being independent of time and place. Every person's psychosocial health is influenced by their life environment; a combination of their work and home environments, their life roles and of their social networks. People who work professionally in the field of ICT or use ICT in their work experience a blurring between their professional and private roles. However, when people's experience of work and leisure becomes blurred, this may impact on their psychosocial health. They need to develop strategies to create ways of allowing time for recovery. In this chapter we present a review of the literature that identifies the effects that cause a blurring of the line between work and leisure. Moreover, we present some examples of strategies for managing the blurring of contexts facilitated by ICT. Presented research combines theories from the fields of psychology, informatics and work science.

DOI: 10.4018/978-1-60960-057-0.ch020

USE OF INFORMATION COMMUNICATION TECHNOLOGY

The presence of ICT (Information Communication Technology) in the psychosocial work environment has increased rapidly during the past 40 years. A development which has provided workers in different organizations with the ability to work even when they are away from the office and on the move. Lately, the presence of ICT has also increased in our personal lives during leisure activities. Therefore, we are not only able to work on the move, but also able to attend to personal needs, such as dental appointments and family matters. This way of interacting with ICT is often characterized in terms of access to information and social networks with the possibility of being independent of time and place; that is, anytime or anywhere (Perry *et al.*, 2001).

When we entered the industrial age, the primary workplace was outside the home; maybe in a factory or an office building. After the workday, the workers would return home or go to another place where they spent their leisure time. Work time and work place were dictated by the employer. With this separation, that is, performing a specific activity at a specific place, the physical and psychological boundaries between home and workplace became easy to define. People went to their place of employment to work and came home to do necessary household tasks and spend their leisure time (Dahlbom, 2003; Jarrick, 2005). However, due to ICT, this separation is less easy to define. One example of this is the use of leisure technologies such as television. At the beginning of the television revolution, programs started at a specific time and ended at a specific time with a limited number of channels. By contrast, today we can watch television whenever we want, regardless of where we are, as long as we have an Internet connection through our mobile phones or computers. The requirement of being at a specific place for a specific length of time has changed.

Figure 1. Past: Work and leisure activities overlapped to a limited degree. Principally, people were able to separate their work time from their leisure time.

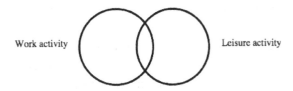

Work and leisure are defined by most as completely different activities, but they are, in reality, bound together, and work could not exist without leisure, and vice versa. Even if leisure provides humans time for recovery, work appears more frequently to squeeze out leisure. Work might be seen as an alienation activity, often referred to as "responsibility', while leisure is defined as a time of freedom, where the activity is chosen by the individual as a means of self-expression and creativity.

Today, being physically away from the workplace does not mean that we are necessarily leaving our work tasks behind in psychological terms. The focus is on completing the work before a deadline, so it does not matter where or during what timeframe the work is done. Today we can use ICT whenever we wish, and some of us may even feel bound to stay connected, not just with our colleagues, but with friends and family, as well. We can manage work, life and other concerns through our use of ICT (Sadler *et al.*, 2006). Regarding of the possibilities of being able to work any time and from any place, the challenge is that one has to plan both work time and leisure time (Allvin *et al.*, 1998). The young people of today have more evening and night-time activities than in the past (e.g., increased availability of television programs, channels, internet, and mobile phones). Moreover, the young people of today not only sleep less, compared to young people 100 years ago, but they are doing it by choice. One might ask how addicted have we become to our mobile phones and computers?

There are numerous benefits from the use of ICT, for example, being able to reach someone regardless of place and time, or the ability to search for information about almost anything. However, there are numerous outcomes that we have come to experience as being psychologically or even physically negative for humans, especially when we are unable to create a boundary between work and leisure. This chapter presents a review of the literature that identifies the effects that cause a blurring of the line between work and leisure, and some examples of strategies for managing the blurring of contexts facilitated by ICT. It combines theories from the fields of psychology, informatics and work science. In this chapter the focus concerns some of the effects that can be found in a review of the literature, and presents a summary of the effects that cause the blurring of boundaries between work and leisure in order to offer some suggestions on how to continue research within this field.

In this chapter we begin by presenting studies concerning psychosocial life environment and life roles in interaction with daily use of ICT. In order to discuss different environments and roles, we present common background theories of how a person performs a number of roles, and how these, together, constitute one's life role. In addition to this, we present results concerning the relationship between ICT and psychosocial health. Finally, we connect identified effects to implications for design in order to further explore the context of life roles and life environment in relation to an individual's use of ICT.

PSYCHOSOCIAL WORK ENVIRONMENT

Since the end of the 1970's, numerous researchers have focused on how work roles and psychosocial environmental work factors are changing

in interaction with ICT, e.g. life roles and life environment (Bradley, 1986); stress as a part of life (Frankenhaeuser and Ödman, 1983); new conditions for life at work (Hanson, 2004); and the individual and life at work (Lennerlöf, 1991; Levi, 2001; Oborne, 1985). According to Bradley, psychosocial work environment is defined as follows:

The term psychosocial work environment is used to signify the course of events or the process that occurs when objective factors in the environment are reflected in the individual's perception (either positive or negative) of work and condition of work. Its essence is the interaction between the environment and the individual. Thus work environment factors exist at different levels – the level of society; the level of the company and level of the individual – and they interact with one another. But there is also a distinction between the objective and the subjective work environment, which also interact (Bradley, 2001, pp 36).

The work environment, as described in the quotation above, can be approached from different levels and perspectives. Concerning the individual that moves between these different environments, one is not only shaped and controlled by one's physical human characteristics, but one can also shape one's life through personal choice and action. Based on this view, Bradley (1986, 2001) illustrates the dual relationship between the objective and subjective work environment. In figure 2, the constant interaction between the objective and subjective work environment is shown.

With the daily use of ICT, our pace of living is increasing, and we are developing new opportunities for flexibility in work and learning, independent of location and time. Bradley (2006) brings forward some examples in various areas of life that are being challenged in the ICT society. She also discusses how to get closer and involve the individual in the ICT society by performing and combining research concerning physical and

Figure 2. Relationship between ICT, objective and subjective work environment and stress. Adapted from Bradley, 1986, 2001.

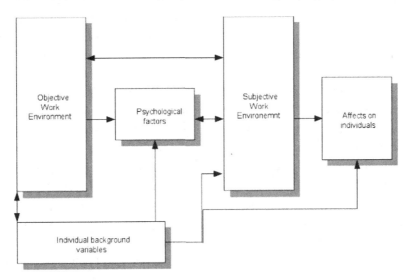

psychosocial life environment, human need, human requirements and human rights.

Life Role and Life Environment

Today, one can carry out different activities in many different environments (home, office, public), but one must "carry out" a *role* to be able to be a part of an environment. These roles are more or less predefined and put the individual in the position of either adjusting to the role or giving up any attempt to enter the profession. According to Goffman (1974), *environment* is described as a stage. We use different stages daily in which we perform roles in order to interact with other people in different situations. A person's life role can be divided into three major sub-roles: the professional role (work life), the private role (private life) and the citizen's role (public life) (Bradley 2001, 2006). Every person embodies different roles (mother, researcher, neighbour), and these, together, constitute a *life role* (see Figure 3).

The concept of *life role* covers the combined *professional* role, *private* role and *citizen* role. The *private role* includes activities that refer to

one's private life (e.g mother, sister, daughter, wife and friend). The *professional role* includes activities that refer to one's work life (the content of one's job and different aspects of the psychosocial work environment, physical and virtual places for performing work, etc.). The *citizen's role* includes activities that refer to life as a citizen

Figure 3. A person's life role can be divided into three major sub-roles: the professional role (work life), the private role (private life) and the citizen's role (public life) (Danielsson & Danielsson, 2008).

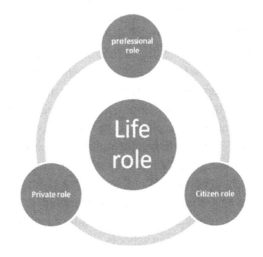

within the larger society (to what extent today's citizens take an active interest in societal issues, e.g., political issues and are active within voluntary, non-profit organizations, etc.).

The "home environment" is the structure within which we live, because it is our base in life, even though we perform activities within other environments during most of our waking hours. Through different ICT's such as the mobile phone, a person becomes mobile, and the home can thereby regain its historic function as a work place, as it was in agrarian society. In this way, we can bring the working solidarity we had in agrarian society back to our homes (Dahlbom, 2003). In today's society, ICT helps us become nomads, and the home, together with other meeting places, becomes our workplace (Bradley, 2006).

The "work environment" could be an office, a factory or a school. It can also be an environment less stationary, like a laptop computer. One major study of office design in relation to psychosocial health presents results concerning workers who did not have a permanent workplace. The study reveals how mobile and non-mobile offices function as a work environment; some of us feel safe at our work desk and/or in front of the computer, because it has become our second home (Danielsson, 2005).

The school environment, another example of a work environment, was earlier seen as an institution with power and status, but today it has lost this aura. As a result, students and teachers can more readily be subject to criticism by the public, because the school has become more human and open to public view (Zeihe, 1986). The school of today is no longer simply a special building, it is also a page on the Internet as more and more education is available online through IT-high schools and IT-universities. Many students today can, in some way, relate more to an activity on the Internet than to a school building (Dahlbom, 2003). By the end of the 1990's, several researchers focused on how a complete education could be achieved with the help of computers in schools, e.g., students' use

of computers and the internet (Bergman, 1999) in learning environments (Danielsson, 1999; Edström and Riis, 1997; Jedeskog, 1994; Pedersen, 1998; Riis and Jedeskog, 1997). The conditions in a work environment can, to a great extent, be compared to and reflect the conditions in a school environment. Some of the common factors are an increased usage of ICT, greater personal responsibility, self-directed work, and a change of the psychosocial work environment (for both the individual and the organization). Research concerning the school system has primarily focused on providing a historical perspective of teachers' health, work, and professional roles (e.g. Carlsson *et al.,* 2004). Although it is relatively easy to find research about students' health (Laurell, 2005; Smedje, 2000) and the use of the internet as a social tool (Gross, 2004), research about how students combine school time and leisure time is still limited.

Use of Mobile Phone

Use of ICT has become an everyday experience, especially mobile technologies. In 2002, the number of mobile phone subscribers overtook the numbers of fixed-line telephone subscribers on a global scale (Srivastava, 2005). In 2005, more than 21 million teenagers between the ages of 12 and 17 had access and routinely used the internet (Lenhart, 2005). Instant messaging has become the most popular online communication function in the United States (Gross, 2004). ICT use for social interaction seems to increase in the younger population.

Mobile phones also provide a medium through which young people can maintain their social network (Taylor and Harper, 2003). By analyzing the various ways young people use their mobile phones, we can understand their lifestyles and their relation to ICT (Licoppe and Heurtin, 2001). Ito (2005) argues that mobile use among Japanese teenagers is structured by the power-geometrics of place, and their usage is highly deferential to the context (home, school, public) in which they find themselves. Mobile communication allows them to create a private place of communication. The evidence suggests that young people are more or less addicted to the mobile phones that play a major role in their daily lives. Kato (2006) has observed that the mobile phone (keitai[1]) has become a seemingly indispensable medium for Japanese youth.

Our extensive use of mobile phones is just one example of how ICT has become an important part of our daily lives. Through the use of the mobile phone, we become available for communication 24/7, that is, 24 hours a day, 7 days a week. While some might find this disturbing, young people often consider it to be more future-oriented and believe themselves to be more open to accepting new ways of using ICT in everyday life compared to adults; it is experienced as a lifestyle (Dalbom, 2003). Therefore, observing children's usage of ICT gives us an understanding of future use, since children frequently innovate and adopt new ways of interacting with technology (Druin, 2009).

Young people do not regard the mobile phone as simply a work tool, they see it as an accessory to show off to their friends and as something that can help them to achieve status (Dahlbom, 2003). Today, many children are growing up with the readiness to accept a range of new technologies, in other words, "born to be wired". Today's youth are often assumed to spend more time online than using any of the other media available to them (radio, DVD, video, television, print, etc.). It is important to notice that as technology develops, various teaching methods are tried (e.g in schools), but they are seldom evaluated until it is time for another method to be tested (Danielsson, 1999).

Diversity already exists among students in today's schools, and this diversity in learning might be supported by the use of different e-learning—that is, electronic learning—technologies (Minton *et al.,* 2004). There will always be individual differences between us and, therefore,

we must avoid considering ICT an object in itself, and instead, look at how we use ICT. That is in line with what Croon Fors (2006) discusses in her thesis: in order to envision the reflexive nature of information technology, the relationship between human experience and information technology must be comprehended as a whole (ibid).

EFFECTS ON INDIVIDUALS

At the beginning of 2000, several studies were conducted on the positive and negative effects of ICT on health and behaviour patterns (see e.g. Allvin *et al.* 1999; Bradley, 2001; Hansson, 2004; Lennerlöf *et al.*, 1991; Sandberg and Augustsson, 2002; Åborg, 2002). Studies have indicated that the boundaries between private and work life could diminish for IT professionals working from home (Ahrentzen, 1990; Ziljstra & Sonnentag, 2006). Ziljstra & Sonnentag (2006) argue that this can even affect the ability to recover from the stress of work. Boundaries between work and home have an important psychological function that can help people to create an essential psychological distance between work and themselves. One of the main findings in Thomée *et al.* (2007) is that a high frequency of combined use of computers and mobile phones was associated with increased risk of experiencing prolonged stress and symptoms of depression (at least for women). Referring to their results, the use of ICT may have an impact on psychosocial health.

According to Söderström *et al.* (2003) and Senge (1990), we need balance in our lives in order to be healthy. This can be both the balance between being active or passive, and being awake or asleep. Stress can occur if there is an imbalance in these states. According to Dahlgren (2005), it is important to achieve a balance between stress and recovery to be able to manage stressful situations. Her studies show that both overtime work and high work-related stress affect the possibility of recovery. Therefore, the research concerning the blurring of the division between work and leisure, and well-being appears to be of importance.

Young Urban Knowledge Workers

Danielsson (2007b) presents in her thesis a research process combining theories from the fields of informatics, psychology, work science and gender theory. She focuses on concepts such as roles, environment, boundaries, work, leisure, health and barriers, as well as conducts interviews with IT-professionals, defined as young urban knowledge workers (Danielsson, 2002, 2003) and high school IT-students, who are likely to become future professionals in the IT-business (Danielsson, 2007a). Her two studies were based on 20 semi-structured interviews that included ten adults and ten teenagers.

The ten people included within the focus group of young urban knowledge workers were people who worked in some kind of IT-company as an employee and/or owner. They were single or co-habiting and had an educational background within an IT-related academic field. Some had finished their degree and some had not. The number of men and women were equal within this group. Moreover, they were understood to be interested in sharing their thoughts and experiences about the subject matter of the study at hand.

The young urban knowledge workers considered themselves to have strong social networks, and their colleagues and friends often turned out to be the same. Both their interest in their work, which allowed their work time to take precedence over their leisure time, and their socialization with friends, who were also their colleagues, created a common experience among them that made it difficult to separate work from leisure (see figure 4). They were constantly accessible by mobile phone or e-mail to discuss work with their colleagues or clients. At the same time, they were pleased about being able to choose the time and

Figure 4. Today: with present ICT, work and leisure activities can easily overlap

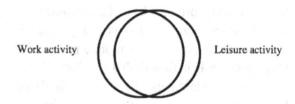

place to conduct their work. The only time they experienced difficulty planning leisure time was when attempting to plan vacation time, because they could not anticipate their workload for any specific timeframe. Working more than 40 hours per week was not considered a problem; rather they appreciated the flexibility of being able to work irrespective of time and place. Consequently, the requirement was that they must be accessible by mobile phone and/or e-mail. With the mobile phone they were always connected to work, whether their workplace was at home or some other place (ibid).

Mobile technology has blurred the boundaries between previously delineated areas of people's lives (Gant and Kiesler, 2001; Harper, 2001). For example, Danielsson (2007b) found that mobile phones allowed knowledge workers to perform their work activities even when they were away from their offices. And in the same way, the use of ICT enabled them to attend to other activities (e.g private) while they were physically absent from an environment. With this blurred separation, the physical and psychological boundaries between home and workplace became harder to define and increased interest in analysing the relationships between ICT, objective and subjective work environment and stress (figure 2). Sadler *et al.* (2006) observed how mobile technology at work is primarily used to manage personal activities and concerns unrelated to current work, for example, planning future work. Observations revealed strategies for managing the blurring of context, for example, local work, personal life, and future work. Strategies such as moving away from fixed resources enabled them to attend to their phones without disrupting their colleagues, but also to handle both current and future work projects, thereby increasing the pace of work (ibid).

These flexible working conditions placed more demands on the individual who was required to define his/her own working conditions and make the distinction between work time and free time (*freedom under responsibility*) (Danielsson, 2007b). This was a distinction that young urban knowledge workers found hard to define, unfortunately. These results agree with the findings of Ahrentzen (1990), Ziljstra & Sonnentag (2006) and Danielsson (2002).

In addition to this, Nyberg (2008) has explored people's attitudes to digital artifacts and identified some strategies people use in order to either *separate* the professional role from the private role, or to *unite* the two. One of the groups she observed resembled the young urban knowledge workers, that is, IT-professionals. Both used the computer and mobile phone to a great extent in their own work. However, her respondents performed research concerning digital artifacts and its consequences in different contexts in contrast to the young urban knowledge workers who developed digital artifacts or worked with ICT services. Moreover, her respondents' work situations were also a form of *freedom under responsibility* in that they could work either from home or at the work place. The professionals Nyberg (ibid) observed changed their behaviors towards ICT, and chose either to separate or unite the two contexts, or both at different times.

At different times in life, they felt a need to either create a clear distinction between the professional role (work context) and the private role (home), or intertwine the two. One respondent considered being an "early adopter" felt "fragmented" and "fed up" with having a day that was too ambivalent. Therefore, he reached the point where he separated the contexts of work and home, being professional and private, and currently considered himself as being more careful in his use of ICT (Nyberg, 2008). Nyberg has posited three categories: (1) private users that have an intense relation to ICT, (2) IT-professionals, and (3) non-users of ICT (people that choose not to use ICT), and what is especially interesting in her research in relation to Danielsson (2007b), is peoples' need for strategies to either merge or separate different contexts of ICT use.

High School IT-Students

The 10 people included within this focus group observed by Danielsson (2007b) were students at an IT- high school. By virtue of their personal interests, they were attending a school with IT emphasis in all major subjects. They did not have any children (same as the young urban knowledge workers that were co-habiting). The number of men and women were equal. Moreover, they were understood to be interested in sharing their thoughts and experiences about the subject matter of the study at hand.

The students' aim was to perform all schoolwork during school hours in order to avoid homework. If they were ill, they choose to do school work at home in order to keep up with the rest of the class. It appeared that they felt a great need to know that schoolwork was completed during school hours so that they could take part in leisure activities. The students preferred to work with their friends, indicating that they were both socializing and working together, mixing their private and professional roles (Danielsson, 2007a).

Free time and leisure activities appeared to be of great importance; they expressed a need to do the things *they* chose to do (*freedom*). However, they had chosen their major subjects because of an interest in the specific fields and, for that reason, they often performed activities outside school that later could be used as school assignments. In short, they failed to notice that schoolwork and leisure interests were virtually one and the same. Moreover, their workplace could be identified as both their school and their computer desk at home (ibid).

Whereas the young urban knowledge workers allowed work time to dominate leisure time, the students did the opposite. For example, their teachers allowed them to read personal e-mails for a few minutes before the lecture began, but during the lecture itself, students could read only e-mails pertaining to the school work (*responsibility*). It is significant to note that the students never turned off their mobile phones, even though they were supposed to during class. It was too stressful for them to turn their mobile phones off out of concern for missing an important call or SMS (ibid), a result similar to the students observed by Ito (2005), who also used their mobile phones during lectures. The phone was not used to receive calls, but in order to send e-mails to friends both present in the classroom and elsewhere (ibid). Results in line with the argument that mobile phones enable us to co-exist in a range of social contexts (Taylor and Harper, 2003; Messeter *et al.*, 2004).

The students in Danielson's (2007a; 2007b) studies experienced both positive and negative stress, as well as physical problems that they blamed on the ergonomically deficient work environment. In today's schools, work and free time are most often clearly separated by time and place. However, the previous clear demarcation between schoolwork and free time is becoming blurred leading students to risk ending up in similar psychosocial environments as the young urban knowledge workers.

SLEEP, RECOVERY AND PSYCHOSOCIAL HEALTH

The size of the workload is negatively correlated to psychological detachment from work during evening hours, and that psychological detachment from work is associated with a positive mood and a low level of fatigue (Sonnentag & Bayer, 2005). There have been major studies that reveal how young people handle stress and maintain psychological health (SOU 2006:77). As has long been known, adequate sleep has a strong relationship to good health. Those people who sleep too little become tired and have a hard time focusing. This naturally affects their ability to perform their jobs effectively.

Numerous studies show that too little sleep for youths increases the risk of psychological problems (e.g., Vignau *et al.,* 1997; LeBourgeois *et al.,* 2005). Sleep is an important factor for our ability to recover and deal with the demands and stimuli of the work day. The length of the work day, as well as the characteristics of the work itself, could affect the possibility of unwinding and recovering after a day of work, as suggested by Zijlstra and Sonnentag (2006). Recent studies show that moderate perceived stress or worry at bedtime is related to decreased sleep efficiency (Åkersted *et al.,* 2007; cf. Sundin, 2009), as well as the function of free-time, in leading to recovery and a sense of well-being (Tucker *et al.,* 2007). According to Lloyd and Auld (2001), people-centered leisure activities are the best predictors of quality of life. However, according to Söderstöm et al. (2003), we need balance in our lives in order to be healthy.

As a theoretical basis for investigating stress, occupational health psychology presents a wide range of different models (Cooper, 1998), such as the "job-demand-control" model (Karasek, 1979, Karasek & Theorell, 1990) and the "effort-reward-imbalance" model (Siegrist, 1996). Many of these models view stress as an effect of the imbalance between the demands that are put on the individual and the insufficient resources the individual has to meet them (cf. Hakanen *et al.,* 2006). Stressful situations with insufficient recovery time can have adverse health effects and can result in burnout over time (Maslach, 1993).

DISCUSSION

Every person's psychosocial health is influenced by their life environment; a combination of their (subjective and objective) work and home environments, life roles (private, professional, civic) and social networks. Recently presented research studies show that moderate perceived stress/worry at bedtime is related to decreased sleep efficiency (Åkerstedt *et al.*, 2007). The function of free-time in aiding recovery and achieving a sense of well-being has also been demonstrated (Tucker *et al.*, 2007). In work environments, learning and human resource development are essential. Therefore, attempts are made to make education more interesting and entertaining in order to make learning more appealing (cf. Danielsson & Wiberg, 2006, Fisch, 2005, Mc Farlane, 2005). However, when people's experience of work and leisure becomes blurred, this may impact on their psychosocial health. One aspect to consider, therefore, is how we can use technology in a more individualized way (Minton *et al.*, 2004) so that people can set their own boundaries when necessary.

Danielsson (2007b) identified some similarities between "young urban knowledge workers" and "high school students" in relation to life role:

- enjoyment of work/school work based on information and communication technologies (ICT)
- accessibility via mobile phone independent of time and location
- blurring of the boundary between work/school time and free time
- goal in life: to "feel good" (both physically and psychologically)
- strong social networks (friends/colleagues very important)
- non-involvement in social issues
- experience of both positive and negative stress

The similarities listed above strengthen the impression of effects of technology in life role on psychosocial health. The subjects presented in Danielson's (2007b) research had no significant control over their use of technology. The extent of their modest amount of control was ability to use different technologies for different tasks. With their mobile phones turned off they felt "out of control". Being out of reach (by ICT) was for the IT-professionals lack of control concerning their work relationships (friends and colleagues were almost the same people), while for the IT-students, it was lack of control concerning friends and family. To help maintain a sense of control, these individuals kept their mobile phones on continually wherever they were (Danielsson, 2002, 2003, 2007a, 2007b).

The workplace can be defined (in many cases) as a second home, where one can socialize, eat, enjoy leisure activities and even sleep (Danielsson, 2002, 2003). These results are in line with Christina Danielson's (2005), showing that when we feel safe behind our work desk (or in front of our computer), the work environment has in effect become a second home.

In Danielsson's (2007b) study, the young people and students interviewed expressed a need for balance, but were less able to find or create ways of allowing the necessary time for recovery. Several of the interviewees experienced worries about their work and some had problems sleeping (ibid). Today, as the use of ICT increase, there is a risk that the experiences identified in the studies presented will emerge among a greater number of people. Communication accessibility, anytime, anywhere, is increasingly important in working life, where talk is central to mobile work and where the telephone is a key tool (Perry *et al.*, 2001). This accessibility is mostly seen as a positive development, but it may also be a factor in increased stress. Apart from sleep, leisure time and the activities we engage in during our leisure time are also important sources of recovery. A common definition of leisure is having time to do what we want to do, thus allowing us to achieve a sense of recovery (Bull *et al.*, 2003).

It appears that people who work professionally in the field of ICT or use ICT in their work experience a blurring between their professional and private roles and need to develop strategies – by themselves or together with friends and family – in order to separate themselves from work. We do not take the position that there should be less use of ICT, but rather that there is *a need to support* the user in drawing a clear distinction between work and leisure activities, particularly, for example, in the case of students, because these are the people who in a few years will leave school and enter working life. If we want them to stay healthy and prepared to manage both work and leisure, it is important to provide them with the possibility to do so. By analyzing the various ways young people use their mobile phones, we can better understand their lifestyle and relation to ICT (Licoppe and Heurtin, 2001).

To try to predict what the future holds, let us consider the development of mobile phone use (*keitai*) among youth in Japan. Katu (2006) asked Japanese university students to produce dramatic visual or radio stories on the theme of *keitai* communication. Through this work, it was found that *keitai* has become a seemingly indispensable medium for Japanese youth. It appears that the same development is occurring among youth in Europe.

There are, of course, always several elements present in a person's experience of stress and other psychosocial problems. ICT is one of the elements that contribute to a blurring of boundaries between work and leisure. When work can be easily performed in any environment (whether private or public), this raises issues about sense of freedom versus sense of responsibility. Moreover, it raises the matter of our need to define a clear boundary between work time and free time. One way of creating a clear distinction between the professional role/work context and private role/home context is to become a less-frequent user or a non-user of ICT (cf. Nyberg, 2008). However, this may not always be a feasible option. Another way, then, to enable individuals to separate leisure from work may be through the design of the media they use.

The focus today on aesthetics and user experience is increasingly in interactive design (see e.g. McCarthy & Wright, 2004, or Norman, 2004). Unlike past technologies that were designed to fit specific contexts of use, the ICT of today are applicable to several activities. Therefore, ICT design should focus on the purpose of the activity and create tools/services that can support the shift between activities (such as work and leisure). A designer should understand the multifaceted and changing nature of the user's experience of an activity, which is dependent on time, place (Preece *et al.*, 2007) and purpose. The young people of today, and especially today's children, are born into a world where we use ICT anytime and anywhere when performing work and leisure activities. For example, we can easily use the same mobile phone for both professional and personal communication and ask for a "split" bill.

Therefore, we emphasize the possibility for users to transit from work to leisure activities using the same ICT, but where support is offered to enable the shift between contexts with a clear demarcation of the separation between them. This support should be a function of the ICT itself, for example through the use of indications – similar to those used in such communication systems as Skype or MSN – which tell others whether we are busy working or available.

We stress that the shift between work and leisure should be supported through software services. Whereas different status modes tell others whether we are working or not, we would point out ways for the user to feel secure in their alternative contexts of work or leisure. Rather than suggesting new ways to inform others about what we are doing, we would instead emphasize ways for the user to experience the separation between work and leisure even though the same ICT is used in both contexts. This proposal is somewhat in line with the research presented by Kohiyama (2006) in a paper discussing the term *personalization in communication* and showing trends in mobile communication in terms of the personalization of devices, connectivity, and services. Kohiyama (2006) explains:

Personalization involves enabling access to the broadest possible range of who, what, where, when and how (4W1H) as well as enabling people to specify and restrict access based on their individual needs (Kohiyama, 2006, p. 71).

The "what" referred to is access to any type of information, while at the same time, through personalization, we are able to filter that information for individual needs. The "where" would initially refer to access from anywhere (work, home, city, countryside, etc.), but in relation to personalization it would enable us to restrict particular communications to particular locations. In terms of the personalization and restriction of the "when", we might consider services where certain types of calls are blocked at certain times or certain information is delivered only at a certain time of day (Kohiyama, 2006).

Messeter *et al.* (2004) highlight that people assume different roles in different contexts, due to usage of ICT. Therefore, designers should be sensitive to the different roles and contexts. In addition to this, Sadler *et al.* (2006) argue that even when people do manage to counter the blurring of contexts, such as between local work, future work and personal life, designers can further facilitate this.

Strategies for division are important not only between work and leisure, but also within work contexts. Harr (2009) has observed the usage of IT systems and our constant availability due to these systems in work situations. He argues that the development of IT, giving us constant access to each other, is not only for the better. At best, we become less efficient, at worst, we become stressed and may experience burnout syndrome. IT creates the experience of constant interruption. Harr (ibid) argues that the development of IT needs to consider our need to be able to control others' ease of access and proposes levels of accessibility, that is, systems that are adjustable according to personal needs. At present, individuals and groups develop their own strategies in relation to the context in order to strike a balance in work. Instead, the technology should be sensitive to the environment in which we are presently active as well as to our specific actions within that environment.

In this approach, ICT – rather than being the initiator of a stressful and unhealthy life environment – is designed to manage these stressful situations and able to support the user in finding time for renewal by drawing a line between work and leisure. This implies the design of services in line with the *personalization of communication* presented by Kohiyama (2006), where we can have the fullest of possibilities, yet can personalize and restrict information and communication to appropriate times and places.

Maybe ICT, instead of creating stressful shifts and endless streams of blurring between work and leisure, can help us recover. The use of ICT both for work and for leisure activities may be designed so as to offer us periods of recovery between periods of work. Our next step is to further explore the possibilities of ICT as a means for recovery. In order to do so, future research concerning our psychosocial life environment should be approached from different levels and from different perspectives using an interdisciplinary research process to analyze broad and important questions such as the ones presented here.

CONCLUSION

An effect of increased use of ICT is the blurring of boundaries between work and leisure. In our present study we have used an interdisciplinary research process that combined theories from the fields of informatics, psychology and work science focusing on the concepts of roles, environment, boundary, work, leisure, health and barriers to explore this issue. In our results, people express a need for balance between work and leisure but are less able to find or create ways of allowing the necessary time for recovery and recuperation. Further, we identified that users create strategies for managing the different roles and environments they shift between. We argued that these strategies may be further facilitated by ICT design. But since the blurring of boundaries appears not yet to be about to cease, a question of importance is how we will relate to these shifts, or this blurring, henceforth.

We have outlined some initial suggestions on how to continue research within this field. In order to clarify the importance of this field of research for our health and, by extension, our productivity, we would like to end with this thought. The directors of today's organizations set rules as to what kind of work employees get paid for doing and during what time frame. The other side of the equation is that it is primarily the *employee* who has the responsibility for getting the assigned work done in the time allotted. At the same time – and this is essential to keep in mind – the employee has both the *freedom* and the *responsibility* of setting aside adequate time in order to *recover* the necessary equilibrium for good health. In short, both parties must work together to assure the best possible result. Therefore, further research should focus on strategies and possibilities for designing ICT as itself a means to enable recovery and recuperation.

ACKNOWLEDGMENT

This chapter is based on a previous paper presented at the working seminar Information systems research seminar in Scandinavia (IRIS) in 2008 (Danielsson and Danielsson, 2008). IRIS is a Scandinavian annual working seminar for PhD students and researchers. The authors would like to take this opportunity to thank previous reviewers of the earlier version of the presented work. Moreover, we are especially thankful for the fruitful discussions at the IRIS seminar.

REFERENCES

Åborg, C. (2002). *How does IT feel @ work? And how to make IT better: Computer use, stress and health in office work.* Ph D Thesis, Department of Information technology, Uppsala University.

Ahrentzen, S. (1990). Managing conflict by managing boundaries: how professional home workers cope with multiple roles at home. *Environment and Behavior, 22*(6), 723–752. doi:10.1177/0013916590226001

Åkerstedt, T., Kecklund, & G., Axelsson, J. (2007). Impaired sleep after bedtime and worries. *Biological Psychology, 76*, 170–173. doi:10.1016/j.biopsycho.2007.07.010

Allvin, M., Aronsson, G., Hagström, T., Johnasson, G., Lundberg, U., & Skärstrand, E. (1998). *Gränslöst arbete eller arbetets nya gränser.* Stockholm: National Institute for Working Life, Arbete och hälsa 21.

Allvin, M., & Wiklund, P. Härenstam, & A., Aronsson, G. (1999). *Frikopplad eller frånkopplad [Disconnected or out of touch].* National Institute for Working Life, Stockholm, Sweden.

Bergman, M. (1999). *På jakt efter högstadieelevers Internetanvändning* [A study of high school students' use of the Internet]. Licentiate of Philosophy. Uppsala: Uppsala University, Sweden.

Bradley, G. (1986). *Psykosocial arbetsmiljö och datorer* [Computers and the Psychosocial Working Environment]. Stockholm, SE: Akademilitteratur.

Bradley, G. (2001). Information and Communication Technology (ICT) and Humans – How we will live, learn and work. In G. Bradley (Ed.) *Humans on the Net. Information and Communication Technology (ICT) Work Organization and Human Beings* (pp. 22-44). Stockholm, SE: Prevent.

Bradley, G. (2006). *Social and Community Informatics. Human on the Net.* New York: Routledge.

Bull, C. Hoose, & J., Weed, M. (2003). *Leisure studies.* London: Pearson Education.

Carlsson, I., Collberg, D., Månsson, E., Greiff, M., Starverski, H., Wigerfelt, B., et al. Klapp Lekholm, & A., Persson, A. (2004) *Nära gränsen? Perspektiv på skolans arbetsliv [Close to the edge? Perspectives of the working life in schools].* National Institute for Working Life, Stockholm, Sweden.

Cooper, C. L. (Ed.). (1998). *Theories of organizational stress.* Oxford: Oxford University Press.

Croon Fors, A. (2006). *Being-with Information Technology: Critical explorations beyond use and design.* PhD Thesis. Umeå University. Sweden: Department of Informatics: Umeå.

Dahlbom, B. (2003). *Makten över framtiden* [Control over the future]. Sweden: Liber Ekonomi.

Dahlgren, A. (2006). *Work stress an overtime work – effects on cortisol, sleep, sleepiness and health.* Thesis: Department of psychology. Stockholm University, Sweden.

Danielsson, C. (2005). *Office environment, health and job satisfaction: an explorative study of office design's influence.* Licentiate Thesis: Royal Institute of Technology, Stockholm, Sweden

Danielsson, K., & Wiberg, C. (2006). Participatory Design of learning media: designing educational computer games with and for teenagers, in ITSE special issue . *Computer Game-based Learning, 3*(4), 4–20.

Danielsson, U. (1999). Learning in Networks. *Proceedings of the Human Computer Interaction International* (pp. 407-411). Munich, Germany.

Danielsson, U. (2002). *Unga IT- Människor i storstad [Young urban knowledge workers].* Fiber Science Communication Network, R-02-34, Sweden.

Danielsson, U. (2003). Young urban knowledge workers – The relationship between ICT and the psychosocial life environment. In *Proceedings of Human Computer Interaction International* (pp. 941-945). Crete, Greece.

Danielsson, U. (2007a). High school students – Relationship between ICT and psychosocial life environment. In *Proceedings of IRIS Information system Research seminar in Scandinavia 30,* Tampere, Finland.

Danielsson, U. (2007b). *Relationships between Information Communication Technology and Psychosocial Life Environment – Students and Young Urban Knowledge Workers in the ICT-Era.* PhD Thesis. Mid Sweden University. Sundsvall, Sweden: Department of Information technology and media.

Danielsson, U., & Danielsson, K. (2008). Boundaries between work and leisure within psychosocial life environment -an interdisciplinary literature review. In *Proceedings of IRIS Information System Research Seminar 31 - Nordic Conference in Informatics.* Åre, Sweden. E-publication

Druin, A. (2009). Mobile technologies for the world's children, talk at *Women in ICT lecture series,* Iowa State University, USA, October 9, 2009. Retrieved March 9, 2010 from http://vimeo.com/6990499

Edström, R., & Riis, U. (1997). *Informationsteknik i skolan [Information technology at school.* En fråga om ekonomi och pedagogik. Uppsala Universitet, Uppsala: Pedagogiska Institutionen: Fisch, S. M. (2005). Making Educational Computer Games "Educational." In *Proceedings of the 2005 conference on Interaction Design and Children* (pp. 56-61). Boulder, Colorado. Frankenhauser, M., & Ödman, M. (1983). *Stress: en del av livet [Stress: a part of life].* Brombergs Bokförlag, Stockholm, Sweden.

Gant, D., & Kiesler, S. (2001). Blurring the Boundaries: Cell Phones, Mobility, and the Line between Work and Personal Live . In Brown, B., Green, N., & Harper, R. (Eds.), *Wireless World: Social and Interactional Aspects of the Mobile Age* (pp. 121–131). London: Springer-Verlag.

Goffman, E. (1974). *Jaget och maskerna* [Eng. The Presentation of Self in Everyday Life]. Stockholm: Rabén & Sjögren.

Gross, E. F. (2004). Adolescent Internet use: What we expect, what teens report. *Journal of Applied Developmental Psychology*, *25*(1), 633–649. doi:10.1016/j.appdev.2004.09.005

Hakanen, J., Bakker, A. B., & Schaullefi, W. B. (2006). Burnout and work engagement among teachers. *Journal of School Psychology*, *43*(3), 495–513. doi:10.1016/j.jsp.2005.11.001

Hanson, M. (2004). *Det flexibla arbetets villkor [The conditions for flexible work].* Doctoral Thesis. National Institute for Working Life. Stockholms University.

Harper, R. (2001). The mobile interface: old technologies and new arguments . In Brown, B., Green, N., & Harper, R. (Eds.), *Wireless World: Social and Interactional Aspects of the Mobile Age* (pp. 207–223). London: Springer-Verlag.

Harr, R. (2009). *Striking a balance: managing collaborative multitasking in computer-supported cooperation.* Doctoral dissertation, Department of Informatics, Umeå University, Sweden.

Ito, M. (2005). Mobile Phones, Japanese Youth, and the Re-Placement of Social Contact . In Ling, R., & Pedersen, P. (Eds.), *Mobile Communications: re-negotiation of the Social Sphere.* London: Springer -Verlag.

Jarrick, A. (2005). *Behovet att behövas* [The need to be needed]. Stockholm, Sweden: SNS Förlag.

Jedeskog, G. (1994). *Datorn i undervisningen [Computers in education]* . Liber Distribution, Stockholm, Skolverket rapport, nr 94:84.

Karasek, R. (1979). Job demands, job decision latitude and mental strain: implications for job redesign. *Administrative Science Quarterly*, *24*(2), 285–308. doi:10.2307/2392498

Karasek, R., & Theorell, T. (1990). *Healthy work: Stress, Productivity and the Reconstruction of working life.* New York: Basic Books.

Kato, H. (2006). Japanese Youth and the Imagining of Keitai . In Ito, M., Okabe, D., & Matsuda, M. (Eds.), *Personal, Portable, Pedestrian: Mobile Phones in Japanese Life* (pp. 103–119). Cambridge, MA: MIT Press.

Kohiyama, K. (2006). A Decade in the Development if Mobile Communications in Japan (1993-2002) . In Ito, M., Okabe, D., & Matsuda, M. (Eds.), *Personal, Portable, Pedestrian: Mobile Phones in Japanese Life* (pp. 61–74). Cambridge, MA: MIT Press.

Laurell, K. (2005). *Headache in school children: Epidemiology, Pain Comorbidity and Psychosocial Factors.* Ph D Thesis. Department of Neuroscience, Uppsala University.

LeBourgeois, MK., Gainnotti, F., Cortesi, F., Wolfson, AR., & Harsch, J. (2005). *The relationship between reported sleep quality and sleep hygiene in Italian and American adolescents* (pp. 257-265). Pediatrics: 115 (1rst).

Lenhart, A. (2005). *Protecting teens online. Pew Internet and American Life Project*. Retrieved March 2010 from www.pewinternet.org

Lennerlöf, L., & Aronsson, G. (1991). *Människan i arbetslivet* [The individual in working life]. Stockholm, Sweden: Nordstedts Juridik AB.

Levi, L. (2001). *Stress och Hälsa [Stress and Health]*. Stockholm, SE: Skandia.

Licoppe, C., & Heurtin, J. P. (2001). Managing One's Availability to Telephone communication through Mobile Phones. *Personal and Ubiquitous Computing, 5*(2), 98–108. doi:10.1007/s007790170013

Lloyd, K. M., & Auld, C. J. (2001). The role of leisure in determining quality of life: issues of content and measurement. *Social Indicators Research, 57*(3), 42–71.

Maslach, C. (1993). *Burnout: A multidimensional perspective. In professional burnout: Recent development in theory and research* (pp 19-32). Series in applied psychology: Social issues and questions. Philadelphia, PA: Taylor & Francis.

McCarthy, J., & Wright, P. (2004). *Technology as Experience*. Cambridge, MA: MIT Press.

McFarlane, A., Sparrowhawk, A., & Heald, Y. (2005). *Report on the educational use of games*. TEEM: Teachers Evaluating Educational Media. Retrieved August 31, 2006 from http://www.teem.org.uk/publications

Messeter, J., Brandt, E., Hasle, J., & Johansson, M. (2004). *Contextualizing mobile IT. Designing Interactive Systems* (pp. 27–36). Cambridge, MA: MIT Press.

Minton, L., Boyle, R., & Dimitrova, V. (2004). If diversity is a problem could e-learning be part of the solution? A case study. In *Proceedings of the ITiCSE '04 Conference* (pp. 42-46). ACM.

Norman, D. (2004). *Emotional design: Why we love (or hate) everyday things*. New York: Basic Books.

Nyberg, A. (2008). *Att studera digitala artefakter i människors vardagsliv*. (English title: On the exploration of people's attitudes to digital artefacts) PhD Thesis. Umeå University. Sweden: Department of Informatics. Umeå.

Oborne, D. (1985). *Computers at work*. London: John Wiley & Sons Ltd.

Pedersen, J. (1998) *Informationstekniken i skolan* [Information technology in school]. Stockholm, SE: Skolverket.

Perry, M., O'Hara, K., Sellen, A., Brown, B., & Harper, R. (2001). Dealing with Mobility: Understanding Access Anytime, Anywhere. *AMC Transaction on Computer-Human Interaction, 8*(4), 323–347. doi:10.1145/504704.504707

Preece, J., Rogers, Y., & Sharp, H. (2007). *Interaction design: beyond human–computer interaction*. New York: Wiley.

Riis, U. Jedeskog, (1997) *Pedagogik, teknik eller ekonomi? [Teaching, technology or economy?]*. Reprocentralen HSC, Uppsala Universitet, Sweden.

Sadler, K., Robertson, T., Kan, M., & Hagen, P. (2006). Balancing Work, Life and Other Concerns: A Study of Mobile Technology Use by Australian Freelancers. In *Proceedings of the 2006 NordiCHI conference: Changing Roles* (pp. 413-416). Oslo, Norway.

Sandberg, Å., & Augustsson, F. (2002). *Interactive Media in Sweden – The Second Interactive Media, Internet and Multimedia Industry Survey*. Stockholm: National Institute for Working Life.

Senge, P. (1990). *The fifth discipline: The art and practices of the learning organization.* New York: Random House.

Siegrist, J. (1996). Adverse health effects of high-effort/low-reward conditions. *Journal of Occupational Health Psychology, 1*(2), 27–41. doi:10.1037/1076-8998.1.1.27

Smedje, G. (2000). *The indoor environment of schools: Respiratory effects and air quality.* Ph D Thesis, Institutionen för medicinska vetenskap, Uppsala University, Uppsala, Sweden.

Söderström, M., Jeding, K., Ekstedt, M., Kecklund, G., & Åkerstedt, T. (2003). *Arbetsmiljö, stress och utbrändhet inom ett företag i IT-branschen.* [The working environment, stress and burnout in a company in the IT sector] 312(pp. 1-54).

Sonnetag, S., & Bayer, U. (2005). Switching off mentally: Predictors and Consequences of Psychological Detachment from Work During off-job time. *Journal of Occupational Health Psychology, 10*(4), 393–414. doi:10.1037/1076-8998.10.4.393

SOU 2006:77. Statens Offentliga Utredningar. Ungdomar, stress och psykisk ohälsa. www.regeringen.se

Srivastava, L. (2005). Mobile phones and the evolution of social behavior. *Behaviour & Information Technology, 24*(2), 111–129. doi:10.1080/01449290512331321910

Sundin, L. (2009). *Work-related social support, job demands and burnout. Studies of Swedish workers, predominantly employed in health care.* Diss. Karolinska Institutet, Stockholm: Universitetsservice.

Taylor, A., & Harper, R. (2003). The Gift of the Gab?: A Design oriented Sociology of young people's use of mobiles. *Computer Supported Cooperative Work,* 267–296. doi:10.1023/A:1025091532662

Thomée, S., Eklöf, M., Gustafsson, E., Nilsson, R., & Hagberg, M. (2007). Prevalence of perceived stress, symptoms of depression and sleep disturbances in relation to information and communication technology (ICT) use among young adults – an explorative prospective study. *Computers in Human Behavior, 23,* 1300–1321. doi:10.1016/j.chb.2004.12.007

Tucker, P., Dahlgren, A., Åkerstedt, T., & Waterhouse, J. (2007). *The impact of free-time activities on sleep, recovery and well-being.* Elsevier.

Vignau, J., Bailly, D., Duhamel, A., & Vervaecke, P., Beuscart, & R., Collinet, C. (1997). Epidemiologic study of sleep quality and troubles in French secoundary school adolescents. *The Journal of Adolescent Health, 21*(5), 343–350. doi:10.1016/S1054-139X(97)00109-2

Zeihe, T. (1986). *Ny ungdom [New youth].* Stockholm, SE: Nordstedts.

Zijlstra, F. R. H., & Sonnentag, S. (2006). After work is done: Psychological perspectives on recovery from work. *European Journal of Work and Organizational Psychology, 15*(2), 129–138. doi:10.1080/13594320500513855

ENDNOTE

[1] Mobile phones are in Japanese called keitai denwa (portable phones). Most often known simply as keitai.

Chapter 21
Services Rendered By Computers and Their Explications

Hans-Erik Nissen
Lund University, Sweden

ABSTRACT

The chapter addresses services rendered by message transforming functions of computer programs. It starts by critically looking at some earlier ways to explicate these. It then presents an alternative approach on which to base such explications. Applying this approach it suggests some explications. The chapter ends with some conclusions.

INTRODUCTION

For quite some time there has been written a lot about information and communication technologies. These are said recently to have been developed to support people's lives and work. To subsume these technologies under one label follows a trend to closely integrate computing and data transmission. Computers can store data and hence be perceived to render the service to transport data over time. The telegraph and the telephone furnish illustrations of technologies rendering services of data transport over space. These technologies are designed, ideally, to reproduce a message left at one point faithfully at

another. However, which services do computers render, when they process input messages to yield quite different output messages. In a number of cases, such as invoicing or wage calculations, they just perform some arithmetic. In other cases, for instance those intended to support decision making: Which service do computers render?

In this chapter I will address the two following and somewhat connected questions. Which services do computers render by transforming messages purported to support decision making, and functions like coordination? How is this service explicated to those affected by it?

The rest of this chapter will be organized in the following way. In section 2 I will present two earlier ways of explaining message transformations by computers. In section 3 I will propose an

DOI: 10.4018/978-1-60960-057-0.ch021

alternative approach, starting from Toulmin's view on argumentation, as a base of such explanations. In section 4 I give some explanations of services rendered by message transformation by computers based on the proposed approach. Finally, in section 5 I will forward a brief summary and a few conclusions.

SOME WAYS TO UNDERSTAND MESSAGE PROCESSING

A Rationalistic Approach

When computers were introduced message processing was understood according to a rationalistic approach. This to a considerable extent is done even today. It should not come as a surprise. The rationalistic tradition follows a common Western and particularly Anglo-Saxon tradition. Resolving a problem, or rather a problematic situation is described as achievable by following these three steps.

a) Circumscribe the situation in terms of identifiable objects exhibiting well defined properties.
b) Look for general rules to this class of recurrent situations in terms of those objects and properties.
c) Apply these rules logically in order to resolve the situation.

These steps are generally applied by analysts and artificial intelligence specialists after brief consultations of a few people concerned. These, and a lot of their colleagues, are intended to act upon the decision support given by a computer. In practice recurrent situations seldom are so homogenous and easy to capture in general laws as this approach presupposes. The approach has been criticized, for instance, in Winograd and Flores (1986).

Simon (1957, chapter 14) suggested a radical revision the optimizing "economic man" of the traditional economic theory. He suggested that an "economic man" only could look for satisfactory solutions to his decision problems. His reason was that man had a limited capacity and time for generating action alternatives and to evaluate them. Still, even Simon's "economic man" belongs to the rationalistic tradition.

A Speech Act Approach

Winograd and Flores (1986) orient the reader about the limitations of a traditional, rationalistic view on computer programming. Here I will focus on a different approach to services computers can render, which they suggest.

They conceive computers as tools for conducting a network of conversations (ibid. pp. 172-173). They "distinguish conversations for action" from "conversations for possibilities" (ibid. pp. 151-152). By this they attempt to safeguard the autonomy of human beings as actors. At the same time they also broaden the view on rationality of human action (ibid. p. 145).

Approaching computer support they focus on coordination of human action. Coordination they identify as the central task of managing broadly understood. They present their description of a conversation for action in the form of a state transition network (ibid. pp. 64 – 66). They end their book by outlining a kind of computer tool, based on their theory of management as conversation (ibid. chapter 11). They call this tool "the coordinator".

How Far Can a Speech Act Approach Help?

How far can a speech act approach help in understanding services rendered by computers? Trying to answer this question I will distinguish a number of domains, which seem to become involved.

Figure 1. Four domains to distinguish. (Adapted from Whitaker (1992, 22 – 24))

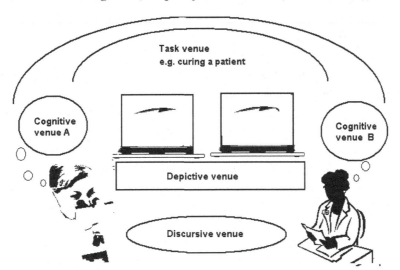

Four Domains to Distinguish

Figure 1 illustrates four domains to distinguish, when discussing services rendered by computers.

Following Whitaker (1992) I will refer to these domains as venues. The term "venue" is based on its legal connotation as "jurisdiction for action". It offers a circumscriptive medium for action. The computers I refer to in this chapter do not intervene directly in the *task venue*. Interventions are left to human beings. These also provide computers with data and/or control structures. Computers influence people by contributing to *depictive venues*. There also exist other depictive venues, for instance using a microscope identifying different types of bacteria. In human activities generally more than one individual is involved. These interact verbally regarding the task venue. This interaction is in Figure 1 called the *discursive venue*. However, each individual in a discursive venue, in a final analysis has her own *cognitive venue* of what she understands and experiences. Against the distinction of these four different venues I will return to how far a speech act approach can be helpful.

What Can A Speech Act Approach Offer?

Austin (1962) founded speech act theory. He distinguished a class of messages, *illocutionary acts*, by which a speaker intends to effect an action in others. Austin, moreover, saw a conventionally circumscribed force imparted to the listener by the message. However, its effect is not deterministically predictable. The outcome of it depends on the listener. Austin was careful in noting this reliance on interactional settings. Searle (1969) refined Austin's observations into a stringently defined framework. (Whitaker, 1992, p. 59.)

Whitaker (1992) discusses the step taken from Austin's seminal exposition of speech acts to Searle's stringent framework. He does so taking Winograd's and Flores' group decision support system (GDSS) the Coordinator as an illustration. To me what Whitaker writes seems to have a broader relevance. It describes the limitations of what speech act theory can offer to explicate services rendered by computers through message processing. As Whitaker writes:

With reference to the GDSS venue framework [see Figure 1], Austin's original theory delin-

eated how activity in the discursive venue could effect changes in the task venue. Searle's logical schematization addressed the manner in which a speaker's intentions for action (cognitive venue) were reflected in her utterances (discursive venue). The Coordinator has applied this schematization through the depictive venue to structure not only the immediate discursive venue (via message protocols), but to impose structure on the available actions beyond the bounds of the communication setting itself – i.e. the task venue. The above-cited experiences with The Coordinator indicate this is a step too far. That it is perhaps only one step too far is illustrated by contrasting positive and negative reactions to The Coordinator. The recorded base of conversations compiled and accessed through The Coordinator has been praised as providing a means for backtracking or tracing threads of communication (cf. Winograd, 1988; Bullen & Bennet, 1990a/b). This constitutes normative intervention in the depictive and/or discursive venues. In contrast, users have reacted negatively to resolution (action) being dictated a priori – i.e. normative intervention in the discursive and task venues. Managers have reacted positively to this arrangement, because the potential for questioning a solicited action is thereby diminished. (Ibid. pp. 60-61. Italics in the original. Text within square brackets added by the current author.)

The theory of speech acts introduced human linguistic interaction using computers or computer networks. By this it opened messages transported and/or processed by computers to be perceived as commitments. The messages support what in Figure 1 has been called the discursive and the depictive venues. However, the schematisms of the speech act theory (Searle) presuppose the cognitive venues of people involved to be consistent. In practice this will never fully be the case. The cognitive venues of people will influence their actions in the task venue. Winograd and Flores (1986) included "conversations for possibilities" in what computers could support. This may be

done by programming them to generate action alternatives for the task venue. However, these will never go outside of what a computer, in beforehand, has been programmed to do. They cannot surpass the potential capacity of redefining a problematic situation or generating new action alternatives for it. In other words they cannot surpass all potential outcomes of the cognitive venues of people involved. Even if speech act theory adds some ways to understand services rendered by computers there remains more to be explicated. In the next section I will suggest an alternative approach. In the introduction I raised two questions: Which services do computers render by transforming messages purported to support decision making, and functions like coordination? How is this service explicated to those affected by it? In the next section I will first present a starting point for answering these questions.

A PROPOSED ALTERNATIVE APPROACH

Figure 2 presents a broad context in which to understand services rendered by computers or computer networks. Here I limit my discussion to cases in which computer applications seriously intend to support people in their lives and work tasks. (This means I will not address computer crimes, information warfare, or infrastructure programs.)

Before answering my first question I will present what Toulmin (1958) and Toulmin et al, (1978) have written about human argumentation. A part of Figure 2 illustrates how Toulmin and his co-authors analyze human argumentation. In this case a medical doctor claims a patient needs treatment with penicillin. She grounds her claim, after speaking with and investigating the patient, diagnosing him having a straightforward upper respiratory infection. At the time of diagnosis, a straightforward respiratory infection warrants treatment by penicillin. Should somebody doubt

Figure 2. A context against which to explicate services rendered by computers (Cf. Toulmin et al. 1978, p. 97, Figure 10-2.) (In order to keep the figure simple it mixes phenomena on different levels of abstraction.)

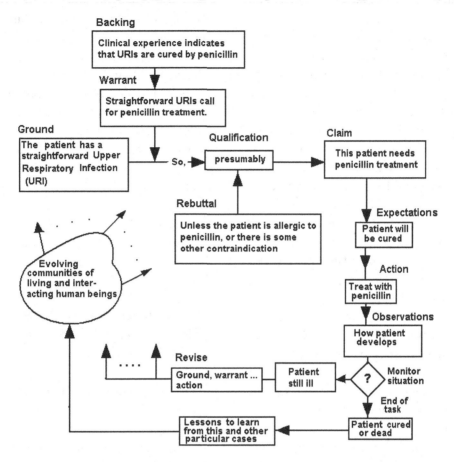

this warrant it can be backed by clinical experience indicating that upper respiratory infections (generally) are cured by penicillin. Still, the claim is qualified by the word "presumably". This marks the awareness of the doctor that there exist contraindications to the presumed treatment. This is called a rebuttal of the warranted treatment. Awareness of possible contraindications will induce the doctor to direct some more questions to the patient. Only after no contraindications seem applicable in the case an action on the claim is undertaken.

In the case illustrated the rebuttal, in a sense, is directed against the warrant as potentially incomplete. A rebuttal, however, also might question or contradict a claim, its ground, or the backing

of a warrant. Anyhow, a rebuttal can introduce a contradiction in the argumentation. This is a feature not admissible in the inference engines of today's computers, which are based on binary logic. Illustrating the qualification by the word "presumably" also indicates that Toulmin's concept of argumentation accepts other logics than binary ones.

The argumentation in this limited case also indicates how much of what people in the situation know becomes interwoven into it. The presentation of argumentation in Toulmin et al. leaves questions about how people arrive at their pre-knowledge. The presentation discussed so far only covers (parts of) what in Figure 1 was called the depictive and the discursive venue. The task venue and the cognitive venues have not been explicitly addressed. This I have attempted to do by the rest of Figure 2.

There I have introduced the *non-verbal action* undertaken in the task venue. This safeguards that the words used in the argumentations are true words. (Cf. Freire (1972) chapter 3). The non-verbal action is performed with the intention to cure the patient. On the way to action I have included the expectations, of the doctor and the patient, about the outcome of the action. These two expectations need not fully to coincide. Further I have added an observation of how the patient develops. This observation may involve the patient himself, the doctor, or perhaps a nurse. The observations may show that the task has been achieved, i.e. the patient has been cured. However, the task also may end if the patient dies. This will generally trigger a post mortem investigation in order to find what caused the death. In both cases there will be lessons to learn. Alternatively the observations may show that the patient still is ill. Then the diagnostic procedure has to start again and some other cure for the patient has to be argued, etc.

So far I have not discussed how arguments used in a particular case are generated. A first indication I have given by writing about "Lessons to learn from this and other particular cases". The generative mechanism cannot be found in any particular case per se. For this reason I have added "Evolving communities of living and interacting human beings". By this I broaden the horizon of observation and simultaneously introduce time in the form of ongoing processes. Figure 2 hence shows phenomena on different levels of abstraction. This entails risks of wrong conclusions being drawn. Figure 2 enables me to start from a concrete case and arrive at generative mechanisms on a higher level in one simple figure. In Figure 3 I attempt to illustrate my approach on the higher level of abstraction which ended my comments to Figure 2.

In the evolving communities of human beings many task venues are going on in parallel. Many of these will only concern sub-communities. Take the case illustrated in Figure 2. In the first instance one sub-community of a patient and his close relatives and friends will be concerned. Moreover, a sub-community of medical professionals will be concerned in this case. Figure 3 illustrates how classes of tasks can be argued and handled. This seems consistent with the purpose of the approach to explicate services rendered by computer applications. These are designed to support classes of tasks.

In section 4 I will use Figures 2 and 3 as stepping stones to answer the two questions raised in the Introduction.

THE NEW APPROACH AND SERVICES RENDERED BY COMPUTERS

Reflections on the First Question

My first question was: Which services do computers render by transforming messages purported to support decision making, and functions like coordination? Reflecting on the contexts shown in Figures 2 and 3 the following answer can be given. They render the service of some *limited* forms of reasoning for a class of tasks. That doing arithmetic, searching in large data bases, and performing logical deductions can be subsumed as reasoning may seem trivial. The importance of the contextual background invoked is that it clearly exposes these forms of reasoning as *limited*. They by far cover all kinds of reasoning and discursive interaction human beings apply in their daily lives and work. Still, reasoning performed by computers may offer forms of reasoning not easily done by human beings. To these forms belong extensive arithmetic calculations, search in huge data bases, and following long (binary) chains of deduction.

Figure 3. The approach illustrated at a uniform level of abstraction

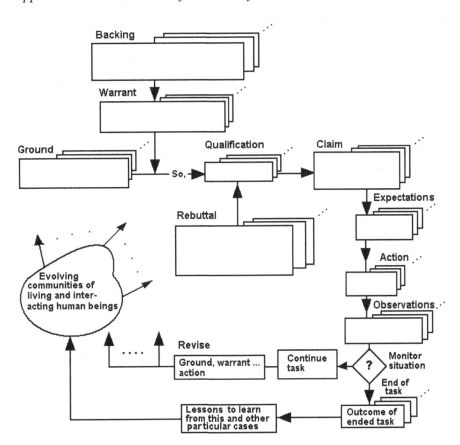

Services rendered by message transforming operations of programmed computers fruitfully can be perceived as *supplementing* human reasoning. The discussions above indicate why such computers never should be understood as *substituting* all kinds of human reasoning.

Figures 2 and 3 explicitly introduce communities of living and interacting human beings. Varela (1979) has presented good reasons for perceiving human beings as autonomous. That means they have the capacity not letting them be controlled from outside (ibid. pp. 58-59). An autonomous actor, ipso facto, has to be described as a responsible actor. An observer, studying people during a limited time period, still could describe many of them as controlled from outside. To perceive human beings as autonomous entails ethical and political implications. Ongoing debates, national and global, how to organize and pay for medical, and health care furnish an illustration. Statements in these can contradict each other. Computers can transport such messages. However, they cannot be used to transform such messages applying their binary logic.

Figures 2 and 3 show that a task needs to be monitored. This follows from the fact that other outcomes of an intervention occur than the expected ones. Weick and Sutcliffe (2007) report the following from studies of *high reliability organizations*. Such organizations are *sensitive to operations*. They are attentive to the front line, where the real work gets done. This indicates an area where message transforming computer programs could help in the form of early warning systems.

The "Outcomes of ended task" in Figure 3 entail both stories of success and of failure. An analysis of the latter and dissemination of its findings contributes to lessons to learn from experience. This ends my reflections on the first question.

Reflections on the Second Question

My second question was: How is this service [of transforming messages] explicated to those affected by it? In designing computer programs much effort is devoted to arrive at adequate requirement specifications. In my discussions of Figures 2 and 3 I have indicated human beings as autonomous and as responsible actors. To act responsibly they must understand how computers transform messages on which they are supposed to base an action. This they have to be informed about in a language they use when discussing their task venue. It entails a rather subtle pedagogical task. It is to understand how categories they use in their natural languages differ from formal categories of message transforming computers. The latter presuppose an objective, observer independent reality. The former presuppose experientially based categories. Only the latter are consistent with individually differing cognitive venues as indicated in Figure 1. Advice given by models imbedded in computers must not be taken as prescriptive for action in the task venue. It has to be taken as adequate if only what is included in the model is important and nothing else. (A comprehensive discussion of the two ways of categorizing in natural languages can be found in Lakoff (1987).)

My suggestion based on the last paragraph is the following. Designers of message transforming computer programs should devote at least as much effort on explaining embedded models as they do on requirement specifications.

CONCLUSION

The rationalistic approach presents the services rendered by message processing in computers as showing how rational people *should* reason. Among others Winograd and Flores (1986) have argued that this view is extremely limited considering the way people in practice act, interact, and reason.

As an alternative to the rationalistic view Winograd and Flores offer the following view. Based on speech act theory they implicitly argue that computers by message transforming services generate new possibilities of action. In conversations for action computers only seem to transmit messages between people. To support conversations for action Winograd and Flores suggest a group decision support tool called "The coordinator".

To analyze how far speech act theory can help I introduced four venues in human action and interaction according to Whitaker (1992). These were task, cognitive, depictive, and discursive venues. Due to Searle's (1979) formalization of the speech act approach it cannot explicate people's potential capacity of redefining a problematic situation. Nor can it explicate the radically different action alternatives people may generate in a particular situation.

Based on Toulmin (1958) and Toulmin et al. (1978) I present a context against which I answer my questions. In this context a computer transforming messages renders the service of a limited form of reasoning about a class of tasks. This service has to be perceived as *supplementing* human reason not as *substituting* it. Only then they can use computer support and remain autonomous and responsible actors. To do so they should be enabled to understand what message transformations by computers offer and what they ignore. This has to be done in the language in which the actors talk about their task venues. This is a design task so far largely neglected. Moreover, as the context in Figure 3 indicates the outcome of actions has to be monitored.

REFERENCES

Austin, J. L. (1962). *How to Do Things with Words*. Cambridge, MA: Harvard University Press.

Bullen, C.,& Bennett. J. (1990a, March). *Groupware in Practice: An Interpretation of Work Experience. Center for Information Systems Research Report*, no. 205. Cambridge, MA.

Bullen, C. (1990b). *Bennett. J* (pp. 291–302). Learning from User Experience with Groupware. CSCW.

Freire, P. (1972). *Pedagogy of the Oppressed*. Middlesex, UK: Penguin Books.

Lakoff, G. (1987). *Women, Fire, and Dangerous Things: What categories reveal about the mind*. Chicago, IL: The University of Chicago Press.

Searle, J. R. (1969). *Speech Acts – An essay in the philosophy of language*. London: Cambridge University Press.

Simon, H. A. (1957). *Models of Man: social and rational*. New York: John Wiley & Sons.

Toulmin, S., Rieke, R., & Janik, A. (1978). *An introduction to reasoning*. (A second edition appeared in 1984, page references to the second edition). New York: Macmillan.

Toulmin, S. E. (1958). *The Uses of Argument*. London: Cambridge University Press.

Varela, F. J. (1979). *Principles of Biological Autonomy*. New York: North Holland.

Weick, K. E., & Sutcliffe, K. M. (2007). *Managing the unexpected: resilient performance in an age of uncertainty* (2nd ed.). San Francisco: Jossey-Bass.

Whitaker, R. (1992). *Venues for Contexture: A critical analysis and enactive reformulation of group decision support systems*. (Diss.) Research Reports in Information Processing and Computer Science: Nr. UMADP-RRIPCS 15.92, Umeå University, Sweden.

Winograd, T. (1988). Where the action is. *BYTE*, *13*(13), 256A–258.

Winograd, T., & Flores, F. (1986). *Understanding Computers and Cognition: A new foundation for design*. New Jersey: Ablex Publishing Corporation.

Section 5
E-Conferences & E-Learning

Chapter 22
Towards a Combined Model for On–Line and Real Conferences:
A Proposal

Pedro Isaías
Universidade Aberta, Portugal

ABSTRACT

This chapter presents a combined model for on-line and real conferences. The chapter introduces Web 2.0 and its importance. Then, using Web 2.0 in real and virtual conferences is discussed since Web 2.0 can make a difference is supporting such a conference model. A past on-line event is analysed and evaluated in order to have lessons learned and make recommendations towards this proposal. The combined model approach is presented and detailed in its components and the importance of Web 2.0 elements is discussed.

INTRODUCTION

Real events have been for years the traditional meeting place for all sorts of professions, ranging from academics to doctors and other professionals. In these sorts of events, participants can interact with each other, see and comment presentations, talk to each other during coffee-breaks, attend all sorts of sessions, etc.

These kind of traditional events have however several limitations:

- Travel and hotel costs;
- Costs linked to rental of physical space and all facilities (i.e. coffee-breaks, lunches);
- Rigid program schedules;
- Limited duration in terms of days;

To overcome these limitations on-line events are a possibility. These have the following main advantages:

- No costs in terms of travelling and hotel;
- Availability during 24 hours a day and for weeks, months or even years;

DOI: 10.4018/978-1-60960-057-0.ch022

- Availability after the end of the event of most of the materials that can be recorded.

A combined model between traditional and on-line conferences may be a solution to overcome the limitations and enhance each other's strengths.

Web 2.0 can play an important role in such combined mode between traditional and on-line events. In the next two sections, Web 2.0 and its possibilities are introduced and using Web 2.0 in real and virtual conferences is discussed.

WEB 2.0

Web 2.0 is now a widespread phenomenon with repercussions in practically all sectors of society. It has evolved so rapidly and so steadily that the decision at this point seems to be either to use it and adapt to it or risk becoming superseded (Kittinger, n.d.: 3).

This term is used freely to define not only websites and applications but online collaborative activities, the exchange of data and the possibility of creating content (Eikelmann, 2007, p. 1). Web 2.0 is based on the principles of simple to use applications, the delivery of software as a service, the use of network effects and the centrality of the role of the user (Constantinides and Fountain, 2008, p. 235-236). It uses collective intelligence and its growth is inherently dependent on the users' collaborative activity (O'Reilly, 2005). Web 2.0 advocates the use of open software and free information flow, so it is based on a code of free delivery of services and users have learn to expect exactly that from the sites they use. Only a reduced number of websites have resorted to commercialising their services (Hoegg et al., 2006, p. 10, 11). Web 2.0 applications can be used both for professional and social matters and the features they offer depend mainly on the nature of the website (Leitner and Grechenig, 2008, p. 189, 190).

Web 2.0 applications are, for example, Blogs, Podcasts, RSS (Really Simple Syndication), Wikis, Social networks (Bughin, 2008, p. 257, 258) and they all have in common the promotion of interactivity between the users and the internet. MySpace, YouTube, Facebook and Wikipedia are some of Web 2.0's websites (Constantinides and Fountain, 2008: 233). Web 2.0 isn't intrinsically connected with a pioneering technology, it is instead a unique blend of existing protocols and languages (Hoegg et al., 2006, p. 5). Its dynamism is in part the responsibility of the programming technologies supporting it: XML, AJAX, Ruby on Rails, Java Script and others (Kittinger, n.d.: 3). These programming languages facilitate the effortless flow of information and data, which adds dynamism to content (Lewis, 2006). AJAX, for example, results in an improvement in the user's experience, because it allows for a reduction in the amount of the information transferred between the user and the server. It ensures that only the changes the user has introduced are updated, rather than the whole page (Hoegg et al., 2006, p. 6). The role of the technologies behind Web 2.0 applications is central, because it is essential to guarantee creative freedom by adding numerous possibilities to the websites, but without compromising their user-friendly nature (Kittinger, n.d.: 7, 8). The software must be straightforward, it is meant be a tool to facilitate the use of Web 2.0 applications and not a disincentive (Zajicek, 2007, p. 35).

The 1.0 version of the web was about people, this improved 2.0 version is set up around the user (Johnson, 2006). Users are no longer limited to their motionless role of information consumers; they assume a different part in this new version of the web, the part of proactive creators of content (Eikelmann, 2007, p. 1). The content generated by users can assume a wide range of formats like audio, video or text (Chai et al, 2007). The time and effort users invest in these applications is compensated by the feeling of belonging to a community, the opportunity to take part in enriching discussions and the access to information (Ewing,

2008: 580). The use of Web 2.0 involves a great amount of trust between its users. The apprehension that was expected from exchanging information online is felt only by a reduced number of users. Most of them do not have privacy concerns over the information they exchange with strangers even if it's private (Eikelmann, 2007, p. 3). Since Web 2.0 is accessible to anyone, people have more information about what is available and can benefit from their peers' knowledge. The users have gained an empowering voice which they can use for many purposes. Anyone can participate, the applications are easy to use, so no sophisticated IT skills are required (Thompson, 2006). There are nonetheless concerns, there is a core scepticism regarding the shift from professionalism to amateurism: "the impact of blogging on traditional journalism and the impact of Wikipedia on traditional scholarship" (Caplan, 2008).

Companies need to acknowledge the importance of this phenomenon and adapt to this reality by using Web 2.0 to their benefit, as a competitive advantage. Those who don't invest in Web 2.0 features will risk becoming obsolete and surmounted by their competitors. Where there is no resistance to use these applications and an investment is made to develop features that will bring their customers closer to the company and more in line with today's technologies, there is a competitive advantage to be gained. The most important stance to adopt, here, is to find ways of including the customer and creating opportunity for them to participate in the improvement of the service (Eikelmann, 2007: 6, 7). It's not only companies that are benefiting from new opportunities to satisfy their consumers. With Web 2.0, consumers have gained a variety of sources where they can get information from (Eccleston and Griseri, 2008: 593).

Content creation is swiftly expanding and this will affect all sectors of society (Kittinger, n.d.: 19, 20). This empowerment of the user has been extended to several different areas like Education 2.0 or Politics 2.0. These concepts refer to the application of Web 2.0 tools to the different sectors they represent, Education and Politics, respectively, and illustrate the effort of adapting to the new demands of students and citizens. In terms of education, Web 2.0 is moulding a more collaborative manner of structuring and delivering education (London Knowledge Lab, 2008: 9). In politics, for example, Web 2.0 is being used to promote political activism, they are creating space and opportunity for people to be politically proactive and they are being used to access political resources, such as speeches and legislation. Web 2.0 is sprouting and impelling civic involvement, by becoming increasingly accessible (Caplan, 2008). There are many other sectors adapting to Web 2.0 and the transformations they make are all based on the precept of engaging with their users and addressing their needs by providing them with opportunity to become more proactive and involved. This is the sort of empowerment Web 2.0 has to offer to anyone who wants to use it.

USING WEB 2.0 IN REAL AND VIRTUAL CONFERENCES

The proliferation of entities organising conferences have made this a very competitive area. Hence, it is important to keep up to date with competitors, adjust to the new demands of the participants and thrive in the delivery of a progressively better service. Web 2.0 provides corporations the possibility to augment their competitive advantage, but it also gives users a more collaborative experience (IBM, 2008, p. 2). The use of Web 2.0 tools in the organisation of conferences can be highly beneficial, especially when it comes to conferences which offer a combination of real and virtual participation. These features can be used before, during and after the conferences.

Web 2.0 works on 'viral marketing', which is a user to user type of advertising (Enders et al, 2008, p. 205) and this can be used in the initial stages of the organisation of conferences to advertise the event and provide more information to potential participants. Web 2.0, in itself has a very limited value, it is the active participation of users that will attract more users and it is the content they bring to the application that will provide quality to that application. It is time and participation that will make a good application. So the only thing providers of Web 2.0 services have to do is to ease this process (Hoegg et al., 2006, p. 14). Conferences are very much like Web 2.0, they depend on participation and they grow with time and an increasing number of participants. It is what the participants bring to the conference that will decide its quality. By the same token, all the organisers can really do is to facilitate the process of participation. This process starts with keeping people informed and for that purpose there are a number of Web 2.0 applications that can contribute to a more successful promotion of the event, like blogs, wikis or social networks. They are excellent for promoting 'viral marketing'.

Especially in conferences that aim to be international and attract the widest variety of countries and contributions possible, it becomes important to facilitate this participation. One of the aspects to take into consideration is access. People from all continents should be able to attend the conference. This is one of the reasons why more and more organisations are resorting to the use of a combination of real and virtual conferences. People with mobility constraints, for example, physical disabilities, can participate if given the right tools. They can interact with the participants and equally present their work, if they use appropriate features. Web 2.0 represents increased opportunities for people with disabilities who use the internet to attain their autonomy (Gibson, 2007, p. 1, 2). Furthermore, participants have other types of limitations which can be impediments to physically attend the conference like prior commitments, budgetary constraints. To introduce a virtual component on a real conference would be to increase immensely the probabilities of people participating in the conference. Web 2.0 rests on

the exchange of information and knowledge and it can be used to improve the participants' virtual experience. People not able to physically attend the conference, rather than sending in a power point presentation or a video with their presentation, which will not provide answers to participants' questions nor create a debate, could use Web 2.0 tools. By using these tools there would be an increased interactivity between the presenter and the remaining audience, even when the presenter is physically absent.

One of the important aspects of conferences is that the participants leave the event with an increased network of contacts. If there is something Web 2.0 is popular for is the creation of communities. Even with the traditional exchange of business cards, sometimes contacts are lost or never established. Web 2.0 applications have the capacity to keep these relationships and to promote the development of collaborative work even when people live in different continents. It is this potential that Web 2.0 has of connecting people that should be optimised by entities organising conferences, themselves platforms for the exchanges of information and knowledge. Web 2.0 helps the maintenance of networks and can be used not only among participants, but between these and the conference organisers. It is very enriching for the conference that the organisers have the possibility to provide and receive feedback about the conference overall. Particularly when the participants were unable to attend it is important to find a way of including them in the event, during and afterwards. These are communication tools and should be used to keep the participants up to date with current and future events and involved with the organisation after the events finish. They hold the potential to create what Wenger (n.d.) calls communities of practice. They are groups with an identity developed around the same areas of interest, where learning is a result of their interactivity and where a common set of rituals and resources are created (Wenger, n.d.). This would be a great achievement for a conference.

Despite the advantages of combining virtual aspects with real conferences and using Web 2.0 applications there are some reservations namely in terms of credibility. The challenge of credibility is pervasive. Efforts must be made to preserve the core scientificity of the event without compromising its capability of adapting to the new demands of authors and participants. The question remains as to how the process of adjusting these new trends will mature and what kind of concessions and transformations both institutions and technologies are ready to accept to make the most of this phenomenon (Bessenyei, 2008).

FROM REAL EVENTS TO ON-LINE CONFERENCES

In 2005, an innovative on-line event has occurred: an on-line (virtual) conference. The virtual conference was called MCCSIS 2005 (Multi Conference on Computer Science and Information Systems) being organised by the International Association for the Development of the Information Society (IADIS) for a period of three weeks and the on-line conference venue was supported by an LMS (Learning Management System) with both asynchronous and synchronous functionalities support and the server is running at the National Sun Yat-sen University, Taiwan.

The conference had the following system architecture to sustain it (see Figure 1) as detailed in Miranda et al. (2005).

The mains components of the IADIS MCCSIS 2005 depicted in Figure 1 were:

1. **The Conference Platform:** The platform was an e-Learning platform that was used to host the conference;
2. **The Conference Forum:** This enabled communication with conference attendees by making it possible to send messages that other participants could comment on;
3. **The Interactive Board:** This enabled upload and presentation of slides with the other participants through interactive broad window. Also had other features like by providing several tools with which annotations could be made on the slides (e.g. pointing to specific parts of a presentation, draw figures). All these actions could be seen by all participants in real-time. The interactive board also allowed to share the desktop with attendees and to browse specific sites and these actually being presented to attendees;
4. **The JoinNet Meeting Room:** This made it possible to hold conversations with other attendees, in audio or text. It was possible to take snapshots using each attendee PC camera for other meeting participants to view, and it was possible to see other people whom are chatting with.
5. **The JoinNet Control Panel:** The control panel showed the audio/video capabilities of all participants. This also was where there were the controls needed for making use of

Figure 1. System Architecture of the system supporting the IADIS, MCCSIS, 2005

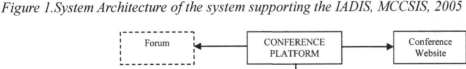
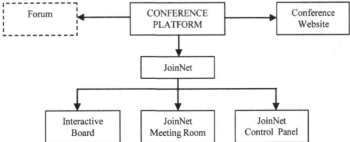

Figure 2. The Conference Platform

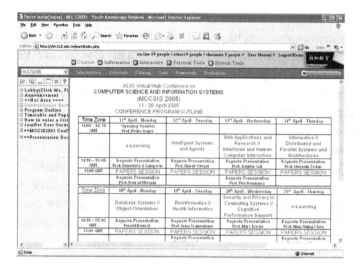

many features like question/answer flow, etc.

6. **The Conference Web Site:** This was aimed firstly to promote the conference with information such as Program Committee, how the conference worked, the call for papers, and so forth, and then at the time of the conference, it made available an up-to-date conference schedule and access to power point presentations from presenters.

In Figure 2 the conference platform is shown. This had a left panel with several conference options (e.g. lobby, announcements, program outline, how to use JoinNet, presentation tips).

In Figure 3 the Interactive Board is presented with a power point of the testing sessions being conducted before the first session in each day started.

In Figure 4 the JoinNet meeting room is presented.

Figure 3. The Interactive Board

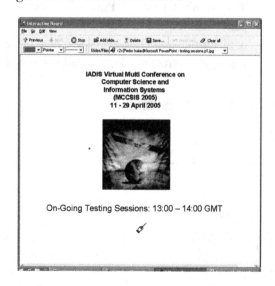

Figure 4. The JoinNet meeting room

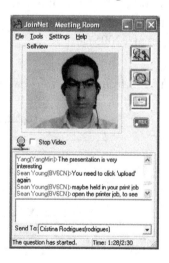

Figure 5. The JoinNet Control Panel

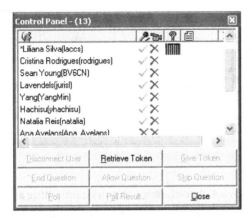

In Figure 5 the JoinNet control panel is presented – this enables to hand over the microphone to a participant allowing the person to make a presentation, retrieve the microphone, allow questions or ending the question, skip a request from a participants' request to speak, and so on.

THE EVALUATION PERFORMED

A thorough evaluation was performed to the IADIS MCCSIS 2005 conference with two goals:

- Assessing that edition;
- Preparing future virtual conferences through lessons learned.

In Miranda et al. (2005) the authors focused only in the assessment of that particular edition of the virtual multi conference. In this book chapter the goal is to take the results of the evaluation performed back at that time and use them to plan and prepare a future edition, already under the combined model, and in this way the goal is to justify some of the options made under this combined model proposal. Tables 1-6 and comments are taken from Miranda et al (2005) and put into perspective as referred.

The evaluation has been conducted through an on-line questionnaire. 27 respondents filled out the questionnaire at the conference platform. Main answers are summarised in the following tables and analysed under this chapters' goal.

Table 1 shows that that the conference was considered as being overall well above average – 85% of the respondents considered it as being excellent or at least good. The quality of the sessions (either Keynotes or regular presentations) was also appreciated (respectively, 71% considered the keynote sessions excellent or at least good, and 78% considered the regular sessions excellent or at least good). The reasons for those participants who ranked as poor might be with limited internet access bandwidth or the difficulty in handing audio/video setting properly on their local computer; these resulted that their online participations were even not possible.

A global analysis of Table 1 also suggests that maybe the small percentage of participants that considered the conference as poor (11%) might have done so for being only an on-line conference. In this combined model those participants could be happier because they could have the option to participate in person at the event. Also the small percentage that classified the quality of the regular sessions as poor or OK could also decrease by having the option of in presence participation of the combined model.

Table 1. Conference in general

Questions	Poor	OK	Good	Excellent	NA
How do you rank the overall quality of the conference?	11%	0%	74%	11%	0%
The quality of the keynote sessions	0%	15%	52%	19%	11%
The quality of the regular sessions	7%	4%	74%	4%	7%

Table 2. Interaction

Questions	Poor	OK	Good	Excellent	NA
The usefulness of the conference forum	15%	37%	26%	7%	11%
The quality of your interaction with participants and speakers	15%	26%	30%	22%	0%
	Short Message	**e-mail**	**Forum**	**Online Chatrrom**	**Other**
How did you interact with the presenters or other participants besides video conferencing? *	26%	44%	4%	41%	4%

• multi responses allowed for this question

Table 2 presents results for interaction in general. Most respondents, 37%, considered the conference forum as ok in terms of usefulness while only 33% considered it good or excellent. The quality of interaction with participants and speakers was considered by most respondents as good (30%), ok (26%) or even excellent (22%). Most participants felt that even the virtual conference environment enable two-way audio/video interaction with each others; they however are not used to talk in front of a computer at the beginning. This would need a few times of practices and custom for overcoming human behaviour nature.

Regarding interaction with other participants (besides video conferencing), a significant 44% signalled e-mail as their alternative method, and also online chatroom (41%) was pointed out by most respondents. Short message (using the platform) was also mentioned by 26% of respondents.

Under the interaction possibilities, there's plenty of room for improvement currently with Web 2.0 tools that can be available for participants

to interact. A conference forum is something available by default but a wide range of other options can be developed or made available.

Comparing to traditional conferences, the virtual multi conference scores very well – see Table 3. Regarding price, a significant 78% of respondents considered it less expensive in overall terms with 15% stating that they somewhat agreeing. In terms of quality, 59% strongly agreed or somewhat agreed that the conference had a similar quality. Regardless, still 22% of respondents considered that the conference did not have similar quality – this might be because in traditional conferences, people seek human contact that might give some sort of future professional or personal reward. In this way, virtual conferences should try to improve forms of people knowing each other; profile matching might be a possibility for this.

By having a combined model those authors that really feel that they should travel to the conference to know other participants in person and auto-reward them in this way will be able to do

Table 3. Comparison with traditional conferences

Questions	Strongly Agree	Somewhat Agree	Neutral	Somewhat Disagree	Strongly Disagree
The virtual conference is less expensive in overall terms (i.e. travel, accommodations and rates)	78%	15%	4%	0%	0%
The virtual conference has similar quality	11%	48%	15%	7%	15%
The virtual conference is more convenient in terms of session availability (including session recordings)	48%	30%	11%	4%	4%
The virtual conference is more convenient in terms of enabling the participant to be at its work or home	70%	15%	7%	0%	4%

Table 4. Positive aspects to participate in the virtual multi conference

Its global contributions.
I think it is good if we can see the participants rather than just reading papers or listening to the presentations but it is hard for the participants to get use to speaking to an audience they cannot see.
The participants will perform better when it is not a first time experience.
Friendly and helpful organizers.
Relaxing atmosphere among participants.
A very good experience.
I had a new experience.
I had the paper published.
I did not spend much energy to present it.
Great experience on virtual collaboration.
It was a new experience for me in such a type of conference.
Ease of participation, I can present my work to others all over the world without travelling expense.
New knowledge, new form of communication.
People from across the world can share ideas, research issues, etc. without having to travel physically to one specific location. Being there without being there.
Good experience of a virtual conference.
Convenience.
I experienced the net meeting and felt it is practical but still not satisfying.

it. But the Web 2.0 tools that can be developed and/or made available can contribute to decrease the dissatisfied percentage of participants with the conference quality (on-line vs traditional conferences compared).

In relation to convenience in terms of session availability, a significant 78% of respondents strongly agreed or somewhat agreed that it was more convenient than traditional conferences. As for convenience in terms of enabling the participant to be at its work or home, 85% of respondents strongly agreed or somewhat agreed that it was more convenient too.

Again the above figures suggest that there are some participants that would prefer to participate in person at the conference and going away from work in this way – this of course leaves people more time for interaction with their peers than being at the office and having to also current daily tasks for example.

Table 4 lists the positive aspects cited by participants. The newness of the experience, easiness and convenience are aspects that come out as most cited – these result from participants being in the office or at home making the presentation or taking part in the event without the need to travel; the costs are obviously much lower and people can still continue their regular work. Some of the aspects of the "virtuality" of the experience are also cited as not totally favourable. Again, the aspect of the audience cannot be seen, because many people did not have a web camera.

Table 4 also shows that participants are open to the experience and that probably under a combined model can have the option to choose what form of participation is better suited for them.

Table 5 shows some of participants' difficulties in participating in the conference. Some difficulties stated like "time differences" are difficult to address whilst others are mainly technical problems that should be addressed in the future

Table 5. Major difficulties experienced to participate in the virtual multi conference

Using the MIC that had not been properly tested because I could not get a response during the testing slot and avoiding distortion of the sound.
Sometimes transmission of presenters' voice is not good, which is frustrating.
If put in a wrong session (in my case, a more pedagogy-oriented paper put in a more technically oriented session), no real sparks between presenter and audience.
The information to upload our power point files should be given before by email.
Video-Audio quality too poor.
Difficult to hear questions.
Need digital tablet for drawing on screen.
To learn how to communicate online with Joinnet the same day to present the paper.
I'm in stage out of my University. I have some problems with my computer.
Get into the meeting. The instructions claimed to select Interactive, but only when I opened the chat room, the JoinNet application launched. So, I was late to enter.
Disability to participate from home (too weak Internet connection).
After explaining how this conference works, everything was clear.
Some people in work interrupt the technological ones.
The feeling of talking to a machine is not very comfortable.
Time difference.
Trouble getting the microphone to work.
Since I was not able to test the system until an hour before I was supposed to speak, this was a problem. I strongly suggest that speakers be able to test their system at least one week before they speak so they can solve any problems they encounter.
The software did not work.
Even late in the conference, some sessions were considerably delayed by participants having microphone or slide upload problems.

with i) more testing sessions and ii) participants training before the conference started. It must be stated that some technical problems relate to having very low bandwidth at participants end. Other difficulties are related to the conference environment and lack of proper testing.

Since four years have passed now from the original experience, one would feel that most of the technical issues encountered have now been addressed, like bandwidth problems in some countries, that are clearly related to some of the mentioned problems. Some of the other problems are issues that can be easily tackled if more time is allowed for testing before the virtual-in presence conference occurs.

Table 6 shows respondents general opinions and suggestions for improvements. For example, session scheduling for participants in different time zones is an issue to consider in the future. Again, technical problems are referred many times and the need to address them in a more effective way with some valid suggestions provided on how to tackle the issues.

As commented for Table 5 results, most of the technical issues should be now solved with increased bandwidth and technical problem address since four years ago.

THE PROPOSED COMBINED MODEL

Considering the evaluation results of the MCCSIS 2005 on-line conference, with both the advantages pointed out and the identified shortcomings, and also the real conferences' history from IADIS, with the evaluation made throughout the years,

Table 6. General comments and suggestions for improvements

Better testing facilities would improve the quality of the conference and the confidence of the participants.
As far as my interest e-learning is concerned, I hope there will be more papers focusing on e-pedagogy, though development and implementation of ICT for learning is equally important.
Please try to make possible uploads of multimedia presentations (flash, small videos etc).
Some social activities where people can meet afterwards, probably forum and discussion for each article in the forum.
Good assistance, some days before, to install and test the microphone and camera. I installed both but realise that only the micro was working in the Joinnet. I think next year I could be more attentive to those aspects before the conference. So, some attention should be given some time before the conference to test all the material, making test sessions, mainly with new participants.
Too much time was spent during scheduled session for resolution of presenters' problems.
It is necessary somehow to provide testing of equipment (mic, etc.) during special sessions prior scheduled presentations.
In the first mail you should explain details about participation in the conference (for viewers as well as speakers).
The only problem I had with the conference was that being in Australia I had to present at 1am, which was a bit difficult. It also made it hard, to participate in other sessions, but the recordings of the sessions is a great idea and I plan to view many of the sessions when time becomes a bit freer.
The conference could include asynchronous presentations where presenters recorded and uploaded their presentations before and, then anyone can watch them at their convenient time. Questions or comments can be posted in the forum, and the presenters can reply at a later date.
The lobby section should have a chat option.
There are not enough audience.
Put more weight on the reviewing process; give the participants the time to change their papers and to take into account the reviewer's comments.
The morning training sessions were a very good idea. But some people did not participate or tried but were unable to resolve their problems in that time, so their problems carried over into the conference sessions.
Consider keeping the training session, monitored by a tech person, running in parallel with the real conference session, so that presented who are still having difficulties could be shifted there to work them out while the conference itself continued.

and having in consideration the original system architecture of the virtual conference, the following combined model is proposed (see Figure 6).

From the proposed model the following components are described:

1. **The conference portal** (this replaces the previous conference platform) – This will host all participants, from authors to keynote speakers, with bio information for each of them and a participant area where all information regarding a paper will be present (i.e. the paper itself in pdf format, the ppt used

Figure 6. System architecture of the combined model of real and on-line conferences

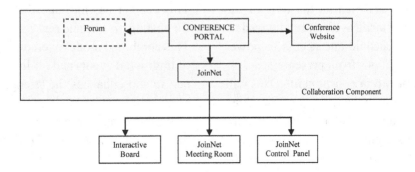

to present it, complimentary elements, links to relevant URLs to the presentation);

2. **The conference Forum** – This enabled communication with conference attendees by making it possible to send messages that other participants could comment on;

3. **The Interactive Board** – This enabled upload and presentation of slides with the other participants through interactive broad window. Also had other features like by providing several tools with which you annotations could be made on the slides (e.g. pointing to specific parts of a presentation, draw figures). All these actions could be seen by all participants in real-time. The interactive board also allowed to share the desktop with attendees and to browse specific sites and these actually being presented to attendees;

4. **The JoinNet meeting room** – This made it possible to hold conversations with other attendees, in audio or text. It was possible to take snapshots using each attendee PC camera for other meeting participants to view, and it was possible to see other people whom are chatting with.

5. **The JoinNet control panel** – The control panel showed the audio/video capabilities of all participants. This also was where there were the controls needed for making use of many features like question/answer flow, etc.

6. **The conference web site** – This was aimed firstly to promote the conference with information such as Program Committee, how the conference worked, the call for papers, and so forth, and then at the time of the conference, it made available an up-to-date conference schedule and access to power point presentations from presenters.

7. **The collaboration component** – This will enable collaboration between all involved participants and will include Web 2.0 subcomponents within the portal component. The collaboration component involves the Conference Portal, Forum, Conference Web site and JoinNet components.

The collaboration component can make a real difference in terms of interaction between conference participants and can integrate several of the following items or tools:

- Author/participant area where papers can be made available (as well as supporting documents such as slides from presentations);
- Matching profiles based on common interest areas;
- Research areas for common developments between participants;
- Forums for group discussions (global, localised);
- Folksonomies to foster content exchange;
- Pre conference developments to make participants acquainted with each other and foster group interaction;
- Post conference developments to keep group interaction.

A deeper study, based on the opinions of past conference participants (both from on-line conferences as well as from real conferences), and also of their future requirements, will help to identify the right items (most desired) to integrate the collaboration component.

CONCLUSION

This chapter has introduced a combined model for hosting on-line and real conferences together. This combined model overcomes the limitations of traditional events and on-line conferences run *per se* and enhances the strengths of each type of event.

In this chapter it has also been defended the importance of Web 2.0 and how it can be used in real and on-line conferences, i.e. in the combined model proposed.

The chapter also presents the evaluation results of a past on-line conference and the respective system architecture, and then from it, derives what can be the system architecture of the combined model.

These type of events have a promising future and the combined model proposed is one of possible solutions that can be found to run these type of events.

ACKNOWLEDGMENT

The author wishes to thank Paula Miranda and Professor Nian-Shing Chen for their participation in a previous paper addressing the on-line conference cited here and also to IADIS for authorising the publication of several excerpts and content from that paper: Miranda, P., Chen, N-S and Isaías, P., 2005. Design, Implementation and Evaluation of a Virtual Conference. *Proceedings of the IADIS International Conference e-Society 2005*, Qawra, Malta, pp. 59-68. Also special thanks to Sara Pífano for the work relating to Web 2.0 research and its role in virtual and on-line conferences that is part of this chapter.

REFERENCES

April 8, 2009 from http://www.time.com/time/business/article/0,8599,1819187,00.html

Bessenyei, I. (2008). Learning and teaching in the information society. *Elearning 2.0 and connectivism. Revista de Informatica Sociala*, 9. Retrieved August 8, 2009 from http://www.ris.uvt.ro/wp-content/uploads/2009/01/ibesseneyi.pdf

Bughin, J. (2008). The rise of enterprise 2.0. *In Direct . Data and Digital Marketing Practice*, *9*(3), 251–259. doi:10.1057/palgrave.dddmp.4350100

Caplan, J. (2008, June 30). The Citizen Watchdogs of Web 2.0. *Time*. Retrieved

Chai, K. (2007). A Survey of Revenue Sharing Social Software's Systems. In *Proceedings of International, Workshop on Social Interaction and Mundane Technologies (Simtech)*, Melbourne. Retrieved August 8, 2009 from http://kevinchai.net/images/resources/survey-of-revenue-sharing-social-software-systems.pdf

Constantinides, E., & Fountain, S. (2008). Web 2.0: Conceptual Foundations and Marketing Issues. *Journal of Direct . Data and Digital Marketing Practice*, *9*(3), 231–244. doi:10.1057/palgrave.dddmp.4350098

Eccleston, D., & Griseri, L. (2008). How does Web2.0 stretch traditional influencing patterns? *International Journal of Market Research*, *50*(5), 591–616. doi:10.2501/S1470785308200055

Eikelmann, S., Peterson, M., Hasbani, G., & Hajj, J. (2007). The Urgent Need for Companies To Adapt to the Web 2.0 – New Models of Online Consumer Behaviour Demand Changes in Corporate Strategy. *Booz Allen Hamilton*. Retrieved May 8, 2009 from http://www.boozallen.co.uk/media/file/The_Urgent_Need_for_Companies_to_Adapt_to_Web_2.0.pdf

Enders, A., Hungenberg, H., Denker, H.-P., & Mauch, S. (2008). The Long Tail of Social Networking - Revenue Models in Social Networking Site. *European Management Journal*, *26*(3), 199–211. doi:10.1016/j.emj.2008.02.002

Ewing, T. (2008). Participation Cycles and Emergent Cultures in an Online Community. *International Journal of Market Research*, *50*(5), 575–590. doi:10.2501/S1470785308200043

Gibson, B. (2007). Enabling an Accessible Web 2.0. *In: W4A2007 - Keynote, Banff, Canada. Co-Located with the 16th International World Wide Web Conference.*

Högg, R., Meckel, M., Stanoevska-Slabeva, K., & Martignoni, R. (2006). 2.0 Communities . In *Proceedings of GeNeMe Conference* (pp. 23–37). Dresden, Germany: Overview of Business Models for Web.

IBM. (2008). *Putting the Power of Web 2.0 into Practice – How Rich Internet Applications can deliver Tangible Business Benefits*. IBM Corporation, Cambridge, USA. Available at: ftp://ftp.software.ibm.com/software/lotus/lotusweb/product/expeditor/LOW14003-USEN-00.pdf [last accessed 04.08.09]

Johnson, S. (2006, December 16). It's All About Us. *Time*. Retrieved from http://www.time.com/time/magazine/article/0,9171,1570717,00.html

Kittinger, R. (n.d.). *Web 2.0 - Social Behavior of Internet Users*. Retrieved May 8, 2009 from http://www.auburnmedia.com/pdf/kittinger_web_2.0.pdf

Leitner, P., & Grechenig, T. (2008). Social Networking Sphere: a Snapshot of trends, functionalities and revenue models. In *Proceedings of the IADIS International Conference on Web Based Communities* (pp. 187-191), Amsterdam, The Netherlands.

Lewis, D. (2006). *What is Web 2.0*. Crossroads ACM Student Magazine.

London Knowledge Lab. (2008). Education 2.0? Designing the web for teaching and learning. A Commentary by the Technology Enhanced Learning phase of the Teaching and Learning Research Programme. Retrieved July 8, 2009 from http://www.tlrp.org/pub/documents/TELcomm.pdf

Miranda, P., Chen, N.-S., & Isaías, P. (2005). Design, Implementation and Evaluation of a Virtual Conference. In *Proceedings of the IADIS International Conference e-Society 2005* (pp. 59-68), Qawra, Malta.

O'Reilly, T. (2005). *What is Web 2.0? Design Patterns and Business Models for the Next Generation of Software*. Retrieved April 8, 2009 from http://oreilly.com/web2/archive/what-is-web-20.html

Thompson, J. (2008, December). Don't Be Afraid to Explore Web 2.0. *The Education Digest*.

Wenger, E. (n.d.). Communities of practice a brief introduction. Retrieved April 8, 2009 from http://www.ewenger.com/theory/index.htm [last accessed 04.08.09

Zajicek, M. (2007). Web 2.0: Hype or Happiness? *W4A2007 – Keynote, May 07–08, 2007*, Banff, Canada. Co-Located with the 16th International World Wide Web Conference.

Chapter 23
Some Experiences of E–Learning in the Moodle E–Learning Environment

Virve Siirak
Tallinn University of Technology (TUT), Estonia

ABSTRACT

In this chapter it is argued that blended learning with web-based support by the Moodle e-learning environment based on social constructivist learning theory is an effective tool for teaching and learning ergonomics and human factor issues for future managers. The author has eight years experience of computer based teaching and learning. The author`s own teaching experience of the Moodle e-learning environment for creating and providing courses in Tallinn University of Technology (TUT), in Tallinn School of Economics and Business Administration at TUT, will be presented. According to the questionnaires given to students at the end of each course, the teaching and learning in the Moodle e-learning environment as blended learning is very useful for development of a learning culture and efficiency. The efficiency and motivation for learning are higher than providing traditional methods of learning. New possibilities and dimensions for teaching and learning are opening.

INTRODUCTION

At 2006 the strategy of e-learning in Tallinn University of Technology (TUT) was approved. According to this strategy for year 2010, 90% of courses have to be provided by support of e-learning environment and the credits obtained by e-learning have to be 50%. Since 2003- 558 courses by support of e-learning environment

(BlackBoard or Moodle) have been created. Of them 188 are created in the Tallinn School of Economics and Business Administration at TUT (TSEBA), using the web support by the Moodle e-learning environment. Since autumn 2006 the courses of Working Environment and Ergonomics by the support of the Moodle e-learning environment have been created by the author.

Before using Moodle software since the year 2001 the computer based learning was used providing this course – materials were available on

DOI: 10.4018/978-1-60960-057-0.ch023

the website. The experience before the Moodle using and after the Moodle using is compared and the advantages of learning by web support of the Moodle e-learning environment are described.

E-LEARNING AS A SOLUTION FOR NEW CHALLENGES

New Challenges for Higher Education

We are living in time of deep global changes. Technology, economy, norms/values and labor market are changing on a global level. New competence requirements in the ICT (information and communication technology) sector and in information and knowledge work mean new challenges for national educational systems. Understanding of human and organizational behaviour, cultural understanding, communication and language skills, and the capacity for conceptual thinking are important competencies needed in the future. The impact of rapid development of Infocommunication Technology (ICT) to all aspects of the society is described by Bradley 2001,2003,2006.

The process of social and psychosocial change and ICT from a global perspective is described in the Convergence Model on ICT and psychosocial life environment. Effects on humans are becoming more multifaceted and complex. Increasing access to more and better information is available by rapidly development of technology. The impact of rapid development of Infocommunication Technology (ICT) to all aspects of the society is described by Bradley by the Convergence Model on ICT and Psychosocial Life Environment (Bradley, 2001, 2006). According to this model it is now very actual to help students turn information into knowledge, teachers need to know and obtain new teaching strategies.

In this situation, new challenges for the higher education are continued. The growing interest of blended learning (combination of traditional

teaching methods of face to face and online media) in higher education is indicated by the increasing number of studies in this area (Poole 2006, Irons et al. 2002; ; O`Toole et al. 2003; Stubbs et al., 2003). In University of Central England in Birmingham (UCE), academic staff are encouraged to incorporate both traditional and web-based ICT (information and communication technology) modes of teaching and learning in the courses they deliver, using Moodle software. Preliminary quantitave evaluations at UCE have releaved that over 70 percent of the 388 students in the sample from across all faculties claimed to have enjoyed using the web-based aspects of blended courses. Over 75 percent of a sample of 329 students felt that Moodle had helped them learn the subject and nearly 80 percent of the sample reported that they would like future modules be blended in this way (Poole, 2006; Staley 2005).

E-Learning in Estonia

The Estonian e-Learning Development Centre was created as a separate structural unit ofthe Estonian Information Technology Foundation (EITF) on 2 May 2006. Before the creation of the Estonian e-Learning Development Centre, e-learning in Estonian higher and vocational education was coordinated by two consortia: the Estonian e-University consortium (founded on 21 February 2003) and the Estonian e-Vocational Schoolconsortium (founded on 16 February 2005). EITF is the legal person of the consortium and the managing bodies are the Council of the Estonian e-University and the Council and General Assembly of the Estonian e-Vocational School, respectively. Now all Estonian universities are networking.

E-Learning in Tallinn University of Technology

At 2006 the strategy of e-learning of Tallinn University of Technology was approved. According to this strategy for year 2010, 90% of courses have to be provided by support of e-learning environment and the credits obtained by e-learning have to be 50%. Since 2003 – 558 courses by the support of e-learning environment (BlackBoard or Moodle) have been created. Of them 188 courses are in the School of Economics and Business Administration at TUT, using the web support by the Moodle e-learning environment.

Tallinn School of Economics and Business Administration (TSEBA) at Tallinn University of Technology (TUT) is one of the most important institutions of higher education in economics and business administration in Estonia. TSEBA is among the biggest by the number of students and one of the leading in respect of teaching quality. Our School is a member of many international organizations like EFMD, CEEMAN, BMDA, EIASM etc. TSEBA offers study programs at bachelor, master's and doctoral level. All TSEBA bachelor, master's and doctoral study programs are fully accredited by the relevant public authorities and international committee.

Since 2006, the web support by Moodle e-learning environment is approved for courses created in TSEBA.

The experience of computer based learning without Moodle software, when the learning materials were only available on the website has described by some articles (Siirak, 2000, 2001, 2002, 2003, 2004, 2005, 2006).

Moodle E-Learning Environment as a Supporting Tool

Since autumn 2006 the courses of Working Environment and Ergonomics were created in the Moodle e-learning environment. All courses are provided as blended learning: the traditional method face-to-face is blended of web-based support by the Moodle e-learning environment. Autumn 2006 the first course of Working Environment and Ergonomics was provided for full-time students of the TSEBA by web-support of the

Moodle e-learning environment. Participated and successfully finished the courses in 2006 – 166 students, in 2007- 229 students, in 2008- 224 students.

AIM OF THE STUDY

The aim of the study is to find out how students appreciate the courses provided by web support of the Moodle e- learning environment.

MATERIAL AND METHOD

At the end of the courses a questionnaire was given to all groups of students. The questionnaires were given for 599 full-time students in the course of Working Environment and Ergonomics (Bachelor level) (82% were filled). The questionnaire was given to the 117 distance learning students (Bachelor level) (80% were filled).

Students had to answer to 5 questions:

1. How do you appreciate the Moodle e-learning environment ?
2. Which part of the course was most interesting for you ?
3. Which part of the course was unclear for you ?
4. How do you will to use obtained knowledge in practice ?
5. What do you like to learn more ?

RESULTS

Of respondents 98% answered that Moodle e-learning environment is very effective learning tool. Students wrote that they are encouraged and motivated to learn more in Moodle e-learning environment and they do not like to learn courses which are not in Moodle e-learning environment. The materials in Moodle e-learning environment are clear. Of respondents 82% answered that their participation in forums and othet activities available in Moodle e-learning environment is very useful for learning from each other obtaining new knowledge. Some students wrote that availability of course materials and activities in Moodle e-learning environment encourage their interest for classroom activities and the face to face contact with teacher is now in a new level. Students appreciate high that they can learn in Moodle e-learning environment the time and place suitable for each student.. Some students wrote that the experience of learning in Moodle e-learning environment is helpful for development of their self- discipline

DISCUSSION

According to my experience with computer based learning since the year 2001, providing of courses in Moodle e-learning environment are more effective than providing the courses where course materials are available on the website. Very effective is that students activities from participation in learning forums and learning from each other are encouraged. The problem is that sometimes students hesitate to participate in learning forums, they are sometimes afraid that other students can read their letters to learning forums. The efficiency of learning process is depending on the style of creation of the course. The course have to be designed simply and clearly encouraging students own activity in the learning process. The assignments encouraging students activity have to be provided. In comparison of previous results before Moodle was introduced (only materials were available on the website), students are more satisfied and motivated to learn the discipline. Students appreciate high that can fill all the assignments in Moodle e-learning environment, what is more suitable for students. Before Moodle was introduced the filling the different assignments was more complicated. There are

no statistical differences of the satisfaction of the courses before Moodle was used. Before Moodle was introduced all the solutions of web based learning were highly appreciated by the students in comparison of traditional courses without using web tools. (Siirak 2007, 2008). After Moodle was used, the motivation of students and their own activity in the learning process, the students interpersonal contacts (learning from each other) were successfully increased. After Moodle was introduced, for the teacher the online contact with students and monitoring their activities is successfully improved.

For me as a teacher, the management of courses where more than 200 students is participating, the Moodle e-learning environment is very useful for more effective management of the students activities and learning process. Before using Moodle software, the management of students learning activities was more complicated.

The advantage of blended learning is that face to face contact with teachers personality is enriching the learning process. According to my experience the activities in the Moodle e-learning environment encourage the students internest to working in the classroom face to face with the teacher.

CONCLUSION

In the 21st century, where structural changes in our industries and economics, globalization of our world need responsible new engineers and scientists, new challenges for the higher education and learning culture are continued, and new possibilities, dimensions and solutions are opening.

One of the new possibilities and solutions is blended learning using the Moodle e-learning environment.

Moodle e-learning environment is a very effective learning tool supporting blended learning which encourages the students motivation for learning activity and interest to the course, developing the learning culture and efficiency. For the teacher the management of students learning activities is more effective.

We have to be open for future development of Moodle e-learning environment according to rapid development of ICT (information and communication technology) dimensions and new possibilities and solutions for developing the learning culture and efficiency. The study is continuining.

ACKNOWLEDGMENT

The author would like to express the gratitude to the European Commission and Estonian National ICT program for Higher Education for supporting the creation of the Course of Working Environment and Ergonomics in Moodle e-learning environment autumn 2006 (EITSA 2 ESF project REDEL).,

REFERENCES

Bradley, G. (2001). *Humans on the Net*. Stockholm, SE: Prevent.

Bradley, G. (2003). Humans on the net: psychosocial life environment and e-society. In *Proceedings of the international Conference Risk and Safety Management in Industry, Logistics, Transport and Military Service: New Solutions for the 21st Century*, (pp. 27-36), Tallinn Technical University, Tallinn, Estonia.

Bradley, G. (2006). *Social and Community Informatics: Humans on the Net*. London: Routledge.

Irons, L. R., Robert, K., & Bielema, Ch. L. (2002). Blended Learning and Learner Satisfaction. Keys to user acceptance. *USDLA Journal, 16*(12). O`Toole, J.M., & Douglas J. A. (2003) The impact of Blended Learning on Student Outcomes: Is there Room on the Horse for Two? *Journal of Educational Media, 28*(2/3), 179–191.

Poole, J. (2006). E- learning and e-learning styles: students'reactions to web-based Language and Style at Blackpool and the Fylde College. *Language and Literature, 15,* 307. doi:10.1177/0963947006066129

Siirak, V. (2000). Influencing behaviour through learning of ergonomics knowledge in Cyberspace: a new millennium strategy to the reduction of health risks and accidents at working environment in Estonia. In K.E. Fostervold & T. Endestad (Eds.), *At the gateway to Cyberspace-ergonomic thinking in a new millennium* (pp. 225-228). Oslo, NO: Nordiska Ergonomisällskapet.

Siirak, V. (2001). New challenge for ergonomics and human factors education in technical universities. In *Proceedings of NES 2001 Nordic Ergonomics Society 33rd Annual Congress* (pp. 210-212). University of Tampere, Finland.

Siirak, V. (2002). Multi-media and the internet as educational tools for solving the problems of ergonomics and safety . In *Human Factors in Transportation, Communication, Health and the Workplace* (pp. 471–472). The Netherlands: Shaker Publishing.

Siirak, V. (2002). Experience of new teaching strategies of occupational health and ergonomics at Tallinn Technical University. In *Proceedings of 6th International Conference Scientific Committee on Education and Training in Occupational Health Ideas that Sizzle* (pp. 224-226). Baltimore, Maryland, USA.

Siirak, V. (2003), Computer Based Learning as an Effective Tool for Prevention of Chemical Risks - CD ROM. In *Proceedings of 8th International Symposium of ISSA Research Section*, Athens, Greece E.L.I.N.Y.A.E. (Hellenic Institute for Occupational Health and Safety)

Siirak, V. (2004). New Challenges for Human Factors and Ergonomics Education in Technical Universities- CD ROM. In *Proceedings of WorkCongress6: 6th International Congress on Work Injuries, Prevention, Rehabilitation and Compensation*, Rome. Italy. INAIL. Italian Workers Compensation Authority. Italian Workcover. Directorate of Communication. External Communication and International Relations Unit. Piazzale Giulio Pastore 6. I-0014 Rome RM, EUROPEAN UNION.

Siirak, V. (2005). Some experience of computer based learning in occupational health and safety education for future engineers. In *Proceedings of the 1st International Conference on Interdisciplinarity in Education ICIE 2005* (pp. 91-96). National Technical University of Athens, Athens, Greece.

Siirak, V. (2006). Some experience of ECTAS education for crossing international, cultural and social borders. Ioannides. In *Proceedings of the 2nd International Conference on Interdisciplinarity in Education ICIE 2006* (pp. 113-117). National Technical University of Athens, Athens, Greece.

Siirak, V. (2007). Experiencing the Computer Based Learning in Occupational Health and Safety Education for Future Engineers. In *Proceedings of 3rd International Conference on Interdisciplinarity in Education ICIE`07 as International Forum for Multi-Culturality, Multi-Ethnicity and Multi-Disciplinarity in European Higher Education and Research MULTIFORUM`07* (pp.276-279). National Technical University of Athens, Athens, Greece.

Siirak, V. (2007). Experiencing Education in Engineering, Computer Technology and Applied Science for Crossing International, Cultural and Social Borders. In *Proceedings of 3rd International Conference on Interdisciplinarity in Education ICIE`07 as International Forum for Multi-Culturality, Multi-Ethnicity and Multi-Disciplinarity in European Higher Education and Research MULTIFORUM`07* (pp. 114-119). Athens, Greece.

Siirak, V. (2008). Moodle e-learning environment – an effective tool for a development of a learning culture. In *Proceedings of International Symposium Hazards XX: Process Safety and Environmental Protection- Harnessing Knowledge _ Challenging Complacency* (pp.290-296). Manchester, UK.

Siirak, V., & Kristjuhan, U. (2000). Changing Paradigms for Ergonomics and Safety Educational Technology in Estonia. In *Proceedings of the Second International Conference ERGON-AXIA 2000 - Ergonomics and Safety for Global Business Quality and Productivity* (pp. 293-296). Warsaw, Poland.

Staley, A. (2005). Students`Perspectives of Moodle, Digital Future. *The Newsletter of the Learning Technology Development Unit, 2*, 2–3.

Stubbs, M., & Martin, I. (2003). Blended Learning One Small Step. *Learning and Teaching in Action, 2*(3).

Chapter 24

The Convergence Model Implements Accessible Information:
Creating Effective ICT Tools for Our Forgotten Ones

Elspeth McKay

RMIT University,School of Business Information Technology and Logistics, Australia

ABSTRACT

In defining 'effective HCI' one may turn to the literature. While there can be no doubt that the 'techno-vista' has changed dramatically in the past decade; there are many new entries in the literature, which still elevate the mechanistic orientation of information communications technology (ICT), placing the social connectedness of human beings in a dependent context. Professor Bradley's voice however shines through revealing her polite yet determined mindset that places human beings in the technological driving seat. This chapter presents a reprinted paper (McKay, 2007b) to acknowledge Professor Bradley's dedicated encouragement for research into the interactive effects of ICT tools and computer literacy on the 'multifaceted' nature of human beings. As Professor Bradley explains that to test her 'Convergence Model', ".... we must develop new concepts to reflect the changes that are occurring, and grasp the latest new phenomena in depth" (Bradley, 2006, p.57). Effective HCI means having a trusted, interactive and communicative computing environment that lets users decide whether to trust it for a particular purpose, or not; furthermore, effective educational HCI is about knowing how to develop a learning design that provides access to an education information system that is easy to use, offering a safe environment for knowledge and cognitive skill development that supports the joy for life-long learning." (McKay, 2007a, p.xii) The following reprinted McKay paper presents two such research projects that tap right into some of the issues that are faced by people through their basic right for unencumbered access to information, as described by Professor Bradley as "psychosocial life environment/quality of life and well being" (Bradley, 2006, p.61). In these funded research projects, McKay highlights the need to enhance access to Web-mediated information for those people who may need special help. Evidence gained through these projects suggests that unless we have input from the corporate sector, little progress will be forthcoming. Sadly however, this is not a new observation; the corporate sector has been on notice for

DOI: 10.4018/978-1-60960-057-0.ch024

several decades: "Family policy was also a part of constructive work environment actions when data processing systems were introduced" (Bradley, 2006, p.199). These two McKay research studies serve to reinforce Professor Bradley's 'Convergence Model' as an effective HCI knowledge developing tool. It is however, incumbent upon the corporate sector to link the interrelating worlds of: globalisation, ICT, life environment, life role and their effects on humans.

PLANNING EFFECTIVE HCI TO ENHANCE ACESS TO EDUCATIONAL APPLICATIONS

Information and communications technologies (ICT) are widely believed to offer new options for Web-mediated courseware design. Multimedia and online courseware development accentuates a belief that highly graphical (or visual) delivery media will meet the individualised instructional requirements of diverse student cohorts. While most electronic courseware may allow the user to proceed at their own pace, two assumptions are commonly made by courseware designers. Firstly, to facilitate learning, all users are assumed capable of assimilating the graphical content with their current experiential knowledge. There is little or no consideration of different cognitive styles. Understanding learner attributes is essential to increasing accessibility to computerized information. Secondly, learning is assumed rather than demonstrated. To deal with this issue, data analysis techniques can be used to differentiate between what an individual knows from what they do not. This chapter presents two research projects that demonstrate the importance of awareness for the human-dimension of human-computer interaction (HCI) in designing effective online experiential learning for special education.

INTRODUCTION

Effective learning is often expressed in measures of knowing. These pieces of knowledge can represent explicit activities required to become an expert in something (Bransford, Nitsch & Franks, 1997). Rarely is the achievement expressed in qualitative terms. Quality may vary according to how a learner feels about a particular learning event (Sonnier, 1989). At best, the results may take a broad view of cognitive performance that cannot be applied to individual learners experiencing learning difficulties. There are suggestions for learning orientation that involve dealing with emotions and intentions, along with cognitive and social factors (Martinez, 2000). Herein lies the first dilemma facing the design of effective learning environments, namely how to create appropriate educational environments for those people who require accessibility assistance.

The notion of effective learning design assumes equal access to instructional strategies. However, the ubiquitous nature of many online learning environments means that people who require enhanced instructional delivery modes cannot become involved. For instance, when decisions are made concerning appropriate training/education/reskilling needs for people after some type of traumatized event, it is important to differentiate what an individual knows, from what they do not. However, for this particularly sensitive group of learners there are currently no means of providing a skills/competency measurement tool that is efficient, reliable, and safe to administer.

This chapter outlines two projects designed to manage this issue. The first of the two projects sought to enhance the evaluation of young peoples' potential to participate in appropriate educational programs following a mental health episode. As both the young people and their support workers require a specialized tool to determine possibilities for educational/academic performance, it was vital to adopt a customized approach for this type of cognitive skills' evaluation. The expected outcomes of this 1-year Telematics Trust funded research project were to provide a useful tool for young people and their Case Managers, called carers, to gauge correctly academic competency in order to offer appropriate skills building programs in the short term, and to enable planning for longer term personal goals. Therefore, it was crucial to determine individual capabilities in terms of intellectual skills, cognitive strategies, verbal information, motor skills, and attitudes (Gagne, 1985).

The second of the two projects sought to enhance the Web-based resources for finding work for disabled people who have never been employed, or for people suffering negative effects of long-term unemployment (van Dongen, 1996). The research team received a small university grant to conduct a 1-year study. The short-term goal of this project was to develop a system that can deliver enough functionality to demonstrate the benefits of customizing a work-searching system to access relevant knowledge building skills in a vocational rehabilitation setting. On the other hand, a middle-term goal was to secure sufficient interest and funding from a community service provider or industry sector to attract more funding to build the complete system for the longer-term goal of providing a fully interactive specialist Web-portal, linking these job seekers with considerate employers.

It is understandable that this group of individuals may suffer lowered self esteem and lack of motivation to try new things. It was anticipated that this project would capture the efficiencies of HCI to enhance job searching outcomes for people undergoing vocational rehabilitation programs. In Australia, there are some Web-based employment services that claim to provide open, flexible and distributed access for people who may experience difficulty in returning to work after a long absence http://www.maxnetwork.com.au/. Therefore, an

immediate challenge for the research team was to provide evidence of the effectiveness of a more specialized Web-mediated work searching system. The first difficulty presented to the design team was to identify the people who will benefit most from such a system. The environmental context of this research project remains unique. Low self-esteem is common amongst the unemployed (Woolston, 2002). Consequently, the system takes on an educative role in order to enhance the self-confidence of people (all age groups) who may have been out of work for many years, or may have never experienced paid employment.

The longer term goal of these research projects is to inform government policy and practice for young Australians with special needs, and reduce the burden for tax payer funded vocational training and rehabilitation programs.

INSTRUCTIONAL DESIGN APPROACH

In any instructional event it is important to identify the learning domain (the instructional content), and to specify the learning tasks for developing the necessary skills and knowledge to achieve the performance outcomes (the instructional goals). To this end, the term cognitive skill acquisition is used to refer to the set of cognitive skills associated with declarative (knowing what) and procedural knowledge (knowing how) (McKay & Merrill, 2003). This type of cognitive skill acquisition can be analysed in four discrete categories (Gagne, 1985):

1. *verbal information* (knowing basic terms).
2. *intellectual skill development* (basic rules, discriminating and understanding concepts and principles).
3. *intellectual skill* (higher-order-rules, problem solving, the ability to apply concepts and principles in new situations).

Figure 1. Cognitive style construct

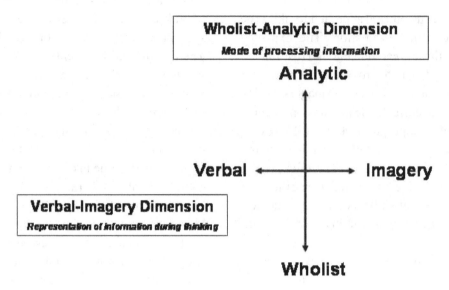

4. two different types of *cognitive strategies* (a) to identify sub-tasks, recognize unstated assumptions, and (b) to recall simple prerequisite rules and concepts, integrating learning from different areas into a plan for solving a problem.

In Project-1, these categories of skill were embedded within the learning content. However, this type of framework was unsuitable for Project-2. Instead, the learning domain concentrated on the intellectual skills associated with problem solving (e.g., deciding which form of public transport to catch to work).

The literature reveals research which distinguishes human ability to process information, as a combination of mode of processing information, and the way people represent information during thinking (see Figure 1) (Riding & Mathais, 1991). Moreover, there are two fundamental cognitive dimensions, Wholist-Analytic and Verbal-Imagery, that affect performance in two ways. The first relates to how information is perceived and interpreted, while the second relates to how already memorised related information is conceptualises (Riding, 1993). Cognitive style is understood to

be an individual's preferred and habitual approach to organizing and representing information. Measurement of an individual's relative right/left hemisphere performance and cognitive style dominance has been a target of researchers from several disciplines over the last decade (Riding & Rayner, 1998). Different theorists make their own distinctions about cognitive differences (Riding & Cheema, 1991). According to Riding and Cheema, for example, the Wholist-Analytic continuum maps to the cognitive categories used by other researchers (see Table 1).

These well known terms are used frequently throughout the literature in a number of different research disciplines.

The Wholist-Analytic dimension defines that Wholist learners are able to understand a concept as a whole, but may find difficulty in disembedding its separate components (McKay, 1999). On the other hand, Analytic learners analyse material into parts, but find difficulty in understanding the whole concept.

The Verbal-Imagery continuum measures whether an individual is inclined to represent information verbally or in mental pictures during thinking (Riding & Rayner, 1998). Verbalisers

Table 1. Researchers' Terms for Processing Information – Mapped to Riding's WA continuum

Terms describing cognitive differences	Researchers
Levellers-sharpeners	Holzman & Klein, 1954
Field dependence-field independence	Witkin, et al, 1962)
Impulsive-reflective	Kagan, 1965
Divergers-convergers	Guilford, 1967
Holists-serialists	Pask & Scott, 1972
Wholist-analytic	Riding & Cheema, 1991

prefer and perform best on verbal tasks, while Imagers are superior on concrete, descriptive and imaginal ones. When there is a mismatch between cognitive style and instructional material or mode of presentation, performance is deemed to be reduced (Riding & Caine, 1993).

Both Projects illustrated this variation in cognitive style, with participants demonstrating preference for verbal or visual representation. For this reason, it is critical to create an instructional environment which caters for the full range of cognitive style preference with delivery options for users to choose from. The Meta-Knowledge Processing Model is proposed here as an effective and robust learning systems' design tool (Figure

Figure 2. Meta-knowledge processing model

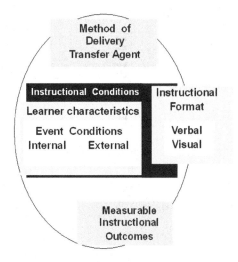

2). This Model provides an adaptive cognitive dimension design-framework, which reflects the user's preference for thinking mode (verbal/imagery), while also providing both wholist/analytic instructional strategies to capture the user's inherent information processing mode.

Every component was described fully to provide detailed system specifications. This was especially important with the production of the visual resources. Each picture was logged with the associated interactions/audio and access location. It was important to keep track of the interrelating resources to ensure a seamless approach that would reduce stress. Contemporary approaches to instructional design often lack an ability to recognise and accommodate the dynamics of cognitive processes necessary for online learning (see Figure 2). This systems' design modelling tool identifies interactive relationships between cognitive style and instructional format, and the need to adapt the instructional format dynamically. It requires a concurrent acquisition of meta-knowledge relating to the learner's cognitive performance with a knowledge-level-analysis of task difficulty (McKay, 2000a).

The instructional environment was described in detail using the Meta-Knowledge Processing Model to define each facet of the system. Consequently, the method of delivery chosen to achieve the measurable instructional outcomes (readiness for study or skills development) utilized touch screen technology. In keeping with the design brief to ensure that the systems were fun to use, the navigation was kept simple. Users were only required to press the screen to navigate forward, backward and exit. The instructional conditions (the learning content) underwent a comprehensive development with subject matter experts and case managers to identify the basic knowledge management issues that surround everyday life-skills. The following were obtained: identification skills (e.g., touching part of a photo that shows a best before date), food preparation (like picking out where the packet of rice was grown), safety (like

Figure 3. Prototype-1 sub-level menu

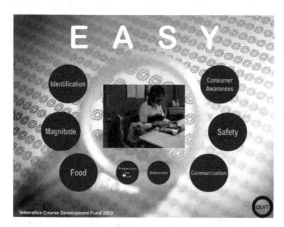

choosing which extinguisher to use for an oil fire in a kitchen), communication (watching the video that involved a young person being interviewed for a job), magnitude (picking the flower that is closest) and consumer awareness (deciding which advertisement was suitable for outdoors work).

The presentation mode or instructional format was pictorial with associated text captions to assist comprehension, and ask questions. Video vignettes with audio explanations were available for demonstrating examples, maintaining the Merrill (2003) 5-star principles of instruction (Problem recognition, Activation, Demonstration, Applica-

tion and Integration). All these principles were designed into the prototypes, including: showing real world problems associated with looking for work, encouraging memory recall by activating some examples of prior experience and integrating new material into everyday life). The vignettes provided examples of everyday activities related to: health and safety, organizing study papers, and preparing for an interview (Figures 3 and 4).

PROTOTYPES

Project-1: EASY

In the first project, the participants were young people who were deemed to have learning difficulties in basic literacy skills (written and oral comprehension and expression), numeracy skills, problem solving and organization, memory and concentration levels. This prototype was built to include a range of tasks that would involve the participants in identifying instances of key elements from safety symbols, diagrams, pictures, tables, or written passages. In addition, the prototype would pose questions relating to magnitudes such as length, width, distance and temperature,

Figure 4. Prototype-2 login screen

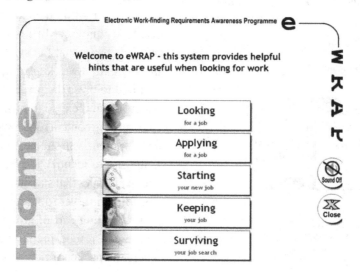

aspects of food purchasing, safe storage of food, interpreting recipes, and calculating purchase prices. The design brief was to make access to the computerised information simple and fun to use. Consequently, the Home Page displayed only the acronym EASY which represents the full name Educational/Academic Skills Evaluation. The six-option menu consisted of 6 large buttons (Identification, Magnitude, Food, Consumer Awareness, Safety and Communication). Pressing these buttons took the participant through the series of cognitive assessment tasks. Pressing the Communication button displayed 2 smaller sub-level buttons; these smaller buttons activated the video vignettes (Figure 3). These videos were produced using young people preparing for an interview, and a day at work.

Project-2: eWRAP

The target learners in the second project were youths and adults who were suffering the negative effects of long-term unemployment. As such this second project takes on an educative role, utilizing ICT to enhance the self-confidence of people (all age groups) who may have been out of work for many years, or may have never experienced paid employment. It was very important therefore to design a tailored learning experience that caters for the special needs of this target audience (people requiring enhanced accessibility to information).

It was important for this project to make access to the information easy. Once again this system utilized touch screen technology with both keyboard and mouse removed during the experiment. Therefore, the method of delivery implemented a Home Page to welcome the user through an audio greeting that is toggled to a textual description as an alternative (Figure 4). The learning content (instructional conditions) consisted of five key job seeking options (Looking, Applying, Starting, Keeping, and Surviving). The navigation was kept simple. Once again Video vignettes offered typical examples of everyday activities that in-

cluded young people in role play performances to depict: health and safety issues, preparing for an interview, typical job environments, and benefits of socializing at work.

EVALUATION

The primary aim of this research was to find ways to enhance the interactive effective of instructional strategies and cognitive style for young people wishing to return to study or work, following a mental health episode. The objective was to develop interactive ICT tools that are safe, accurate and easy to use. At the core of this work is the ability to provide adaptive technology that can differentiate users' expectations. In particular cognitive preferences, motivation levels towards the task at hand.

Participants

The 25 participants were attending a special education unit or community-based centre offering vocational programs. They aged between 15-25 years and represented a range of scholastic experiential awareness. The sample was grouped according to Project. The Project cohort varied in their catchment areas from suburban to poor urban. There were more school aged participants attending the special education unit than the community-centre, while the number of participants with a working background was low compared with the number of those attending the community-centre. In each Project, all the participants were given the opportunity to decide whether to participate or not. Many of them of them had no previous computer related experience.

Materials

Both Projects involved a computerized prototype system, preloaded onto one standalone IBM compatible computer. Each prototype employed a touch screen to reduce the likelihood of reluctance to access a computer (McKay & Izard, 2004). The participants were not expected to access the prototype using a mouse or keyboard; the processing unit was placed away from the screen. Due to the need to respect the privacy of the participants, the prototypes were not designed to capture and store any data. The cognitive performance data-capture instruments were hard-copy. A performance coding sheet was used to collect the data for Project-1, while a simple feedback sheet was used for Project-2.

PROCEDURE

The research team conducted a thorough task analysis of the knowledge acquisition environment relating to young people wishing to return to study or participate in community-based vocational rehabilitation programs.

For Project-1, the experiment tested the participants to determine the level of remedial intervention required for vocational re-training/rehabilitation. The Australian benchmark, Curriculum and Standards Framework (2000), (CFS), was used to devise the learning outcomes as key English literacy learning areas/strands (speaking and listing, reading and writing). The CFS is structured in key learning areas, strands and levels, describing what students should know and be able to do in eight key areas of learning at regular intervals. Each strand was divided into sub-strands (texts, contextual understanding, linguistics, and strategies). A cognitive performance matrix was developed by the lead researcher to fill the gaps found in existing systems, which currently adopt the CFS framework (CFS, 2000). This matrix identified educational and academic tasks in terms of basic to complex (see the left-hand, vertical rows in Table 2), and measurable cognitive performance outcomes in terms of declarative (knowing that – verbal information) to procedural knowledge (or knowing how – a cognitive strat-

egy) (Izard & McKay, 2004). These categories are shown on the horizontal rows in Table 2. This framework formed the basis of the educational/academic skill's performance testing instrument, along with a series of visual (pictorial) and text-based information sequences to depict everyday life experiences, including: identifying factual detail, examples of magnitude, food preparation, consumer awareness, safety and communication. In order to evaluate the cognitive performance of each participant, the QUEST Interactive Test Analysis System was used. The QUEST software application was written by Raymon J. Adams & Siek-Toon Khoo, and published by The Australian Council for Educational Research Limited in 1993 (Adams & Khoo, 1996). Central to QUEST is a measurement model developed in 1960 by the Danish statistician George Rasch. QUEST develops a uni dimensional scale with equal intervals along each axis, to measure individuals' performance and test items together (Adams & Khoo, 1996). The resultant cognitive performance measurement instrument was calibrated to ensure validity (Izard, 1999).

However, for the job search prototype (Project-2), the performance matrix had limited value. Instead, a series of meetings were held with subject matter experts to develop a typical user profile (McKay, Thomas & Martin, 2004). A number of characteristics were identified by the involved experts, including: confidence and self esteem, revaluating personal goals, experienced some break from employment, education and training (can be several years), last experience of employment education or training may have ended negatively. Consequently, a list of key work-seeking skills were identified: finding appropriate work (indoors/outdoors), preparing an application, dealing with rejection, planning for the first day (travel/food/clothing), how to stay employed, and what to do when the work ended. Visual (pictorial) metaphors were devised to facilitate the learning content to include: self-confidence, motivation, managing food, travel, per-

Table 2. Cognitive Performance Capability Matrix

Instructional Objectives: Measuring Academic Performance: Concentration and Attitude						
	Declarative Knowledge		Procedural Knowledge			
	Band-A	**Band-B**	**Band-C**	**Band-D**	**Band-E**	
Automated Educational/ Academic Skills Evaluation for Young People: (EASY) system Proof-of-Concept	Verbal information skill	Intellectual skill	Intellectual skill	Cognitive strategy		
	Concrete concept	Basic rule	Higher-order-rule	Identify sub-tasks	Knowing the "how"	
	Knows basic terms	Discriminates	Problem solving		Recall simple pre-requisite rules & concepts	
	Knows "that"	Understands concepts & principles	Applies concepts & principles to new situations	Recognizes un-stated assumptions	Integrates learning from different areas into plan for solving a problem	
Learning Domain Task Code = R	Texts	Aspects of Language				Totals
		Contextual understanding	Linguistics		Strategies	
Reading (constructing meaning from print & non-print)	Literature (books, etc)	Everyday texts (telephone conversations, notices)	Media texts (newspapers, Internet, TV, Video, CD-ROM)		Workplace texts (letters, resumes, reports, etc)	

sonal budgeting and managing social welfare benefits. Textual representation was kept to a minimum; instead, voice clips were available to provide appropriate information. Not enough is known yet about how people respond to hypertext in a Web-based instructional environment. Research is needed to establish a taxonomy of tasks to analyse and compare usability issues (Chen & Rada, 1996). Video vignettes were used to depict examples of real world instances of deciding on which type of public transport to catch, preparing food and clothes, and a sample job interview (both examples and non-examples). It is sound instructional design practice to contrast the good example (of a concept of thing) and show the non-example to increase the effectiveness of the demonstration (Merrill, 2003).

The data gathering process was different for each Project. The data gathered for Project-1 occurred during a pre-arranged consultation session. This session was facilitated by the participant's regular teacher. The participant's performance was recorded by the teacher on the performance coding sheet during the session. Project-2 captured participants' answers on the feedback sheet that they were asked to complete at the end of their session. In addition, in Project-2, a research team-member sat in the room while the participant used the prototype, to answer any questions from the participant.

RESULTS

Analysis of the test item data for Project-1 used the QUEST interactive test software (Adams & Khoo, 1996) in order to avoid measurement errors in the testing instruments. The QUEST estimate allows for improved analysis of an individual's performance relative to other participants (Izard, 1995), and relative to the test-item difficulty (McKay, 2000b). This analysis was able to calibrate the responses to the cognitive performance measurement instrument, providing a basis for assessing the participants' progress towards returning to study or vocational training. The analysis of the data showed a clear differentiation of test-item difficulty and user skill levels (Izard & McKay, 2004). The QUEST tool, combined with the teacher's observations, was also able to identify that some participants performed well with visual tasks (select the closest flower, pick the largest building block, etc), where they had difficulty with text/numeric test-items (find an ingredient from a recipe, calculate the cost of several grocery items, etc). Conversely, those participants able to quickly calculate purchases, often pondered over visual perception tasks. In summary, an analysis of the test item data reveals there were 56 right/wrong and partial credit test items (with a maximum possible score of 64), suitable for the evaluation of educational and academic skills of young adults, were able to be calibrated to form the basis of assessing progress made towards returning to study or vocational training (Izard & McKay, 2004).

Testing of the systems for Project-2 was executed over a four month period during 2003. Preliminary qualitative feedback, including that of several non-computer users, was very positive. The users found the system easy to use, informative; they could relate to the characters in the various video vignettes. An example of the comments from the participants included: *"the person applying for the computer position reminded me of people I know, it made me think that behaving like that is not good"* and *"I can see that wearing suitable clothing is important for an interview"*. As with Project-1, there was differentiation between participants' usage of the system. Some participants preferred listening to the verbal descriptions of menu items, whereas others turned the voice toggled option off, and read the textual descriptions. Many of the participants enjoyed the videos and comic metaphors. However, a few preferred just to read through lists and descriptions.

ACCESS TO INFORMATION

There can be no doubt that interest in learning has shifted from an insular approach to school-based education to participation in a global knowledge sharing environment. As a result, a turning point has been reached in the design and development of multimodal courseware. For instance, within the context of online asynchronous learning platforms, there is a noticeable shift from traditional teaching methods, which provide for a sole learning-content provider (class-room teacher) (Axmann, 2002), towards a multiple mentor-guiding approach (multiple facilitators on duty to answer questions) (Axmann, 2004). However, in adopting this newer approach, it is assumed that the knowledge management process during the learning event will appeal to all learners Axmann et al, (2006). Sadly, this type of online instructional strategy reflects a lack of understanding of the effects of computerized learning on the population at large, rather than reaching the individuals who may require increased assistance with access to information.

The design process of a computer-human interface is complex, and instructional designers need to ensure that careful attention is paid to sound and well-founded instructional design principles Preece et al, (1994). In general terms, online courseware designers need to be aware of a meta-knowledge acquisition process, relevant adaptive instructional strategies, the need to articulate the conditions-of-the-learner, which relate to information processing preferences and learning content environmental factors (McKay, 2000a), and to demonstrate that the desired learning has occurred. This combination of design processes formulate a comprehensive HCI model to direct the online learning experience that best achieves a high quality instructional outcome McKay (2000b). The advent of ICTs has perhaps introduced a false sense of making life easier for the educational systems designers. While multi-sensory instruction is known to improve a student's capacity to learn effectively (as judged from appropriate

Table 3. Human Factors in HCI (adapted from Preece et al, (1994, p.31)

ORGANISATIONAL FACTORS training, job design, politics, roles, work organisation		ENVIRONMENTAL FACTORS noise, heating, lighting, ventilation
HEALTH 7 SAFETY FACTORS stress, headaches, muscular-skeletal disorders	cognitive processes & capabilities THE USER motivation, enjoyment, satisfaction personality, experience-level	COMFORT FACTORS Seating, equipment layout
USER INTERFACE input devices, output displays, dialogue structures, use of colour, icons, commands, Graphics, natural language, 3-D, user support materials, multi-media		
TASK INTERFACE easy, complex, novel, task allocation, repetitive, monitoring, skills, components		
CONSTRAINTS costs, timescales, budgets, staff, equipment, building structure		
SYSTEM FUNCTIONALITY hardware, software, application		
PRODUCTIVITY FACTORS increase output, increase quality, decrease costs, decrease errors		

evidence), the overarching role of knowledge-mediated HCI has been poorly understood in the design of instructional strategies that integrate contextual components in asynchronous learning frameworks. The limitations of contemporary approaches to instructional design appear to lie in the failure to recognise and accommodate learning process dynamics, specifically the interactive effects between cognitive style and instructional format and the need to adapt the instructional format dynamically. It may be concluded that the mechanism to achieve such dynamics lies in the concurrent acquisition of knowledge about the learner's cognitive performance within a contextual framework defined by a knowledge level analysis of task difficulty.

Customising learning environments draws together the inter-disciplinary nature of HCI. Aspects of instructional science, cognitive psychology and educational research are combined to articulate these meta-knowledge requirements. Consider the interactive relationships that occur between the environmental factors of an online work-space that, for example, includes general noise that surrounds the work-space, and health and safety factors that may directly induce stress

through unwise choice of colour in the user interface design (Table 3, adapted from (Preece et al, (1994).

There are few instances of online courseware design where these relationships are maximised. For instance, in a recent study of adult learners in Mexico (Santos, 2004), where special circumstances relating to access to educational technology were identified, the courseware designers neglected to address many of the HCI components listed in Table 3. In that nationwide qualitative diagnostic study, which involved community based adult education centres, the researchers were hoping to provide online educational facilities for disadvantaged adults without a basic education. It was known beforehand that these adult learners may also suffer from socio-economic marginalization, and may not have access to educational content relating to work-based training using printed, audiovisual and electronic media. Surprisingly, the study was not planned with an emphasis on any of these necessary HCI inter-relationships. Consequently, constructive learning or practical application was not achieved.

HCI relationships are magnified in the special education environment that has been described earlier in this paper. They involve people who require enhanced accessibility to information that is to be found on the Internet. Special education is now further defined here in a broader sense, as pedagogical practice especially designed as assistive technology for people with learning disabilities (Atkinson & Walmsley, 2003), which include the residual effects of recovering from an episode of mental illness (McKay, Thomas & Martin, 2004). While a special education literature on computerized learning programs has emerged in the last decade, mapping this type of HCI in terms of utilizing new knowledge in new situations has not been achieved. However, at this point, computerised learning systems that would monitor how teenagers and young adults engage in knowledge development, would implement HCI in a manner akin to a revolution in conceptual change (Thargard, 1992). Currently there are no assessment instruments that adapt according to the interactive effects of cognitive style and instructional format.

CONCLUSION

The two projects outlined in this paper have provided valuable experiential knowledge of the educational systems' design process. The EASY Project evaluated the effectiveness of an innovative testing tool, which enables differentiated teaching, provides adaptive cognitive skills measurement, correctly identifies different levels of competency, promotes self-confidence and enhances motivation towards learning abilities. The eWRAP Project evaluated an online job seeking prototype designed to assist the long-term unemployed.

To offer new options for Web-based courseware designers, this paper has presented examples of practical ICT applications that promote the principles of sound instructional design implemented through HCI. The essence of this work reflects the importance of the interacting relationships

amongst the various HCI components as identified by Preece et al (1994). While it is suspected that these variables form dependent relationships online; it is still early days. More research is needed to understand how these interacting variables behave within a Web-mediated context. Progress may be slow, as it does take time to disseminate researchers' findings through to the community to solve real world problems.

ACKNOWLEDGMENT

The reprint of the journal article: 'Planning Effective HCI to Enhance Accessibility,' is with kind permission of Springer Science and Business Media. Telematics Fund Trust (Project-1), RMIT Foundation/Macromedia Inc. (Professor David Merrill's visiting Fellowship - 2003), RMIT VRI Small Grants Scheme (Project-2). 3M Touch Systems Pty Ltd kindly provided the touch technology as in kind support for the project.

REFERENCES

Adams, R. J., & Khoo, S.-T. (1996). *QUEST: The interactive test analysis system (Vol. 1)*. Melbourne: Australian Council for Educational Research.

Atkinson, D., & Walmsley, J. (2003). Time to make up your mind: Why choosing is difficult. *British Journal of Learning Disabilities, 31*(1), 3–8. doi:10.1046/j.1468-3156.2003.00181.x

Axmann, M. (2002). An online mentorship programme for the online educator: Patterning for success. In *Proceedings of the Australian Society for Educational Technology International and Technology Conference (ASET 2002): Untangling the Web-Establishing Learning Links*. Melbourne, Australia.

Axmann, M. (2004). *Human capital development in an online mentoring system*. MA Thesis, University of Pretoria.

Axmann, M., McKay, E., Banjanin, N., & Howat, A. (2006). Towards web-mediated learning reinforcement: Promoting effective human-computer interaction. In *Proceedings of Web-Based Education (WBE 2007), International Association of Science and Technology for Development (IASTED)* (pp.210-215), Chamonix, France.

Bradley, G. (2006). *Social and Community Informatics: Humans on the net*. London: Routledge.

Bransford, J. D., Nitsch, K., & Franks, J. J. (1977). Schooling and the facilitation of knowing . In Anderson, R. C., Spiro, R., & Montague, W. (Eds.), *Schooling and the acquisition of knowledge*. New Jersey: Erlbaum.

Chen, C., & Rada, R. (1996). Interacting with hypertext: A meta-analysis of experimental studies. *Human-Computer Interaction*, *11*(2), 125–156. doi:10.1207/s15327051hci1102_2

English curriculum and standards framework II. (2000). 375.0009945.

Gagne, R. M. (1985). *The conditions of learning: And the theory of instruction* (4th ed.). New York: Holt/Rinehart/Winston.

Guilford, J. (1967). *The nature of human intelligence*. New York: McGraw-Hill.

Holzman, P., & Klein, G. (1954). Cognitive-system principles of levelling and sharpening: Individual differences in visual time-error assimilation effects. *The Journal of Psychology*, *37*, 105–122.

Izard, J. (1995). *Trial testing and item analysis*. Victoria, Australia: International Institute of Educational Planning.

Izard, J. (1999). *Some potential difficulties in educational research studies (and how to avoid them)*. Philippines: The Third Elementary Education Project.

Izard, J., & McKay, E. (2004). Automated educational/academic skills screening: Using technology to avoid or minimise effects of more formal assessment. In P.L. Jeffrey (Ed.), *Proceedings of the Australian Association for Research Education (AARE 2004): Positioning education research*. Melbourne. Retrieved from http://www.aare.edu.au/04pap/iza04951.pdf

Kagan, J. (1965). Individual differences in the resolution of response uncertainty. *Journal of Personality and Social Psychology*, *2*(2), 154–160. doi:10.1037/h0022199

Martinez, M. (2000). Foundations for personalized web learning environments. *ALN Magazine - A publication of the Sloan Consortium, 4*(2).

McKay, E. (1999). An investigation of text-based instructional materials enhanced with graphics. *Educational Psychology*, *19*(3), 323–335. doi:10.1080/0144341990190306

McKay, E. (2000a). *Instructional strategies integrating the cognitive style construct: A meta-knowledge processing model (contextual components that facilitate spatial/logical task performance)*. Unpublished PhD Thesis, Deakin Univ., Australia. Retrieved from http://tux.lib.deakin.edu.au/adt-VDU/public/adt-VDU20061011.122556/.

McKay, E. (2000b). Measurement of cognitive performance in computer programming concept acquisition: Interactive effects of visual metaphors and the cognitive style construct. *Journal of Applied Measurement, 1*(3), 257–286.

McKay, E. (Ed.). (2007a). *Enhancing learning through human-computer interaction*. Hershey, PA: Idea Group Reference.

325

McKay, E. (2007b). Planning effective HCI to enhance accessibility. *Universal Access in the Information Society*, *6*, 77–85. doi:10.1007/s10209-007-0070-3

McKay, E., & Izard, J. (2004). Automated educational skills evaluation: A systems design case study. In E. McKay (Ed.), *Proceedings of the International Conference on Computers in Education - Acquiring and Constructing Knowledge through Human-Computer Interaction: Creating new visions for the future of learning*. Melbourne Exhibition Centre, Australia: Common Ground Publishing, *1*(3), 1051-1061.

McKay, E., & Merrill, M. D. (2003). Cognitive skill and web-based educational systems. In E. McKay (Ed.), *Proceedings of the eLearning Conference on Design and Development: Instructional Design - Applying first principles of instruction*, (pp.96-108). Melbourne: Informit Library: Australasian Publications. Retrieved from http://www.informit.com.au/

McKay, E., Thomas, T., & Martin, J. (2004). Work search prototype design: Human-computer interaction for vocational rehabilitation. In V. Uskov (Ed.), Paper presented at the *International Association of Science and Technology for Development - Computers and Advanced Technology in Education (CATE 2004)* (pp.167-172). Anaheim: ACTA Press.

Merrill, M. D. (2003). Keynote address: Does your instruction rate 5 stars? In E. McKay, (Ed.), *Proceedings of the eLearning Conference on Design and Development: Instructional Design - Applying first principles of instruction*, (pp.13-14). Melbourne: Informit Library: Australasian Publications. Retrieved from http://www.informit.com.au/

Pask, G., & Scott, B. C. E. (1972). Learning strategies and individual competence. *International Journal of Man-Machine Studies*, *4*, 217–253. doi:10.1016/S0020-7373(72)80004-X

Preece, J., Rogers, Y., Sharp, H., Benyon, D., Holland, S., & Carey, T. (1994). *Human-computer interaction*. Harlow, UK: Addison-Wesley.

Riding, R. (1993). *A trainer's guide to learning design: Learning methods project report, Assessment Research Unit*. Birmingham, UK: University of Birmingham.

Riding, R., & Cheema, I. (1991). Cognitive styles - an overview and integration. *Educational Psychology*, *11*(3&4), 193–215. doi:10.1080/0144341910110301

Riding, R. J., & Caine, R. (1993). Cognitive style and GCSE performance in mathematics, English language and French. *Educational Psychology*, *13*(1), 59–67. doi:10.1080/0144341930130107

Riding, R. J., & Mathais, D. (1991). Cognitive styles and preferred learning mode, reading attainment and cognitive ability in 11-year-old children. *Educational Psychology*, *11*(3 & 4), 383–393. doi:10.1080/0144341910110312

Riding, R. J., & Rayner, S. (1998). *Cognitive styles and learning strategies*. UK: Fulton.

Santos, A. (2004). Do community technology centers decrease social inequities? Results of a nationwide qualitative study to evaluate the plazas communitarieas project in Mexico. In E. McKay, (Ed.), *Proceedings of the International Conference on Computers in Education - Acquiring and Constructing Knowledge Through Human-Computer Interaction: Creating new visions for the future of learning* (pp.1133-1144.), Melbourne Exhibition Centre, Australia: Common Ground Publishing.

Sonnier, I. L. (1989). *Affective education: Methods and techniques*. New Jersey: Educational Technology Publications.

Thargard, P. (1992). *Conceptual revolutions*. New Jersey: Princeton University Press.

van Dongen, C. (1996). Quality of life and self-esteem in working and non-working persons with mental illness. Community . *Mental Health, 32*(6), 535–549.

Witkin, H. A., Dyke, R. B., Patterson, H. F., Goodman, D. R., & Kemp, D. R. (1962). *Psychological differentiation*. New York: Wiley.

Woolston, C. (2002). *Why unemployment is bad for your health*. Principle Health News.

Section 6
The Information and Communication Society

Chapter 25
Information Integrity in the Information Age

Simon Rogerson
De Montfort University, UK

ABSTRACT

The converging technologies have changed the way we should look at information. Illustrations are used to discuss how we create, communicate and consume information in many different forms. The relationship between information and technology can be both beneficial and problematical. A set of fresh issues has been raised which needs to be fully explored and addressed if we are going to realise the full potential of the information society. The nature of information, the concept of information integrity and the use of information provenance are discussed. It is argued that in the information society there is a moral obligation to address information integrity. Information provenance offers a normative instrument for turning this moral obligation into ethical practice.

INTRODUCTION

Converging technologies have changed the way we should look at information. They have raised a set of fresh issues which need to be fully explored and addressed if we are going to realise the full potential of the Information Age. The growing dependency on information and communication technologies (ICT) to publish, consume and manipulate information has impacted upon economic and cultural life. The Information Age has spawned

a new society – the Information Society. The Information Society crosses traditional boundaries and as such comprises individuals from many different cultures. This cultural variability means that the expectations of individual cybercitizens can differ considerably.

Everyone belongs to one or more cultural communities and so, as Hongladarom and Ess (2007) point out, it is impossible to consider the Information Society from a culturally neutral perspective. For example, Brey (2006) describes a positive view of the internet from a libertarian ideology which is in marked contrast with the

DOI: 10.4018/978-1-60960-057-0.ch025

negative view he describes from the perspective of Orthodox Judaism. This cultural variability has been explored by Nance and Strohmaier (1994). They suggest there are two important dimensions to consider regarding cultural variability. The first dimension is the continuum from individualism to collectivism. Individualism emphasises self-interest and promotes the self-realisation of talent and potential. Its demands are universal. Collectivism emphasises pursuit of common interests and belonging to a set of hierarchical groups where, for example, the family group might be placed above the job group. The demands on group members are different to those on non-group members. The second dimension concerns cultural differences in communication referred to as low context communication and high context communication. In the former the majority of the information resides in the message itself whilst in the latter the communication is implicit. Nance and Strohmaier (1994) suggest that the USA utilises low context communication whilst Japan uses high context. So even with a shift towards cultural homogenisation through ICT usage, the variability that remains makes it very challenging to provide information or conduct a debate in a way that is acceptable to all (Fairweather and Rogerson, 2003). It involves establishing a set of common behavioural standards whilst ensuring that there is no dominant participant. The current internet seems a long distance from this position. Indeed, given such cultural variability it is clear that there are great difficulties in providing information in a form that is acceptable to all. This is certainly one of the great challenges of the Information Age where we all create, communicate and consume information.

THE NATURE OF INFORMATION

But what is information? Eaton and Bawden (1991) suggest that information exhibits five intangible characteristics which differentiate it from other types of resource. The value of information is difficult to quantify and its value is relative in terms of both time and information users. Information has a multiplicative quality in that it is not lost or decreased if it is consumed and indeed using information often causes it to increase in value and size. Information is a dynamic force within the system it resides which causes that system to flex. There is no predictable life cycle of information, indeed once dormant information can become current and valuable in changed circumstances. Finally information manifests itself in different forms relating to particular situations. Meyer (2005) extends this list to include other characteristics. Information has the attribute of alleviating uncertainty. Information is always an essential intrinsic component of technology. Information is a catalyst to enhance economic growth. Information extends the knowledge base. As Macgregor (2005) states, "Ultimately information behaves in a unique manner when compared to other resources because it essentially represents the genesis of human thought, and is heterogeneous and intrinsically intangible."

Technological maturity has reached a point where information of nearly every form is available at the touch of a button, the click of a mouse or the pointing of a cursor. Never before has it been possible to support many-to-many or many-to-one information publication and consumption. Existing new information conduits such as blogs, podcasts and wikis offer so much. Access is now possible to all forms of information including music, moving images, literary works and art. Consider the following example of information conveyed in different forms. This has been used by the author to explore the relationship between ICT and information with students at different levels and in different countries.

On 26 April 1937 the Basque town of Guernica was subjected to the first carpet bombing of a civilian population during the Spanish Civil war. The raid was conducted by the German Luftwaffe "Condor Legion" and the Italian Fascist Aviazione

Legionaria. The attack destroyed the majority of Guernica and there were widespread civilian deaths. The attack is recorded in military books as an example of terror bombing. It is still a source of emotion, revulsion and public recrimination. In 1937 Picasso painted his famous anti-war painting. This 3.5 metres by 8 metres canvas in black and white depicts the horrors of war in a way never seen before.

The events of Guernica are an invaluable information source for the education of future generations. The challenge is how to use it. Can ICT be used to assist in its educational value? Here are some suggestions.

- Picasso's Guernica is accessible in electronic form and therefore can be displayed using PowerPoint and a data projector. Against this backdrop the story of Guernica can be told and the audience given a sense of what it was like to be there by introducing the sound of bombing as the story unfolds.

- There is an evocative song by Katie Melua called *Market Day in Guernica* which tells the story of the day of the bombing. This can be used as a sound track to accompany a set of still photographs of the destruction including pictures of distraught children in the bombed out streets. A period of silent reflection follows for the audience to think about what they have seen.

- There are many accounts of Guernica on the web which can be used as sources to deliver a more factual account of the events. This can be used to explore, in an objective way, the reasons the bombing took place, its impact on the civil war and how it has been used since to promote particular causes.

These three, very different approaches provide information to the audience. Two make use of converging media to capture the attention of the audience and shock them into thinking more deeply. It is information but not in a form that we perhaps recognise. The last version is a traditional way of information dissemination. ICT-based information has a history of text and words and this final approach relies upon this.

This example and its use by the author in a variety of settings illustrate how ICT can be used to create and convey information in a variety of ways. But what does the introduction of ICT do to the meaning of information? Does the reduction of a 3.5 metres by 8 metres canvas into a small projected image in a lecture theatre detract from the painting's impact? Does the adding of sound detract or add to the impact? Is the creation of a slide show with a popular song accompaniment simply an emotional trick or does it have informational value? Will the bullet-pointed objective presentation tease out the real information rather than dwell on the emotional hype and retain the audience's attention?

These questions lead to some general statements about ICT and information. ICT offers new forms of access to information. However, ICT has the potential to add value as well as subtract value to existing informational forms. The consumption of information and the resulting value derived are greatly influenced by individual perception and learning styles. Often the perceptions of the information creator are different from those of the information consumer. It is concerning that these types of issues are rarely considered when "enhancing" information provision through ICT.

It is the power and versatility of ICT which can change the nature of information and how we perceive it. Borgman (1999) suggests there are three types of information. There is information about reality in which reports disclose what is distant in space and remote in time. There is information for reality in which recipes transform reality and make it richer materially and morally. Finally there is information as reality in which recording information through the power of technology steps forward as a rival of reality.

It is the latter which challenges the traditional view of information. Borgman illustrates this third form with classical music. "The technological information on a compact disc is so detailed and controlled that it addresses us virtually as reality. What comes from a recording of a Bach cantata on a CD is neither a report about the cantata nor a recipe (the score) for performing the cantata; it is in the common understanding of music itself."

THE INFORMATION DICHOTOMY

There is an interesting dichotomy in the technologically dependent Information Society. Information is the lifeblood of organisations in the information age (Rogerson and Bynum, 1995). The veins of data communications along which this blood circulates are the new utility of the Information Society. Without communicated information organisations cannot interact with individuals and other organisations along the supply chain. However, with the advent of computer technology and more significantly the convergence of this technology with other technologies such as media, the amount and type and amount of information available has exploded. Tofler (1970) predicted this information overload where individuals and organisations were swamped with so much information that it prevented decision making and actually reduced knowledge. This problem continues to grow at a seemingly accelerating rate. Indeed Nielsen (2003) argues that we are reaching the point of saturation; "Information pollution is information overload taken to the extreme. It is where it stops being a burden and becomes an impediment to your ability to get your work done."

If humankind is going to survive this mutation of information lifeblood into information pollution a new way of thinking and an associated new way of operating has to be derived. As Evans remarks (1979), "Computers, in other words, have not arrived on the scene for aesthetic reasons, but because they are essential to the survival of a complex society, in a way that food, clothing, housing, education and health services are essential to a slightly simpler one. The truth is that one of the main problems - perhaps the main problem - of the time is that our world suffers from information overload, and we can no longer handle it unaided."

INTEGRITY AND PROVENANCE

One aid that could reverse this mutation is explicit guidance as to the status of information as it is presented. In other words, to provide a rating of the integrity of the information before it is consumed. Information integrity is about accuracy, consistency and reliability of information content (Mandke and Madhavan, 2003) and information systems. If information is questionable then decisions and actions which are based upon it could be flawed and unsafe. The expectation that information has integrity and therefore is dependable and trustworthy is reasonable. But how can dependability and trustworthiness be demonstrated? Trustworthiness is an intrinsic reality. Its perception, particularly in the beginning, depends critically on the perception of certain extrinsic forms (signs, labels, messages, etc) that are understood to represent the presence of underlying trustworthiness (McRobb and Rogerson, 2004). It is these extrinsic messages which would provide the much needed guide to information integrity.

If such messages were recorded over time then the information would exhibit a provenance. In general provenance defines the place of origin and is a proof of authenticity or of past ownership. Therefore, information provenance fixes the origin and network of ownership thus providing a measure of integrity, authenticity and trustworthiness. It provides an audit trail showing where information originated, where it has been and how it has been altered. In this way people would be able to consider how much credence they would give to a piece of information before acting upon it. For any piece of information people should be able to answer "Can this information be believed to be true? Who created it? Can its creator be trusted? What does it depend on? Can the information it depends on be believed to be true?" (Huang and Fox, 2004). According to Huang and Fox (2004) information provenance has four levels; Static, Dynamic, Uncertain and Judgement-based. The Static level focuses on provenance of static and certain information. The Dynamic level considers how the validity of information may change over time. The Uncertain level considers information whose validity is inherently uncertain. Finally, the Judgment-based level focuses on social processes necessary to support provenance. This model enables information to be categorised which in turn provides integrity guidance. Moreau et al (2008) suggest that ICT applications must be provenance-aware so the information's provenance can be retrieved, analysed and reasoned over. This seems to be regardless at which of the four levels the information resides. They cite the example of an organ transplant management system which comprises a complex process involving medical decision making, data collection, organ analysis and eventual surgery. If this system was provenance-aware and had embedded in it a provenance life cycle then on demand queries such as: list all doctors involved in a decision; find all blood-test results for a donation decision; or find all data that led to a decision, could be easily satisfied. This would ensure system integrity and increase trustworthiness.

Advances in ICT provide an even stronger argument for information provenance. Groth (2004) explains that advances in computer visualisation have promoted human capabilities to recognise interesting aspects of data. How people undertake this recognition is variable and difficult to express. This results in an inability to define the discovery process and hence calls into question the integrity of the discovery. For this reason Goth argues that an information provenance system is mandatory which tracks the human activity so that the knowledge discovery process using visualisa-

tion can be captured automatically. In a second example, Pinheiro et al (2003) discuss the need for information provenance in the Semantic Web because more answers are derived from automatic information manipulation rather than simple information retrieval. In addition they explain that users of information are both humans and agents and as such common sense cannot be relieved upon to judge information integrity.

Therefore information provenance is a powerful instrument in improving information integrity. Consider this example. In the course of its enquiries a police authority collects information about an individual. This information is held within the police authority's information systems. Such information is allowed to be shared with a number of other authorised agencies across a secure network. Access is instigated by the agencies so no track is kept of where the information has been shared. Once this happens the copies of this information become legally owned by the recipient agencies. Agencies update this information for their own purposes and based upon their own intelligence. These new versions of the information are passed onto other authorised agencies. The police authority then updates the information about the individual based on new evidence. Agencies are not aware of this and continue to use their own version of the information. In this situation there exist multiple copies of the information across a complex network of agencies. Copies are not the same and there is no mechanism in place to ensure that they are the same. Clearly the integrity of the information is questionable but those receiving it are likely to be unaware of this. Decisions may be made are based on this untrustworthy information, that have detrimental effects on the individual. If the information had been accompanied by the information provenance then decision makers would be able to see how the information had changed and therefore consider how safe it was. Also provenance would provide a method to track back to the provenance of original information held in the information systems of the police authority to check whether the original information had altered since it was first accessed.

A second example is discussed by Morozov (2009) and concerns the informational power of the internet. There are many who would argue that the internet has empowered people and allowed the free flow of information. It is a deterministic argument claiming that the introduction of the internet with its many new forms of communication, such as social networking and twitter, will increase the likelihood of democratic dialogue, freedom of speech and transparency. Morozov advocates caution. He explains that the new media not only empowers activists and human rights defenders but also nationalists, anti democratic movements and openly extremist forces. He suggests that authoritarian governments are using new media to create propaganda via a network of "government-friendly bloggers and commentators who are paid to spin the discussion and pretend to be the voice of the people". Blog aggregators and wikis enable regimes to harvest information about emerging threats. Fake deliberative mechanisms are used to propagate unfounded confidence in growing liberalisation. This cynical information manipulation of the internet is problematic but such manipulation of the internet without provenance is both problematic and unacceptable because the questions of why, how, when and who go unanswered.

These two examples illustrate that in the information society there is a moral obligation to address information integrity. Information provenance offers a normative instrument for turning this moral obligation into ethical practice.

INFORMATION MELTDOWN

We all need information all of the time. It is information that enables us to exist and flourish as humans. The converging technologies are transforming information and its access at an accelerating speed. Our traditional information bearings have been demolished which in turn threatens to send us into information meltdown. This meltdown can be avoided if we can curtail our insatiable appetite for information junk replacing it with a controlled diet of quality information in an acceptable form and delivery on demand. ICT allows us to blend forms such as prose, poetry, music and pictures and deliver them using, for example, writing and singing in either a serious or humorous fashion. We need to learn how to benefit from this varied diet of fit-for-purpose information and how to judge information is trustworthy. The Information Age offers so much but only if we master the technological keys to the informational Pandora's Box.

REFERENCES

Borgmann, A. (1999). *Holding On to Reality: The Nature of Information at the Turn of the Millennium*. Chicago, IL: University of Chicago Press.

Brey, P. (2006). Evaluating The Social And Cultural Implications Of The Internet. *Computers & Society, 36*(3), 41–48. doi:10.1145/1195716.1195721

Eaton, J. J., & Bawden, D. (1991). What kind of resource is information? *International Journal of Information Management, 11*(2), 156–165. doi:10.1016/0268-4012(91)90006-X

Evans, C. (1979). *The Mighty Micro: The Impact of the Computer Revolution*. London: Victor Gollancz Ltd.

Fairweather, N. B., & Rogerson, S. (2003). The Problems of Global Cultural Homogenisation in a Technologically Dependant World. *Information . Communication & Ethics in Society, 1*(1), 7–12. doi:10.1108/14779960380000221

Groth, D. P. (2004). Information Provenance and the Knowledge Rediscovery Problem. In *Proceedings of the Eighth International Conference on Information Visualization*, (pp. 345-351). Washington: IEEE Computer Society.

Hongladarom, S., & Ess, C. (Eds.). (2007). *Information Technology Ethics: Cultural Perspectives.* Hershey, PA: Idea Group Inc.

Huang, J., & Fox, M. S. (2004, May). Uncertainty in Knowledge Provenance. In *Proceedings of the 1st European Semantic Web Symposium*, Heraklion, Greece (LNCS).

Macgregor, G. (2005). The nature of information in the twenty-first century: Conundrums for the informatics community? *Library Review, 54*(1), 10–23. doi:10.1108/00242530510574129

Mandke, V. V., & Nayar, M. K. (2004). Beyond Quality: the Information Integrity Imperative. *Total Quality Management and Business Excellence, 15*(5-6), 645–654. doi:10.1080/14783360 410001680134

McRobb, S., & Rogerson, S. (2004). Are They Really Listening? An investigation into published online privacy policies. *Information Technology & People, 17*(4), 442–461. doi:10.1108/09593840410570285

Meyer, H. (2005, January). The nature of information and its effective use in rural development. *Information Research, 10*(2). Retrieved October 20, 2006 from http://informationr.net/ir/10-2/paper214.html

Moreau, L., Groth, P., Miles, S., Vazquez-Salceda, J., Ibbotson, J., & Jiang, S. (2008). The provenance of electronic data. *Communications of the ACM, 51*(4), 52–58. doi:10.1145/1330311.1330323

Morozov, E. (2009). Censoring cyberspace. *RSA Journal*, 20-23.

Nance, K. L., & Strohmaier, M. (1994). *Ethical accountability in the cyberspace. Ethics in the computer age* (pp. 115–118). New York: ACM.

Nielsen, J. (2003, October 13). Web guru fights info pollution. *BBC News Online.* Retrieved October 24, 2006 from http://news.bbc.co.uk/2/hi/technology/3171376.stm

Pinheiro da Silva, P., Deborah, S., McGuinness, D. L., & McCool, R. (2003). Knowledge Provenance Infrastructure. *A Quarterly Bulletin of the Computer Society of the IEEE Technical Committee on Data Engineering, 26*(4), 26–32.

Rogerson, S., & Bynum, T. W. (1995). Cyberspace: The Ethical Frontier . *Times Higher Education Supplement, 1179*(9), 4.

Toffler, A. (1970). *Future Shock.* New York: Bantam Books.

ENDNOTE

[1]   A shorter, earlier version of this chapter appeared as Rogerson, S. (2007). Information and integrity in the information age. *Ethical Space, The International Journal of Communication Ethics, 4*(1&2), 10-12.

Chapter 26

Community Informatics, Civil Society & Capability Approaches Converging to Cope With 'Bifurcation Challenges' in Current Societal Development

Peter Crowley
Deputy Chairperson, Vienna NGO Committee on the Family

ABSTRACT

This chapter maps out various 'bifurcation challenges' to societal development, such as, (a) climate change (b) demographic change (c) the increasing urbanisation of society and (d) 'food security.' The research encapsulates a basic Human Rights approach to foster the acquirement of the necessary 'capabilities' to make informed discriminate choices, with regard to one's personal development and to one's community of reference. It further offers a concept of Civil Society of committed individuals, facilitating the discovery of new aspects of their identity, through their commitment to societal development. The three main concepts, in this chapter: 1. The 'Community Informatics' Concept, 2. The 'Civil Society' Concept and 3. The 'Capabilities' Concept, could, with the aid of Information and Communication Technologies (ICTs), converge, to cope with the current discernable bifurcation challenges to societal development.

INTRODUCTION

The global community is confronted with a number of challenges, mapped out below, leading to a bifurcation stage (Hofkirchner & Maier-Rabler, 2004), which offers the opportunity of a rare new window of decision making. The challenges re-ferred to apply concurrently to the following areas of; (a) climate change (b) demographic change (c) the increasing urbanisation of society and (d) 'food security'.

Robert Frost wrote the following lines in 1920 which can be seen as an allegory for the bifurcation challenges facing societal development and which demand discerned choice, not only by governments, but also by individuals.

DOI: 10.4018/978-1-60960-057-0.ch026

Two roads diverged in a wood and I –
I took the one less traveled by,
And that has made all the difference

(Robert Frost, 1920)

It will be argued that convergence of endeavors will be necessary, in the sense conceived by Bradley (2006, 53); 'Convergence means a move towards a common point', to cope with the outlined bifurcational challenges, and that when such convergence occurs, it is further conceivable that the process of societal development will be more comprehensively fostered.

'BIFURCATION CHALLENGES'

Climate Change

While the Copenhagen Climate Change Conference in 2009 did not reach binding protocols to replace those of Kyoto, a consensus is building world-wide as to the need for bifurcational choice, with regard to climate change. The Intergovernmental Panel on Climate Change (IPCC) Report, (United Nations, 2007 p.2) stated; "Eleven of the last twelve years (1995-2006) rank among the twelve warmest years in the instrumental record of global surface temperature (since 1850)." While dissenting voices exist, the consensus would seem to be that climate change is indeed unequivocal and decisive decisions are inevitable.

The Report of the Global Humanitarian Forum 2009, (11), states that; "Science is now unequivocal as to the reality of climate change. Human activities, in particular emissions of greenhouse gases like carbon dioxide are recognized as its principle cause." The report goes on to point out (14) that; "Solutions do also exist for reducing greenhouse gas emissions, some even with multiple benefits. For instance, black carbon from soot, released by staple energy sources in poor communities, is likely causing as much as 18 percent of warming.

The provision of affordable alternative cooking stoves to the poor can, therefore, have both positive health results, since smoke is eliminated and an immediate impact on reducing emissions, since soot only remains in the atmosphere for a few weeks."

The United Nations Environment Program maintains that; "The changing climate is pushing many Earth systems towards critical thresholds that will alter regional and global environmental balances and threaten stability at multiple scales. Alarmingly, we may have already passed tipping points that are irreversible within the time span of our current civilization." (UNEP Report 2009, p.21)

Demographic Change

Demographic change refers to the three areas of; (a) the aging of society (b) the decline in the birth rate and (c) migration. The aging of society is attracting increased attention and research. Aging is in effect a positive result of e.g. advances in both medical and economic fields. However relatively little attention is being give to the fact of the increasing cost of medical care for the elderly. 'The Global Burden of Disease and Risk Factors' study, carried out by the World Health Organisation of the United Nations and published by the World Bank (2006), forecasts that disabilities caused by increases in age and related chronic disease will soon be greater than those from accidents, as well as infectious and childhood diseases, and hence increase the demand for more health care considerations for the ageing. The U.S. National Institute on Aging, of the United States government, issued: "Why Population Aging Matters: A Global Perspective" in 2007, which highlights the fact that the impact of population aging has yet to be fully understood and preparing financially for longer living and seeking ways to reduce aging related disability should become national and global priorities. (cf. Crowley, 2010, 30)

The Urbanisation of Society

The United Nations estimated that in 2008, for the first time, more that 50 percent of the world population is living in an urban environment. Urban populations are further projected to grow quickest in the poorest countries (United Nations 2007). The United Nations projects that 4.9 billion people, or 60% of the global population, are expected to be urban dwellers in 2030. (United Nations, World Urbanization Prospects: The 2005 Revision).

The United Nations Human Development Report (2006) points to the fact that life expectancy at birth in the Europe of the 1820s was still only 40 years. From the late 19th century on, this situation changed appreciably though the development of new medicines, improved nutrition, better housing and increased income. One of the most powerful triggers of change was adequate sanitation. At present ca. 1.1 billion people lack access to safe water, and 2.4 billion people access to what would be regarded as basic sanitation. Water and sanitation are both important for slum upgrading. (United Nations, Habitat, 2006). Habitat further points out that, slums could become a predominant type of settlement in the 21st century and may become characteristic of cities in many parts of the developing world. Urbanization is becoming synonymous with the occurrence of slums, especially in Sub-Saharan Africa, Southern and Western Asia. The United Nations 2007 Report on the State of World Cities shows how shelter conditions impact human development, including child mortality, education and employment. The question remains as to whether architects and city planners, especially in so-called 'developing countries' are adequately prepared, and in sufficient numbers, for these challenges. (cf. Crowley, 2010, 33)

A consequence of the increasing urbanisation of global society is the problem of producing adequate food for city dwellers. The rural and maritime communities have traditionally nourished the urban communities.

'Food Security'

The United Nations Food and Agricultural Organisation [FAO] (2001, 1) stated that: "As cities grow in population and area, they require more extensive structures to bring food to consumers, including distribution systems and wholesale and retail markets. At the moment, markets in most of the developing world's cities are unplanned, which leads to environmental problems and increasing losses".

Securing world food security in light of the impact of climate change may be one of the biggest challenges we face in this century. More than 860 million people in the world today suffer from hunger. Of those, about 830 million live in developing countries, the very countries expected to be most affected by climate change. (FAO 2009, 1)

Food security exists when all people, at all times, have access to sufficient, safe and nutritious food to meet their dietary needs and food preferences for an active and healthy life. (FAO 2006, 1)

Food security has the following dimensions:

- **Food Availability:** The availability of sufficient quantities of food of appropriate quality, supplied through domestic production or imports (including food aid).
- **Food Access:** Access by individuals to adequate resources (entitlements) for acquiring appropriate foods for a nutritious diet. Entitlements are defined as the set of all commodity bundles over which a person can establish command given the legal, political, economic and social arrangements of the community in which they live (including traditional rights such as access to common resources).

- **Utilization:** Utilization of food through adequate diet, clean water, sanitation and health care to reach a state of nutritional well-being where all physiological needs are met. This brings out the importance of non-food inputs in food security.
- **Stability:** To be food secure, a population, household or individual must have access to adequate food at all times. They should not risk losing access to food as a consequence of sudden shocks (e.g. an economic or climatic crisis) or cyclical events (e.g. seasonal food insecurity). The concept of stability can therefore refer to both the availability and access dimensions of food security." (United Nations FAO, 2006, 1).

Other authors would perhaps include other bifurcation challenges, such as the energy demand of an increasingly developing world or e.g. the present financial crisis (cf. Beck, 2009). The above outlined list is meant to document the need to strive for societal development before it becomes irrevocably challenged. It has already become evident how various bifurcation challenges are interwoven and only a comprehensive approach can attempt to deal with such interconnected issues. To deal with these bifurcation challenges convergence of approaches by government policies and Civil Society (CS) will be necessary.

Civil Society

Civil Society (CS) has come to be mostly defined through active Non Governmental Organisations (NGOs). The definition of CS offered by The Centre for Civil Society at the London School of Economics (2009, 1) states: 'Civil society refers to the arena of uncoerced collective action around shared interests, purposes and values. In theory, its institutional forms are distinct from those of the state, family and market, though in practice, the boundaries between state, civil society, family and market are often complex, blurred and negotiated.

Civil society commonly embraces a diversity of spaces, actors and institutional forms, varying in their degree of formality, autonomy and power. Civil societies are often populated by organisations such as registered charities, development non-governmental organisations, community groups, women's organisations, faith-based organisations, professional associations, trades unions, self-help groups, social movements, business associations, coalitions and advocacy groups." Malena & Finn Heinrich, (2007, 340) regard CS "as the arena, outside the family, the government, and the market, where people associate to advance their interests. […] In conceptualising civil society as an arena, we wish to emphasise the importance of its role in providing a public space where diverse societal values and interests interact, i.e. where people come together to discuss, associate, and seek to influence broader society. […] Conceptualising civil society as a public arena allows us to take a holistic view of it and to explore critical factors that a narrower definition, such as an organisation-focused civil society, would not detect." (Malena & Finn Heinrich, 2007).

Castells (1998) would seem to imply, similar to de Tocqueville, that CS provides a source of identity for individuals, which underlines the involvement of an emotional aspect. The approach to Civil Society as an arena of commitment would also seem to reinforce the ideas of Sen, (2002) with regard to commitment and identity. Commitment is in effect more than mere sympathy or compassion, because it implies identifying with others and encompasses action, as otherwise it would remain on a level of compassion. New aspects of identity through actions out of commitment to various communities of identification can be discovered as well as various identities. (cf. Crowley, 2010, 86)

The United Nations and the European Union would seem to be signaling towards CSOs, a participating-partnership approach in the search for solutions to the challenges to societal development. Olson (United Nations, 2006, 5) states; "The

United Nations takes the notion of partnership with civil society.[…] This has evolved greatly over the years into a two-way partnership with civil society, […] making civil society a major contributing factor to the international debates, as well as helping to increase the understanding of governments and the United Nations system. This has been a tremendous advance." The European Union underlines in its 7th Research Framework Programme, 'Science in Society' (2006): "The Programme should contribute to looking at civil society not as a constraint but as a driver and locus for innovation and therefore an active player in building a democratic knowledge society."

'Capabilities' Approach

The Nobel Laureate for Economics in 1998, Amartya Sen, wishes to move beyond development in economic terms of GNP or GDP and sees development as a cluster of freedoms and emphasizes five types: "*political freedoms*, include civil rights, an uncensored press and free democratic elections; *economic facilities* include both free markets and access to the resources necessary to participate in a market economy; *social opportunities*, refer to the arrangements society makes for education, health care, etc., which greatly affect a person's ability to improve his situation; *transparency guarantees*, which require that people deal openly with each other under guarantees of disclosure and lucidity, and help to prevent corruption and financial irresponsibility; *protective security*, refers to the social safety net (e.g., unemployment benefits, income supplements for the poor) that prevents abject poverty." (Sider, 2001, 1).

These freedoms are interrelated in Sen's understanding of development, which he calls a "capability approach." Sen was one of the more instrumental figures behind the United Nations 'Human Development Index' and (2003, vii) quotes Dante's The Divine Comedy, "Born to ascend on the wings, / Why do ye fall at such a little wind?" and mentions that: "The contrast between

what great things human beings can achieve and what limited lives most women and men end up living is truly remarkable. […] The potentialities of human beings far exceed what we actually manage to do, and that general contrast characterizes the human predicament in contemporary as well as classical understanding." He regards this as a metaphor for the discrepancy between the human potentiality, and what could be achieved e.g. by the presence of adequate education, health care, economic opportunities, and civil rights. (cf. Crowley, 2010, 77)

'Development as Freedom' was a series of lectures to the World Bank (Sen, 1999) and the Internet receives exiguous attention. However in (2000, 5) Sen maintains that: "The role of information technology and the communicational revolution must be considered in this context, [human security] since they are among the major sources of strength in improving the quality of living across the world." He regards the lack of access not only as a result of "economic penury" but also from "educational inadequacy." Sen also emphasizes the importance of improving efforts, both globally and locally to facilitate the access to these "new opportunities that can radically transform human lives."

The approach of Civil Society availing of ICTs, as facilitating tools for the acquirement of 'capabilities' could become a converging factor with Community Informatics, to empower humanity, both in developed and developing regions, as the examples below endeavor to indicate.

Community Informatics in Practice

McIver (2003, 1) states that: "Community informatics is an emerging, interdisciplinary field concerned with the development, deployment and management of information systems designed with and by communities to solve their own problems." In 2006, (5) McIver emphasizes the practical application of Community Informatics when he states that: "This definition is not enough, however. Community informatics must be seen clearly to inform and encourage a praxis. That is, teaching and research within the discipline must be directed more vigorously to the practical application of its knowledge. Such a praxis should be focused, in particular, on major societal issues such as those represented by the MDGs." [Millennium Development Goals].

The United Nations, where the MDGs were defined and set in 2000, with 1990 benchmarks, for achievement by 2015, would seem to concur with this view, through the following: "It is now well established that the capacity to generate, assimilate, disseminate and effectively use knowledge to enhance economic development is crucial for sustainable growth and development, since knowledge forms the basis of technology innovations." (United Nations Information Economy Report, 2007-2008, 1)

The UNESCO World Report (2005): "Toward Knowledge Societies" would seem to reiterate the above when it states that: "A knowledge society puts more emphasis on the ability to produce and integrate new knowledge and to access information, knowledge, data and a huge range of know-how." The UNESCO Report continues (27): "The new information and communication technologies have created new conditions for the emergence of knowledge societies. Added to this, the emerging global information society only finds its raison d'être if it serves to bring about a higher and more desirable goal, namely the building, on a global scale, of knowledge societies that are a source of development for all, first and foremost for the least developed countries." […]

Knowledge societies are about capabilities to identify, produce, process, transform, disseminate and use information to build and apply knowledge for human development. They require an empowering social vision that encompasses plurality, inclusion, solidarity and participation. […]

The human-development and empowerment-centred approach, implicit in the concept of knowledge societies, should ensure that human rights and fundamental freedoms are implemented more fully, while making for greater effectiveness in the fight against poverty and the framing of development policies. (UNESCO 2005).

The following could be regarded as examples of knowledge systems and communities, which are converging with the aid of ICT tools to facilitate committed individuals and organizations to make informed choices for their individual and societal well-being and, in effect, foster societal development, and as a consequence, positively contribute to reaching the required bifurcation decisions as listed above.

System of United Nations Cyber Libraries: http://www.un.org/ depts/dhl/sflib/libnet.htm

The United Nations system has increased its information and knowledge resources (United Nations, 2007) which include 56 electronically accessible libraries, 250 Websites, as well as a world-wide accessible, 'Cyber-School Bus' [http://cyberschoolbus.un.org/] which complement the building of knowledge communities. Aims of the Cyber-School Bus, inter alia, are; to create an on-line global education community, demonstrate to students that they have a role in finding solutions to global problems, and give them a voice in global issues as well as to provide high-quality teaching resources.

The University of South Africa (UNISA): http://www.unisa.ac.za/

The University of South Africa is a comprehensive, open learning and distance education institution, which, in response to the diverse needs of society

- *provides quality general academic and career-focused learning opportunities underpinned by principles of lifelong learning, flexibility and student centredness;*
- *undertakes research and knowledge development guided by integrity, quality and rigour; participates in community development by utilising its resources and capacities for the upliftment of the disadvantaged;*
- *is accessible to all learners, specifically those on the African continent, and the marginalised, by way of a barrier-free environment, while responding to the needs of the global market;*
- *addresses the needs of a diverse student profile by offering relevant learner support, facilitated by appropriate information and communications technology;*
- *develops and retains high-quality capacities among its staff members to achieve human development, by using the resources at its disposal efficiently and effectively;*
- *cultivates and promotes an institutional ethos, intellectual culture and educational experience that is conducive to critical discourse, intellectual curiosity, tolerance and a diversity of views;*
- *contributes to good and responsible society by graduating individuals of sound character and versatile ability;*
- *meets the needs of the global competitive society by nurturing collaborative relationships with its stakeholders and other partners." (http://www.unisa.ac.za/Default.asp?Cmd=ViewContent&ContentID=20551)*

SANGONet: http://www.ngopulse.org/about

The Southern African NGO Network (SANGONeT) was founded in 1987. Over the past 22 years it has developed into a dynamic civil society organisation with a history closely linked to the social and political changes experienced by South Africa during its transition to democracy. (http://www.ngopulse.org/about)

The NGO Pulse Portal (first established as the SANGONeT NGO Portal on 24 October 2005) represents our strategic response to the challenges facing the local NGO sector. It is the culmination of SANGONeT's years of experience of working in the online environment. Since our inception, we have developed a wide range of online resources to highlight development issues in South Africa, the wider Southern African region and the African continent in general. The NGO Pulse Portal and the weekly NGO Pulse e-newsletter provide a gateway to the South African NGO sector. Its four main objectives are to develop the institutional capacity of the NGO sector through providing information that supports stronger management practises; map NGOs and their activities through Prodder, the most comprehensive database of its kind in Africa; create a community space for civil society exchange; and promote the benefits of ICTs in support of the work of civil society through the SANGOTeCH Technology Donation Portal. The portal provides NGOs with a mechanism to air their views, while also creating the opportunity for other stakeholders to critique and evaluate the sector. It has become a marketplace where services can be procured and exchanged. It also provides SANGONeT with a strategic mechanism to communicate its activities and services to the NGO sector and other development stakeholders. NGO Pulse provides a gateway to the NGO sector in South Africa, raising the profile of South African NGOs both locally and internationally, and supporting the process of repositioning and strengthening the sector in response to the development challenges facing South Africa. (http://www.ngopulse.org/group/home-page/about-ngopulse)

The Container Project Jamaica: http://www.container-project.net/

The Container Project is a not-for-profit Community Multimedia Center providing access to new technology for marginalised and under-educated people in rural communities. The Project promotes the use of the Internet and other multimedia platform as a new and innovative means of learning and creative development for career boosting activity and empowerment through the use of information communication technology and computers. Our main strategy lies in the introduction of the use of computer related technology to grassroots communities, empowering the youths and long-term unemployed in developing and improving their ability to successfully interact with the new and emerging technologies. The "Container" is a phisically a 40ft shipping container unit, equipped with computers and other forms of communication media (http://www.container-project.net/)

CONCLUSION

ICTs are becoming the fulcrum and lynchpin of knowledge communities with global reach. The widespread, and ever increasing, use of ICTs by Civil Society, both individually and as organisations, is facilitating the establishment and impact of such truly global knowledge communities. To tackle the above identified, and outlined bifurcation challenges, evolving in societal development, convergence of Community Informatics and Civil Society is becoming increasingly indispensible to facilitate the acquirement of the necessary capabilities of citizens globally, to be sufficiently informed, in order to be able to make meaningful personal choices for their individual well-being, as well as collectively, for society, and to enable them to participate freely in increasingly interdependent globalising communities and societies.

Collaborative cooperation and partnerships by Civil Society, Governments, international organizations, such as the United Nations, and Academia, will continue to become indispensable, to stimulate and motivate individuals and groups to achieve these 'capabilities', which are intricately interwoven with societal development.

It is however necessary to be mindful of avoiding merely 'technology push' approaches and to incorporate those which are based on literacy advancement. "Basic human needs and 'people-push' technology not 'technology push' should be a leading principle." (Bradley, 2006, 60). Convergence of governments and International Organisations programmes to provide adequate literacy structures, as well as affordable and accessible technology infrastructures, along with civil society endeavors, both local and global, is desirable and necessary. This convergence and synergy could enable the acquirement of life enhancing capabilities to reach that 'common point' (cf. Bradley, 2006) and cope with the concurrent discernable bifurcation challenges to societal development.

REFERENCES

Beck, U. (2009). *World at Risk*. Cambridge, UK: Polity Press.

Bradley, G. (2006). *Social and Community Informatics: Humans on the Net*. London: Routledge.

Castells, M. (1998). *The Rise of the Network Society: The Information Age: economy, society and culture*. Malden, MA: Blackwell.

Centre for Civil Society. (2009). *What is Civil Society?* Retrieved June 11, 2009 from http://www.lse.ac.uk/collections/CCS/introduction/what_is_civil_society.htm

Crowley, P. (2010). *Information and Communication Technologies Enabling to Create a Self-Organising Civil Society 'Knowledge and Service Commons' and 'Capability' Capacities to Counteract 'Chaos Points*. Ph.D. University of Salzburg.

Frost, R. (1920). *Collected Poems, prose and plays, 7.* New York: Library of America.

Global Humanitarian Forum. (2009). *The Anatomy of a Silent Crisis*. Geneva. Retrieved June 2, 2009 from http://www.ghf-geneva.org/

Hofkirchner, W., & Maier-Rabler, U. (2004). The Ethos of the Great Bifurcation. *International Journal of Information Ethics*, *2*(11), 1–11.

Malena, C., & Finn Heinrich, V. (2007). Can we measure civil society? A proposed methodology for international comparative research. *Development in Practice*, *17*(3), 338–352. doi:10.1080/09614520701336766

McIver, W., Jr. (2003). A Community Informatics for the Information Society. In S. O'Siochrú and B. Girard (Eds.) *Communicating in the Information Society*. Geneva, Switzerland: United Nations Research Institute for Social Development (UNRISD), 2003. Retrieved May 12, 2008 from http://www.unrisd.org/80256B3C005BCCF9/(ht tpPublications)/5DCA28E932BB8CFDC1256E2 40029A075?OpenDocument&panel=additional

McIver, W., Jr. (2006, November). Community Informatics and Human Development. In *Proceedings International Workshop on Community Informatics*, (COMINF'06). Montpellier, France. NRC 48767.

National Institute on Aging & National Institutes of Health. Washington. (2007). Why Population Aging Matters: A Global Perspective. Retrieved February 12, 2008 from http://www.nia.nih.gov/NR/rdonlyres/9E91407E-CFE8-4903-9875-D5AA75BD1D50/0/WPAM.pdf

Olson, E. (2006). Families-Agents of Social Development . In *Proceedings of International Seminar*. Vienna, Austria: Families Agents of Social Development.

Sen, A. (1999). *Development as Freedom*. Oxford: Oxford University Press.

Sen, A. (2000). *Why Human Security. International Symposium Human Security*, Tokyo, 28 July, 2000. Retrieved June 17, 2009 http://indh.pnud.org.co/files/rec/SenWhyHS.pdf

Sen, A. (2002). *Rationality and Freedom*. Cambridge, MA: Harvard University Press.

Sen, A. (2003). Development and Capability Expansion . In Fukuda-Parr, S., & Shiva Kumar, A. K. (Eds.), *Readings in Human Development*. Oxford: Oxford University Press.

Sider, R. (2001). Book review: *Development as Freedom Amarta Sen*. Retrieved June 12, 2009 from http://www.leaderu.org/ftissues/ft0101/reviews/sider.html

The European Union. (2006). *7th Research Framework Programme, 'Science in Society'*. Brussels. Retrieved February 19, 2008 from http://cordis.europa.eu/fp7/home_en.html

UNESCO. (2005). *Towards Knowledge Societies*. Paris, France. Retrieved October 11, 2007 from http://unesdoc.unesco.org/images/0014/001418/141843e.pdf

United Nations. (2005). *World Urbanization Prospects*. Retrieved February 7, 2008 from http://www.un.org/esa/population/publications/WUP2005/2005wup.htm

United Nations. (2007). *Human Development Report 2006*. New York. Retrieved November 28, 2007 from http://hdr.undp.org/en/media/hdr06-complete.pdf

United Nations. (2007). *Inter Government Panel on Climate Change*. Fourth Assessment Report. Valencia. Summary for Policy Makers. Retrieved June 3, 2009 from http://www.ipcc.ch/pdf/assessment-report/ar4/syr/ar4_syr_spm.pdf

United Nations. (2007). *State of the World's Cities*. New York. Retrieved May 12, 2008 from http://www.un.org/Pubs/chronicle/2006/issue2/0206p24.htm

United Nations. (2007). *Resolution 62 / 111A General Assembly*. New York. Retrieved May 12, 2008 from http://daccessdds.un.org/doc/UNDOC/GEN/N07/470/43/PDF/N0747043.pdf?OpenElement

United Nations. (2008). *Information Economy Report* 2007-2008 Science & technology for development: the new paradigm of ICT. New York. Retrieved February 13, 2008 from http://www.unctad.org/Templates/webflyer.asp?docid=9479&intItemID=1397&lang=1&mode=toc

United Nations Environment Programme. (2009). *UNEP Year Book* 2009. Nairobi. Retrieved June 3, 2009 from http://www.unep.org/geo/yearbook

United Nations Food and Agricultural Organisation. (2001). *Feeding the Cities*. Rome. Retrieved June 3, 2009 from http://www.fao.org/fcit/docs/introduction_en.pdf

United Nations Food and Agricultural Organisation. (2006). *Food Security*. Retrieved June 5, 2009 from ftp://ftp.fao.org/es/ESA/policybriefs/pb_02.pdf

United Nations Food and Agricultural Organisation. (2009). *Climate Change and Food Safety*, Rome. Retrieved June 7, 2009 from http://www.fao.org/ag/agn/agns/files/HLC1_Climate_Change_and_Food_Safety.pdf

United Nations Habitat. (2006). *Report World Urban Forum*. Retrieved February 4, 2008 http://www.unhabitat.org/downloads/docs/4077_70142_WUF3-Report-final%20%20dm1%2023%20june.REV.1.pdf

World Bank. (2006). *The Global Burden of Disease and Risk Factors*. Oxford: Oxford University Press.

Chapter 27
Connection, Coupling, and Persistence in Online Social Networks

Barrett S. Caldwell
Purdue University, USA

ABSTRACT

The rise of multiple online social network sites represents a new set of opportunities for persons to develop and sustain a variety of personal and professional personas with increasing ranges of access. In some cases, these sites allow individuals to enable or re-establish connections with members of a social network that are separated over time and distance. For instance, the author's children are now able to find friends from elementary school, and reconnect with them as they enter into adulthood, providing renewals of relationships from childhood that in past eras might have dissolved. One child is also demonstrating professional development in an online social network community for musicians. New rules and considerations for social interaction and management reflect changing uses of information and communication technologies (ICTs) in a richly integrated Information Society. These considerations can be described in terms of mathematical properties of coupling, persistence, and work functions associated with accessing, sharing, and transitioning among multiple social representations that evolve and diverge over time.

INTRODUCTION

The growth of social networks and other means of connecting "humans on the net" (Bradley, 2006) has become a substantial, and perhaps even transformational, phenomenon affecting social interaction and culture in the Information Society.

DOI: 10.4018/978-1-60960-057-0.ch027

Systematic methods to describe, compare, and manage changing models of social interactions are important for the scientific examination of social network information and communication technologies (ICTs). However, the quantitative tools for describing this phenomenon are still at an early stage of development. Without such tools, information society researchers are limited in their ability to interact effectively with computer science and engineering disciplines in the design and improvement of ICTs. The search for quantitative tools that reflect both the psychological and social complexity of the Information Society, and the underlying rigor of the mathematical frameworks that drive engineering system development, has been an ongoing goal for this author. In fact, one of these initial attempts represents the original context for my meeting Prof. Gunilla Bradley at the ODAM Conference in Stockholm in 1994 (Caldwell, 1994).

A common challenge as one grows older is the negotiation and shift of social affiliations and self-identity. Even as one's sense of self evolves, there is a potential for changing the subcultural groupings to which one wishes to belong. For those who manage to live happily within a single community that fits well and is stable throughout one's life, such discomforts might be minimized. However, for a growing number of people in the economically developed and developing world, there is a need to manage one's presence and participation in a variety of communities of place, interest, or practice. Historically, those who moved to another home far away from one's birthplace or prior residence, or those who shift from one social class or reference group to another, could find it relatively easy to leave that "prior self" behind as one managed a new set of activities, affiliations, and associations.

Examples of the changing role of ICT in creating and managing communities affect my own children. After moving away from their childhood hometown in Wisconsin, they are now returning to that same hometown as young adults. Despite living nearly half of their lives in another place, they were able to continue connections with friends from primary school using social networking sites such as MySpace and Facebook. In a more professional social network, my son's career as a musician has blossomed over the past year because of a new ICT interaction medium. Beginning in Fall, 2008, he began to participate in Soundcloud, an international social network / community of practice site for musicians with growing popularity in that community (Von Buskirk, 2009). Soundcloud was created by several Swedish musicians and technology developers who wanted to be able to share and collaborate on music more easily than in existing tools (Soundcloud, 2009). What makes Soundcloud useful includes several elements of the function of a social network for musicians, and not simply the structure of a site. These elements will be discussed in the following sections.

ELEMENTS OF FUNCTIONAL ICT BENEFITS

The growth of online communities and social network technologies has substantially influenced the ability to find another person through multiple channels and mutual personal connections. The advent of widespread internet-based ICTs in the 1980s and 1990s, including the development of bulletin boards and discussion groups, allowed the creation of professional and personal communities of practice or social affiliation that no longer aligned with an individual's current physical community of place. Some researchers decried this phenomenon as the harbinger of a new era of social isolation and breakdown of interpersonal interactions. Others, such as the author's Group Performance Environments Research (GROUPER) laboratory, emphasized the ability of internet communications to support a greater variety of social interactions and self-identified communities not tied to communities of place (Taha & Caldwell, 1993). This might be seen as especially valuable for members of minority or alternative subcultures, who might be unable to find others with similar interests and values nearby; those without options to routinely use other channels to socially interact with others due to infirmity or illness also found value in social reintegration (Brennan. Moore, & Smyth, 1995; Brennan et al., 2001).

Growth in electronic means of interaction also provides opportunities for social connections to a previously hidden group: those who found unmediated social interactions difficult or overwhelming to manage. Some authors (Daft & Lengel, 1986; Rice, 1992; Rice & Shook, 1990) used theories such as Media Richness Theory to complain that computer-mediated communications were always inferior to face to face interactions due to the reductions in social cues. GROUPER research had shown that situational factors strongly influenced the value and relative benefits of computer-mediated communications in a variety of users (Caldwell & Paradkar, 1995; Caldwell, Uang, & Taha, 1995). However, the reduced complexity and richness of ICT compared to face to face interactions might become, in themselves, an advantage to using ICT-based social interaction technologies.

Previous discussions of electronic social interactions assuming a superiority of face to face, unmediated interactions, make a primary assumption that is demonstrably incorrect in a number of situations. This assumption takes the form, *Social actors have the cognitive, language, and social skills to access, manage and prefer the complexity of unmediated interpersonal dynamics.* Insight into at least three distinct groups for whom this assumption might not be true came from the author's interactions as a university faculty member in the mid 1990s, as electronic mail systems became a common method of faculty-student interactions. When I began to encourage students to send email questions based on lecture, and consider them equally in evaluations of class participation, one student expressed appreciation for this policy. As an international student at an American university, this student did not feel sufficiently comfortable with their command of spoken English to speak aloud in class. When communicating via email, the student had more time to consider the use of idiom and specific technical terms, and use a dictionary as required. (Similar techniques were useful to me when attempting to utilize some

terms in Swedish when lecturing in Sweden.) An email query, or an electronic bulletin board discussion of critical points raised in class, allows for additional time to review and incorporate the use of the complexities of both informal technical language of communication.

A second consideration, more cultural than language, reflected the student's reluctance to be seen as questioning the professor during class. For many East Asian or other cultures with both strong respect for elders, and reverence for teachers, asking a potentially challenging question and "disrupting" class would be considered highly taboo. A question phrased in electronic form, when does not interfere with the flow of an in-class presentation, has fewer perceived social violations of appropriate behavior for such students.

Introduction to a third group of those uniquely disadvantaged by unmediated communications came from other students. In at least two cases, I worked with students who expressed considerable discomfort with free-flowing social interactions. With additional interactions (both unmediated and mediated), the issues became evident: both students had conditions placing them on the autistic neurological spectrum of information processing. (Because of the focus on information processing, and debates among the Asperger's syndrome and autism communities about the status of such conditions as disorders, these conditions will be discussed here as issues of autistic spectrum interactions, or ASI.) For ASI individuals, the complexity of verbal, paraverbal, and non-verbal forms of unmediated communication can represent a potentially overwhelming complexity of input which is extremely difficult to process and respond effectively in real time. These difficulties can be multiplied in complex social environments with a great deal of peripheral activity. In such environments, background activity can also reduce the ratio between the "signal" of the primary conversation and the "noise" of the social environment. (Those with sensory disorders have similar problems, such as picking out a single conversation in a noisy restaurant, or looking at a visual display in a highly reflective, low contrast setting.) Electronic interactions effectively moderate this signal-noise ratio, by reducing the number of confusing social cues and background, and making many paraverbal or nonverbal cues more explicit (through the use of emoticons or tags: <sarcasm>, for example). Thus, someone with a sensory or speech production disorder, or an individual with ASI or social anxiety, the advantage of well-utilized electronic interactions is precisely *because* of the reduced social cues and richness decried in prior media richness theories. However, there is another element of mediated ICT use that has a significant advantage over unmediated interactions: the property of persistence.

The experiences of the email that can be re-read, the discussion list that threads contributions from group members across the world, and the social network site that allows for searching of past colleagues and classmates all demonstrate persistence of electronic access over multiple time scales. For unmediated communications, the decay of information access is known and well studied by cognitive psychologists. Sensory decay of non-repeating input signals is approximately .3 – 3 seconds (in log scale, from -0.5 to 0.5). The limits of working memory are approximately 30 seconds (in log scale, 1.5) (Bailey, 1996; Wickens, Lee, Liu, & Gordon Becker, 2004). Thus, in a heavily task loaded environment (where activity exceeds the ability to reliably recognize and encode inputs), information decay represents two orders of magnitude of persistence, from -0.5 to 1.5 log seconds. However, the use of a social network site to retrieve and update interactions with a classmate for one's 30th year high school reunion represents a potential persistence of nearly one billion seconds (9.0 log seconds).

Persistence in a social networking or other ICT context provides another difference in social interaction: the ability to reconnect to another person days, months, or years later, with relatively little awareness of what events have affected that person during the intervening period. While this can be seen as an advantage for those whose lives have taken different paths, there are both positive and negative elements to such reconnection. The process of updating interpersonal contacts is one of sharing knowledge about another person, and improving the efficiency of information exchange and mutual understanding based on those shared experiences. As the period of time without interaction increases, the likelihood increases that the strength of any previously shared information or experience will decay. There are two major sources of decay: a) due to degraded memory of past experience; and b) increasing influence of other events and information that are used in other social contexts. For those whose social networks are constrained to a small group over a long period of time, shared events and information is maintained within a small circle of actors who mutually update each other's knowledge and experience. In these cases, social networking interactions may increase the rate of interaction, but not change its overall scope or range. (This is the same process that occurs with those who live their lives in a small neighborhood throughout one's life, where social mobility and changing interaction groups is limited. The range of interactions is limited, no matter how tightly connected those interactions are maintained over time.)

ENGINEERING MEASURES OF SOCIAL NETWORK COMMUNITY INTERACTIONS

Based on the above discussions, there are three fundamental concepts that affect the value of an ICT community to its members. Each of these concepts not simply suggests an engineering analogy, but directly indicates quantitative measures derived from their use in engineering disciplines. These measures will be described here, using the Soundcloud example.

Persistence: Robustness to Information Decay over Time

Persistence can be measured over time scales from seconds to decades, and represents the likelihood that information available at time t_0 can be retrieved again at some later time t. The most popularly recognized measure of the decay of some information or signal is usually that of the "half-life" measure of radioactive decay (when half of the original concentration of a radioactive energy source is still present). However, persistence in ICT need not be restricted to this exponential decay function. The author's previous work has demonstrated that information decay can take several forms, including linear, exponential, and second-order decay models. Two second-order decay models represent both synchronous (real-time) and asynchronous (delayed) interaction styles.

Members of the Soundcloud community can post music compositions that are days, weeks, or even years old, and allow them to remain visible to members of the community for an arbitrary period of time (limited more by the longevity of the site). Membership levels are based on number of compositions uploaded in a given month, more than the total storage space used. Thus, both my son and his peers have access to prior music projects done by members of the community over time, allowing previously unused compositions to be revived and reintegrated in novel ways.

Work: Effort Required to Flow Across a Distance

In a variety of engineering disciplines, work is the fundamental measure of force applied across a distance. When operating in a complex environment, it is not simply the net distance travelled, but the force applied along a particular path. The value of an ICT is often described as reducing the work required for members of a community to interact—either in terms of reducing the total

path travelled, or in reducing the force required to move along that path.

Soundcloud operates to reduce both the force and path requirements to connect musicians. Members of the community are not required to go to music concerts and clubs on five continents in order to discover each other, or release tracks on traditional music production labels in order to gather a following. In addition, the design of the Soundcloud interface allows music tracks to be shared easily, including time-based commenting on specific dynamic and sonic elements. Thus, the Soundcloud site permits reduced work by shortening the path (connecting distant users) and reducing the force (an easy interface for the flow of music information) required to effectively share among musicians. (My son has been able to have over 1500 community members around the world following his work without leaving the US. During the week of 5 July 2009, his area of the site experienced over 1350 downloads of music tracks in five days without any advertising or promotion on his part. By 18 July 2010, at least 34 tracks had been played over 250 times, including pieces written before the start of the Soundcloud site. One seven-minute piece has received over 16,500 plays, and over 50 time-stamped comments, in approximately 10 months of persistent availability on the site.)

Coupling: Transmission of Valuable Information without Loss

The engineering concept of coupling refers specifically to the ability to have energy information flow from one node or component to another with a minimum of distortion due to loss or noise. Some metaphoric uses of coupling may suggest that loose coupling is superior to tight coupling. However, from a technical perspective, complex systems are much more difficult to manage (and take a great deal more energy) if much of the input to the system is lost before it results in effective transmission to the output. From the perspective of information sharing in a social network, coupling can be described as the probability that two individuals exchanging a message would have the same understanding of the message after it has been received. This coupling relies on both the structural aspects of having pathways available to exchange the message, and the functional elements of shared cultural meanings appropriate to interpret the message in compatible ways.

The focus of Soundcloud is on music sharing, with an efficient interface for exchanging the critical elements of activity for that community. Thus, members of the community are able to ensure that the important aspects of their community of practice are shared efficiently, without losses due to translations (between languages, or between language descriptions of music and the music itself) or difficulty in making the music available to others. Clearly, coupling in Soundcloud cannot achieve the theoretical limit of 1.0 because of the unique experiences and references that each person has to music. However, music, with metadata tags, shared among a community of musicians exchanges much more shared cultural meaning than instant message or email pathways that primarily transmit words and support music exchange poorly or not at all.

Summary: Paths to Quantifying Connections

Using the concepts of persistence, work, and coupling, existing engineering and mathematical definitions can be used to describe the behavior of social connections using ICTs. Social network communities exist because they are known to their members, and because members find benefit in using them. The case of members of a single physical community where all members interact with each other regularly over a period of time represents one special case of such connections. The persistence of the community is refreshed with each new social interaction, which for a small community happens routinely over the course of

each day until the members of the community die. Whether a community is considered isolated can be defined by the ratio of contacts its members have within the community to the total number of contacts (Caldwell, 1990). This ratio might also be described as the participation ratio of a member to a community. If no one in the community interacts with anyone outside of the community, its isolation ratio is one. (A person who has no social interactions with other members of a community may still consider themselves a part of that community, but would be invisible to those other members and thus not actively included as one of those members. This is the issue associated with "lurkers" in online communities.)

If the members of a small community only interact with each other, they do not manage social interactions with the world beyond the boundaries of that community. Thus, the coupling of the community to the rest of the world must be zero, as there is no mechanism for social interactions or information to be transferred between the community and others. Similarly, the work required to connect that community to the world is infinite (because the lack of a path requires infinite force to connect).

The more realistic situations of ICT-based social connections and networks suggest much more complexity in terms of the actual measures of interaction. However, the principles defined in this paper remain valid. For persons who maintain most of their social interactions through a particular social network community, their relative participation ratios to those communities are high compared to other possible community affiliations. One benefit that members of online communities often find is that, because the work paths of connecting to one or more communities is lower, they can participate more readily in multiple communities. Persistence is refreshed when new community interactions occur (such as discussion group or blog postings, or even individual messages from one community member to another). Although the work for connecting may be reduced in these situations, coupling remains a complex consideration.

As a person interacts as a member of a particular community (online or physical, in communities of affiliation, practice or any other characteristic), they adopt communication styles and language uses that evolve to be distinctive to that community. However, different communities may use the same terms and words (or even acronyms) to have distinct, community-specific meanings. As such, the use of a particular term as an "efficient" form of communication could demonstrate instead possible confusion between meanings in different community contexts (such as "TMI" referring to "too much information," or a nuclear plant mishap in the 1970s at the Three Mile Island power plant in the United States, or a Scandinavian consultancy firm with projects and offices in Denmark and Sweden). This increased probability of confusion, of course, reflects lower coupling between individuals who participate with each other in one community, but also have non-overlapping sets of participation in other social network communities.

These characteristics of social networks based on ICTs can even explain apparent violations of previous theories of media richness assuming the superiority of face to face communications. Let us return to the discussion of ASI or other individuals for whom real-time social interactions in a socially complex context represent traumatic overload, rather than desired integration. An ICT-based social network community has several advantages, including increased persistence (individual messages can be processed and reviewed many times over a period of days) and coupling (queries and miscommunications can be explicitly addressed in the network, with clarifications made available to the community as a whole to further confirm and codify shared meanings). The work of such connections is drastically reduced, because of the relatively lower barriers of accessing the community via a website from home rather than physical travel to a social setting. Once the communities

are identified (perhaps using a search engine), the participation ratio of an individual within that community is likely to be higher than for other social interaction contexts.

CONCLUSION

The growth of ICT support for a variety of social and community networks has allowed for a rich and complex range of interactions and methods of participation. The use of such networks, rather than being seen as a poor substitute for face to face interactions, can be also considered as an enabling technology to support previously difficult social interactions. Members of communities who were previously separated by time, loss of physical proximity, or difficulties in managing complex social dynamics, now have additional opportunities to create and re-establish fulfilling interpersonal connections.

This author believes that the progress of our understanding of these social and technological dynamics in the Information Society will be enhanced through the development and application of appropriate quantitative tools to describe social network behaviors. Primarily, social network communities are about paths that maintain both structural connections and functional processes of shared social meanings. Thus, three new quantitative measures are suggested that can help to analyze individual and social aspects of social interactions in ICTs. Coupling, persistence, and work are based on engineering measures of efficiency and effort required to sustain connections between entities, and all can be seen to describe important features of participation in social network environments. (Another measure, the participation ratio, actually represents aspects of the author's work that predates the 15 years of collaboration between the author and Prof. Gunilla Bradley.)

Of course, critical questions of *how to manage* social aspects of connections in an enriched context of ICT-based networks will not be answered by tools that describe *characteristics* of those connections. For instance, the persistence of Facebook and MySpace pages, and the concept of reduced work in accessing prior personal information, explains the existence of new social questions raised about adolescents finding documentation of their youthful behaviors causing difficulties in their professional lives. These issues may have always been true to some extent, but creating access to one's past via a much lower work function represents a more extensive and common expression of the concerns involved. A retreat from physical interactions to a different network of ICT-based interactions may be seen by some as an unhealthy and unwarranted restriction of social contacts.

However, for those who have moved away from their childhood homes and friends, the ability to rediscover old connections via reduced work functions can be seen as a tremendous benefit. ICT-based interactions can provide substantial improvements for members of communities that can be more easily managed and enjoyed than the complexity of some face to face interactions. For nearly all participants in the Information Society, the reduced work functions and increased persistence available in long-term access to social networks allow for greater variety and flexibility of participation in multiple affiliative, professional, and special interest networks. These opportunities will further increase the rarity of the completely isolated physical community whose members continually and exclusively interact with each other. The challenges of effective coupling between members will increase as participation in one social network can be further affected by social interpretations and meanings from other networks. More importantly, these dynamics will not be seen as mysterious phenomena outside of the realm of systematic study and evaluation. Quantitative descriptions of important characteristics of social network participation do permit more and better connections to other communities of technology developers and systems engineers with whom ICT researchers can effectively interact and share knowledge about the changing functions and dynamics of the Information Society.

REFERENCES

Bailey, R. W. (1996). *Human Performance Engineering: Using human factors / ergonomics to achieve computer system usability* (3rd ed.). Englewood Cliffs, NJ: Prentice Hall.

Bradley, G. (2006). *Social and Community Informatics: Humans on the Net*. London: Routledge.

Brennan, P. F., Moore, S. M., Bjornsdottir, G., Jones, J., Visovsky, C., & Rogers, M. (2001). HeartCare: an Internet-based information and support system for patient home recovery after coronary artery bypass graft (CABG) surgery. *Journal of Advanced Nursing, 35*(5), 699–708. doi:10.1046/j.1365-2648.2001.01902.x

Brennan, P. F., Moore, S. M., & Smyth, K. A. (1995). The Effects of a Special Computer Network on Caregivers of Persons with Alzheimer's Disease. *Nursing Research, 44*(3), 166–172. doi:10.1097/00006199-199505000-00007

Caldwell, B. S. (1990). Development of Models for Park Rangers' Perceived Isolation of National Park Service Areas. *Environment and Behavior, 22*(5), 636–649. doi:10.1177/0013916590225004

Caldwell, B. S. (1994). Developing Robust Mathematical Models of Information Technology Use in Organizations Human Factors in Organizational Design and Management – IV: In *Proceedings of the Fourth International Symposium on Human Factors in Organizational Design and Management* held in Stockholm, Sweden (pp. 526-530). Amsterdam, NL: North-Holland.

Caldwell, B. S., & Paradkar, P. V. (1995). Factors Affecting User Tolerance for Voice Mail Message Transmission Delays. *International Journal of Human-Computer Interaction, 7*(3), 235–248. doi:10.1080/10447319509526123

Caldwell, B. S., Uang, S.-T., & Taha, L. H. (1995). Appropriateness of communications media use in organizations: Situation requirements and media characteristics. *Behaviour & Information Technology*, *14*(4), 199–207. doi:10.1080/01449299508914633

Daft, R. L., & Lengel, R. H. (1986). Organizational Information Requirements, Media Richness and Structural Design. *Management Science*, *32*(5), 554–571. doi:10.1287/mnsc.32.5.554

Rice, R. E. (1992). Task analyzability, use of new media, and effectiveness: A multi-site exploration of media richness. *Organization Science*, *3*(4), 475–500. doi:10.1287/orsc.3.4.475

Rice, R. E., & Shook, D. E. (1990). Voice messaging, coordination, and communication . In Galegher, J., Kraut, R. E., & Egido, C. (Eds.), *Intellectual Teamwork: Social and Technological Foundations of Cooperative Work* (pp. 327–350). Hillsdale, NJ: Lawrence Erlbaum Associates.

Soundcloud (2009). *Who We Are*. Retrieved July 11, 2009, from http://soundcloud.com/pages/who-we-are

Taha, L. H., & Caldwell, B. S. (1993). Social Isolation and Integration in Electronic Environments. *Behaviour & Information Technology*, *12*(5), 276–283. doi:10.1080/01449299308924391

Von Buskirk, E. (2009). SoundCloud Threatens MySpace as Music Destination for Twitter Era. *Wired*. Retrieved from http://www.wired.com/epicenter/2009/07/soundcloud-threatens-myspace-as-music-destination-for-twitter-era/

Wickens, C. D., Lee, J. D., Liu, Y., & Gordon Becker, S. E. (2004). *An Introduction to Human Factors Engineering*. Upper Saddle River, NJ: Pearson Prentice Hall.

Chapter 28
The Community Event Research Method

Sarai Lastra
Universidad del Turabo, Puerto Rico

ABSTRACT

During the process of designing a community information system for my dissertation study using ethnographic and grounded theory methods in a Latino diasporic community from Paseo Boricua in Chicago, Illinois, between 1999 and 2001, I experienced the efficacy of community events as tools for educating me about the essence that was organizing a community's way of life. The process of achieving the dissertation goal generated a new method based on the traditions of community informatics (CI) and participatory design (PD). This chapter presents the method—the Community Event Research Method (CERM)—and explores issues in developing and applying it. CERM reasons that community events are knowledge objects which embody social processes, cultural meanings and information needs of a community and that a selected set of community events, which are related in some larger cultural context (in one way or another), can serve as a valuable unit of analysis for systematically uncovering strong and weak voices in a community. The method not only focuses on understanding the community ethos, but also presents alternatives for recasting knowledge into design.

INTRODUCTION

Whatever we observe is impregnated by assumptions (Silverman 2001, p.2).

The tradition of community informatics shows an emerging field of research and practice that is at a

point where social informatics was in the late 20th century with respect to mapping out its borders. Community informatics (CI) is a technology-based discipline devoted to understanding "social factors influencing ICT utilization"(O'Neil 2001, p.3) in local communities. CI "pays attention to physical communities and the design and implementation of technologies and applications, which enhance and promote their objectives" (Gurstein 2000, p.2).

DOI: 10.4018/978-1-60960-057-0.ch028

An inspection of the CI literature illustrates the difficulties of the research and practice in CI because of a need to integrate various methods, research goals, community programs, potentially conflicting assumptions, multiple voices, theories and practices. The shortcomings in the evolution of community informatics' doxa relate to a gap in the establishment of a common ground of principles, methods and theoretical frameworks needed to bring coherence and establish disciplinary boundaries for CI (Bishop, personal communication, 2001; Gurstein 2003, 2007; Pitkin 2001). For instance, concerning a critical aspect such as "effective use of ICTs," Gurstein notes, that the term "has been widely employed [with] little or no systematic analysis" (2003, p.8).

Although CI is slowly meeting its challenges of closing its theoretical and methodological gap, as Pitkin recommends, "head on" (2001, p.10), the nature of the CI discipline calls for its researchers and practitioners to be forever engaged with a "diffusion of methods, ideas and approaches from field to field."[1] This need for multidisciplinarity in CI's doxa raises a number of critical issues and research problems related to the maturation of a common rhetoric for an emergent discipline. For one, the complexity of understanding community ICT projects requires CI researchers to go beyond just describing success stories (or failures) to analyzing the principles underlying the various ICT developmental case studies. Yet, going beyond just describing stories will require CI to work on providing a common ground of principles, methods, constructs and theories.

To the extent that CI closes its theoretical and methodological gap, more sense making CI research that contributes to a steady evolution of the discipline and that brings insights into the relationship between ICTs and community development projects should appear in the future.

Along these lines, this study looks at the research problem of developing a method based on community events helpful to community informat-

ics for uncovering the "local knowledge" (Geertz 1983) of a marginalized diasporic community, and beyond that, for exploring ways of recasting this local knowledge into designing more socially inclusive community ICTs.

The development of this method focuses on mapping the action of the research activity as what happens when various methods, theories, practices and goals integrate and adjust into a unit of analysis of community events, producing an interpretation which is useful for designing more socially inclusive community ICTs.

In general, the concept of "community" is defined in this study as a dynamic and constitutive group that can develop tenacious coalitions that work towards a particular end while dealing with internal tensions, inconsistencies and contradictions that may hinder the development of a particular goal. Specifically, the research problem situates the development of the method in the Latino community of Paseo Boricua, Chicago, Illinois, during the years 1999 through 2003 (Lastra 2006).

Community Events

Every local community has problems. Some local communities have problems that are worse than others. Every local community has some form of social capital that influences how it deals with its problems. The premise of the argument that informs the construction of this asset-based, participatory design method comes from an analogy between scholarly communities and marginalized communities. Just as it is possible to study the behavior of scholarly communities by focusing on how they create knowledge objects (books, articles, research papers, conferences, etc.)[2], similarly it is possible to study a community's behavior (how it organizes, creates local knowledge, what are its information needs) by focusing on community events. I summarize the importance of the premise for this study as follows: *Community events are community assets that represent collective knowledge products.*

This method explores the concept of community events as symbolic objects useful for carrying out concrete analysis that would be of interest to community informatics. The empirical analysis provided by CERM is useful for enabling an engagement process between designers and community people, a component of the design process that is crucial for building a participatory object. Alternatively, it is possible that CERM could be developed into an evaluative tool for community informatics. This study, however, focuses on developing and applying its capabilities as a prescriptive method for building more socially inclusive ICTs.

As a research method, the community event research method grows its methodological roots from an assemblage of multiple methods: the "dimensions of the folk event" (Bauman 1986; Toelken 1996, pp.157-182), grounded theory (Strauss and Corbin 1997), reciprocal ethnography (Lawless 1993; 2000) and interpretive interactionism (Denzin 2001). With respect to its categorization, CERM falls under the umbrella of event-driven analysis, a series of methods that have been used in various disciplines and for quite different purposes. For example, event-driven analysis has proved itself highly useful in other disciplines such as Folklore, Software Programming and Sociology. In Folklore, for example, it is used to study particular events that provide insights into a culture (Toelken 1996). In the area of software programming, Ruble (1997, pp. 79-115) describes an event-driven model for collecting data on user transactions as guides for designing the prototypes of graphical user interfaces (GUI). In sociology, Abbott (1995) has developed a statistical technique (OPTIMIZE) that analyzes a sequential list of events using scaling, clustering and other categorical methods to "uncover actual categories of patterns" (pp.108-109) of data about careers, welfare states, or dances.

Community Ethos

It is Bourdieu's concept of habitus that helps this research frame an operational definition for community ethos. Using the construct of habitus, community events can be defined not only as "symbolic systems" (Bourdieu 1977; Geertz 1983; Toelken 1996) that have a shape, place, form, but also as "systems of durable dispositions" (Bourdieu 1977; 1993) that speak on behalf (are informants) of the various mind sets brought by community people. When a community is creating and supporting its community events, it is learning, producing, reproducing, co-constructing, transmitting and promoting its community ethos. By focusing analyses on community events, it is possible to gain understanding on the essence that informs a community's belief system, not as an agentless source of community energy, but rather as a social and cultural practice. Community events help us understand this process of "community ethos" socialization—that is, how a local community learns and reproduces its community ethos. Thus, spotlighting community events is an alternative way of collecting data on community ethos. This study proposes the following operational definition for community ethos based on the concept of habitus and symbolic systems. *Community ethos is the set of collective belief systems that influence community actions and relationships.*

In no way am I proposing that the construct of community ethos can be measured or defined univocally using community events as a unit of analysis. The community ethos as a latent structure is not measurable by indicators set by methods.

Yet I am proposing that *beliefs*, *actions* and *relationships* are elements of a whole called community ethos. Community events are like kaleidoscopes. They can help us scope elements that reflect a community ethos.

The theoretical framework that informs this community event research method comes from the theory of social capital, a best practice asset-based approach for rebuilding communities, and from an argument based on the work of Geertz (1983), Toelken (1996) and Bourdieu (1977; 1993) framing how community events are symbolic systems that capture local knowledge. I argue in this study that by focusing on community events it is possible to get valuable insights into the ethos of a local community. Moreover, based on an understanding of "what is right" in a community instead of focusing the beginning of the analytical process on understanding "what is wrong" (the pathos), it is then likelier that a more socially inclusive community ICT will emerge from the designing process.

In sum, this participatory design process selects community events, key participants and codifies community ethos with the purpose of aligning the ICT being designed with the community ethos. CERM codifies an unstructured construct (community ethos) into discrete themes, relations, beliefs and actions which are hypothesized to be informing a community's day to day practice. Community events are the unit of analysis because this method argues that an implicit structure resides in this genre that can speak on behalf of what is important in a community. The usefulness of an idea about community ethos, within the context of participatory design, is meaningless without people and becomes real through the actions of community people evolving into community relationships. Thus, the method is effective for spotlighting who are the key people within a local community doing most of the work.

This multi-method approach has deep roots in democratic principles of participation. The research process is influenced by action research (Reason and Bradbury 2002) and assumptions are rooted in the theory of asset management (Kretzman and McKnight 1993). The task of *knowing what to design* (Armour 2000) is driven by insights related to understanding how the ethos is woven through a locality's community events.

THE CERM RECIPE

This study proposes an event-driven analysis based on community events as a framework that can help a participatory community ICT designer capture a community's assets, actions, and beliefs as well as its social relations. The process of discovery of this insight into the power of community events for CI is chronicled through the analysis of four community events presented in the dissertation study (Lastra 2006). The premise guiding CERM is that acquiring knowledge *in situ* of the *community ethos* (versus the pathos) is pivotal for enabling the engagement process between designers and community people, and for ultimately designing more socially inclusive community ICT projects. Due to scope, this chapter presents examples from one community event.

CERM has three basic steps: representation, alignment, and engagement. The representation step focuses on developing fundamental knowledge on the main elements (e.g., community ethos, beliefs, actions, relationships, key participants— identified in this method as *Los Mismos*—community members who do most of the work). The alignment step applies firm insights gained on community ethos to closing the gap of knowing what to build (Fadel and Tanniru 2005). The engagement step or "performance outcome" looks at how the designed space converts into a place recognized by locals as another community event. Closure means that some level of redundancy or consensus in functionalities and constraints being suggested for the ICT has been reached. The CERM recipe is presented next.

Total Preparation Time: To Be Determined Locally
Relative Costs: To Be Determined Locally
Ingredients/Elements: Time and geographic place will influence final results.

    i.   Community Events (past, present, in the making)
    ii.   Beliefs, Actions, Relationships (main elements)

iii. Community Ethos (codification of main elements into aspects or themes vital to a locality)

iv. *Los Mismos* or Same Ones (key people who perform most of the community work)

Participatory Processes

1. *Representation:* Identify and select community events; define community ethos; select and invite "Los Mismos" to participate in the project.
2. *Alignment:* Align goals of community ICT to community ethos.
3. *Engagement:* Mediate or negotiate the conversion of the design project into another community event.

The Participatory Design Method

a. *Representation:* This step focuses on community events as a way of uncovering insights related to the selection of participants (key people who do most of the volunteer work), the community ethos (main elements), and the system functionalities and constraints (users' wants and needs).
- Selection of Community Events
  i. Focus the analysis on community events that occurred in the past, in the present and in the making. Select as representative of the predominant culture of a locality a few (e.g. three to four) events that are common in a community's way of life but also prominent in community dialogues or discussions. Select community events designed and implemented by a collectivity. Observe and inquire: *What are community members talking about?*

ii. Conduct participant observations on these community events. As units of analysis, community events are informants of collaboration and cooperation patterns by helping PD observe, inquire, identify who is participating in the pre-during-post-planning of various community events, or who is just participating as a member of the general audience. Observe and inquire: *What are people saying versus what are community events showing?*

iii. Avoid narrowing the view to only the community events initially selected. It is crucial to this method to adopt a relational view on community events versus observing them as discrete events because this relational view on events is what makes them powerful tools for reducing information overload when the task at hand is to identify key voices, to understand predominant or competing belief systems, to understand community actions, and to spot inclusive (or exclusive) social relationships working within a local geographic community.

iv. One of the goals of this Representation step is to begin discerning key voices and collaboration patterns. Community events help uncover the paradoxes between wants, needs, uses—i.e., inconsistencies in beliefs and actions, "user-perceived sensitivities"[3] in a locality that must be considered and respected when designing a socially inclusive community ICT.

v. Observe and inquire: *What is the set of collective belief systems that is influencing community actions and relationships?*

vi. Observe and inquire: *Who are the key players in the planning, executing and post-planning of the community events?*

○ Selection of Participants

i. Select participants who are active in community work.

ii. Select participants who have first-hand knowledge or experience on the community events selected for analysis.

iii. Contact participants directly and "ask for his or her permission for the interview. Don't work through the family…Always get a yes or no answer directly from the prospective narrator" (Ericson 2001, p. 2).

○ Develop Interview Questions

i. Conduct research on the community events selected for analysis.

ii. Develop interview questions about community events that uncover understandings about the past, present, and future status of the event in the locality. Ask participant if there are any other community events he or she feels should also be included in the study? Why? Ask about historical perspectives and information, communication and technology needs related to the events. Avoid starting the interviewing process by focusing on the pathos. Establish the interviewing pace by spotlighting community assets, passions, goals, interests, accomplishments of the locality. *How did they bring about the community events? Who was involved?*

iii. Conduct formal interviews. Begin by verifying that community events selected are indeed considered by the participant as representative of the community's culture and way of life.

iv. Continue observing key players in the local geographic community (through direct observations, participant observations) regarding their involvement in community work (collaboration and cooperation patterns)

v. Identify a sample of community activists performing most of the work. These activists may eventually be coded by CERM as Los Mismos—the Same Ones. Los Mismos are community members that end-up doing most of the work whatever kind of work needs to get done. They will vary in roles in different community events. In some events they function as key planners while in others they assume the role of basic workers—e.g., are responsible for cleaning-up after the event has finished. Be sensitive to the difference between key voices in the community and project participants. Selection of key community voices is an ongoing process throughout the entire design cycle. The selection of the key voices should not be restricted to those who agreed to participate in the formal interviews.

○ Codification of Community Ethos

i. Transcribe interviews, analyze fieldnotes, and examine documents.

Table 1. Community event: Humboldt Park empowerment plan

A Sample Coding Table Community Event: Humboldt Park Empowerment Plan – HPEP (Present)			
Participant/Role	**Actions**	**Beliefs**	**Relationships**
P1/NGO volunteer P2/NGO director P3/NGO director	Community observer Community observer Active participant in its imple- mentation	A good strategic plan A good strategic plan An important plan	Indirect; weak Indirect; weak

Note: In general, data in this table is collected through informal/formal interviews, participant and direct observations, newspaper articles and NGO reports. [For a detailed description of the process used to create the coding tables, the reader is referred to Lastra (2006).]

ii. Code interviews by identifying information, communication and technology needs, beliefs, actions, and relationships. Look for repeating themes or patterns in interviews using techniques such as Grounded Theory Methods (Strauss and Corbin 1997).

iii. Validate the commonness of themes that are emerging using techniques such as the Delphi Method.[4]

b. *Alignment:* This step aligns or reprioritizes the goals of the community ICT to the common themes emerging (community ethos). As participatory designers gain insights into community ethos it is easier to recognize and respect user-perceived sensitivities that can eventually affect usability of a community ICT.

i. Codify functionalities, constraints and community ethos (see table below).

ii. While constructing the paper model (table) align or reprioritize system functionalities and constraints to the uncovered beliefs, actions and relationships.

iii. Use the Delphi Method to reach consensus on functionalities and constraints being suggested. This step should include all of *Los Mismos* identified so far if by any chance or reason *Los Mismos* have not participated in the formal interviews.

iv. Construct scenarios with the help of key participants basing the stories on functionalities and constraints that are being suggested as useful features for the community ICT.

v. Involve participants in the testing of scenarios with community members.

vi. Adjust the paper model as needed in light of the data being collected through the use of scenarios and formal interviews.

vii. *Putting it All Together: The coding tables of CERM.* The tables below (1 and 2) show an example for coding for community beliefs ("a good strategic plan"). In this case the Humboldt Park Empowerment Plan (HPEP) was developed as an alternative plan to an initial empowerment application that was submitted to the USA federal government that was rejected. The table captures the beliefs of community members to direct action and their relationship to the development of the community event.

EVENT: An Anti-Deterritorialization Tool and Community Builder
Community ICT Functionalities suggested:

Table 2. A Community wellness ICT for Latinos of Humboldt Park

Sample Coding Table A Community Wellness ICT for Latinos of Humboldt Park		
Community Ethos	**Functionalities/Constraints**	**Multiple Frames of reference**
Direct Community Action	1. Communication tool-chats & discussion boards 2. Media tool: webcams and virtual tours of Paseo Boricua	1. Paseo Boricua community has a non-violent *"organized response"* to community problems. 2. PB and HP are exemplars of a Minority Civil Society

Note: data in this table was collected (2001) through informal/formal interviews, participant observations, NGO reports and newspaper articles. PB means Paseo Boricua; HP means Humboldt Park.

1. Demographic information and analysis of Latino census data
2. Provide maps of Chicago wards with mobility data for different Latino groups
3. Showcase businesses within the Paseo Boricua economic/cultural corridor
4. Provide housing information
5. Provide immigration information
6. Provide information on grants and grant writing strategies
7. Communication tool – chats & discussion boards
8. Media tool: webcams and virtual tours of Paseo Boricua
9. *"see* what others are doing"; "share annual reports & strategic plans to avoid duplication of efforts"

A Sample Designed Space

The paper model presented below shows multiple frames of reference considered side by side with functionalities, constraints and community ethos.

System constraints are used in the Sample Coding Table to denote the selection of components that could potentially be included in a community ICT and their possible alignment with the community ethos. System constraints reflect the complexities of the *wants* and *needs* of the participants gathered in the data collection stages.

c. *Engagement:* This step focuses on negotiating and mediating the socially inclusive process while aligning goals of the tool to areas highly sensitive to the community ethos.

i. Engagement occurs throughout the entire life cycle of CERM.
ii. Decide how broad and deep to recast the themes on community ethos into the system functionalities and constraints.
iii. At this step the art and science is to observe how the notion of the community ICT is being transferred back and forth between participants (e.g., researcher-designer, community members, *Los Mismos*).
iv. It is also a crucial step where local participants could disengage from the design project if interest or trust either in the designer or project's goals is compromised.
v. The engagement process sheds light on becoming a good listener and on negotiating disputes.
vi. The key question to monitor and answer throughout this step: *Who really has (or is gradually having) the power to shape the functionalities and constraints of the tool.*

The fundamental question of how to engage a community to participate in designing a community ICT system remains open and requires a depth and breadth of understandings of interactions, negotiations among a community of users, stakeholders, designers, and a melange of cooperative work relationships. Community Informatics needs to develop alternative methods that help participatory ICT designers understand the community as the unit of analysis (Day 1999; Gurstein 2003), as well as facilitate an inquiry into the socially inclusive process that allows (or excludes) a community's opportunity to actively influence the technology being designed.

CONCLUSION

When to Use This Method?

CERM is particularly useful within a PD learning context where the focus of the tool has not been established or the design team does not have clarity about the tool's possible uses or who could be potential candidates to interview or to involve in the design project. CERM's research logic allows for participatory designers to collect and analyze community behavior that is useful for shaping ICT requirements and constraints precisely when the focus of the design project is vague.

The method is useful if the goal is to convert the tool with its related processes into another community event. The design process for CERM, similar to the process for cooking an Enchilada, can be confusing because ingredients are mixed and wrapped together, apparently, all at once. This successful conversion of a community ICT into a place of community action will take time, effort and involve unknown risks because as more people become involved there are risks of longer completion times, more arguing, and of the design project actually becoming a highly contested space, as most democratic deliberation places and/or processes become, but the ultimate payoff will be a participatory community ICT.

Community informatics is in need of developing participatory action research methods and frameworks devoted to the problem of understanding how to uncover hidden communities (Gurstein, 2003) and how to design more socially inclusive community ICT projects (Day 1999). This study explores the development of an event driven framework useful in assisting participatory action research methods in ways to improve its methods of engaging participants in research and development (R/D) intervention design projects.

Concerning participatory design issues and, ultimately, addressing the open problem of how to recast the capturing of local knowledge into designing more socially inclusive community ICTs, this method recasts the design process as a three-step concurrent process grounded in participatory action research methods, prototyping design techniques, and knowledge management perspectives.

CERM provides an alternative way to build participatory community ICTs. It addresses design challenges of finding the right members, detecting *"user perceived sensitivities"*, and helps build a low-cost paper prototype model.

ACKNOWLEDGMENT

The development and application of CERM for designing socially inclusive community ICTs is indebted to the guidance and encouragement I received from my dissertation research committee, Dr. Linda C. Smith (advisor), Dr. Ann P. Bishop, Dr. Michael Twidale, and Dr. Elizabeth Hearne of the Graduate School of Library and Information Science from the University of Illinois at Urbana-Champaign. I also acknowledge here the contribution of the Paseo Boricua community of Chicago, Illinois, for their participation, cooperation, encouragement, insightful comments and interest throughout the various data collection stages of this research project.

REFERENCES

Abbott, A. (1995). Sequence analysis: New methods for old ideas. *Annual Review of Sociology*, *21*(4), 93–113. doi:10.1146/annurev.so.21.080195.000521

Armour, P. G. (2000). The five orders of ignorance: Viewing software development as knowledge acquisition and ignorance reduction . *Communications of the ACM*, *43*(10), 17–20. doi:10.1145/352183.352194

Bauman, R. (1986). *Story, Performance, and Event: Contextual Studies of Oral Narrative*. New York: Cambridge University Press.

Berkenkotter, C. (1995). Theoretical issues surrounding interdisciplinary interpretation . *Social Epistemology*, *9*(2), 175–187. doi:10.1080/02691729508578784

Bourdieu, P. (1977). *Outline of a Theory of Practice* (pp. 143–158). New York: Cambridge University Press.

Bourdieu, P. (1993). *The Field of Cultural Production: Essays on Art and Literature*. New York: Columbia University Press.

Day, P. (1999). Information Policy and Promoting Active Communities in the Information Society. Retrieved from http://www.scn.org/tech/the_network/Proj/ws99/day-pp.html

Delphi Method. Techniques and Applications. Retrieved from http://is.njit.edu/pubs/delphibook/delphibook.pdf

Denzin, N. K. (2001). *Interpretive Interactionism: Applied Social Research Methods*. Thousand Oaks, CA: SAGE Publications.

Ericson, S. (2001). *A Field Notebook for Oral History* (4th ed.). Idaho Oral History Center. Boise, Idaho: Idaho State Historical Society.

Fadel, K. J., & Tanniru, M. (2005). A Knowledge-centric framework for process redesign [Atlanta, Georgia.]. *SIGMIS-CPR*, *05*(April), 14–16.

Fielding, R. T., & Taylor, R. N. (2000). Principled Design of the Modern Web Architecture. Retrieved from http://www.ics.uci.edu/~fielding/pubs/webarch_icse2000.pdf

Geertz, C. (1983). *Local Knowledge: Further Essays in Interpretive Anthropology*. Basic Books.

Gurstein, M. (2000). *Community Informatics: Enabling Communities with Information and Communication Technologies*. Hershey, PA: Idea Group Publishing.

Gurstein, M. (2003). Effective use: A community informatics strategy beyond the digital divide. *First Monday*, *8*(12). Retrieved from http://firstmonday.org/htbin/cgiwrap/bin/ojs/index.php/fm/article/view/1107/1027.

Gurstein, M. (2007). What is Community informatics? (And Why Does It Matter). Polimetrica, Milan. Retrieved from http://eprints.rclis.org/12372/1/WHAT_IS_COMMUNITY_IN-FORMATICS_reading.pdf

Haythornthwaite, C., Bowker, G., Bruce, B., Lunsford, K., Kazmer, M., Brown, J., et al. (2003). Technical Report: *Challenges in the Practice and Study of Distributed, Interdisciplinary, Collaboration*. Retrieved from http://www.igi-global.com/Bookstore/Chapter.aspx?TitleId=27290

Kretzman, J. P., & McKnight, J. L. (1993). *Building Communities From The Inside Out: A Path Toward Finding and Mobilizing A Community's Assets*. Chicago, IL: ACTA Publication.

Lastra, S. (2001). Harvesting community knowledge. In *Proceedings of the 34th Hawaii International Conference on System Sciences*, Los Alamitos CA, IEEE Computer Society.

Lastra, S. (2004). The Power of Community Events for Designing Participatory Community ICTs. *PDC04: The Eighth Participatory Design Conference*, July 27 – 31 Toronto, Canada.

Lastra, S. (2006). *Making sense of community informatics: The development and application of the Community Event Research Method*. Ph.D. dissertation, University of Illinois at Urbana-Champaign, United States -- Illinois. Retrieved October 4, 2009, from Dissertations & Theses: Full Text. (Publication No. AAT 3242911).

Lawless, E. (1993). *Holy Women, Wholly Women: Sharing Ministries of Wholeness through Life Stories and Reciprocal Ethnography*. Philadelphia, PA: University of Pennsylvania Press.

Lawless, E. (2000). Reciprocal ethnography: No one said it was easy. *Journal of Folklore Research, 37*(2/3), 197–205.

O'Neil, D. (2001). Merging theory with practice: Toward an evaluation framework for community informatics. *Internet Research 2.0*: INTERconnections. The Second International Conference of the Association of Internet Researchers, University of Minnesota. Available at http://www.ehealthstrategies.com/files/eval_comm_inf.pdf.

Pitkin, B. (2001). Community Informatics: hope or hype. In *Proceedings of the 34th Hawaii International Conference on System Sciences*. Retrieved from http://csdl.computer.org/comp/proceedings/hicss/2001/0981/08/09818005.pdf

Reason, P., & Bradbury, H. (2002). Introduction: Inquiry and participation in search of a world worthy of human aspiration . In Reason, P., & Bradbury, H. (Eds.), *Handbook of Action Research: Participative Inquiry and Practice* (pp. 1–14). Thousand Oaks, CA: SAGE Publications.

Ruble, D. A. (1997). *The Event Model, Practical Analysis and Design for Client Server & GUI Systems* (pp. 79–115). Upper Saddle River, NJ: Prentice Hall.

Silverman, D. (2001). *Interpreting Qualitative Data: Methods for Analysing Talk, Text and Interaction*. Thousand Oaks, CA: SAGE Publications.

Strauss, A., & Corbin, J. (Eds.). (1997). *Grounded Theory in Practice*. London: SAGE Publications.

Toelken, B. (1996). *The Dynamics of Folklore*. Utah: Utah State University Press.

ENDNOTES

[1]   Berkenkotter argues on the difficulties of conducting interdisciplinary research (1995, p.175).

[2]   For further understanding on this argument, see the work of the Distributed Knowledge Initiative at http://www.dkrc.org and in particular research espoused by Haythornthwaite et al. (2003) on the creation of knowledge products by scientists in distributed communities.

[3]   Fielding, R. T. and Taylor, R. N. "Principled Design of the Modern Web Architecture", http://www.ics.uci.edu/~fielding/pubs/webarch_icse2000.pdf

[4]   A basic description of the technique is available at http://is.njit.edu/pubs/delphibook/delphibook.pdf

Chapter 29
The Ethics Driven Spatial Management in Multiculturalism through ICTs

Sangeeta Sharma
University of Rajasthan, India

ABSTRACT

The new inclusive social dynamics is refocusing the intricacies of formation of social structures. The process of globalization is unifying various cultures leading to the creation of Multiculturalists society. As a corollary to this various ethnic groups are expanding their boundaries to form the larger social structures. The concept of spatial management relates to the management of spaces of various ethno-cultural formations into single social unit. This merging can be facilitated by building up mutual trust and respect for each other, which in turn can be reinforced by communicating with the help of Information and Communication Technologies. Hence the role of ICT in enhancing the process of unification is crucial as it pierces through the tightened boundaries of ethnic groups to develop the newer identities. This unveiled dimension is explored in this article, which focuses on the use of the technology in social reconfiguration.

INTRODUCTION

The social relevance of Information and Communication Technologies in reducing the value-gaps prevalent in different ethnically configured societies is the less explored research area, which needs attention from academia. The divisive tones set by the strict adherences to respective sets of ethnicity are leading to alienation causing turbulent undercurrents. The concept of 'universal whole' has been thrashed out in the recent writings on moral philosophy as the important component of constructing Universal Ethics (see Rachels, 1995; Fleishacker, 1999; Goertzel, 2004). The man-machine interface to build values is yet to find a place in academics. The role of ICT is very distinct in achieving the goal of constructing the Universal ethics and can be identified at three levels, first preparing Database of philosophical, professional and personal values on the basis of

DOI: 10.4018/978-1-60960-057-0.ch029

doctrines perpetuated from time to time; second applying Data mining to excavate the needed ethical patterns and third converting excavated ethics into adaptable value packages. Hence in the times when ethics are eroded despite the Data material available on web nets, reflect the inability of scribbled doctrines to reduce the gap of philosophy and practicing ethics. The ICT interventions can help in locating areas of feasibility amongst various ethnic groups to convert differences into productive alliances due to pervasive nature of such technologies.

The Multiculturalism often conceived as an applied ideology of racial, cultural and ethnic diversity within the demographics of specified place, surfaced in 1970s did provide some normative solutions for accepting the coexistence of various communities in a particular society. It had been adopted as the official policy in many Western nations. This is most debatable discourse, which came under criticism by questioning certain fundamentals and impacts of such policy. (Blainey 1984; Cliteur,1999; Ellian 2002). It is clear that inclusion is not possible within some parochial forms of liberalism (Modood 2007).

The social structures are constellation of various cultures aligned to form the ethical axis with which a particular social identity is associated. However the proliferation of technology in every sphere is building up renewed systems with much larger perspectives congregate to form a universal ethical axis. It will be interesting to explore the possibilities of transforming the communities where people hold on to captivity of their belief systems so much so that they refuse to respond to any movement of evolving a 'universal ethics', because they never evinced any inclination to merging process. It will be pertinent to see the effects of the two simultaneous processes one of retaining individual societal identities and another of merging individual identities into a 'universal whole' in the process of societal restructuring at the global level. The major efforts are needed to evolve a conceptual framework of unifying differ-

ent ethnic value patterns through effective spatial management by providing respectful spaces to communities within the integrated socio-ethical frames. Two means of evolving universal ethics are religious faith and rational thought (Gellner 1992; Ahmed 1992). As autonomous moral agents we have personal responsibility to constantly question the veracity of our own beliefs. The cultural diversity that now surrounds us helps us in this process, by equipping us to obtain an insiders' feel for world views other than our own (Sheikh, 2000). James H. Svara, posits three ways to resolve the ethical dilemmas first, duty ethics or deontology, applies rules to achieve justice; second utilitarianism focuses upon the greatest good for greatest number and third virtue ethics argues that the moral sense should guide the ethical choices (Svara, 1997). The deliberations regarding unification have been brought out in many forums but convertibility of these into practical domains through ICT has not been in focus. This presentation is an addition to visualize ethics as the tool of cohesion with the help of technology.

The technological dimension thus remains at the pinnacle of this analysis, as it is the essential tool of unifying various cultures by perforating the tight boundaries via circulating messages with more humane contents. The unwieldy system will become non-existent either due to not responding or if there is slow pace of response to the humane purpose. In spatial management all three **P**'s are important viz., **pace, perspective, and projection**. The trajectory of social formation at world level is needed to design future. The genesis of future knowledge society lies in evolving a new social matrix based on symbiotic relationship between various ethnic communities to occupy space within integrated whole. This in turn requires perfecting the human minds to nurture relationships beyond the self-driven interests.

The social structures replicate the peoples' psyche in the form of bonding that gives the society a definitive shape and also the fluidity to keep the pace with changes through adaptations. The interlocking of many ethnic groups is redesigning social structures and blurring the boundaries of otherwise separated and closed societies. The emerging socio-ethical configuration all over the world is creating a new social order. The fundamentals are changing, the merging of various cultures is affecting the process of conglomeration, technological proliferations are helping in evolving the new identities, the transition is gripping the world with more worries and commitment to resolve the conflicts, voices of dissents are paving their ways, forces of globalization are acting on so called marginalized societies and such others indicate prognosis towards formation of future society where the humaneness has to be given the right impetus.

This paper addresses the focal research problem of how ICT can help in formation of socio-ethically inclusive societies with universal ethics as the epicenter. This is a normative rationalization of evolving the conceptual construct to envision the potential role of ICT in Spatial Management by creating a congenial environment that will nurture the culture of togetherness as indispensable ground for Multiculturalism by dissolving non-important differences. It also addresses the question of using ICT to enable person to lead life free of parochial visions by agreeing to pursue the exposure of collaborative coexistence. Precisely this paper explores the connectivity between four concepts i.e. Multiculturalism, Spatial Management, Ethical Framework and ICT. The basic premiss is that ICTs can help in mobilizing spaces of ethnic groups in the multicultural society by building up humane-bond by integrating various individual identities within the universal socio-ethical framework.

REVIEW OF LITERATURE

The topical advances in the field of Information Communications and Technology are opening new vistas. In many fields ethically driven decision-making will be presented as unprecedented new

tool for development in future. In such field as agriculture, health, education, human resource, environmental management, transport, and bureaucratic development the consequences could really be revolutionary. The Information and Communication Technology has enormous potential specially in furthering sustainable development with humane core. (UN Secretary General, Kofi Anan, 1997, p.1). The role of ICT in managing ethnic spaces in the multi-culturally stratified social structure is supportive. The collaborative bond can be strengthened by increasing the pace of sharing discourses between various group-constituents including intelligentsia, professional, peasants, younger generation and other marginalized groups. Such frequently structured dialogues bring out tangible areas where process of unification can be maneuvered. The productive exchanges of discourses in the Workshop organized by European Commission led to the advocacy of including the ethical aspects in Information Society. The ICTs are advancing rapidly and are changing the society profoundly (Simon Rogerson, 2007). Workshop organized by French Commission for UNESCO in collaboration with Council of Europe from 13-14 September 2007 brainstormed the issue of using technical tool to mobilize the participation of people to work for collective development of society in addition to the universalization of rights and freedom. Thus its usage to configure society is quite penetrative. Simone Henriqueta Cossetin Scholze in the presentation made in Workshop on Ethics and ICT held in Brussels from 14-15 October, 2004 tried to find out how can we envisage ethically oriented approach through ICTs (UNESCO Division of Ethics of Science and Technology, 2004). It has been pointed out that refined understanding of essential part in describing and explaining social, ethical and political dimensions of IT is needed (Helen Nissebaum,2004). The contribution of Enid Mumford to the discipline of Information Society is enormous; her researches also extend to the field of socio-technical design, and action researches that are well placed in the academia. She promoted the humanization of work and aimed to enlist technology as a tool in this endeavor. Her socio-technical work is predicated on the idea that technology can be used for ethical purpose of improving social reality and explicitly focused on ethics and ICT (Stah, 2007). Mostly the researches in the field of IT and ethics relate to the 'computer ethics' and 'information ethics' (Floridi 1999; Floridi & Sanders, 2002; Bynum & Rogerson, 2004). Jeroen van den Hoven has analyzed the approach to software engineering and system development which is referred as 'value sensitive design' presents the ways in which our accepted moral values can be operationalized and incorporated in IT designs (van den Hoven, 2007). However the center theme of this paper is how ICTs can contribute in building up virtues and can incubate ethical sensitivity in people by designing universal ethical framework which looks beyond the individualized value patterns which have restricted utility in propagating humanity. How the virtuous practices can be designed and perpetuated through technological interventions to sensitize people in general towards kindliness is the basic purpose of this paper. To get an insight into this constructive role of ICTs it will be pertinent to construct a framework to propose an operationally viable solution of managing ethnic spaces in the given society collaboratively. This paper explores and discusses the role of ICTs in attaining the unification of various groups in society through a conceptual construct of 3P framework for spatial management, each P stands for pace, perspective and projection respectively.

3PS-FRAMEWORK FOR SPATIAL MANAGEMENT

The world is undergoing transformation and transitional period for any society is getting over in the era of globalization. The visibility of certain universal trends such as urge for mega markets or emergence of corporate culture or adopting alternative medicine systems or inter-dependability of resources and like others are clustering the individualized social composition into larger units. The retention of individual ethnic identity is becoming increasingly difficult due to emerging compulsions to unite. The experimentation with intermixing of the different communities to amalgamate in combination must be encouraged. The created divides are bridging up for the compulsive and non-compulsive reasons. The individual spaces though are important but so is the creation of collaborative spaces. The creation of collaborative spaces can provide the actual answer as to how to have peace and manage the differences. To group together the conventional rivals into a team can be motivating example for spatial management. This can be used as the mechanism to develop as a 'whole'. It will be pertinent to analyze how the collaborative spaces can be evolved. The logistics of having such spaces involve,

- Identifying those cohesive factors that essentially bind various communities into a social fabric. These are fundamental to the socio-ethical axis of a particular society. Thus forming the nucleus of society encircled by the values, norms, traditions, and conventions that eventually become its guiding ethos. The fundamental axis can also be restructured only if these values come in the way of transformation.

- Identifying those factors, which are neutral and as such do not have much role in shaping the society. But with the planned interventions these passive factors can be activated to have collaborative spaces. These are the areas from where changes can be introduced. The system of education for instance can be one such circle, which has enormous capacity to mould the society, with the well-connected e-networks.

- Identifying those areas of social feasibility where possible alliances can be made to dissolve individual characteristics to form a larger social structure with much more productive perspectives and bigger visions.

There are confluences of seen or unseen factors that are acting on society leaving very few options but to reconfigure the system with visionary mission of internalizing ethical patterns at every level. The process of reconfiguration needs to be in consonance with the process of developing unified ethics. The process of polarization is getting a peculiar focus as a result of two seemingly incongruous processes, one of unification and another of discordance acting at the same time giving rise to unexpected relational equations which is well evident from the recent political transmutations. For instance traditional allies are enlarging the orbit of alliances with new partners thus issues are acquiring central position in relationship. In global sharing the role of three P's that is Pace, Perspective and Projection in managing spaces within the given social structure is very important. It will be interesting to see how individual social structures can be webbed into a complete socio-ethical frame.

Pace- the technological proliferations, which are becoming increasingly diffusive and affecting the human minds, can be used as the source of transformation. The technological advancements are inevitable hence the social pace has to be kept at par with these developments so that positive impacts can be created. The IT has enormous potentiality to draw consensus on introducing eufunctional changes irrespective of the tightened boundaries of few societies by mobilizing public participation through e-discussions. The purpose of this is to know about those ethical patterns, which have been subdued so far, and to open various options before the closed social structures. This is a potential tool of bringing world together and also Vivekananda's initial vision of universal brotherhood a utopian view now seems possible due to better electronic con-

nectivity. Many discourses of awakenings and of soul transformation are already disseminated on web-nets thus uniting all like-minded people from all spheres of life at the world level. The variety is now emerging into a striking unity and there cannot a better time to look back and to prepare a balance sheet of losses and gains in terms of humanity. The literature has to be compiled and shared at a greater pace so that new idealizations can be converted into reality. The pace can help various ethnic groups to,

- Know the positive and negative aspects of their identities;
- Learn to accommodate other ethnic groups with their limitations
- Broaden the myopic visions which may be self-driven thus less productive to make tolerant structures necessary for the buoyant coexistence.
- Visualize the possibility of becoming potential partners in the process of universal transformation and brotherhood to protect humanity at large.

*Perspective-*the increased pace of social transformation with the help of technology is gradually changing the perspective. The perspectives are constructed by the perception any society holds about itself. The inherited norms of culture play an important role in developing the perspectives. The different path to develop an ideal focus, becomes the guiding spirit to act, converges into perspectives and can refurbish the regimented opinions. What individual perceives is within one's limitation but at the same time limitations are also affected by the perception of ideal global society, which can revitalize the basics of humanity through educational institutions. New innovations in the form of digital games and simulations to stimulate classroom dynamics for pre-service teachers giving them an authentic context within which to practice and experience ethical dilemmas and critical thinking to decision making are path-breaking works coming up in ethics through ICT (Schrier and Kinzer, 2008).As the institutions of dissemination of moral values their contribution is of the utmost significance. Seed sown in present will build the future; hence inculcation of right thrust will create a just society, which eventually will metamorphose into a just world. This world will need development of right vision and perspective. The role of changing perspectives in evolving a unified socio-ethical framework is crucial as,

- It will help in internalizing the tolerant attitude.
- It will become inclusive of more ethnic groups thereby converging into a larger social base.
- It will maneuver the equity amongst the groups of diverged nature thereby managing conflicting situations in a constructive mode.
- It will help in upholding the trust-based gesticulation thereby creating a congenial environment for collaborative alliances.

The merging of various communities or classes or groups is not possible without re-molding the perspective with right core. Thus use of ICT in dissemination of right learning might deconstruct some of the inhibitions about other ethnic group and can make them more understandable about each other.

Projection- evolving a different but secured future for the present generation is the most pertinent and obvious question that needs a pressing response. The permutation and combination of inputs to idealize tomorrow's world and then planning the creation of realistic world of future is possible with the help of technological tools. Certain forces will remain even when the society progresses, hence will continue to act in future too, however there are many other forces, which can be molded to deliver the desirable results. The inputs essential for projection are,

- Ethical patterns based on patience, sympathy, purity, perseverance, free of ill practices, endurance, compassion etc. need to be recycled into the social system at a regular interval with the help technological tools so that future becomes coherent with the humane fundamentals.
- The database on ethics can be categorized as Transformative information has capacity of producing positive impact without getting trapped into parochial formations; Transcendental information is capable of building up humane essence by evolving a developmental vision to form universal social structure; Technological information which is capable of upgrading the instruments so as to keep pace with the scientific know-how; Transmittable information which is gathered after close surveillance regarding the kind of information generated need to be put to use by the knowledge based society.
- Internalization of right perspective to have productive alliances with various groups so as to have mega social structures on the basis of principle of equality thereby exhibiting the virtuous conduct and exercise of reason to construct the system.
- Transparent and trust based institutions to minimize the deceptive actions by powerful people against the righteous person.

This 3Ps framework needs ICT impetus to optimize the effectiveness of all Ps included in the framework. The ultimate aim is to design a cohesive ethical frame that might help in changing the mindset of people. It will be pertinent to explore the making of such a frame.

TOWARDS A UNIFIED SOCIO-ETHICAL FRAME

The analysis so far has conceptual ambience but there is no conceptual construct that cannot be operationalized. The prerequisites of operational dynamics would be the existent ethnic groups in a particular society; the core of social identity; the possible junctures of bonds; and the unified socio-ethical frames. The construction of this frame needs excavation and incorporation of sacred virtues that guide people to overcome their vices that are compiled on web nets. For instance the works on consciousness depicted in little book 'The Voice of the Silence' by H.P. Blavatsky,(1889) in which Helena Petrovna Blavasky has said that before the soul can see, the harmony within must be attained and fleshly eyes be rendered blind to all illusions, similarly 'Viveka-Chudamani' - an eighth century philosophical treatise by Adi Shankarachrya, (Chateerji 1932), can be a valuable book source, Ramana Maharshi and the Path of Self Knowledge,(Arthur Osborne 1906; 1995) and such innumerous works of Great Rishis of spiritual geniuses can liberate us from parochial vision. Hence true liberation and salvation can take us to the development of right socio-ethical frame, which can potentially unify divergent personalities and societies by ethically driven human-bonds. This frame, which is based on eternal truths, can manage the spaces of seemingly discordant groups by dissolving the tightened boundaries of religiosity between them and converging into a harmonious group with peace at the centre stage.

The future society would be formed with the knowledge as its epicenter. The right knowledge will have enormous impact in generating renewed thrust in the world relational equations with human face. The proper assimilation and dissemination of true knowledge is possible by optimal deployment of technological tools in collecting, compiling and building productive connectivity within various group components. The E-forums are inexhaustible platforms of liberation from the identity driven socialization. The varieties of subjects included for the conversation are redefining the notional domains of existent concepts thereby helping in deconstruction of the obsolete contents. The web-communities/dg-communities are emerging as potential force of affecting the social dynamics by rediscovering the primary relationships between the partners of the eco-systems. The advantage of this era is technological propagation, which facilitates accessibility of knowledge to people across the cross-boundaries. There is merging of diverse ideologies and doctrines to discover the essentials of universal consciousness. The debates on ethics, morality, and corruption on web-net are infusing newer viewpoints to understand their ramification on social dynamics.

The schema explains the process of conversion of discordant groups into harmonious groups and virtual formation of future society where technology has to fulfill the objective of evolving transcendental humane society.

The operational mechanics with the help of ICT would include the following steps,

- Preparing the complete database about the major and minor ethnic groups including information regarding their mores, customs and value patterns.
- Separating the particularistic and universalistic traits of individual ethnic group.
- Constituting the zone of universal value contents drawn from the various groups.
- Perpetuating these contents at every level of social structures.
- Designing a computer-aided trajectory on the basis of various inputs fed for the spatial management for spacing the various groups.
- Taking policy initiatives to incorporate the required components to get the desirable and projected effects.
- Constructing a precise transcendental road map for achieving and sustaining the redesigned spaces.

Figure 1. Towards Unified Socio-Ethical Frame. (Source: Author herself, 2009)

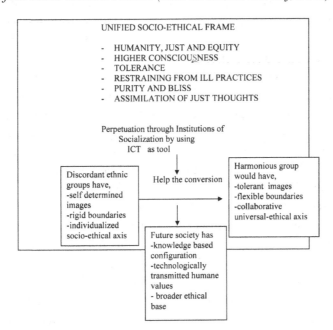

The prerequisites for operability of this frame include, inviting public opinion on values through web nets; organizing workshops to churn out ideas related to inculcation of humane values; designing uniform ethnical code by including values enshrined in different ethic communities; devising the mechanisms to control variances in particular society and involving people around the globe to implement these value designs to combat destructive tendencies. The cyclic schema can explain the process of unification and spatial management.

The role of ICT in exploring the conventions and practices of ethnic groups; in diffusing inhibitions about various ethnic groups; in building up of mutual trust for each other and the last forming the zone of functional space by accommodating various groups in a multiculturalists society is imperative. To imbue the respect for every ethnic group through proper web- networking can resolve the conflicts prevailing in the present times. The continuous perpetuation of the need to nurture the symbiotic relationship in ecosphere is made effortless by the modern technology. The transmission of the redesigned transcendental patterns is feasible through e- connectivity.

The ethics are the spirit of conscientious actions without which no activity can lead to humanity. Humanity comes from humane orientation for the mankind capable of managing the miseries. What causes misery is the pertinent question, which can also answer why is it necessary to build ethics. There can be various ways to look at this sensitive issue for instance psychological way might find it the repercussion of attitudes which in turn comes from cognition, so making one's life miserable gives few people immense satisfaction; the sociological explanation extends to the emerging class differences because of different configuration of social structure that becomes divisive; economical perspective relates to the difference of wealth which gives some people more buying power over the others and so on so forth. Most of these justifications have unreasonable reasoning that makes society more fragile. This in totality leads to the erosion of morality and values thereby damaging the socio-ethical axis. This dysfunctional aspect of social structuring needs to be addressed. Eckhart Tolle in his exposition of 'New Earth' refers to the inherited dysfunction by pointing out that normal state of mind of most human beings contains a strong element of what we might call dysfunction. He further mentions that the science and technology have magnified the destructive impact that the dysfunction of human mind has upon the human himself or herself. That is why according to him the history of twentieth century is where that dysfunction, collective insanity can be most clearly recognized. (Tolle 2000; 2005). In subtle manner one gets apprehensive about the fact that dysfunction of egoist human mind posing potential threats to the planet has now been magnified by science and technology. There are many discourses, which are pointing toward this threat and if not addressed properly might converge into irreparable crisis. The technological progression has to be accurately premeditated to uplift the human face before the race becomes faceless. The management of such dysfunctional actions is only possible when ethics are recycled into the society. The science and technology has enormous capacity to transform the generations, provided, a right thrust gets right direction. The science is capable of creating just society due to its penetrative power, provided that wider issues of humane enrichment are ascertained. The process of unification of ethics can be divided into many stages such as,

- Identification of individual socio-ethical patterns prevailing in the particular society, which extends into the identity. The sources of such patterns may be cultural, religious, traditional, and customs.
- Confluence of similar ethical patterns, which can be collectively identified from the individual society to construct a more tolerant social structure. The role of IT can be more crucial at this level due to its impact capacity.

- Evolving the universal ethical patterns, which will transcend the man created boundaries and differences.

Each stage has very specific focus, which subsequently shifts as we move on to the other stages. This process of converting divergent patterns into convergent patterns is the most fundamental for humankind. Norbert Weiner (1950; 54) developed a method for identifying the enormous impact of ICT upon human values. According to his views the integration of ICT into society will constitute the remaking of society. In his Principle of Minimum Infringement of Freedom he propels an idea that any demand must be exercised in such a way that it does not produce any unnecessary infringement of freedom (Weiner 1954, p.106). In similar exposition it has been spelt out that for any society there will be a cluster of existing laws, rules, principles and practices to govern human behavior within that society (Bynum and Schubert, 1997). The people make the society; if people at large are unhappy then it will lead to violence and eventually towards the destruction. The need of postmodern society is to perpetuate egalitarian aphorism into the social arena with the help of these Technologies.

DISCUSSION

This paper reinforces the renaissance of humanity through ICT to build up such values that can maneuver collaborative alliances for coexistence. There is a need to look beyond rites, rituals, and scriptural knowledge to be able to peruse goals of higher existence. The post modernist mind is receptive to the idea of evolving an objective, standard and rational mechanism of converting ethical disagreements into amicable ethical agreements regarding what must constitute the universal belief system. This paper discusses how ICT can help in deconstruction of mythical connotations and unproductive dictums attached to particular social structure and reconstruct the new transcendental belief system. The concrete examples of benefits have been offered by the Committee on the Ethics of Scientific Knowledge and Technology, COMEST (Kweku Appiah, Chair of Ghana Group, 2004).Macklin anti-relativist opines " who amongst us would defend intolerance and insensitivity as virtues?" (R.Macklin, 1999:268). This paper is a small step forward in discovering the role of ethics building through e- technologies. It raises a very fundamental question- can trust in humanity be restored and perpetuated thereafter through ICT? To this it proposes 3P framework, which is normative in its contention and prognostic in application. This construct the argument that data mining on morality, value and ethics will reconfigure the future knowledge based society with pragmatic solution, provided value contents are converted into packages to endow with road map for inculcating ethics in all sphere of activities. The adherences to ethnicity-based value patterns may not find place in future society. This would mean realignment of ethical axis around which conglomerates the global society. The problem of discordance amongst people of different ethnicities has been manifested at global level can be resolved by creating socially inclusive larger group through spatial management. The term spatial management refers to the mechanism of incorporating various communities in a manner which prepares people to leave aside the coercive elements of their ideological dictums and adapt more amicable ethical frameworks with only core of humanity. The use of ICTs in tracing information on virtues enshrined in philosophical discourses through data mining can help in designing value packages that are free of dogmatic adherences. The prominent characteristics would include value content of universal ethical framework. Thus role of ICT in Spatial Management is important at three levels, one in preparing the data base, two in incorporating the values of every great spiritual traditions into unified value content and third outreaching the people through technological

Figure 2. Pathways of Inclusive Ethics through e- inclusion. (Source: Author, 2009)

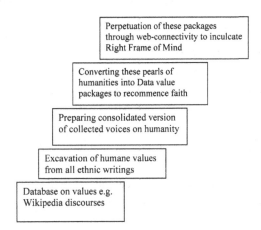

intercession to reset the minds with righteous attitudes instilled with compassion. This paper also conceptually advocates that the emergent trends of negativity which are gripping the world today can be reversed if man-machine interface is used in a productive manner for nurturing the forgotten humane values. Across the religiosity every religion teaches the path of enlightenments then why not to make an effort to liberate individuals from the frigidity of ethnicity. All teachings are rooted in simple, life-patterns filled with unconditional affection for humanity. These are not unattainable but continuous recharging in value-ridden ethics is needed. The ICTs can be the tools of transmission of such values to remind everyone to relive their life without getting trapped into exuberant desires, which deprive many of us of human dignity. Who would resolve the conflict? If people have to resolve than the purity of ideas need to be strengthened. The ways are through social inclusion, ethnic inclusion and e-inclusion that carry every step towards creating violence free societies. The stepwise pathways for inclusive ethics building can be depicted as

The perpetuation of humanity by building-up universal values needs strategic interventions, which are beyond time and space. It will be interesting to explore the role of ICT in not only restoring the trust in humane values but in understanding how technological tools can facilitate this process of building up universal ethics. Parochial interests are driving world towards turbulence. The reversal is possible by redesigning the 'root thoughts of purity' to trigger right feeling and actions thereafter. A structured discussion on How 'Right Frame of Mind' can be evolved through better ICT connectivity to carry out conscientious actions can help in managing confusions at subliminal level. The role of IT in compiling works on ethics is complete but the next phase of designing the set of universal values still need important forum to research out what might be the value content and then percolating at all societal level of world with the help of technologies.

CONCLUSION

The ethical issues relate to the various functional domains of activities. This article takes some steps toward highlighting the potential dynamics of information flow due to emergence of technology into dealing with the ethical dilemmas that might concern the individuals. This paper lends credence to the urgency of designing value- packages to restore the faith in peace by integrating the data available on web nets on philosophies, professional and personal ethics. The ancient doctrines have emphasized that those persons who transcendent the religious boundaries, are tolerant and can recommence the faith in humanity are also the embodiment of giver of unconditional love. Such people will make the society more tolerant and receptive to the ideological adjustments thus contributing to the formation of mega society. Two simultaneous processes must be designed to have a desired impact on the structuring of the future society. First, how much retention of the social identity is required in the process of integration and second, how much intermixing of deviant ethnic groups is possible to evolve the new collaborative identity. The pace of these two processes initially

will need some stimuli such as globalizations, emerging threats of terrorism, reduction in the levels of differences of economic divides, dissolving the extreme ideologies around which the individual social structures have conglomerated or mixing of various races to have hybrid generation before getting the resultant output of the unification processes. Thus the unification can be an alternative for survival rather than retaining the polarized societies with highly individualized identities. The social mixing can be activated with the help of technology, which in turn can help in designing the socio-ethical frames with humane centric index and can also perpetuate the same. The 'better tomorrow' so far is a catchphrase, needs a very rigorous planning before a better tomorrow is really created. The mission of unanimity amongst various groups has to be the core focus. These are manmade groups and can only be disintegrated by man made efforts to evolve a unified social whole. The unity is the key that holds for future revolution. The man created differences in terms of ideologies or status or unintentional injustices have to be put to equality with redefined notion of existing concepts. The ethical patterns are viable cohesive force to build society, which is free of apprehensions giving every individual the space to elevate his consciousness, and eventually converging into a divine. The peace has to come from within that is not dependent on the life's circumstances and this is a profound eternal peace, which can be enabled by ICTs. The ways to attain a balance between inner-self and outer social-self has to be ascertained, as a consequences of which the compassion would become the hallmark of our outer lives. Living in conflicts and dilemmas cannot assure the ethical sustenance. This needs applying academics and esotericism in to action relying on the innate strength. Adopting the Ethical Pathways can resolve the conflicting demands of self and society, selfishness and altruism. The role of ICTs in perpetuation of thoughts proceeding from philosophical anecdotes can provide the basic inspiration to have socio-cultural unification with ethical epicenter.

REFERENCES

Blavasky, H. P. (1889). *The Voice of Silence*. New York: J.W.Bouton. Centenary Edition of the book is published in 1992 by Quest Books Publishers.

Buchman, J. M. (1985). *Liberty, Market and State: Political Economy in the 1980 New York*. New York: New York University Press.

Burjor, A. (2007). *India: The Ancient Past*. London: Routledge.

Bynum, T., & Rogerson, S. (Eds.). (1996). *Global Information Ethics*. Opragon Press.

Bynum, T., & Schubert, P. (1997). In van den Hover, J. (Ed.), *How To Do Computer Ethics- A Case Study* (pp. 85–95). Erasmus University Press.

Chateerji, M. M. (1932). *Viveka Chudamani or Jewel of Wisdom of Sri Shankaracharya*. Whitefish, MT: Kessinger Publishing Company.

Colero, L. (2007). *A Framework for Universal Principles of Ethics*. UBC Center for Applied Ethics. Retrieved from www.ethics.ubc.ca

Drucker, P. (1954). *The Practice of Management*. New York: Harper Business Reissue.

Ethics and Human Rights in IT organized by French Commission for UNESCO. Retrieved from portal.unesco.org/ci/en/ev.php-URL

Fleishacker, S. (1999). From Cultural Diversity to Universal Ethics: Three Models. *Cultural Dynamics, 11*(1), 105–128. doi:10.1177/092137409901100107

Fort, T. (2001). *Ethics and Governance: Business as Mediating Institutions*. New York: Oxford University Press.

Godman, D. (1991). *Be as You Are: The Teachings of Sri Ramana Maharshi*. New York: Penguin Book.

Goertzel, B. (2004). Universal Ethics: The Foundations of Compassion in Pattern Dynamics. Retrieved from www.goertzel.org.

Goniak, K. (1996). The Computer Revolution and Problem of Global Ethics. *Science and Engineering Ethics, 2*(2), 177–190. doi:10.1007/BF02583552

Green, H. (1971). Human Values in Technological Society. *Dimensions of American Judaism, 5*, 19–23.

Hongladarom, S. (2001). Cultures and Global Justice. *Polylog: Forum for Intercultural Philosophizing, 2*, 1–34.

Hongladarom, S. (2007). Information Divie, Information Flow and Global Justice. *International Review of Information Ethics, 7*, 1–5.

Hutcheson, F. (1729). *An Inquiry Concerning Moral Good and Evil*. Retrieved from www.encylopedia.com/doc/1E1-Hutcheso.html

Kalin, J. (1970). In Defense of Egoism. In D. Gauthin (Ed.) *Morality and Rational Self-Interest*, New York: Prentice Hall.

Macklin, R. (1999). *Against Relativism*. New York: Oxford University Press.

Pye, G., & Warren, M. J. (2006). Striking a Balance Between Ethics and ICT Governance. *Australian Journal of Information System, 13*(2), 201–207.

Radhakrishnan, S., & Moore, Ch. A. (1957). *A Sourcebook in Indian Philosophy*. Princeton, NJ: Princeton University Press.

Rogerson, S. (2007). E- Inclusion Ethics. *ETHICOLinthe IMIS Journal, 17*(7).

Schrier, K., & Kinzer, Ch. (2008). Using Digital Games to Develop Ethical Teachers . In Glibson, D., & Baek, Y. (Eds.), *Digital Simulations for Improving Education: Learning Through Artifial Teaching Environment* (pp. 308–333). Hershey, PA: IGI Global.

Sheikh, A., & Gatrad, A. R. (Eds.). (2000). *Caring for Muslim Patients*. Oxford, UK: Radcliffe Medical Press.

Smith, A. (1759). The Theory of Moral Sentiments. In A. Smith (Ed.), *Moral and Political Philosophy* (hH. Schneider, New York, NY: Harper & Row. (1948 & 1978).

Strasnick, T. (1981). Neo-Utilitarian Ethics and Ordinal Representation Assumption. In by J.Pitt. (Ed.) *Philosophy in Economics*, Reidel Publishing.

Sugden, R. (1986). *An Introduction to Game Theory and the Spontaneous Emergence of Cooperation in the Economics of Rights, Cooperation and Welfare*. Oxford, UK: Basil Blackwell.

Svara, J. H. (1997). The Ethical Triangle . In Bowman, J. S. (Ed.), *Public Integrity Annual* (pp. 33–42). Lexington, Ky.: CSG/ASPA.

Toll, E. (2000). *A Power of Now: A Guide to Spiritual Enlightenment*. UK: Hodder and Stoughton.

Toll, E. (2005). *A New Earth: Awakening to Your Life's Purpose*. UK: Dotton.

Van den Hoven, J. (1996). Computer Ethics and Moral Methodology. In P. Barroso, S. Rogerson & T. Bynum (Eds.) *Values and Social Responsibilities of Computer Science,* Proceedings of ETHICOMP 96. Computence Univesity Press: pp.444-453.

Van den Hoven, J. (2007). *The Information Society: Innovations, Legitimacy, Ethics and Democracy. IFIP International Federation for Information Processing, 233* (Goujon, P., Lavelle, S., Duquenoy, P., Kimppa, K., & Laurent, V., Eds.). Boston, MA: Springer.

Wiener, N. (1948). *Cybernetics: Control and Communication in Animal and the Machine*. London/New York, UK/NY: John Wiley & Sons.

Wiener, N. (1954). *The Human Use of Human being*. Boston, MA: Houghton Miffins.

Chapter 30
From Social Capital to Social Production:
Implications for Individuals, Organisations and Nations

Margaret Tan
Nanyang Technological University, Singapore

ABSTRACT

In recent years, the advancing and sophisticated interconnectivity of the fast-evolving interactive digital technologies have dramatically created a new space that is both virtual as well as physical, that is both conceptual as well as real. This new collaborative space known as the 'co-space' provides a new paradigm shift to the economic and social ecology of information and knowledge creation. For instance, various social networking tools and technologies that enable individuals and the communities to express, communicate, and interact to share their creative works and knowledge in the new 'co-space' can facilitate profound networks of relationships that not only constitute a valuable conduit for the conduct of social affairs but also the social production of intellectual capital. In other words, as social production becomes a critical contributor in the knowledge-based economy, it is important to recognize that the key to today's innovations may be developing the organizational ability to harness such social production efforts so as to use them in the formulation of competitive actions at the individual, organizational as well as national level.

THE IMPORTANCE OF SOCIAL CAPITAL

Although the concept of social capital has been much discussed in the past by researchers, such as the sociologists and economists, it is important to revisit the concept in the new context of the fast-evolving interactive digital and media technologies which have dramatically created a new collaborative space called the "co-space" – that is both virtual and physical, and that is also both conceptual and real. Defined by Cohen and Prusack (2001), social capital consists of "the stock of active connections among people, such as the trust, mutual understanding, and sharing of values and behaviors that bind the members

DOI: 10.4018/978-1-60960-057-0.ch030

of the human networks and communities, which in turn, make cooperative actions possible". The structure of social capital can take several forms in terms of social norms and relationships. For instance, some may be close-knit and exclusive while others may be in the form of loose ties and yet share some commonalities (Carilli et al. 2008). In other words, in cultivating the various relationships, individuals interact with each other using certain signals like membership in a group or association, the adoption of a language, or other cultural practices, as such signals are accepted in conveying their credibility and trustworthiness to each other (Leeson, 2007).

In this context, a society is said to have strong social capital when there is a high level of information and knowledge sharing in an environment of close and trusted relationships. Thus, the building of social capital is posited to be more likely to develop "in collectives characterized by a shared history, high interdependence, frequent interaction, and closed structures" (Wasko and Faraj, 2005). The central thesis is that networks of such close and trusted relationships constitute a valuable conduit for the conduct of social affairs, which in turn facilitates the creation of new intellectual capital. In short, when there is a high level of social capital in a particular network, it acts as "the fabric around which knowledge and intelligence and activities spin" (Rothberg and Erickson, 2005).

In recent years however, the ability to express and communicate information and knowledge has been dramatically facilitated across space and time by the advent of easy interconnectivity tools and digital media applications. Indeed, and coincidentally so, a modern-day social phenomenon has been quietly developing in the virtual space. Whether one should be alarmed or not, it appears that many individuals and even communities are increasingly looking to cues from one another rather than from the traditional institutional sources. This is because the new interactive and digital media technologies are allowing individuals to bypass conventional conduits to readily and voluntarily produce and share ideas, opinions, information and creative works in innovative ways.

THE RISE OF SOCIAL PRODUCTION

Various enabling interactive digital media such as blogs, forums, email, instant messaging, twitter, social bookmarking and other instances of what is often called 'social networking' software can be intriguing for researchers to understand how individuals mobilize information and knowledge in the collaborative virtual space. The simplicity of using such media has led to the creation of a critical mass of adopters or users. For instance, setting up and maintaining a blog is an excellent example of how easy the social networking process can be. A person can simply sign up for a free account at any blog-publishing sites, such as WordPress or Blogger. Videos and photos can be easily inserted into the blog by uploading and then linking to the free YouTube video-sharing service and Flickr photo-sharing service for example. Tracking visitors can be readily done by signing up with MyBlogLog (again a free service) while allowing visitors to subscribe to regular blog postings can be simply accomplished by opening a free account with Feedburner to use its RSS technology (Carr, 2008). Online chats and comments can also be easily enabled to facilitate interaction with visitors on such blogs. Beyond blogging, Facebook and MySpace are also examples of free-access social networking websites whereby users can form and/ or join specific community networks to connect and interact with other people.

The rapid evolution of social networking technologies has also made it possible to have varied collaboration on an unprecedented scale. This is because the electronic network can scale quite seamlessly to very large numbers of participants and efficiently bypass the traditional limitations associated with complex large-scale cooperation (Hansen et al. 2006). Let's take for example, Wikipedia. It is based on the premise that anyone or everyone can participate as peers in contributing their knowledge, expertise and resources to an overall project. More important, such collaboration can take place asynchronously and instantaneously across time and space.

On close reflection, what is particularly surprising about this growing phenomenon are the scope, scale and sophistication of collaborative peer production of knowledge within the respective electronic networks of practice (Carr, 2008). This rather sudden rise in social production of knowledge poses an interesting question about the motivations of such people when they energetically and jointly participate in contributing their knowledge on a voluntary basis (Benkler, 2006). Recent research has shown that such social production occurs for a variety of reasons including people's perceptions that it enhances their professional reputations to contribute their expertise, especially when they are structurally embedded in the peer network. Interestingly, these voluntary contributions are made "without regard to expectations of reciprocity from others or high levels of commitment to the network" (Waswo & Faraj, 2005). This is somewhat contrary to the traditional assumptions of social capital. In other words, with the radical changes in electronic networks of practice that fast-evolving information and communications technologies have engendered, social production (rather than exclusive focus on social capital) may be the new phenomenon that researchers should increasingly pay attention to. Importantly, this recent rise of social production in today's knowledge-based society has profound implications for individuals, organizations and nations.

IMPLICATIONS FOR INDIVIDUALS

In a society that is increasingly characterized by the rise of social production, what will make a person more likely to be successful or influential

in the future? Traditionally, it is posited that such individuals would typically possess a high level of intellectual intelligence (IQ) and/or emotional intelligence (EQ) (Goleman 1995; 1998). In the future however, it is likely that people will increasingly also need a different kind of intelligence in order to participate effectively and responsibly in a world in which both the physical and virtual spheres overlap – in the new world of 'co-space' where collaboration will increasingly be the focal point of human endeavor.

In the physical world, for example, it has long been acknowledged that human beings are gregarious and sociable. Humans have been argued to possess a built-in bias toward empathy, cooperation, and altruism, and as such, "social intelligence" may be what makes one person better able than oth\ers in nurturing these capabilities to be successful and/or influential in society (Goleman, 2006). In the virtual sphere which is still taking shape and where networking can have a dramatic multiplier impact, a similar kind of social intelligence – which can be termed as "social networking intelligence" - is needed. Successful individuals are likely to be those who are network-savvy and who also have the sense of empathy, cooperation and altruism to see themselves as potential contributors to public discourse and as potential actors in chosen arenas (Benkler, 2006). Although, the ordinary person would be largely content to be just passive recipients of knowledge flows, some bloggers today command high respect and their regular blog postings attract a big and faithful following on the Internet, in spite of the continuing dominance of mainstream media. It appears that such bloggers intuitively understand that a different kind of intelligence is needed to be successful on the Internet. A good example is Michael Arrington's Techcrunch blog which began in 2005 and has quickly become one of the most influential news websites dedicated to profiling and reviewing new Internet products and companies. This site is now ranked one of the world's most popular blogs by Technorati, with

Business Week magazine naming Arrington one of the most influential people on the Web.

Against this backdrop, a couple of questions come to mind. How would the educational systems prepare the new generations of young minds to participate and collaborate responsibly and effectively in the new co-space? How would we prepare the education curricula to take into account the new dynamics of students interacting and living in the 'co-space', that is, both physical as well as virtual?

IMPLICATIONS FOR ORGANIZATIONS

Driven by the traditional emphasis on social capital, sociologists and other researchers have long studied social networks of individuals within organizations and in society at large. Accordingly, corporate best practices in knowledge management have traditionally revolved around the provision of a variety of trusted environments for communication and collaboration to facilitate knowledge creation and sharing (Keen & Tan 2007). However, traditional knowledge management often excels at gathering, codifying, and storing knowledge but it is not as effective in enabling employees at all levels to seek out pertinent knowledge on an on-demand basis (Rothberg & Erickson, 2005).

In recognizing the rising importance of social production, it can be argued that there is a need to move beyond traditional focus on knowledge management towards greater understanding of the dynamics of knowledge mobilization. While traditional knowledge management addresses the supply side of information organization (ie., the institutional mechanisms to encourage knowledge creation and sharing), knowledge mobilization reflects the demand side that is dominated by knowledge being part of individual identity and hence personal choice of whether, where, why and with whom to share knowledge and expertise (Qureshi & Keen 2005; Keen & Tan 2007). For

example, corporate blogs are largely driven by personal initiative and have the potential to become a significant force in mobilizing knowledge production and sharing within, across and beyond the organizations. In fact, several world-class companies such as Microsoft, Sun Microsystems, Infosys, for example, claim that these blogs have significantly improved their ability to reach, influence and communicate with the community, partners as well as their customers. This concept seems to hold true as noted by Technoratic CEO, David Sifry, who commented that "Bloggers are an incredibly influential consumer segment. These people are hugh networkers. They get the word out quickly on products they like – and they don't like" (Kline & Burstein, 2005). In the same vein, Catherine Paker, a marketing guru explains, "If your company is releasing a new product or service, no formal marketing method meant to increase its exposure can match the power of people talking to each other." And that is because most people are immune to marketing hype, thus, a referral from an unbiased blogger can often have more impact than the expensive advertising (ibid).

If blogs are indeed powerful platforms that may make or break a company, it is alarming to note that most companies do not yet have official blogging policies. In a study of some Fortune 500 organizations, Lee, Hwang and Lee (2006) found that many organizations attempt to balance autonomy and control in determining their corporate blogging strategies. Organizations with a bottom-up blogging strategy tend to focus on product development and customer service content, while those with top-down blogging strategy tend to focus on thought leadership. This search for the "ideal" balance between bottom-up and top-down and between autonomy and control continues to be an important concern in the corporate world of today. Thus, if blogs represent big business opportunity, for the corporations, the new key to today's competitive advantage may be in developing the "mobilizing" ability of the workers to leverage the social production efforts and use them in the ongoing formulation of competitive actions.

Against this backdrop, several questions come to mind. Will traditional organizational structures still be effective in the dynamism of the fast evolving co-space? What are some possible new ways to organize employees to better exploit the social production phenomenon for innovations and competitive advantage? Will social production lead to increases in business productivity and economic growth?

IMPLICATIONS FOR COUNTRIES

Over the years, the debate over what makes one country more successful than another has evolved into the search for the economic system, policies and the role of the government that can sustain international competitiveness over the long term. Porter (1996) notes that such competitiveness is "the degree to which a nation can, under free and fair market conditions, produce goods and services that meet the test of international markets while simultaneously maintaining or expanding the real incomes of its citizens". Specifically, it includes the ability of the nation to sustain future growth relative to that of rival countries.

According to Porter (1994), favorable factor conditions may yield sustainable competitive advantage for a firm based in the particular country, because determinants such as education, industry networks and social structures are less permeable across national boundaries and thus, is country-specific. In today's knowledge-based economy, such factor conditions will increasingly include the capacity of the nation's citizens to engage in social production for national competitive advantage. In the government machinery of most countries however, there appears a lack of appreciation of the future impact and potential value arising from the sudden rise of collaborative peer production of knowledge which can even be across-borders. Many countries do not seem to have policies to

encourage and manage (responsible) social production for (active) knowledge mobilization. This lack of attention to the rise of social production is not surprising especially in countries where independent websites, unrestrained blogging and online forums are viewed with a certain degree of ambivalence and caution by the institutional authorities. Since the dynamism of the modern knowledge-intensive economy makes it difficult for one person or an elite group of persons (however outstanding) to lead everything from the top, this lack of recognition of the potential value of social production (and the need to channel it appropriately) may impact a country's future competitiveness vis-à-vis other nations. On the other hand, failure to channel such energies to productive and constructive use may allow the emergence of increasingly unexpected outcomes that may run out of control. This is because the downside to the virtual world is that it is also vulnerable to falsehoods and untruths being propagated rapidly throughout electronic communities, sometimes with the objective of rallying certain segments of the population to stir unrest.

In a sign that traditional institutions are recognizing the increasing influence of activities in the virtual world, authorities in many countries throughout the world are gradually paying attention to the blogging phenomenon with regards to its possible impact on election outcomes, for example. In the United States, it was reported that both the Democratic and Republican parties issued press credentials to certain citizen bloggers during the U.S. presidential election in 2004 so that they (the bloggers) can cover their respective national conventions. Indeed, the social networking tools were effectively deployed in the 2009 presidential election. In the recent 2008 elections in Malaysia, political postings by bloggers appeared to be widely followed by the general populace and were acknowledged by the Malaysian Prime Minister to have some impact on the final election results (with the ruling coalition suffering unexpected shock defeats in several states).

Against this backdrop, several questions come to mind. Should the social production phenomenon be allowed to grow in an unfettered way? Is it possible or desirable for governments to channel such energies towards productive ends, and can such intervention be made without trying to exploit the situation for political advantage?

CONCLUSION

In closing, Benkler (2006) documents the revolutionary and fundamental changes in the ways in which global citizens today are producing and sharing - aided by social networking technologies - ideas, information and creative works. To put it succinctly, this new world of 'co-space' may shift the economic and social ecology of information and knowledge creation, with profound impact on the global economy and society. In turn, this has important implications at the individual, organizational and national levels.

At the individual level, citizens must increasingly reflect on how they can participate effectively and responsibly in a world in which both the physical and virtual spheres increasingly intersect. At the organizational level, companies need to be cognizant that the value of information and communication technologies (ICT) goes beyond just management, sharing and analysis of data and information, and that the strategic value of IT may instead lie in its ability to facilitate knowledge mobilization and innovations. Finally, at the national level, governments must begin to encourage responsible social production – in line with enhancing national competitiveness and building nationhood - while being alert to possible unexpected consequences of new and unprecedented citizen participation in political and social arenas.

Currently being propelled forward by a confluence of several forces including fast-evolving networking technologies, new interactive digital media applications and intensifying human collaboration, this rise of social production - beyond traditional focus on social capital - deserves greater attention on the part of researchers and practitioners alike in the new knowledge-based economy.

REFERENCES

Benkler, Y. (2006). *The Wealth of Networks: How Social Production Transforms Markets and Freedom.* New Haven, CT: Yale University Press.

Carilli, A. M., Coyne, C. J., & Leeson, P. T. (2008). Government intervention and the structure of social capital. *The Review of Austrian Economics, 21,* 209–218. doi:10.1007/s11138-007-0035-z

Carr, N. (2008). *The Big Switch: Rewiring the World, from Edison to Google.* New York: WW Norton & Company.

Cohen, D., & Prusak, L. (2001). *In Good Company: How Social Capital Makes Organizations Work.* Cambridge, MA: Harvard Business School Press.

Goleman, D. (1995). *Emotional Intelligence.* New York: Bantam Books.

Goleman, D. (2006). *Social Intelligence.* New York: Bantam Books.

Hansen, K. K., Larsen, C. F., & Olsen, J. B. (2006). P2P: Information Exchange & Knowledge Production. Retrieved from http://rudar.ruc.dk/bitstream/1800/2941/1/P2P%20Production.pdf

Keen, P., & Tan, M. (2007). Knowledge Fusion: A framework for extending the rigor of knowledge management. *International Journal of Knowledge Management, 3*(4), 1–17.

Kline, D., & Burstein, D. (2005). *Blog! How the newest media revolution is changing politics, business, and culture.* New York: CDS Books.

Lee, S., Hwang, T., & Lee, H. H. (2006). Corporate blogging strategies of the Fortune 500 companies. *Management Decision, 44*(3), 316–334. doi:10.1108/00251740610656232

Leeson, P. T. (2007). Balkanization and assimilation: Examining the effects of state-created Homogeneity. *Review of Social Economy, 65*(2), 141–164. doi:10.1080/00346760600709960

Qureshi, S., & Keen, P. (2005). Activating Knowledge through Electronic Collaboration: vanquishing the knowledge paradox. *IEEE Transactions on Professional Communication, 48*(1), 40–54. doi:10.1109/TPC.2004.843296

Rothberg, H. N., & Erickson, G. S. (2004). *From Knowledge to Intelligence: Creating Competitive Advantage in the Next Economy.* Oxford, UK: Elsevier Butterworth-Heinemann.

Wasko, M. M., & Faraj, S. (2005). Why should I share? Examing Social Capital and Knowledge Contribution in Electronic Networks of Practice. *Management Information Systems Quarterly, 29*(1), 35–37.

Chapter 31
Seeking Utopia:
Communities and the Commons in the Contemporary Media Environment

Natalie Pang
Nanyang Technological University, Singapore

ABSTRACT

The chapter starts by elucidating the concept of the contemporary media environment as a complex interaction of two computing variables: the growth of personal computers, and the popularity of the Internet and World Wide Web. This environment is then analysed for its impacts on collective processes in both virtual and physical communities. It is argued that these collective processes contain multiplier effects; and one of these effects lies in the subtractability of resources; an important concept in the knowledge commons. Examples are used to illustrate these perspectives. The author maintains, throughout the chapter, that it is essential to see all of these interactions as two-way, dialogical relationships and structuration theory is used in support of this argument. As a concluding note, the chapter makes a number of forecasts on the benefits and potential pitfalls for the society as a result of these relationships.

INTRODUCTION

As far back in 380 BC, philosophers have thought about, and debated about the ideal community. Thinking around such work was perhaps best captured in Plato's *The Republic*, where he began with the attempt to define justice – highlighting that 'it concerns the way we ought to live' (Ferrari, 2000, p 28). In that light, he also lamented that 'the unjust man enjoys life better than the just'

(ibid, p 35) and argued for the need to address these issues in order to achieve a 'just' community.

These thoughts by Plato were later made popular by Sir Thomas More's *Utopia* in 1516, describing a fictional island with an outwardly perfect social system. Since this famous work, communities, philosophers, researchers, writers, and the like – have used *Utopia* to refer to the desire for an ideal society. The study and desire for the commons today (Pang et al, 2008) reflect a core belief in such epitomes. Likewise, Hardin's (1968)

DOI: 10.4018/978-1-60960-057-0.ch031

Figure 1. Dimensions of the duality of structure (Giddens, 1984, p. 29)

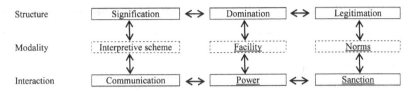

famous essay on the 'tragedy' of the commons also summarises criticisms against the commons.

Does it remain an unrealistic dream? Or have people, communities, the society at large – been defining and refining their own *Utopia*, even if unconsciously? The criticism that it is unrealistic aside, *Utopia* captures the essence of Plato's *Republic*, where a society ruled on principles of equality, peace, and tolerance was also sustainable because of its focus on collective instead of self interests. At the core of these ideals is the fabric of collective processes governing communities, and an inquiry on how it has evolved together with changes in the contemporary media environment is important.

This is the key objective of this chapter, and the chapter endeavours to achieve this goal by discussing structural forces shaping, and are shaped by communities – at the same time making distinctions between the key collective processes governing communities of today.

THE DUALITY OF STRUCTURE

Giddens argued that structures, together with meanings and actions are continuously interdependent:

The best and most interesting ideas in the social sciences (a) participate in fostering the climate of opinion and the social processes which give rise to them, (b) are in greater or lesser degree entwined with theories-in-use which help to constitute those processes and (c) are thus unlikely to be clearly distinct from considered reflection which lay actors may bring to bear in so far as they discursively articulate, or improve upon, theories-in-use (Giddens, 1984, p. 34).

This clearly articulated the recursive nature of human relationships in communities. In the everyday exchanges between human actions and structures, people are also constantly transforming the very same structures that empower or constrain their actions. This insight is essential in realising that the study of people and their interactions with various political, technological, social, or economic structures there is the inevitable dilemma of structure and agency. In other words, studies involving human communities must account for both objective and subjective realities.

The central notion of structuration theory focuses on how the conflict between objective and subjective realities can be resolved. Structures are viewed as 'both the medium and outcome of the reproduction of practices' (Giddens, 1979, p. 5). Given this insight, cultural context can thus be understood as being generated and regenerated through the interplay of actions and structures. This is known as the duality of structure, which is explained as:

Structure as the medium and outcome of the conduct it recursively organizes; the structural properties of social systems do not exist outside of action but are chronically implicated in its production and reproduction (Giddens, 1984, p. 374).

Using three analytical structures, such duality can be illustrated (Figure 1). Structures of *signification*[1], *domination* and *legitimation* are termed as analytical – as in reality these are not dichotomies. However, for the purpose of illustration they are clearly distinguished as in Figure 1. At the level of interaction are three residing actions which are constrained or empowered by their structures. In the middle row are three modalities, acting as mediators between the three analytical structures and actions. For example, a structure of signification can be changed using the action of *communication*, through the use of *interpretive schemes*.

Structuration theory is a highly complex conceptualization and must be understood in the contexts it is applied to. For the purpose of this discussion, it is sufficient to draw from structuration theory the two-way, dialogical relationships between humans and objects. At the same time, it is essential to recognise that institutional properties shape, and can be altered by human actions.

In this chapter the social system within which institutional properties are embedded is the contemporary media environment. The next discussion will examine how it has come about, and their implications for communities.

THE CONTEXT OF THE CONTEMPORARY MEDIA ENVIRONMENT

Using historical research, Pang and Schauder (2007) made the observation that the intense 'growth of personal computing in the late 20th century' and the 'potentially decentralised, self-organising technology of the Internet' were developed (p. 209). This was termed the 'PC/I (Personal Computing/Internet) threshold', explained as:

the transition from large centralised computing with non-interoperable networking arrangements to autonomous decentralised computing with a globally interoperative Internet (Pang and Schauder, 2007, p. 209).

Operating as a structural environment, the PC/I threshold led to the growth of the World Wide Web (WWW), a complex medium by which people connected to the Internet can access and contribute knowledge using their personal computers (including mobile devices). The decentralised nature of such an environment has important implications; especially in the growth of user-generated content – quickly produced and exchanged. Due to such increased velocities of production and exchange content can be circulated at a nominal cost over the WWW; making up a significant portion of the knowledge commons. Much attention has also been given to the rise of participation within this context, with the help of computing devices.

An example is Twitter, a social messaging and micro-blogging application allowing users to post messages and follow the updates of others. This is simple enough; but the interfaces that are linked to a user's page are complex and multi-faceted. For example, a user can update his Twitter page using 'Twitterrific', an application on the iPhone, the Web, or via 'Tweeter', a Facebook application. Figure 2 and 3 shows examples of the common applications available on two media platforms to help users post and read updates on Twitter.

There are other examples of changes that have come about due to the PC/I threshold. The increased need for global communication, coupled with progresses in internet connectivity – faster, clearer, and cheaper – led to the growth in Internet telephony. Applications such as Skype, allow users to utilise their existing Internet connections to communicate with others around the world at only a fraction of the prices they used to have to pay using a landline.

The developments of personal computers and broadband connectivity revolutionised the ways music, television, and movies are now consumed. Other technological applications such as iTunes, or web portals have been developed to allow consumers to pay for entertainment on a per-view or per-piece basis from the comforts of their homes instead of having to go to a record store

Figure 2. By adding 'Tweeter' in Facebook, users will be able to update their Facebook statuses whenever they post to Twitter. Likewise, status updates to Facebook will also update their Twitter pages. In addition, users will also be able to follow Twitter updates of their social networks from the Facebook application.

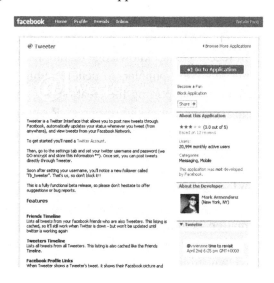

Figure 3. Twitterrific can be added to the iPhone via iTunes, as a free application from Apple. With this application, users are able to post messages and micro-blogs to Twitter whenever they connect to the Web or the third generation network using their iPhones.

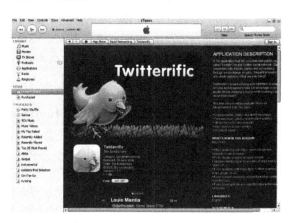

to purchase whole albums. Of course, there are pitfalls with such development – digital copies are also more susceptible to being illegally copied or manipulated.

The examples are not limited to consumption. Distinct practices have also emerged from various disciplines such as the creation of music and art, curator practices in library and museum collections, and politics – all involving bigger bandwidths and better equipped personal computing devices. Rural library and museum collections in Australia have begun to make use of communication technologies to engage the participation of stakeholder communities that were otherwise disconnected because of their remoteness (Pang et al. 2008; Pang et al. 2006). In recent years, the use of social networking applications such as blogs, YouTube and Twitter have penetrated political scenes in countries such as the United States, Malaysia, Thailand, Australia, Israel, and Netherlands.

It would be a mistake to view the advances in computing devices and the Internet as two disparate but coincidental developments. With structuration theory, it is convincing to posit that these two trends had all along been shaping each other. In other words, growths in Internet connectivity have also impacted progressions of computing devices, and vice versa. As Giddens noted, the human agent is one of the keys behind all these changes. In their groups and mass communities, they are powerful catalysts and shapers of the media environment that compels and at the same time, provides sanctions for their actions.

COLLECTIVE PROCESSES IN THE CONTEMPORARY MEDIA ENVIRONMENT

Whenever individuals come together in a community, even if such a community is virtual, issues inevitably arise about individual and collective interests. This is the principal driver of Olson's collective action theory (Olson, 1965). Asserting that individuals will not work together to contribute to a common good, or common resources without coercion or incentives, collective action theory sets up clear conditions for individuals to cooperate:

Unless the number of individuals in a group is quite small, or unless there is coercion or some other special device to make individuals act in their common interest, rational, self-interested individuals will not act to achieve their common or group interests (Olson, 1965, p.2).

This argument provided support for Hardin's (1968, 1971, 1982) reasonings on 'the tragedy of the commons and problems of collective action' (Lichbach, 1996). The pessimistic view of the commons in this case suggests that if resources are freely available to everyone, people won't behave in a sharing way. In other words, people abuse what's free. The issue of 'free-riding' in communities is universal, regardless of the types of communities, and whether they are bounded by market mechanisms, instrumental reasons, or social bonds.

Ostrom provided empirical evidence that communities in fact invest voluntarily in resources for the purpose of 'monitoring and sanctioning the actions of each other so as to reduce the probability of free-riding' (Ostrom, 2000, p.138).

Ostrom (2000) also pointed out that the theory of collection action and the probability of free-riding is often contradicted by everyday observations of people behaving as individuals or in groups. For example, many people tend to vote in elections without coercion; people do not, and accept that, as a general rule, cheat on their taxes (and likewise, those who do cheat on their taxes are punished by legitimate structures in the form of moral sanctions); and people do voluntarily contribute to associations and charities.

Motivations aside, such observations highlight that there are different layers and levels of collective processes driving actions within a community. The chapter will explore and distinguish these processes; but it is crucial to introduce the knowledge commons first, as it is an important dynamic and entail different collective processes at various stages in the development, or use of a common resource.

The Knowledge Commons

Historically, the term 'commons' refers to the use of common land used by people in communities. In recent years, 'knowledge commons' has become relatively popular, to denote public or shared spaces supporting the creation, use, and storage of public knowledge resources. Resources created under such conditions are therefore free from market constraints, and are accessible to everyone in the community.

Understandably, the study of the commons has thus given rise to a range of terms including the information commons, the learning commons, the creative commons, the cultural commons, and so on. Ownership is a constantly recurring issue: are resources that are collaboratively created, shared and used – owned by everyone, no-one, or something in between?

This is an ongoing issue of debate, especially with regards to accountability and control. An analogy is seen with the problem described by Hardin (1968) as the 'Tragedy of the commons'. His classic essay in the journal 'Science', Hardin articulated anew the conflict between public and private good in the exploitation of a finite resource. This conflict was a highly political issue in England in the early 18th century, when common land was systematically transferred to private ownership or 'enclosed'. At that time one of the key arguments in favour of such enclosures was that in private ownership the land would be well maintained and productively used, whereas in common ownership an increasing population would merely exploit the land for personal advantage with no incentive to maintain it (Linebaugh, 2001; Lloyd, 1833).

Stories such as these suggest that there are varying degrees of availability of resources to communities. In other words, certain resources are, or only become common, to the defined community congregating around them. This is referred to as 'subtractability' – first formally conceptualised by Ostrom, Gardner and Walker (1995) and further studied by others (Carpenter, 1998; Schlager, 2002). A working definition of 'subtractability' is put forward by Carpenter:

Subtractability deals with whether or not one person's appropriation of a resource reduces the availability of that resources for others (1998, p. 38).

High subtractability is characterized by well defined boundaries offering resources only to specific communities; in their creation, sharing and use of these resources. Low subtractability on the other hand, has loose or easily permeable boundaries that can be easily accessed to others beyond a specific community. Because they are often shared widely, such resources are the most difficult to exclude, and their appropriations does not result in unavailability to others.

The contemporary media environment not only includes to the increased importance of knowledge processing characterized by information and communication technologies; it is also driven by the existence of abundant networks of people who are connected by strong and weak bonds, sharing and creating knowledge resources together. The earlier examples, along with many examples in the contemporary society, show that the media environment enables the transformation of resources to take on different characteristics: reducing their subtractability and increasing the scope of participation in communities.

Without coercion or centralized directives, people are creating and undertaking actions towards collective interests in large groups. What this also implies is that collective action as conceived by traditional collective action theory by Olson, 1965) may warrant further work with the goal of conceptualizing more complex and varied forms of collective action with contemporary media.

The relationship between participation and subtractability is therefore inverse and recursive. The greater the participation, the lower the subtractability of common resources. At the same time, resources with low subtractability can also enable greater participation. The self-created blogs and 'tweets' (as discussed earlier) containing book reviews, stories, and thoughts in general, trigger people to comment, share and submit their own contributions through the same or other communication technologies – thereby facilitating participation in the creation and sharing of resources with others.

Borrowing perspectives from structuration theory, such communication facilities inherent in contemporary media contributes to a structure of signification, through shared interpretive schemes. This is an important insight to the picture of the knowledge commons, as not every resource is in the knowledge commons – only the ones that are shared and communicated are considered significant to the communities that create, share and use them.

No community, however, can claim to possess collective knowledge without the involvement of others, especially in the process of collaboration. The production of knowledge in a community is never an isolated process: without the inspiration of others, whether they are remote or direct. De Angelis (2006) argued that without communities Hardin's (1968) proposition of a tragedy of the commons would be true. In the context of the knowledge commons, it is put forward here that without communities there will be no commons. This leads on to the suggestion that the relationship between the commons and the collective processes driving its creation, sharing and use is an intricate one. Three key collective processes are explained.

Three Key Processes

With communication tools that enable people to easily participate in the creation, sharing and use

Figure 4. A vision of collective processes

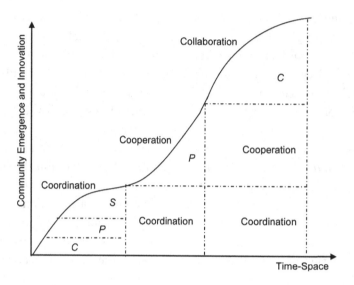

of resources, these resources change in terms of their extents or degrees of subtractability. The community therefore provides sustainability to the commons, as collective resources in the commons will deteriorate over time due to high subtractability. Such effects are recursive. With resources characterised by high subtractability, communities cannot evolve to the state of collaboration; implying a lack of emergence and innovation. While the tragedy of the commons argued in 1968 (Hardin, 1968) had the pursuit of self-interests of individual property owners as its premise, the tragedy of the knowledge commons of today will be caused when a community halts its progress and evolution, and stops negotiating its boundaries. This is the reason why the state or public institutions alone are not sufficient: the community is necessary to sustain a healthy and vibrant commons; often with the aid of the contemporary media environment.

This insight has been made clear with the examination of public institutions. In six case studies of cultural institutions in Australia and Singapore, the involvement of the museums was crucial to the sustainability of resources in a collection. Yet, as recognised by the cultural institu-

tions themselves, the collections also cannot be without the communities that identify with them and are motivated to contribute positively to them. Collective processes that drive such contributions are therefore significant in their associations with the types of characteristics arising from resources in the knowledge commons.

The evolution of collective processes involved in the knowledge commons is envisioned through the time and space analogy of Giddens (1979). This is compared on a vertical axis of community emergence and innovation. A high level of community emergence and innovation is less prescriptive and the community is characterised by self-organising attributes.

A representation of this relationship is illustrated in Figure 4. As seen from the figure, the relationship between collective processes over time and space, versus the total emergence and innovation of the community resulted in an S curve. Interactional practices outlined by structuration theory (Giddens, 1979) – sanctions (S), power (P), and communication (C) – are represented in each collective process, with the interdependencies between coordination, cooperation, and collaboration highlighted via underlying areas under the curve.

The dependencies of community emergence and innovation versus the time and space continuum of social practices are represented as concave and convex curves. In this figure, coordination (represented by a gradual concave curve) stipulates a basic level of community emergence over a rapid collective process of coordination in order for communities to collectively produce and use common knowledge resources. Cooperation, which implies procedural compliance, is reflected as a convex curve – indicating the growth of cooperation on a diminishing (but still increasing) level of community emergence and innovation. The highest level of collective process, collaboration, is represented at the top part of the curve – a steeper concave curve – highlighting the emergent and dynamic networks that are constructed and de-constructed in the case of collaboration.

The factor of defection is defined as the departure of one or more community members from the original goals of the community. Defection for all three collective processes is not included in this picture, as they are independent of time and space, and the impact of defection on collective emergence and innovation in a community can be insignificant depending on the community. A tightly coordinated community can have minimal defection and still emerge over time and space and become creative. A collaborating community in producing and using knowledge resources, such as the open source movement of software development, can have high rates of defecting but still remain innovative in terms of contributing and using knowledge resources from the community. This is perhaps best manifested by many virtual communities, such as those that congregate around open source projects.

The implications of defection are varied and dependent on a wide number of variables, such as group dynamics, communication devices, the strength of social networks, and so on; and

although it is not examined here in considering collective processes of knowledge production and use, further work is required to study their implications in greater details.

Collaboration is therefore the most desired form of collective process in the context of producing and using knowledge in communities. It should not be misunderstood as a collective process without cooperation and coordination – because if viewed independently as a dichotomy on its own it would only stand as a vague and abstract concept that is hard to achieve in communities. Although it is significantly different from coordination and cooperation, it is an evolved form of collective process – and in the context of contemporary media where time and space are highly dynamic and continuously redefined and renegotiated, the evolution of collaboration is similarly vibrant, characterised by a rapid rate of knowledge transfer and sharing, highly unpredictable community networks that are bounded together for multiple reasons, emergent relationships and high levels of creativity. Examples such as Wikipedia and the many peer to peer networks purposed for knowledge production and use are testimonies to collaboration.

Time-Space Influence on Collective Processes

As Giddens (1979, p. 54) argued, time-space intersections are 'essentially involved in all social existence'. While all three proposed types of collective processes can be observed in everyday life and in institutional case studies, they were not dichotomies and evolve in many different ways. In other words, the collective processes did not exist in isolation and are shaped over the time-space continuum.

The greater the complexity of collective processes such as cooperation and collaboration, the more likely they need time to evolve and with certain forms of space. For example, in one library, the use of online spaces (i.e. blogs and shared

Figure 5. A vision of collective processes (revised from Figure 4)

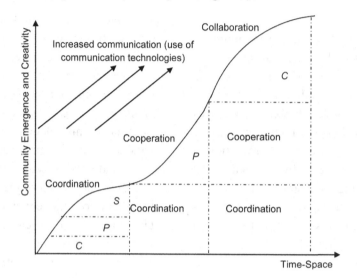

book reviews) provided people with a platform to create dialogue on thematic areas of interests. In another case of a museum in Australia, an online portal helped to facilitate contributions and sustain cooperation with a rural women community. In such examples, the institution and communication technologies were both powerful catalysts in engaging, over time, with communities who were challenged with potential internal disconnections by physical distances, inter-generational values, and a rapidly changing societal structure.

Such examples reinforced the relevance of the time-space continuum to collective processes, thereby in congruence with Giddens' (1979) assertion that the time-space intersections are omnipresent in social existences. In addition, the role of contemporary media in shaping the emergent collective processes from communities was clear – informing the picture further as an additional insight. Depending on the types of media, institutions and organisations could engage their communities in certain collective processes, and they evolve over the time-space intersection.

This insight is also consistent with Figure 1, where collaboration is envisioned as predominantly characterised by communication at its

core of interaction. With communication facilities embedded in contemporary media, it is therefore not surprising that collaboration occurs when institutions utilise contemporary media technologies in their interactions with their communities.

Where communication facilities are not present, collective processes that emerge from communities are characterised by power relations and established sanctions – cooperation and coordination – reinforcing the earlier proposed picture (Figure 4) of collective processes. The figure is revised in Figure 5, this time reflecting the effect of increasing the use of communication technologies.

As shown in the figure, increases in communication can shift collective processes towards greater cooperation and collaboration. However, this intersection should not be perceived in isolation or misunderstood as implying a technological determinism of the various collective processes. Increased communication should be viewed as interacting with the time-space continuum and at the same time can be shaped by, or shape the overall emergence and innovation of the community.

This has implications for both cultural institutions and communities, in that communication technologies may be considered to draw or engage communities in deeper interactions. This finding also adds an additional perspective to the concept of collaboration (Schneider, 2006; John-Steiner, 1998), which contends that collaborators can work with one another without being directly connected. The use of communication technologies can facilitate collaboration in the absence of direct connections between potential collaborators.

In terms of participation, the finding distinguishes communication as a key factor in transforming collective processes towards collaboration. In instances of cooperation, power relations between the cultural institution and their communities become a key enabling factor.

Coordination, on the other hand, is seen as the most fundamental form of collective process; resting largely on established sanctions and norms. Coordination is argued to be the most basic process underlying different collective energies from communities. Although it is the least complex, it is a fundamental component: without which, other collective processes which are more complex in nature – are not sustainable over time.

IMPLICATIONS FOR CIVIL SOCIETIES

The implications for societies are diverse; and this will be explained in light of three types of structural forces in a civil society: public institutions, social networks, and the public sphere.

There have been many arguments for the erosion of institutional structures and their influences on civil society. While it is conceivable to say that institutions have indeed changed in contemporary times, it is argued here that they pose an important dynamic to the bonds and eventual collective action in a society. Quite often, they set up power relations with their communities, and when power distances were perceived differently in dissimilar cultural contexts, the accepted power relations between the cultural institution and their communities also differed.

What this means for institutions, therefore, is this: utilizing contemporary media technologies is not a clear-cut decision. However, it needs not be complicated, as the first question public institutions need to ask themselves is whether or not their communities are already empowered adequately to participate and engage. Some cases have shown that certain cultural institutions are often the proactive initiator of cooperative projects with communities. This however, does not imply that the potential of cultural institutions in initiating cooperation with their communities would be undermined in cultures that are less self-organising and are more likely to view great power distances between public institutions and local communities. It is essential for institutions to realize that collective processes are constantly negotiated over time and shared spaces, and institutions as much as communities shape such evolution.

As a matter of contrast, in cultures demonstrating a shorter distance of power, institutions would be more likely to leverage on the already empowered community for collective action. In such cases these communities are also more likely to proactively interact with cultural institutions in cooperative arrangements.

The increased use and integration of technologies in everyday life presents a dialogical paradox. Communication technologies allow individuals to interact with one another with greater velocities and spaces. In this sense, individuals will be able to form tighter bonds with people that were not previously possible with cultural, proximity and language factors.

This presents an isolation at the same time. A simple one can be understood by pointing to communities who, for various reasons, have limited or no access to communication technologies that enable them to connect with others. So these communities may live in isolation, but may have strong bonds within their own groups. A more complex issue of isolation lies with the first group – those who have access to communication technologies and are intense participants. This level of isolation is individualistic in nature. As they form social networks across wide spaces with unlikely people, they may become increasingly disconnected from their own immediate, local community. Therein the paradox: and it remains a salient issue that governments, social institutions, and individuals must all confront and address.

The last implication is associated with the public sphere. One of the greatest impacts of the contemporary media environment is that it has made everything 'flatter' (Friedman, 2006). So there is, in essence, greater communicative freedom that is enabled by communication technologies. As already witnessed this has brought about benefits in the sense that there is a greater amount of information and knowledge resources that are available, either freely or at affordable expense to anyone who desires them.

This however, also brings with it the challenge of managing information integrity, quality, security and privacy issues. There is also greater democratization in politics, as manifested by the online presences of many prominent political leaders in recent years. The ease of communication has resulted in a trend of decreasing deliberations by individuals, communities, and institutions. In other words, it is argued here that the public sphere is undergoing a great transformation, with the contemporary media environment as one of its key drivers.

This chapter sets out as one of its key goals to engage readers in a discourse about distinct collective processes, bearing in mind that such processes are never in isolation and are constantly in negotiation (and renegotiation) with structural forces such as their institutional frameworks, and the contemporary media environment. Though it remains a pilot framework to be improved, these insights are essential to provide important perspectives to the commons. At the same time, it argues that communities are connected today in diverse forms of collective actions. While this picture is not exactly the Utopia that More envisioned, it is necessary to acknowledge that there is now an evolution towards their ideals. Further work is required to develop this framework deeper, such as the inclusion of the self and collective interests (which may provide a tension to a community), and the implications of defection.

REFERENCES

Carpenter, S. R. (1998). Sustainability and common-pool resources: Alternatives to tragedy. *Philosophy and Technology*, *3*(4), 36–57.

De Angelis, M. (2006, November 1*). On the "tragedy of the commons* (that is, the tragedy of commons without communities). The Commoner. Retrieved December 4, 2006, from http://www.commoner.org.uk/blog/?p=79

Ferrari, G. F. F. (2000). *Plato: The Republic.* (T. Griffith, Translation - Original work published 380 BC. New York: Cambridge University Press.

Friedman, T. L. (2006). *The world is flat* (2nd ed.). London: Penguin Books Limited.

Giddens, A. (1979). *Central problems in social theory: action, structure and contradiction in social analysis*. Berkeley: University of California Press.

Giddens, A. (1984). *The constitution of society: Outline of the theory of structuration*. Cambridge, UK: Polity Press.

Hardin, G. (1968). The Tragedy of the Commons. *Science*, *62*, 1243–1248.

John-Steiner, V., Weber, R., & Minnis, M. (1998). The challenge of studying collaboration. *American Educational Research Journal*, *35*(4), 773–783.

Lichbach, M. I. (1996). *The cooperator's dilemma*. Ann Arbor: University of Michigan Press.

Linebaugh, P. (2001). 'The Red-Crested Bird and Black Duck'—a Story of 1802: Historical Materialism, Indigenous People, and the Failed Republic. *The Republic Journal*, 2(Spring/Summer), 104–125.

Lloyd, W. F. (1833). *Two lectures on the checks to population*. Oxford, UK: Michaelmas.

More, T. (1961). *Utopia*. (P. Turner, Translation - Original work published 1516). London: Penguin Books.

Olson, M. (1965). *The logic of collective action*. Cambridge, MA: Harvard University Press.

Ostrom, E. (2000). Collective action and the evolution of social norms. *The Journal of Economic Perspectives*, *14*, 137–158. doi:10.1257/jep.14.3.137

Ostrom, E., Gardner, R., & Walker, J. (1995). *Analysing long-enduring, self-organised, and self-governing CPRs*. Ann Arbor, MI: University of Michigan Press.

Pang, N., Denison, T., Williamson, K., Johanson, G., & Schauder, D. (2008). Augmenting Communities with Knowledge Resources: The Case of the Knowledge Commons in Public Libraries . In Aurigi, A., & De Cindio, F. (Eds.), *Augmented Public Spaces: Articulating the Physical and Electronic City* (pp. 185–199). Ashgate Publishing.

Pang, N., & Schauder, D. (2007). The Culture of Information Systems in Knowledge-Creating Contexts: The Role of User-Centred Design. *Informing Science: The International Journal of an Emerging Discipline*, *10*(Monograph), 203-235.

Pang, N., Schauder, D., Quartly, M., & Dale-Hallett, L. (2006). User-centred design, e-research, and adaptive capacity in cultural institutions: The case of the women on farms gathering collection. In C. Khoo, D. Singh & A. Chaudhry (Eds.), *Proceedings of the Asia-Pacific Conference on Library & Information Education & Practice* (A-LIEP 2006) (pp. 526-535). Singapore.

Schlager, E. (2002). Rationality, cooperation, and common pool resources. *The American Behavioral Scientist*, *45*(5), 801–819. doi:10.1177/0002764202045005005

Schneider, F. (2006, November 6). *Collaboration - some thoughts concerning new ways of learning and working together*. Centre for Research Architecture. Retrieved March 7, 2007, from http://roundtable.kein.org/node/525

KEY TERMS AND DEFINITIONS

Communication: regarded as a 'general element of interaction, and is a more inclusive concept than communicative intent (i.e. what an actor means to say or do)' (Giddens, 1984, p. 29). In other words, communication is regarded as an interaction or action between people – rather than simply intending to communicate. Communication between humans agents draw from and also shapes interpretive schemes (modality).

Community emergence and innovation: refers to communities who displays high levels of this are less prescriptive, more creative and innovation.

Domination: as conceived by Giddens 'is the very condition of existence of codes of signification' (Giddens, 1984, p. 31) and is dependent 'upon the mobilisation of [authoritative] and [allocative] resources. This is an analytical structure that is shaped by, and shapes in turn the use of power in the interactions between people and facilities allocating resources.

Facility: a modality that refers to the ways by which both allocative and authoritative resources are allocated. Facility is reflexively applied in the sustaining or distribution of power, or it is caused by the exercising of power relations in interactions. It shapes and is shaped by the structure of domination. For example, an administrator of a website is granted certain rights (facility) and this may also shape, or be shaped by his position in the community.

Interpretive schemes: 'are the modes of typification incorporated within actors' stock of knowledge, applied reflexively in the sustaining of communication' (Giddens, 1984, p. 29). Unlike the other two modalities (facility, norm), interpretive schemes are not explicated through written documents or acknowledgements. Giddens claimed that most discourse in communities are in fact characterised by this modality, given the need to apply knowledge in social encounters. In other words, becomes practical rather than theoretical within this modality.

Legitimation: refers to formally accepted social orders and codes of conduct, are enshrined within the norms and the use of sanctions in interactions.

Norms: refer to sanctions that have been normalised and formal legitimations that have resulted in norms. In structuration theory, norms exist as a modality that mediates and is shaped by both legitimation and sanctions.

Power: seen by Giddens as 'inherent in social association or human action' (Giddens, 1984, p. 32). It is 'not just the capacity to say no' but includes the capacity to transform how resources are allocated. The use of power in the interactions between people is shaping and shaped by structures of domination through the modality of facility.

Sanctions: refer to 'the constraining aspects of power...ranging from the direction application of force or violence, or the threat of such application, to the mild expression of disapproval.' (Giddens, 1984, p. 175). Sanctions are felt as coercion, which culminates as norms, or are shaped by these norms. As interactions, sanctions have a recursive relationship with the structure of legitimation.

Signification: is mediated by the modality of interpretative schemes as signs and knowledge that has been 'the medium and outcome of communicative processes in interaction' (Giddens, 1984, p. 31).

ENDNOTE

[1]   Selected terms which are defined in the glossary section appear in this form, when they are mentioned in their contexts for the first time in this paper.

Chapter 32

Convergent Media Policy Issues for the Developing World:
The Need for Digital Independence

Eduardo Villanueva Mansilla
Pontificia Universidad Católica del Perú, Perú

ABSTRACT

ICT4D policies tend to present two problems: they are designed without consideration of the larger role ICT play in society, especially regarding communication and cultural issues; and they are based on local effects, not considering the potential society-wide effects. This paper analyses this set of issues and proposes an approach that shifts the focus from the institutional focus of policy making to societal considerations that include the potential for cultural development, with emphasis in the need for digital independence, not just in terms of infrastructure, but also of production and consumption of media products based on a dynamic and dialogic community of users.

DEVELOPMENTAL SHORTCOMINGS

Information and communication technologies (ICT) have been the object of many debates regarding national policies in the last twenty years, with a surge corresponding to the successful expansion of the Internet outside of its original area of education and academia, towards almost all aspects of society. The policies proposed and pursued during the last decade have been transformed from "information society" ones to more specific, subject oriented ones, with emphasis in the intellectual

property, free and open software promotion, and educational aspects of the perceived benefits of ICT implementation, at all levels of society.

In the Global South / Developing World / Third World, the emphasis has not changed: policies, being general ones like the "information society" approach, or subject specific ones, have been focused on development. This particular term is an elusive one, that is not the purpose of this paper to define. However, it may be broadly considered as a significant change of a set of economic, social and cultural conditions that will align living conditions of a given country with the standards of the Developed World, as measured by standard

DOI: 10.4018/978-1-60960-057-0.ch032

indicators, including per capita income, or more recent ones, like the Human Development Index promoted by the UNDP.

Ignoring for the moment the practical, economical, cultural or even the ethical implications of development as understood in the industrialized countries of the world, this specific goal has been present, in many specific forms, in a large numbers of national policies, international agreements, and programs and projects, drafted by the countries involved, by national or private donors, by international bodies and even by individuals and collectives interested in the advancement of human conditions all around the world. In many cases if not the full majority of those, the intentions are sincere and honest. In too many cases, the actual results have come appallingly short of the expected outcomes.

In the area of ICT, the abundance of development agendas and plans for developing information / knowledge societies is quite significant. Development has taken the route of the full set of information policies to more specific approaches towards economic and industrial development, infrastructure building, educational reform, basic social services, e-government, and lately, specific hardware initiatives for educational purposes. But two main sets of shortcomings may be identified as part of the reason why these projects haven't brought the desired development to the poor nations of the world, besides the fact that the money spent, no matter how large the numbers appear, is actually small.

The first set of shortcomings is directly related to the structure of project-based development, with its priorities set by donor agencies, its calendar-based schedules and their sets of structured goals, that oftentimes have a weak relation with actual social or economic transformations, and a strong link with donor satisfaction. This collection of problems is well documented, and has a long tradition that is not reserved for ICT projects, but present in many different areas.

The second set is more directly related with ICT, both with its main characteristics and the illusions brought by their potential, by what has been called its transformational nature. ICT, being very flexible and user-transformable technologies, with global reach but easy to be perceived as "localizable", are extremely tempting as a perfect tool for almost any problem. Development is seen as just one of many problems to be dealt with ICT, and being new and "sexy" they are the *plat-du-jour* for those interested in not losing the current or forthcoming bandwagon.

The problem lies in the reality of ICT-based development, that has acted in many occasions as the proverbial hypodermic needle. Introducing ICT does not bring development, especially when the problems created by the introduction are sometimes larger and more complex than those that should have been (and sometimes are not even remotely close to been) solved through technology.

It is a matter of scales and a matter of pertinence. Scale, because in many cases the transformation that ICT may bring is too small and unrelated to the actual causes of the problems being addressed, since the existence of ICT as a manifestation of economic success is just that, a manifestation of a complete societal stage where the combination of productive forces, market agents, human capacities and social, cultural and educational conditions have not only brought the actual ICT but have created the environment where they flourish and are an ingredient of success, a commercially-viable proposition or a tool reachable by all. Even successful projects are too small to transform all the aspects that may turn one specific case into an engine for growth.

But it may the case that the pertinence of technological projects is even more critical to success than the scale. Pertinence, a more complex issue, is related to the role ICT may play in different levels of society and in facing actual problems, that in each case, may be better confronted through the use of different tools. It may be the case that ICT is not a pertinent solution, or that digital media is not pertinent, is disruptive or too difficult to use as a component in development strategies. The experiences so far are not necessarily conclusive, and there are many different areas of government action that are being proposed as the ideal grounds for ICT projects; but it may be stated that there are many different subjects and issues where technology-based solutions compete with other, non-ICT based ones, that may be better or at least equal to the task, with less investment needed.

The crux of the matter lies in establishing exactly what is to be developed: specific solutions to very concrete problems, or something more elusive but actually more important, like human capacities, not just skills, for taking control of ICT and making it a part of locally-defined strategies for growth. Both at the individual and the organizational level, these capacities are present, certainly in less than adequate levels, in many if not all the developing world; problem is, they are not available to all the members of society, nor are attainable for all, since they are costly, complex and in many cases, not even taught at local schools or businesses.

It is ultimately a matter of agency, that is, the capacity to appropriate ICT towards self-defined ends. Being individual agency, organizational agency, or social agency, it is a significant resource, and as defined by Amartya Sen, among others, the inequality of agency, that is, the less-than-equal distribution of agency all along a society, is at the basis of poverty and underdevelopment. Creating conditions for agency building should be one of the main goals of development policy, specially ICT-based policy; its absence as a consideration in many policies is thus critical.

ACCESS AND CONTENT

One of the main issues to be addressed in the fight against poverty and for development is the structural disadvantages that the poor inhabitants of a given community or country are facing. Not just poverty measured in income terms, but also structural poverty, based on structural inequalities of which income disparities are just an indicator, and this whole subject may be one of those where ICT solutions have to be thought again to see if they are the right ones. From a wider perspective, there has been little if any recognition of inequality, in its many different meanings, as a critical issue to be attacked from as many angles as possible. ICTs, digital media or mass media are not seen as part of strategies of development that may change not only specific economic indexes but the general conditions of any developing / poor society. The fight against inequality should not be just a question of macroeconomic indexes, but an attempt to change the conditions of individual and social development, providing opportunities for all.

Following this reasoning, what we should be concerned about is not only income inequality, but also *agency* inequality, as a result of structural conditions of inequality derived from the existence of entrenched poverty. As such, agency inequality needs to be addressed at the same time than other forms of inequality; the best possible avenue for addressing this form of inequality is through complex media and technological policies that develop the potential of the population beyond their current conditions, including the use of ICT for economic and cultural development. The Peruvian example serves to call attention to two of the main problems coming from these failed approaches, and may serve as an starting point for developing an inclusive analytical framework. These two problems are the access to technology emphasis and the disconnection between media and new media / digital content in policy making[1].

While many Peruvians are able to participate in the external manifestations of the global economy, as buyers of legal or illegal digital content and able users of digital media, interpersonal or otherwise, the actual way that this participation is taking place is not as creative and engaged members of a global community, but as secondary players, consuming content and finding ways to take advantage of digital resources to gain advantage, in economic and social terms, inside the unconnected part of Peruvian society. The end result is a wider gap between those who have access not only to technology but to knowledge and know-how about the practices, values and possibilities of the global economy and those who not.

A clear effort to promote a different approach to policy-making have to consider this gap (or "divide", if so preferred) and the strategies to close it. Accessing the vast potential of information available through digital media present a specific challenge, since usage of this information towards creation of knowledge demands understanding of the role information plays in the current global economy, not just access. And here we have a significant problem. But, as stated before, older, mass media has to play a part, because the problem itself is both of an economic and cultural nature, and has to be addressed from these two angles.

However, there is a problem with the digital media part of the equation. Despite any promise thus far, or many attempts to reverse current trends, market forces and cultural fads have combined to create wide-ranging access mechanisms to ICT, in the form of many variants of the cybercafes existing all around the world, while not promoting any change in the overwhelming dominance of First World-produced content. Thus, the cybercafes and the Internet in general are wonderful channels for accessing non-local content and not necessarily much more. Those beyond the reach of the cybercafe, due to economic, geographical or language/cultural reasons, or a combination of them, are left with the access mechanisms provided by development projects, or without any access at all.

Curiously enough, those who are not the subject for development projects, have less-than-ideal access to the Internet, on their own terms and for their own purposes, and probably will continue to access digital media, with only those under the poverty line or under institutionalized access (at

school, perhaps at tertiary-level education) will have contents fitted for purpose. But those accessing those contents may not be able to access digital media outside of the controlled environment of project-created access mechanisms, with all the potential issues about sustainability and continuity in time.

The previous argument should not be read as denying any role for ICT in development, but rather that the focus should be slightly shifted, both in terms of the target population and of the issues confronted. ICT is a powerful tool for fighting inequality, to promote economic development and to enhance individual opportunities, but not necessarily for all and every member of society at the same time and at the same rate. The following will try both to assert this point and to propose a different, more complex focus.

CONCEPTUALIZING INEQUALITIES

Just recently, some researchers from economics and social science backgrounds have started to replace the much abused *digital divide* with *digital poverty* (Borja and Gigler 2005). This new term assumes that the question to be researched is not accessibility or usage of technologies, but the impact these technologies have as a component of poverty analysis and poverty reduction / alleviation strategies. Assuming that, although the easiest to measure, demand for technologies is just the means for estimating and reducing digital poverty (Barrantes 2005), this approach actually tries to establish a link between digital poverty and agency, being the issue here actual income poverty, generational gaps or discriminatory situations that impinge on the possibility of individuals to try and find ways to take advantage of technology and digital information towards the personal (and ultimately social) goal of reducing poverty.

Digital poverty is a complex concept, not only multi variable both also combining different realms of social and economic analysis. Including people effectively under the standard, income-defined poverty line will not be enough, since there are many occasions when those individuals are actually using digital information as a way out of poverty, as many community-based experiences with telecenters have shown(Delgadillo, Gómez and Stoll 2005). Therefore, it may be considered that the absence of technological supply is the first level of digital poverty, if this absence is due to personal or specific social conditions (lack of sufficient income or lack of aggregated demand in the area of residence / work to bring operators interested in providing service); a second level of digital poverty is one of ability, when both the services and the conditions are in place but the individual is not capable of using the media. And finally, there is also a demand issue, when having both access to the media and the basic abilities, and income to use for this, the potential customers are not interested in digital information.

However, any category as wide as "digital information" requires clarification. Apart from the standard critique, as in Winner (1989) or Valovic (2000), of "digital" as inherently better than "paper" information, there is also the issue of what exactly is information for those using digital sources. At least three big possible conceptions of information are simultaneously used by different players, and sometimes the resulting confusion obscures the discussion even more than it normally is.

A *cabina* is a place where any kind of signals are provided to all kinds of users. The nature of the predominant user creates a market that drives development of a specific kind of *cabina*, that strives to provide the best possible service for the primary or predominant user. Neighborhood *cabinas* are inhabited by throngs of teenagers playing *Counterstrike* or *Doom*; *cabinas* in the vicinity of universities offer services for students; *cabinas* in high-street areas offer services for young professionals, families, youngsters looking for music or IM-ing opportunities. The nature of these specific markets creates a specific *cabina* supply [2].

Information, in the *symbolic* sense, is the manifestation of human agency as communicative agents, and allows us to exist in society and to increase our common knowledge stock. It is the result of our cultural exchanges too, and any society creates information as part of its cultural processes. The significant change that the 20th century brought was the conversion of the cultural manifestations of popular western culture into a commodity, the product and commercial value of the cultural industries. The mass media was created to deal with this kind of information, and still does, and presents a powerful image of what is culturally desirable to the masses of the world, including the developing world, even if they already have a significant culture scene with manifestations available on its own media.

What is normally understood as information is the one that serves as *data* in large databases and may be used for productive purposes, being running a factory or writing a paper for a conference; it may be actual data, or the capacity for processing such data into end-user services, middleware or backroom services, or basic data for research. This kind of information, traditionally stored in libraries or archives or maybe handbooks and manuals, is now being made available on the Internet and other digital media. The usual understanding of the Internet as the realm of information as productive data is shown when it is stressed that social agents will use the Internet as rational agents to make the best possible decisions towards the best possible course for their own interests; it is interesting to notice that many of those that actually use digital media do not act as rational agents but as consumers of information in the symbolic sense. Even more so: the abilities and capacities of those that usually access the Internet for symbolic exchange purposes can be construed as different, maybe even as opposite, to the abilities and capacities that information as *productive data* demand.

Finally, there is a third aspect under which information may be considered. The flow of data across the world is basically a collection of rather undifferentiated *signals* that have, traditionally, been separated by its being mainly a cultural product (as media) or interpersonal or institutionally relevant data (telecommunications). Convergence brings a generalized carrier, the Internet, that may serve as a vast system of delivery of all kinds of signals, being them created by cultural industries or conventional telecommunications services or institutional data services. The success of the Internet lies, amongst other things, in making it possible to have access to any kind of information, as the pipes bring signals without much concern of its initial or final purpose. Signals are a second level notion of information, characterized by its technical nature, not by its usage or cultural origins.

Seen as a solution for the access issue, places like the *cabinas* are supposedly also a place to obtain abilities and capacities for getting the best out of the digital content available. Certainly, there are two main categories of telecenters, the *cabinas* as private business running under commercial objectives, and the community based telecenters, as community organizations with a clear communal purposes[3]. Then again, most of the telecenters are commercial in nature, so the basic access model to be considered is the *cabina*, notwithstanding the specificities mentioned regarding the markets being served.

As the recent debates about fair use and copyright protection have shown, the two information categories mentioned are normally considered as one, with the protections to pop cultural industries being passed on to other kinds of information and vice versa (Verhulst 2004). Technically, those interested in using ICT and new media should submit themselves to the whole set of rules that international corporations are trying to establish to control usage of content. This situation clashes with the reality of widespread, rampant content piracy in the developing world, which would not be stopped through legislative or punitive ways, but taints all the approaches to accessing information and cultural products, in more ways than normally considered. The existence of widespread access facilities (the *cabinas*) create not only the means for accessing content, but also a simple way to avoid taking responsibility for respecting these rules, since it is not a personal or institutional responsibility, but rather a customer relationship where the onus of enforcing regulations are in the hands of the *cabina* managers, who may decide it is easier for them to look the other way instead of losing customers to less law-abiding *cabinas*.

As they currently exist, the *cabinas* are successful when they provide information as *signals*: they are not really concerned on the nature of the usage of the information made available through them. If the provision of signals is adequate, for the intended uses envisioned by the imagined market, then the *cabinas* have a future, while the absence of good service, i.e. good access to signals, make them a failure. There is little relationship with the results of accessing information in the cultural / economic sense. As such, the *cabinas* provide a very focused but primary service, and this it is possible, as it happens in Peru and arguably in many other places, to have wonderful and successful mechanisms of signals access without an impact in the areas where information is allegedly more critical, like for instance developing a new economy or strengthening cultural expression.

While many of those that use *cabinas* as their primary way to access digital information do it because they are looking after symbolic, pop culture content, the abilities and practices they acquire are shaped by the *cabina* experience. This situation is certainly interesting since it allows for more cultural consumption that normal levels of income would allow, creating a sort of equality mechanism. The long term problems created by this kind of equality of consumption are, on the other hand, quite interesting to look after and significantly complicated in the long run, both for development as a whole and for A2K policies specifically; they also put the concept of digital poverty into a lot of stress.

Many of those that are able to take themselves off digital poverty do it thanks to the *cabinas*, mostly because they provide an inexpensive, quick way to access ICT, the Internet and the breadth of digital media. As the *cabina* becomes the favored method of access for those who are in income brackets that do not allow for personal access at home, nor have the facilities at their work place or school, the socially shaped practices prevalent at the *cabinas* take hold of most of the experience, since the main reason to access the Internet is not the demands generated by a competitive educational or economic marketplace, but rather a more diffuse cultural consumption and interpersonal communications. The approach taken to the Internet is thus shaped by the prevalent "piracy-oriented" consumption of content, most of it generated by the big global conglomerates. The Internet becomes a free-for-all not in the original sense of an end-to-end, innovation-friendly network, but in the sense that there are no restrictions to content access and no interest in working inside the regulated sphere of content as designed by the international IP discussion or the open access movement. Even the implications of Creative Commons licenses and other public policy issues may be ignored, since they are not relevant in an environment where there is no concern at all to the moral as well as the economic and legal reasons behind IP. Everything is "free", so why bother?

Of course, there could be many among the users of the *cabinas* that do develop links with the formal economy or the open access alternatives. But the *cabinas* are part and parcel of the informal, second economy, as they exist, among other reasons, to provide a solution to a poverty-induced problem: how to consume content without the means to pay. Not only in terms of accessing the media, but also of accessing protected content. So there is no surprise when, with the same ease that a song is downloaded for free, a school paper or an official document is downloaded for free, in the widest possible interpretation of free.

Therefore, the social practices acquired in the *cabinas* are not useful in the formal economy, nor in the formal educational sector. Those that are forced to act in the formal economy have to fight against attitudes shaped in the informal sector, and information is quite similar in this respect. In other words: piracy and informality begets a different sense of agency than formality and respect for IP rules engender, even if the end result is the need to fight the restrictions such rules imply. The kind of fight that someone in the informal sector will put against IP regulations will not necessarily be similar as the one expressed by someone who recognizes the need for respecting other peoples' work and creativity.

Also, those in the formal economy, approaching digital content in a formal way, end up having higher operating costs and charging higher prices and rates that those that do not act formally, having to pay licenses for software, or subscription fees for content. This increases the wedge between the formal and the informal sectors, making the whole economy of a country less competitive since those that act "formally" have higher costs than those that do not; it is less attractive, and certainly financially quite daunting, to become formal. The end result is a perverse incentive to stay outside of formality, even if formality presents a set of advantages only attainable through acceptance of its rules, like participation in the global economy or not being hassled by enforcing agencies, acting on behalf of the providers of "formal" content. For a small university, it may become a significant technical and organizational hurdle to make sure that all its computers are used in a legal way, without downloading illegal content, so "farming-out" computer access to the *cabinas* may seemed a neat solution of compromise. In this fashion, informality and piracy become a hindrance to equality of agency, and actually entrench digital poverty.

COMPLEMENTARY PERSPECTIVES: DIGITAL INDEPENDENCE

The ideas expressed in the previous paragraphs are an attempt to present the existence of a specific form of inequality, that may be directly related to digital poverty and to structural agency inequality. This *digital inequality* is more than a question of accessing technologies or capabilities to use ICT and digital, but a complicated set of social practices that separates the social agents that engage the global media and information environment to the ones that rely on parallel social practices, as piracy in its many incarnations appears to be.

Piracy and the general informal approach to digital content create a divide between those able to connect to the world and those that are not aware of the potential benefits of such connection. It is not a question of choosing to be disconnected, or to fight the connection, as happens with the different and very disparate groups engaged in the anti globalization protests movement. It is a fact of being separated and thus, exposed to a very specific form of inequality, one that is quite difficult to notice but that may be as harmful as income inequality.

To confront and maybe win over this digital inequality, communities and nations need to fight it with the same zeal that income inequality is –or at least should be– fought against. Since the acquisition of digital capabilities is one of the definition of competitiveness and social participation in the coming years, absence of these capabilities may result in entrenching inequality, and thus turning social conflicts into unmanageable conditions. Policies for A2K should be drafted as levers towards reducing digital agency inequality and to dissolve the separation between the formally connected and the informally connected.

Going beyond access, the need for developing digital media and content should be a goal. Not only because there are benefits in participating in the global digital economy, but also, and maybe more critically, because creating content is the

only way to enhance public participation in the "proper" digital culture.

This may be called *digital independence*: the achievement of sufficient capacities and social abilities to produce both content and set of rules that allow enough content to reach all those who need it, empowering them to approach digital technologies, media and content from a locally grounded perspective of what is at stake globally, and specially what is fair and what is good for the whole of the community, not just for individual satisfaction or achievement. Instead of trying to promote accessing digital media, the goal should be creating digital content relevant for the needs, all the needs of information.

Digital independence may express itself in country specific A2K policies: promoting creation of local content, or making services and content available to education, health or local government; preparing specific sets of legislation that promote commons-based and open access IP, and that allow specific government or civil society agents to negotiate in better terms for accessing information under control of global media corporations. But also, digital independence should take into consideration policies to promote a healthy, competitive mass media environment, both as provider of content that could be made available through digital means, and also as a countermove against the overpowering presence of global cultural products. This discussion is to be considered in more detail in the next section.

Good government policies should not be just for enabling a good content production environment, but should also take the form of specific public services geared towards providing better opportunities for all. Most of the efforts on e-government have tried to digitalize almost all the services in government, ending up just making "digitally aware" services in the areas where economic incentives are the highest[4]. In Peru, this include most of the services provided by quasi-independent organisms, that have the potential to charge for the provision of information; such a development creates great information services for the formal economy, but little if any services for those outside the formal economy or for the common citizen. Compounded with a general distrust of electronic means (completely understandable since the usage of these means is based on the premise that formal content is to be breached and that nothing is really secure on the Internet), e-government ends up being a perfect excuse for augmenting the capabilities of the formal economy and putting away the rest of the social and economic players.

There is a debt that e-government has not paid yet: it has not significantly improved the lives of the citizenry nor has changed the conditions to leap forward and break the cycle of informality. It may be a wonderful tool for competitive participation in the global economy for those *already in it*. The "other half" is still waiting for digital independence.

CULTURAL REPRESENTATION IN DEMOCRATIC SOCIETIES THROUGH DEMOCRATIC MEDIA

One of the issues that have to be considered together when dealing with A2K matters and the *digital independence* proposal mentioned herewith is the need for cultural affirmation. This could be understood as the need for all communities and nations to develop in the digital realm as a way of securing a future, not as museum pieces but as dynamic participants in the international exchange of ideas. This is a particularly significant defect of the current digital media discussion, one that is based on a technocratic perspective of the role of technology and on an understanding of globalization as a juggernaut that can not be appeased by half-measures, but has to be allowed to suppress all that cannot defend itself against the onslaught of global cultural industries.

Without the cultural component, there is little chance for A2K policies to succeed beyond the restricted area of those already connected to the global arena. As long as bringing as many people into the benefits of global economy is accepted as a desirable goal, there is a clear demand for fighting inequality of agency; this requires social agents to engage into an intense discussion of the issues brought by globalization in the many realms it affects, participating in a dialog with the rest of digital content producers of the world. This cannot be achieved only as a rhetorical digital policy, but as a promotion of content production of all kinds. Cultural policies should promote that all the people able to have the means to produce and publish the content they wish to; certainly, there are economic reasons weighing in favor of digital content, but there are plenty of intellectual and artistic pursuits that may have a better way of expression through conventional media.

Thus, mass media has to play a role. It cannot be hoped that societies dependent on mass media for information and culture in wider sense may find a way for development through the recourse of a different set of media, especially when the reason why they use these other media is the attraction of finding content related to the old, mass media content, or when usage of new media, even interpersonal one, brings a barrage of promotion and advertising for mass media products. Good quality, critical mass media is just as relevant now as it was fifty years, as a means to produce the *grand public* explained by Dominique Wolton (1999), or to allow for the search of transparency that Gianni Vattimo (1990) considers as a critical component of modern societies. Societies like Peru's cannot imagine themselves as one without recourse to some social "glue" that put in center stage the issues we share and the rich culture we live with.

Then again, mass media as it exists right now is barely able to fill this role. The preeminence of private broadcasters and the poor market capitalization of the networks and stations leave them quite feeble in front of the coming technological changes, from the new convergence driven by web based video *a la* Google Video o iTunes Video Store, or digital terrestrial television, further ahead in time. The structural weaknesses of mass media in Peru are very orders of magnitude more severe than those of the rest of Latin America, but nevertheless the presence of a growing media sector geared towards the Latin American market in cable television, and the divide opened between those with access to current content through any form of pay media and those left with old, free-to-air mass media, are growing, and are specially critical in Peru.

The only kind of broadcaster able to fill both the role of competitive and national mass media is the public one (Galbi 2003, McChesney 2004). Here, Peruvian situation is similar to the common one in the region, with a weak public broadcaster subject to the whims of political appointees (Fuenzalida 2000). This weakness is one of the issues to be faced if any attempt to promote a local media sphere that allows *space* and *place* to coincide again.

Empowering public media is a must, then. A combined radio / television / new media conglomerate, responsive to market and popular culture demands but also aware of the need for a critical and community-based appraisal of the need for developing local answers to the demands of the hour could be a powerful voice for change, positive and necessary change. It could also be a lever for engaging expatriate communities, always growing in Latin America and especially critical in Peru after many years of disenchantment with the perceived future of the country.

Also, a powerful public broadcaster could act as a barrier to the undemocratic tendencies current in many areas of Latin America, and also as proof that approaches not entirely based on profit making are viable, as the open source movement is trying to demonstrate. The basis of the open source movement is an idea of democratic community, allowing the sharing of ideas, predicated on the premise that ideas are, in the long run, a creation of the community. It is not possible to promote community ideals only through media that does not have a wide, national appeal, in the countries where those ideals are scarce, questioned by many or simply under attack from different sides, historically and currently, as is the case of Peru. A nation-wide appeal is needed, and that is the role of mass media.

ACKNOWLEDGMENT

A shorter, earlier version of this paper was presented at the Prato 2007 conference, and it is available at http://www.ccnr.net/prato2007/archive/villanueva-prato-1.pdf. .... My thanks to Michael Gurstein, Scott Robinson and Larry Stillman for their individual help in different moments of the development of this paper.

REFERENCES

Barrantes, R. (2005). Analysis of ICT demand: what is digital poverty and how to measure it? In Galperin, H., & Mariscal, J. (Eds.), *Digital poverty: Latin American and Caribbean perspectives* (pp. 29–53). Lima, PE: Practical Action Publishing.

Borja, G., & Björn-Sören, G. (2005). The concept of information poverty and how to measure it in the Latin American context . In Galperin, H., & Mariscal, J. (Eds.), *Digital poverty: Latin American and Caribbean perspectives* (pp. 11–28). Lima, PE: Practical Action Publishing.

Delgadillo, K., Ricardo, G., & Klaus, S. (2005) Telecentros… ¿para qué? *Lecciones sobre telecentros comunitarios en América Latina y el Caribe*. Quito: Somos@telecentros.

Fuenzalida, V. (2000). *La television pública en América Latina: reforma o privatización*. México: FCE.

Galbi, D. A. (2003). *Communications policy, media development, and convergence.* Retrieved from http://www.galbithink.org/media.htm

McChesney, R. (2004). *The problem of the media: U.S. Communication politics in the 21st century.* Chicago, IL: Monthly review.

Valovic, Th. (2000). *Digital Mythologies: the hidden complexities of the Internet.* New Jersey: Rutgers.

Vattimo, G. (1990). *La sociedad transparente.* Barcelona, ES: E: Paidos.

Verhulst, S. G. (2004). About scarcities and intermediaries: the regulatory paradigm shift of digital content reviewed . In Lievwrouv, L., & Livingstone, S. (Eds.), *Handbook of new media* (pp. 432–437). New York: Sage Publications.

Winner, L. (1989). *The whale and the reactor: a search for limits in the age of high technology.* Chicago, IL: Chicago University Press.

Wolton, D. (1999). *Internet et après? Une théorie critique des nouveaux medias.* Paris, FR: Flammarion.

ENDNOTES

[1] There should be more research into the actual connection in developing societies between knowledge for wealth creation and cultural expression; this connection appears to be prominent in societies that are able to establish "cultural industries" that both create a cultural imagination that most of the population finds pertinent to their own image, as well as a business that brings economic opportunities for creators and intellectual innovators. This connection exists in societies with a certain critical mass of both popular expression and markets for the products of this expression, as India, Brazil or Mexico; societies and countries like Peru have this confluence of market and creation at a significantly smaller scale.

[2] These statements are based on data collected during coursework by students of the paper's author.

[3] The third possible way is the *cybercafe*, as a commercial business oriented to tourists and transient customers. It is not similar at all to the *cabinas*, since the emphasis is not on creating a long term relationship with a community, but to serve the needs of specific customers that demand occasional access. It has to be stated that this is just a semantic, uniquely Peruvian difference.

[4] A perverse incentive to government electronic services has been the need for self-financing of e-government programs, since they are geared towards specific segments of the economy that are able to pay for the information provided, while leaving outside those that cannot afford them. This is the situation in Peru, where large services of great quality have been designed under the premise of paid usage, while some less competitive but otherwise socially relevant ones, like health or educational ones, are still waiting for implementation.

Chapter 33
Information and Communication Technologies for a More Sustainable World

Lorenz M. Hilty

University of Zurich, Switzerland & Empa, Swiss Federal Laboratories for Materials Science and Technology, Switzerland

ABSTRACT

As has been discussed for decades, a reduction of the input of natural resources into industrial production and consumption by a factor of 4-10 is a necessary condition for Sustainable Development. This paper discusses the potential contribution of Information and Communication Technology (ICT) to such a dematerialization of the industrial societies and introduces a conceptual framework which accounts for positive and negative impacts of ICT on physical flows. This framework addresses three levels: the ICT life cycle itself, life cycles of other products influenced by ICT applications, and patterns of production and consumption. The conclusion is that ICT will only contribute to Sustainable Development if this technology is recognized and used as an enabler of a deep structural change; a transition towards an economic system in which value-creation is mainly based on information processing while keeping the physical properties of material within some limits that ensure that it can be recycled. This structural change will include the transition from a material-property-transfer mode to a service-transfer mode of consumption in areas where this is technically feasible and beneficial in terms of resource productivity. In such a post-industrial society, which may also be called a sustainable information society, open technological standards will play a crucial role, since they allow for complexity reduction while keeping competition alive, thus minimizing the risk of unmastered complexity in new critical infrastructures.

INTRODUCTION

The most prominent definition of Sustainable Development was given by the World Commission on Environment and Development, also known as the "Brundtland definition": In order to be considered sustainable, a pattern of development has to ensure "that it meets the needs of the present without compromising the ability of future generations to meet their own needs" (WCED, 1987).

DOI: 10.4018/978-1-60960-057-0.ch033

Read as a normative statement, this definition combines two ethical claims, intragenerational justice (meeting the needs of the present) and *inter*generational justice (not compromising future generations). This double claim leads to a dilemma, since it is impossible to extend the present consumption patterns of the rich industrialized countries to all parts of the world without putting a great burden on future generations.

In order to solve or at least mitigate the dilemma, the global economy will have to learn to produce more quality of life with less input of material and energy.

It is apparent that the widespread use of Information and Communication Technology (ICT) is changing our world, a development taking place even faster than political decision makers can react to the changes. The Internet (with e-mail, the Web, VOIP and unlimited future applications), the mobile networks (with 4 billion subscribers world-wide), Radio Frequency Identification (RFID) systems and embedded ICT systems (to which 98% of all microprocessors belong) have massive economic, social and ecological effects on a global scale.

This chapter brings together the issue of Sustainable Development with perspectives of an information society that is post-industrial in the sense that the throughput of material and energy needed to satisfy human needs would be much lower than today. The chapter also presents a conceptual framework to assess the material effects of ICT, providing a basis for political strategies towards a sustainable information society.

PERSPECTIVES OF ICT AND SUSTAINABILITY

Starting from the issue of economic dematerialization as a necessary condition for Sustainable Development, a conceptual framework will be presented and exemplified which accounts for positive and negative impacts of ICT on material and energy flows at different levels: the ICT life cycle itself (first-order effects), life cycles of other products influenced by ICT (second-order effects), and patterns of production and consumption (third-order effects).

The Dematerialization Issue

The dematerialization discourse was started about two decades ago with statements such as the following:

"Considering the fact that for every person in the United States we mobilize 10 tons of materials and create a few tons of waste per year, it is clearly important to gain a better understanding of the potential forces for dematerialization. Such an understanding is essential for devising strategies to maintain and enhance environmental quality, especially in a nation and a world where population and the desire for economic growth are ever increasing" (Herman et al., 1990, p. 346).

At the global level, 58 billion metric tons of resources were extracted from nature in 2005 (OECD, 2008). This includes fossil fuels, metals, industrial and construction materials as well as biomass. Although the current rate of resource extraction seriously affects the global ecosystem, the increase is expected to continue. This even includes the use of fossil fuels, although that is supposed to be limited by climate policies. The OECD estimates that global resource extraction will exceed 80 billion tons in 2020. This means that mankind will have doubled the annual global rate of resource extraction within only 40 years (1980-2020).

Let us look at some more specific examples: The *per capita* consumption of aluminum in industrialized countries today is higher that in a typical developing country by a factor of 14 and that of steel by a factor of 130. An average North American consumes about 340 kg of paper per year, whereas an Ethiopian – on the other end of the scale – about 300 g. This list could be continued almost indefinitely. Even if the figures are only snapshots, very imprecise and some of them out-dated, their magnitude reveals the basic dilemma of all sustainability policies: the lifestyle of the rich industrialized countries cannot be adopted in its present form by the whole globe, nor can any lifestyle that is as material-intensive as that of today's richest countries.

Since the mid-1990s estimates have been discussed according to which the material intensity per service unit must be reduced by a factor of 4 to 10 if the lifestyle of the rich North is to be applied across the whole globe. By and large, there are no doubts as to the technical feasibility of such a big leap in resource productivity (Von Weizsäcker et al., 1997; Schmidt-Bleek, 2009).

Viewed from this perspective, there is only one relevant role ICT can play in supporting Sustainable Development: enabling or facilitating the dematerialization of production and consumption processes, i.e. to contribute to a drastic increase in resource productivity. This idea leads to the vision of an ICT-enabled 'weightless economy' or 'sustainable information society', as suggested by Heiskanen et al. (2001), Schauer (2003), Isenmann (2008), as well as by the author (Hilty, 2008a).

The Role of ICT in Dematerialization

Given that dematerialization is so important, the next question we must address is whether and under what conditions ICT can contribute to this change.

Unfortunately, we have to face the fact that the richest economies – which also have the highest penetration of ICT – are not the most dematerialized ones. For example, the consumption of an average inhabitant of Switzerland causes a material flow through the global economy of roughly 48 tons per year, which is about five times the current global average (based on data provided by FSO, 2008, and OECD, 2008). It is remarkable that the material throughput per capita is highest in rich societies in which 'light' and 'virtual' are attributes with positive connotations.

The sobering observation that ICT does not automatically create a dematerialized society, however, does not imply that this is impossible in principle. The following two arguments shall explain why there is still a chance to unleash the dematerialization potential of ICT.

The *first argument* is based on an analogy, replacing resource productivity with labour productivity for a moment. In the 1980s and 1990s, the so-called 'IT productivity paradox' was discussed in economics and management literature for a long time. Robert Solow, the 1987 Nobel laureate in economics, initiated the debate by stating that "we see the computer age everywhere except in the productivity statistics" (Solow 1987). The common belief that computers increase labour productivity was surprisingly not supported by macro-economic data (just as it is the case for resource productivity today). The subsequent controversy motivated a range of interesting research projects on the question as to how computers affect the productivity of organizations. The firm-level data showed substantial variation across firms, leading to the conclusion that the effect of introducing the new technology was depending of the organizational conditions under which it was applied (Brynjolfsson and Hitt, 1998).

In a very similar way, it may turn out in the near future that ICT does enable massive increases in resource productivity under specific organizational conditions; conditions which are not common so far, but may spread in the future.

The *second argument* is based on the idea that positive effects of ICT are already there, but cancelled out by negative ones when all effects are aggregated to the macro level. To create a 'selective environment' for ICT applications, one which clearly prefers the 'truly dematerializing' ones, would then be the silver bullet to dematerialize the economy. A simulation study commissioned by the Institute for Prospective Technological Studies (IPTS) of the European Commission concluded that, under conditions generally conducive to environmental protection, ICT reduced the overall environmental impact by around 20% (from 2000-2020), whereas under the least favourable conditions ICT was responsible for 30% of the additional environmental impact. However, under business as usual conditions, the positive and negative effects of ICT on the environment had the tendency to cancel each other out, so that no clear effect at the macro level occurred (Erdmann et al., 2004; Hilty et al., 2006a).

It is therefore possible that the dematerializing effect of ICT would dominate if there would be a selective environment (the framework conditions set by politics) encouraging the "dematerializing" applications and to inhibit the others. In particular, rising prices for materials and energy can be expected to create dematerializing changes in production and consumption patterns, using (and as well needing) ICT as an enabling technology.

However, there will only be room for big leaps if people's view of material goods changes: In many fields, consumption patterns will have to change from purchasing *material goods* (transferring material property), which are then used and destroyed, to purchasing *services* instead. Since the material goods needed to produce the service are owned by the service provider, this company has a strong incentive to see them being put to optimal use and to maximize service life (which slows down material flows). ICT is an enabling technology to implement the business models needed for this type of change.

The Full Picture of Material ICT Effects

In general, there are three levels of material ICT effects that must be taken into account (Erdmann and Hilty, 2010):

- 'First-order' or 'primary' effects: effects of the physical existence of ICT (environmental impacts of the production, use, recycling and disposal of ICT hardware).

- 'Second-order' or 'secondary' effects: indirect effects of ICT due to its power to change processes (such as production, transport or consumption processes), resulting in a decrease or increase of the material impacts of these processes.
- 'Third-order' or 'tertiary' effects: effects of the medium- or long-term adaptation of behavior (e.g. consumption patterns) and economic structures to the availability of ICT and the services it provides.

The third-order effects include the widely discussed rebound effect. A rebound effect occurs if and when the efficiency of providing a service is increased but there is no factor limiting the demand for this service, such as the price to be paid or the time needed for consuming it. The economic system adapts to the higher efficiency level at which the service is provided by increasing the demand for the service (Hilty, 2008a).

Linked Life Cycles: A Framework to Assess First- and Second-Order Effects

Figure 1 shows how the service provided by using an ICT product can have an effect on the life cycle of another product. There are three types of effects: optimization (dotted arrows), induction (straight arrow), and substitution (bent arrow).

Optimization effects (denoted by the four dotted arrows) may occur in all phases of the life cycle, as well as in the design phase. CAD tools, for example, can be used to optimize a product for environmental criteria (eco-design). Design has a strong impact of the life cycle because it constrains the optimization potentials that will exist in the production, use and end-of-life phases. For example, if the variety of materials or the complexity of the product can be reduced in the design phase, it will be possible to reach a higher efficiency level in end-of-life treatment.

Induction effects (denoted by the arrow in the middle) occur when an ICT service stimulates

Figure 1. How ICT products influence the design, production, use, and disposal of other products (Hilty 2008a)

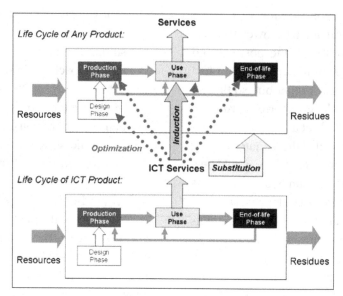

the use of the other product, i.e. more functional units per unit of time are consumed (e.g. the text-processing service provided by a PC system with a printer may stimulate paper consumption).

Substitution effects (denoted by the bent arrow) occur when an ICT service replaces the use of a physical product, e.g. when e-mail replaces the use of conventional paper-based mail.

With Life Cycle Assessment (LCA) methodology, it is possible to quantify the potential environmental benefit of specific optimization and substitution effects. For example, a given conference can be hypothetically virtualized and the difference in environmental impacts assessed (see Figure 2). We did so for *EnviroInfo 2001*, which was held at ETH Zurich, assuming that all travel of participants would have been replaced by Internet connections for video streaming, online discussions, upload and download of presentations, etc., including the estimated environmental

Figure 2. CO2 emissions caused by an international conference, physically or virtually (Hischier and Hilty, 2002)

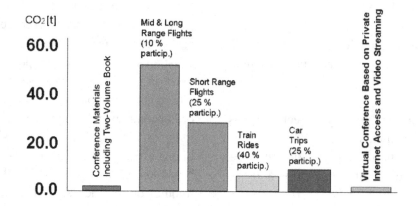

Figure 3. The idea of a largely dematerialized closed-loop economy. The transformations of material resources at nodes denoted 'S/H' add value by creating structure without devaluating the material. Each value-creating node is driven by renewable energy (symbolized by a solar panel) and consists of a hardware part H (capital goods for transforming material and energy) and a software part S (the knowledge of how to control these transformations in a manner that adds value).

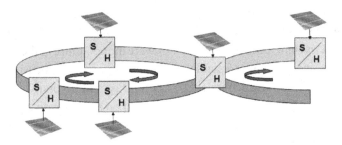

impact of the Internet connections. It turned out that the virtual conference would only have caused 2-3% of the actual CO_2 emissions of the physical conference.

The main part of the total emission was due to travel activities, as can be seen in Figure 2. Only 6% of the participants who had to take a long-range flight accounted for 60% of the overall emission of the conference (Hischier and Hilty, 2002).

Positive Third-Order Effects

What is needed from the perspective of sustainability is a deep structural change which would make the above-mentioned substitution effects into an essential feature of the economy. In an economy that has been dematerialized in this way, value-added would depend a lot more than it does today on the creation of structures at the symbolic level and not on the churning of material and energy.

Figure 3 sketches the basic idea of such an economy. In such an economic system, all scarce substances are carried in closed cycles which are maintained by renewable energy. All value creation takes place alongside these closed cycles, transforming the (symbolic) structure of material while keeping its physical properties within

some limits that ensure that it can be recycled. The whole system consists of a network of such closed cycles.

The hardware/software dichotomy of the ICT sector is generalized to the whole economy: Each node of the network consists of hardware (capital goods for transforming material and energy) and software (the knowledge of how to control these transformations in a manner that adds value). Today's distinctions among raw materials, product and waste will become obsolete, since there is no beginning or end of the cycles. Innovation will mean the introduction of new nodes into the system.

Negative Third-Order Effects

There are two types of negative effects at the systemic level that should be counteracted by policies for a sustainable information society:

- rebound effects and
- dependability on highly complex infrastructures.

Rebound effects occur if and when the efficiency of providing a service is increased but there is no factor limiting the demand for this service, such as the price to be paid or the time needed for consuming it. The economic system (as a functional system of society) adapts to the higher efficiency level at which the service is provided by increasing the demand for the service (Hilty et al,. 2006b). Therefore, as pointed out above, ICT will only succeed as an enabler of dematerialization if an adequate selection environment is in place.

But, even worse, the system does not only adapt to higher efficiency, it also adapts to stable availability of a service – by becoming dependent on it. The Internet and other ICT infrastructures such as mobile phone networks are therefore becoming critical infrastructures for society and should be applied with precaution in order to maintain a margin for future developments (Som et al., 2004). ICT has also "has pervaded other infrastructures, rendering them more intelligent, increasingly interconnected, complex, interdependent, and therefore more vulnerable" (IRRIIS Consortium, 2006). These other infrastructures include transport, energy, water, finance, and national security (Hilty, 2008b).

The actual level of vulnerability of an ICT system is almost impossible to assess due to the problem of "unmastered complexity". This term was coined by one of the world's most influential computer scientists, Edsger W. Dijkstra. He repeatedly warned the community of computer professionals against the complexity of their own artifacts: "Computing's core challenge is how not to make a mess of it. … Because we are dealing with artifacts, all unmastered complexity is of our own making; there is no one else to blame and so we had better learn how not to introduce the complexity in the first place." (Dijkstra, n.d., pp. 1 f). No single programmer has a truly comprehensive grasp of the code that has been written for even one of today's operating systems or large application programs. If these systems are connected via networks, systems of an even higher level of complexity are created the behavior of which is no longer predictable.

Dijkstra's warning hasn't been heeded much in commercial practice, as shown by today's most popular systems. It is because of this general and deeply rooted flaw that catastrophic attacks against ICT infrastructure can't be ruled out. For the same reason, the risk of such attacks cannot be quantified in advance. What we do know for sure is that software diversity mitigates the vulnerability of critical information infrastructures, whereas software monoculture makes them more fragile. Open standards make it possible to reconcile interoperability and diversity: They specify the 'What' based on a cooperative process and leave it to the market to find the best solution for the 'How'. By contrast, so-called proprietary standards (which are no standards, *de-facto* standards at the best) are used to create consumer lock-in effects and lead to technological monocultures.

So-called proprietary standards have even more disadvantages with regard to sustainability: They are not based on a consensus and can be modified arbitrarily by their proprietor: Even small changes may invalidate capital invested in the standard, such as fully operational equipment (with all its ecological backpack), skills created by adaptation to the standard (human capital), and confidence in infrastructures, institutions and people (social capital). Since an open standard is defined in a consensual process, it can usually not be changed arbitrarily to the disadvantage of parties who have made investments based on the present version. Proprietary *de facto* standards thus concentrate destructive power, bearing a high risk for society and nature.

From the perspective of complexity reduction, it is clearly better to have a reliable and stable specification (the definition of the 'What') and a variety of competing approaches to the implementation (the 'How') – which is then irrelevant and may be hidden – than to have an unreliable specification with only one implementation, which is then replicated millions of times with all its errors and security holes.

Information infrastructures based on proprietary standards are therefore not sustainable. The fact that many commercial software products are peppered with errors and consequently depend on regular updates creates an additional problem because this leads to a concentration of power in the hands of any actor who is recognized as the legitimate provider of an update.

CONCLUSION

We have shown that the Brundtland definition of Sustainable Development, read as a normative statement, leads to a fundamental dilemma at the metabolic level of the economy for which we introduced the term 'sustainability dilemma'. If ICT is to solve or at least mitigate this dilemma, it is vital to purposefully deploy this technology for the dematerialization of production and consumption processes.

ICT will grow into this role if and when the economic incentives pass a certain threshold to change behaviour and trigger innovation towards dematerialization, which has not been the case so far.

While many activities to use ICT for Sustainable Development focus on first- or second- order effects, it is particularly important to use the enabling potential of ICT for long-term structural change. This means to use ICT with the awareness that "doing more of the same" with the help of this technology (e.g. guide more cars though a congested road) will not solve the critical problems the world is facing, because it will not contribute to solving the sustainability dilemma. It could even create rebound effects and consolidate old structures.

What we need is a deep structural change towards an economic system in which value-creation is mainly based on information processing while keeping the physical properties of material within some limits that ensure that it can be recycled. This structural change will include the transition from a material-property-transfer mode to a service-transfer mode of consumption in areas where this is technically possible and leads to a higher resource productivity (assessed from a life-cycle perspective).

In such a post-industrial society, which may also be called a sustainable information society, open technological standards will play a crucial role, since they allow for complexity reduction while keeping competition alive, thus minimizing the risk of unmastered complexity in emerging critical infrastructures.

ACKNOWLEDGMENT

The author would like to thank Thomas Ruddy from the Technology and Society Lab at Empa for his long-standing collaboration on the topic discussed in this chapter, and the members of the IFIP Working Group 9.9 'ICT and Sustainable Development' (http://www.ict-sd.org) for creating awareness of sustainability issues among the ICT community.

REFERENCES

Brynjolfsson, E., & Hitt, L. (1998). Beyond the Productivity Paradox. *Communications of the ACM, 41*(8), 49–55. doi:10.1145/280324.280332

Dijkstra, E. W. (n.d). The next fifty years. Retrieved April 12, 2008 from http://www.cs.utexas.edu/~EWD/ewd12xx/EWD1243.PDF

Erdmann, L., & Hilty, L. M. (2010). (accepted for publication). Scenario Analysis: Exploring the Macroeconomic Impacts of Information and Communication Technologies on Greenhouse Gas Emissions. *Journal of Industrial Ecology*.

Erdmann, L., Hilty, L. M., Goodman, J., & Arnfalk, P. (2004). *The future impact of ICT on environmental sustainability. Synthesis report. Institute for Prospective Technology Studies*. Sevilla, Spain: IPTS.

FSO - Federal Statistical Office. (2008). *Environmental Accounting. Swiss Confederation*. Neuchatel.

Heiskanen, E., Halme, M., Jalas, M., Kärnä, A., & Lovio, R. (2001). *Dematerialisation: The Potential of ICT and Services*. Helsinki, Finland: Ministry of the Environment.

Herman, R., Ardeni, S. A., & Ausubel, J. H. (1990). Dematerialization. *Technological Forecasting and Social Change, 38*, 333–347. doi:10.1016/0040-1625(90)90003-E

Hilty, L. M. (2008a). *Information Technology and Sustainability: Essays on the Relationship between ICT and Sustainable Development*. Norderstedt, DE: Books on Demand.

Hilty, L. M. (2008b). Emerging Risks in Information Infrastructures – A Technology Assessment Perspective. In *Proceedings of IDRC 2008, International Disaster Reduction Conference*, Davos, Switzerland.

Hilty, L. M., Arnfalk, P., Erdmann, L., Goodman, J., Lehmann, M., & Wäger, A. P. (2006a). The Relevance of Information and Communication Technologies for Environmental Sustainability - A Prospective Simulation Study. *Environmental Modelling & Software, 21*(11), 1618–1629. doi:10.1016/j.envsoft.2006.05.007

Hilty, L. M., & Köhler, A., Von Schéele, F., Zah, F., & Ruddy, T. (2006b). Rebound Effects of Progress in Information Technology. *Poiesis & Praxis . International Journal of Technology Assessment and Ethics of Science, 4*(1), 19–38.

Hischier, R., & Hilty, L. M. (2002). Environmental Impacts of an International Conference. *Environmental Impact Assessment Review, 22*(5), 543–557. doi:10.1016/S0195-9255(02)00027-6

IRRIIS Consortium. (2006). *Integrated Risk Reduction of Information-based Infrastructure Systems*. Retrieved May 18, 2008 from http://www.irriis.eu

Isenmann, R. (2008). Sustainable Information Society . In Quingley, M. (Ed.), *Encyclopedia of Information Ethics* (pp. 622–630). Hershey, PA: IGI Global.

OECD. (2008). *Measuring material flows and resource productivity. Synthesis report*. Paris, France: Organisation for Economic Cooperation and Development.

Schauer, T. (2003). *The Sustainable Information Society: Vision and Risks*. Ulm, DE: Universitätsverlag.

Schmidt-Bleek, F. (2009). *The Earth: Natural Resources and Human Intervention*. London: Haus Publishing Limited.

Solow, R. M. (1987). We'd better watch out. *New York Times Book Review, 12*(2), 36-50.

Som, C., Hilty, L. M., & Ruddy, T. F. (2004). The Precautionary Principle in the Information Society. *Human and Ecological Risk Assessment, 10*(8), 787–799. doi:10.1080/10807030490513801

Von Weizsäcker, E. U., & Lovins, A. B. L., & Lovins, L. H. (1997). *Factor Four: Doubling Wealth, Halving Resource Use – A Report to the Club of Rome*. London: Earthscan.

WCED – World Commission on Environment and Development. (1987). *Our Common Future*. London: Oxford University Press.

Chapter 34

Why Do the Orders Go Wrong All the Time?
Exploring Sustainability in an E-Commerce Application in Swedish Public School Kitchens

Christina Mörtberg
University of Umeå, Sweden & University of Oslo, Norway

Dagny Stuedahl
University of Oslo, Norway

Sara Alander
Independent Scholar, Norway

ABSTRACT

In this paper we discuss sustainability, particularly social and cultural sustainability, in relation to an e-commerce application used in the kitchen of a Swedish public school. The notion of sustainability got its public definition through the Brundtland Commission and the report Our Common Future in which ecological as well as economic and social dimensions were underlined. An additional dimension, culture, has recently unfolded. The data reported in this paper were collected in public school and pre-school meal production. This is a large, institutional, tax-funded activity in Sweden as all pre-schools, compulsory schools and most upper secondary schools serve free lunch to the children and students. We discuss how an e-commerce application complicated the daily routines in the school kitchen rather than making the ordering of food stuff easier or more flexible and how small things that mattered in the staff's day-to-day activities shed light on the application's problems and weaknesses. Following Agenda 21, we relate these shortcomings to sustainability and also to participation. The discussion builds on social and cultural sustainability and participatory design with a focus on the involvement of users in design and implementation of IT systems and services.

DOI: 10.4018/978-1-60960-057-0.ch034

INTRODUCTION

Today, green or sustainable design is given particular attention in architecture and urban planning, industrial development and development of energy systems. Central issues are physical and technological principles, environmental and health considerations. Other aspects include choice of low-impact materials, energy efficiency, quality and durability, reuse and recycling, as well as service substitution, standardization and modularity. The technological focus has primarily been on the development of appropriate technologies that create an overlap between technology and context, as well as cutting the use of resources.

In information systems (IS) design or design of information technology (IT) sustainability has, above all, been used with a focus on durability (Braa et al. 2004; Byrne 2005; Byrne & Sahay 2007) or how IT can support a sustainable development of future societies – and less on how the principles of sustainable development can be integrated into the design of future IT services and systems. To use sustainability in this way is probably a consequence of its general meaning. Cheney et al. (2004, p. 226) argue, for example, that sustainability was about 'permanence and implies notion of durability, stability and eternalness'. Although durability is part of the dominant discourse, others also exist. For example Blevis (2006, 2007) has moved beyond durability when he integrates sustainability into interaction design. His rationale is to reduce the use of materials in order to minimize ecological footprints.1 While Blevis's focus is on ecological issues, Mörtberg et al. (forthcoming) also include the concepts social and cultural sustainability in IT design. Their focus is on standards, formats, and routines in digital design and how to find sustainable ways of living with technologies (Mörtberg et al. forthcoming). The exploration builds on two research projects: e-government in municipalities in Sweden and the reconstruction of a Viking boat in Norway. Mörtberg et al. discuss how a standard identifier

(OCR number) of the invoices causes additional work for the person in a municipal account office responsible for the invoicing process – the design based on the identifier was not sustainable enough without manual interventions to correct inappropriate functionalities of the systems. In the reconstruction of the Viking boat, Mörtberg et al. also illustrate the necessity of paying attention to the users' creation of meanings and values in order to design connections between present understandings and the standards used for archiving cultural objects, narratives and knowledge. They conclude how important it is to also integrate social and cultural sustainability in the design of sustainable IS/IT and services – i.e., as a prerequisite in the creation of sustainable societies.

Shapiro (2005) argues that it is estimated that large scale IT systems are either not used or they do not work according to the specification in around 75 per cent of cases. Shapiro does not discuss the high rate of failures in terms of sustainability, but he argues for the use of participatory design (PD) approaches in order to reduce the rate of failure. The main focus in PD is on participation and how to involve a range of practitioners in IT design in order to design a system that is based on those who work with it in practice. Our argument to tie together PD and sustainability is based on what PD researchers emphasize:

[Accordingly,] IT usage is regarded sustainable to the extent that it contributes to a balance in the development, use, and protection of a company's resources. This should be done in ways that accommodate the company's existing goals and needs, without jeopardizing its future development potentials (Bødker et al. 2004, p. 54).

And:

Good IT design requires knowledge of work practices in order to determine which company traditions are fundamental and sustainable, and which are outdated. Put in a different way, only

when a design team has fundamental knowledge of existing work practices can it arrive at what we call a 'sustain- able design' (Bødker et al. 2004, pp. 140–141).

The social and cultural sustainability that we explore here proposes a focus on an e-commerce application used in municipal meal production in Swedish institutional kitchens. We pay particular attention to participation and PD as enablers to involve employees in IT design in order to make social and cultural sustain- ability visible, and to integrate them in the design and implementation of IS/IT.

In the next section, we present the notion of sustainable development, Agenda 21, and the four dimensions of sustainability. This is followed by a description of PD and participation. The setting, context, and methods are then described and the empirical data collected in the meal production for schools are presented. We will end with some concluding thoughts.

SUSTAINABLE DEVELOPMENT AND AGENDA 21

Sustainability has not always been connected to ecological issues but derives from the emerging environmentalism in the 1960s and 1970s. Eco-logical dimensions were reinforced when sustainable development was given its public definition in the Brundtland Commission and its outcome, Our Common Future (WCED 1987). The liveable and sustainable futures with 'a development that meets the needs of the present without compromising the ability of future generations to meet their own needs' were highlighted in the report (see http://www.un-documents.net/ocf-02.htm). Further, sustainability was extended with the inclusion of a social and economic dimension to the existing focus on ecological dimensions. There is not, however, an existing common understanding of the notion of sustainability because it has been

unfolding since the 1960s and, today, it is used in a variety of ways and settings. Eichler (1999, p. 189) concludes that the notion 'gives most of us a warm and fuzzy feeling but we don't know what it means'. Others claim that the concepts of strength, flexibility and possibilities are shown by continuous discussions and debates about its meaning (Lafferty et al. 2006).

The notion may not stable and fixed, but the Brundtland Commission's outcome documented in the report Our Common Future (WCED 1987) was a starting point for integrating social, economic, and ecological dimensions in the objective of achieving sustainable futures. This work continued at the United Nations Conference on Environment and Development in Rio de Janeiro in 1992. A result of this was a plan for actions, Agenda 21, in which the three dimensions of sustainable development: ecological, economic, and social, were reinforced. Agenda 21 also emphasizes the need for grass-root- level involvement in development projects which reinforces people's opportunities to become involved in the creation and implementation of sustainable futures. Participation was one normative principle in Our Common Future and it was strengthened in the action plan, Agenda 21, through the emphasis on local action. In addition to local actions, Agenda 21 also emphasized that actions should be integrated into the whole society, globally and nationally, in order to support sustainable development. Further, specific groups are designated in Agenda 21, such as women, NGOs, business, industry, and scientific communities. (It is noteworthy that women, as a group, are singled out but not men.) Agenda 21 also focuses on innovative and system-changing attempts in the development of technologies, in particular in relation to inclusion of groups that are neither the most dominant participants in the development processes nor are generally involved in decision-making positions. The focus on technology is in continuation of the work of the Brundtland Commission, with its requirements for the development of sustainable technologies: 'a technical system that can search continuously for new solutions' (WCED 1987, p. 65). The focus on technology has, however, been discussed and criticized because of its tendencies to fall back on technological optimism and also because it is yet an additional expression of western countries' domination over other cultures (Visvanathan 1991; Escobar 1995). Despite the criticism, the commission's statement about technology can still be used as a point of departure in explorations of sustainability in IT design.

While Our Common Future and its followers focused on sustainable development in general, the United Nations plan of action shed light on information and communication technologies (ICT) and its relation to sustainability. Cultural diversity and identity, linguistic, and local content are examples of the 11 key principles for the sustainable development of an Information Society (WSIS 2003). Hence, stimulating respect for cultural identity, traditions and religions are defined as essential. Among the principles, cultural diversity is defined as diversity of cultural expression, indigenous knowledge and traditions, on institutional, national and private levels. The focus on diversity calls for a better understanding of how to integrate diversity in IT design particularly, with a focus on social interactions and social life in the development of information societies, and, in our case, how cultural diversity and identity can influence social interactions with technologies. This needs a more distinct notion of what cultural diversity consists of – and how to analyse it in real-life situations.

The four dimensions of sustainability have been extended to include social and economic rather than just ecological issues in order to create viable futures. The ecological dimension is discussed in terms of responsibility and not preying too much upon our common resources. Health and viability are related to economic sustainability, and equity and justice to social sustainability. A fourth dimension, cultural sustainability, has emerged out of social sustainability (Hawkes 2001). Cultural

sustainability has its focus on the development, renewal and maintenance of human cultures in order to create positive, enduring relationships with other people in the immediate neighbourhood but also throughout the world (Hawkes 2001). Cultural sustainability embodies new approaches to be integrated in design in terms of identity, values, norms, diversity, and tradition, among both users and designers. This gives valuable knowledge that can be of help in the design of sustainable products and systems. Our focus will be on how these traditions, identities, norms and values in school and pre-school kitchens are considered in the e-commerce application. We will also argue that ecological, economic, social, and cultural sustainability are valuable dimensions to be integrated in sustainable IS development. Such dimensions intersect in people's everyday lives, consequently it is not always possible to figure out where one dimension (ecological, economic, social, cultural) stops and where the other starts (Alander 2007). It is, however, valuable for analytical reasons to separate the dimensions.

PARTICIPATION IN DESIGN AND IMPLEMENTATION OF INFORMATION TECHNOLOGIES

In Our Common Future the dimension of sustainability was developed, along with the development of technologies as a way to create sustainable lives. These lines of thought have been developed in the action plan, Agenda 21, in which actions and participation with a particular focus on the local was underscored. Enhancing participation and fostering cooperation and common responsibility are all obvious social efforts in the work for sustainable development. But transitions towards sustainability will also affect every dimension of the sociotechnical system in which we live (Alander 2007). We argue that when the principles of sustainability are translated into IT design, additional principles are required in order to enhance participation – so that the IT systems will be adapted to the work practice or that the system will support citizens and prospective users in their everyday activities. This is underlined by the key principles for an information society for all: 'Applications should be user-friendly, accessible to all, affordable, adapted to local needs in languages and cultures, and support sustainable development' (WSIS 2003, p. 7).

Participation is emphasized by both the WSIS and Agenda 21; PD is an approach with a focus on participation in IT design, enabling the involvement of various stakeholders and practitioners in the IT design and implementation process. Participation and participation on equal terms are elementary principles in PD. Further, rather than IT systems and applications being designed and implemented in isolation, 'decisions about technology also involve decisions about work content and job design' (Greenbaum 1993, p. 28). Hence, in PD projects, a range of people with different experiences and knowledge are involved in the design and implementation of IT systems. Consequently, their visions and ideas intervene in the design of the system, but the question is whether equity can be achieved, even where the intention is to work on equal terms. A range of methods and techniques have been developed by the PD community in order to enable various stakeholders to get first hand experi- ences of a practice, and to try and obtain equality in the co-operation. Examples are future works, participant observations, interviews, scenarios, story-boards, prototypes, etc. (Bødker et al. 2004). This also includes more creative and experimental methods such as games (Brandt 2006), probes (Gaver et al. 2003), cartographies (Mörtberg & Elovaara 2010 in press), and performances (Jacucci et al. 2005).

The involvement of practitioners or users in IT design has a long tradition in Scandinavian countries. This tradition can be described with its two main trajectories: one to democratize the working life and the other to democratize the design process in order to get a better understanding

of the practice and to involve those who work in the practice (Bjerknes & Bratteteig 1995). The aim of involving prospective users has been based on the ambition to support those at the margins. Today, various practitioners are involved in order to contribute inspiration and creative ideas to the design process (Kanstrup & Christiansen 2006). Kanstrup and Christiansen (2006, p. 328) emphasize how the Scandinavian tradition of PD builds on phronesis (practical wisdom) when they write: 'designers strive to serve the common good and avoid harming people's possibilities to develop a life of their own'. Hence, participation has a particular meaning in this tradition with its focus not only on participation but on participation on equal terms – that is, to be actors based on equality in the design of IT systems and services. Participation on equal terms is not an easy goal to achieve because asymmetrical power relations, such as gender, age, expert/non-expert, etc., are intertwined with the design process. The rationale for being involved in a PD project is not always the same: some try to obtain cooperation as equals, others to get their product adapted to a new customer. No matter why and how people participate, their motive of being involved has an impact on the process (Jansson et al. 2008).

In participatory approaches, it is also important to identify activities that are not always visible or obvious to others not involved in the day-to-day activity because they take place backstage, or have low status and are considered as routine work (Karasti 2001). The meal production explored in this paper is a sector with low status, dominated by women, and in which IT systems and services have recently been implemented.

Design From Somewhere Or Nowhere?

Design is a practice with the potential to learn from each other. That is, the designers learn from the users and the users learn from the designers: mutual learning (see, for example, Bratteteig

2004). Design and implementation processes are thus sites for knowledge production. Suchman (2002) locates design with the use of three positions: 'design from nowhere', 'detached intimacy', and 'design from somewhere'. In the position of 'design from nowhere', the designers distance themselves from the practice where the system will be used, from the prospective users and their activities. This can be compared with what Haraway (1991) calls 'the view from nowhere'. In this position, knowledge is regarded as universal and uniform, without impact from the individuals involved in the research or in the design project. In 'design from nowhere', the designers can see everything but not how their own position, knowledge, and understandings intervene in how the design is conducted, and also in the system's functionality. Further, designers think they are able to design IT systems and services without the involvement of prospective users or other practitioners in the process. Features of the second position, 'detached intimacy', include building alliances with professional colleagues in order to create intimate relationships with them while, at the same time, keeping their distance from prospective users and their work practice.

In 'design from somewhere', designers consider themselves as actors in practices with a range of experiences and knowledge but also consider that their own visions and ideas are created 'somewhere' because knowledge is not complete but is always partial and situated (Haraway 1991). Designers who are located in this position understand that it is impossible to capture everything but, with involvement of various competences and views, it is possible to extend their understanding in order to take responsibility for the design process and its outcome. Basic principles in PD locate the approach in this position as 'design from somewhere' or located accountability (Suchman 2002).

PD strives for a design process on equal terms and to find out fundamental traditions and values in a practice. Equity is an aspect in social sustainability, tradition, identity, norms and values in cultural sustainability, and in Agenda 21's focus on local activities. We argue that PD is useful in the development of sustainable design practices, methodologies and methods.

RESEARCH METHODS AND CONTEXT

The empirical data used in this paper were collected in public-sector-meal production in a municipality in northernmost Sweden during 2002–2005.2 Interviews with two municipal managers of the meal production for children, participation observations in kitchens, and literature studies, including texts and documents concerning the municipality and public sector meal production, were used. In this paper we use data from participant observations in a pre-school kitchen and two interviews conducted with the municipal manager of meal production for schools, manager A, and her successor, manager B.

The participant observation was carried out in 2002 in a pre-school kitchen. The first interview was conducted in February 2003 and the second in October 2005. A range of projects had been conducted in school kitchen meal production with the goal of changing the practice. Manager A had been involved in these projects and it was the reason why she was interviewed: she had an overview of the transformations that had taken place, on both the municipality and school-kitchen level. The second interview was conducted in order to follow up the transformation that had taken place in the municipality described by manager A in the first interview. As manager A had been replaced, the second interview was conducted with the new manager, manager B. The interviews were semi-structured, audio-recorded and transcribed verbatim. They lasted for approximately 90 minutes and were carried out in the managers' offices.

Public Meal Production in Sweden

In Sweden, all children in compulsory school (from the age of 6 until they are 16) get free lunch that is tax-funded. This is also the normal situation in the majority of upper secondary schools. Free school lunches have been served in compulsory schools since 1946 and became a legal right in 1998. The legislation was approved after this right had been questioned during the economic crisis of the early 1990s. Together with the meals served in day-care centres, school lunches make up almost 2,100,000 of the 2,600,000 meals that are produced in the Swedish public sector every weekday. The public sector's meal production is extensive, tax-funded, and dependent on a range of technologies. Thus, the meal production has an impact on most Swedish people and it is an extensive activity not only in terms of economy and technology but also related to social and cultural aspects. Consequently, the sector is of interest both in relation to design and implementation of IT-based information systems and to sustainable development.

The Swedish public sector is in a transformation or modernization process where rationalization and effectiveness are more or less explicit goals. Therefore public meal production is also under transformation. This is, among other things, carried out with the implementation of large-scale systems, such as cook-and-chill, where the preparation and cooking is concentrated to a few kitchens where the meal is chilled before it is transported to the local kitchens. This transportation takes place a number of times each week. Another trans- formation is the implementation of a range of IT systems and services such as, for example, the application used in the school kitchens that we report on here.

The work on meal production is distributed over the whole day, though probably it is more intensive on some occasions than others, e.g.,

during lunch. In school restaurants, though, the workload is more concentrated around lunchtime, some school kitchens serving lunch for up to 500 pupils during a few lunch hours. The work in kitchens and restaurants includes, of course, keeping the kitchen in order: washing up, taking care of the waste and ordering, unpacking and storing the food-stuffs, and so forth. On weekdays, approximately 25 per cent of the inhabitants have at least one meal from the institutional kitchens in the municipality (elder-care included) (Alander 2007). The work in school kitchens and restaurants is mobile in terms of responsibility for who does what around the kitchen and in the restaurants, particularly in pre-school kitchens.

A Pre-School Kitchen

In pre-school kitchens, normally, one person works alone. In the school studied, Lisbeth (the name is fictitious), (the majority of kitchen staff are female) was responsible for preparing, cooking and serving breakfast, lunch and afternoon snacks or sandwiches to 20–80 people. Besides cooking, she ordered, received, unpacked and stored the food-stuffs, dished up and took care of waste. Once a week, foodstuffs and other things required in the work practice were delivered by a small truck and then stored in a room connected to the kitchen. The kitchen was rather small with just enough space to move around between the different technologies and equipment placed along the walls. A cooking island was placed in the middle of the room with an oven, sink, chopping board, and four stove plates. Lisbeth had arranged a small office area with a telephone, files, and a notepad. The office area was just by the only window in the kitchen. At the time of the observation, an e-commerce application had been implemented and was in use in the municipality's kitchens. The computer was placed in a room beside the kitchen.

ALL THE PROBLEMS: ARTICLES, QUANTITIES AND FRESH FRUIT

The main argument for the purchase and implementation of the e-commerce application was to make the municipal invoicing process more efficient. One part in the rationalization was to integrate the meal production, invoices, and the orders for food-stuff and other goods into the application. Every school kitchen was equipped with a stationary computer, with Internet access, to be used to order foodstuff for the school restaurant. The orders were carried out with the use of a web-based interactive form. The e-commerce application was thus a web-based, standard application developed by an external software company. The co-operative distribution and the municipal's new agreement on purchasing were introduced simultaneously with the e-commerce application. The structures of the new purchase agreement and the co-operative distribution technology were integrated in the e-commerce application, although not dependent on it.

The employees in the kitchens were not familiar with the use of computers and IT systems in their day-to-day practices. Meal production has a low status, is dominated by women, and has not been given priority when IT systems and services have been designed and implemented. In order to know how to use the application and the functionalities, all those responsible for ordering (or at least one person in every kitchen) participated in a training course. An employee in the municipality was appointed to do the training. Manager B was responsible for the training before she replaced manager A as the manager of the municipal meal production for schools.

We have chosen to focus on problems and shortcomings with the e-commerce application. The argument is that in 2005, three years after the implementation, 10 out of 21 kitchens had returned to manual ordering. We start with a brief description of the transformations in the school kitchens that took place with the new e-services.

Transformations in the School Kitchens

In the interview, manager A explained that the meal production's complexity was the reason why it had been chosen to be the first sector in which the e-commerce application was implemented. This complexity was supposed to be simplified and made more effective with the use of the IT application. Manager A also explained that this municipality was a pioneer compared with other municipalities in implementing IT in meal production. Manager A said the application had both advantages and disadvantages. Both the user's adaptation to the application and the contextualization of the application to the specific practice could be bedevilled by 'teething troubles'. Manager A explained that the system would be an advantage if 'the ordering goes faster' and 'one becomes more aware of the prices'. She was also clear that 'it is necessary to get the systems to work' in order 'to do the order- ing more quickly' because the employees in kitchens do not have spare time to sit in front of the computer. Efficiency was also the main argument for implementing the application. But did the assumptions prove true and did Lisbeth share manager A's optimism? We will illustrate the experiences with some examples of how small things matter in the day-to-day activities.

Before the e-commerce application was implemented Lisbeth carried out the food orders by phoning producers and suppliers. Lisbeth worked alone in the pre-school kitchen, consequently she had to plan her tasks in the kitchen in order to be able to leave it long enough to order the stuff. Lisbeth tried also to plan for the requirements for one week in just a single order. If there were problems with the system it would of course take longer than she had estimated and, if this was the case, she would have to take a break, return to the kitchen, and continue with the order later – a change compared with the manual system, where it was possible to continue with some tasks in the kitchen and she, at least, had better control of the cooking process.

The deliveries were also confirmed by the application. The task of control-ling and comparing the delivery order with the goods listed on the invoice was not changed by the IT application. Other manual tasks related to the invoices were, however, replaced through the application. Further, the e-commerce application had caused transformations in how the work was organized and conducted in the school kitchens. The staff had to deal with the transformation, the new tasks and the use of computers, which were a novelty for many in the school kitchens. They used a range of technologies but not, however, computers. Lisbeth's equipment was placed in a room apart from the kitchen – a stationary computer with an Internet connection. Thus she had to leave the kitchen to use the e-service while manual routines had allowed her to remain in the kitchen to control the cooking and also to continue with her tasks in cooking the food.

Riven' and 'Batteridriven'

The articles in the provider agreement were stored in a database to be used in the meal production units when they ordered stuff. Lisbeth and her colleagues ordered the foodstuff or other things with the use of a form on a web page. A browser was also available. She was able to search for an article with its article number or its article name: abbreviated or with the complete name. Although abbreviation was possible it was not always easy to figure out the search function's logic. This was illustrated with an example from manager B who explained that if one wanted to order grated cheese (*riven ost*) one has to register the whole term – '*riven ost*' – because batteridriven (a battery-operated thing) comes up if one only registers '*riven*'. The result was not wrong but it was not always self-explanatory, particularly if one was unfamiliar with the application and also had limited time for ordering. Manager B explained

that the fastest way to carry out the orders was to use the article number – something the staff in the kitchen were at first unfamiliar with but which they found out after some time. She also recounted that one way to deal with the unfamiliarity was to create one's own paper-based list of the most commonly used article numbers to be placed next to the computer. The quantity was also something the person had to ponder on before s/he made the order: whether it was two bottles of ketchup or two boxes of bottles; if the bags of potatoes were 10 kilos or 25 kilos. Hence, quantity registration had caused problems and annoyance in the kitchens not only for Lisbeth but also in other kitchens.

Fresh Fruit Or?

Lisbeth, who worked alone in the kitchen, was proud that she had been able to learn how to work with the computer and even gave the impression that she was almost surprised that she could actually do it. Lisbeth said, however, that stress in the kitchen had increased due to all the problems with the electronic ordering system. Sometimes she created problems by punching the wrong key; other times the errors were attributed to the software or the product list. The latter resulted in wrong deliveries. Lisbeth told how she had realized that if something went wrong it was not necessarily her fault. Lisbeth gave as an example her decision to order several kilos of mandarin oranges. They were categorized under the heading of fresh fruit in the product list. Lisbeth made the order but was, however, surprised when the truck arrived with the ordered food stuff: it appeared she had got the whole amount as canned mandarins instead of fresh fruit. Lisbeth said she felt a little silly and thought she must have done something wrong when she registered the order. She repeated the order, this time carefully checking that she ordered fresh fruit. But what happened after the order was sub-mitted? The following week when the truck arrived with the stuff the delivered mandarins again were not fresh but canned. This time, Lisbeth said, she was sure that there had to be something wrong with the system and the order forms. Lisbeth had made the order correctly but the delivered stuff was not in accordance with what she had ordered. The information presented on the webpage and the content in the database diverged. Manager B explained that such problems were well known and also those with ordered quantities.

Small Things Matter

The meal production manager, manager B, was on leave from her ordinary job as an accountant when the e-commerce application was implemented with the need for her to train all the necessary kitchen staff in how to use the application: 21 people in total. By the time of the interview, manager B indicated that only around 10 out of the 21 she had trained still used the e-commerce application. The majority of the staff in the kitchens had returned to manual ordering due to a deeply-felt irritation with all the problems. For example, some bugs that had been corrected appeared again after a new version had been installed. Manager B explained the latter problems:

a small thing matters and it only has to be a minor thing but it explodes... it is very annoying, it will be difficult to gain acceptance of a new e-commerce application – the functionality must be much better.

Manager B had experience of e-commerce applications other than the one used in the municipality and none was apparently better than the other; they all had their pros and cons. Manager B commented on her experiences: 'those who construct the system do not visit the kitchens to find out how it really is or to listen to the cooks who have not experience of computers'. In spite of this, manager B was enthusiastic over the possibilities that an e-commerce application could bring into the work practice. In the present system, she highlighted the account-coding that facilitated the ordering process in the kitchens as something positive. Manager B had also made suggestions about how to improve the functionalities. As the manager of the meal production, she was also aware of the disadvantages in the present application. One general aspect was the usability, she said: 'it should be easy for the staff; an application should improve the day-to-day work'. Usability issues should be considered in the light of the limited time the staff has because no extra time was assigned to conduct the ordering and associated tasks that had appeared with the IT application. Manager B also expressed doubt as to whether the reported bugs or the suggested improvements had actually reached the software company, though she knew that they had been reported to the person who was the municipality's contact with the supplier. Manager B also pondered whether it had become a matter of prestige, or a need for those responsible for the purchase of the system to minimize the problems. Despite all the problems they had had with the application, manager B was convinced that e-commerce could improve the work in the school kitchens. However, her enthusiasm with the present application had dwindled to mistrust.

CONCLUDING THOUGHTS

We have explored in this article social and cultural sustainability, with a particular focus on participation, in a discussion of problems related to the implementation of a web-based application in the school meal production in a municipality in northernmost Sweden, where, three years after the start, 10 out of 21 kitchens had returned to the manual routines.

Arguments about effectiveness, or how to make a practice more efficient in order to justify design and implementation of IT systems and services in organizations, are usual. The question is whether the e-commerce application can be considered as effective or sustainable when 10 out of 21 kitchens had returned to manual routines. Shapiro (2005) argues for a use of PD in order to decrease failures related to design and implementation of IT systems and services. Participation, and participation on equal terms, in design and implementation of IT/ IS is also an argument for sustainability, and particularly social sustainability.

Equity is one aspect of social sustainability, dignity another. Problems with quantities, with categories, and with the wrong products delivered, were things the staff in the school kitchens had to deal with. To find out that one's orders result in incorrect quantities or in canned fruit instead of fresh fruit does not increase one's self-respect and confidence, particularly if one is unfamiliar with IT systems and services. Initially, Lisbeth assumed that she had made mistakes before she realized the system's shortcomings. The bugs and problems seem not to be too complicated; however, they appear to have caused annoyances and stress. Further, that some bugs returned after new versions had been installed increased the annoyance and prevented the work process in the kitchens. Design and implementation of IT services without the involvement of those who work in the school kitchens, and that, in addition, cause a deterioration in the staff's working conditions, is not sustainable enough in regard to either social or economic dimensions.

It did not appear from either Lisbeth's narratives or from those of the managers whether the co-operative distribution and agreement on purchasing integrated in the ordering of foodstuff could explain some of the delivery problems. It was, however, obvious that the employees in the municipality's school kitchen did not participate in either the purchasing or in the design of the application. One of the managers of the meal production for schools expressed an existing gap between those who design the application and those who work in the kitchens where the system was used. The designers have neither the experience nor the knowledge about the work practice and the day-to-day activities. The manager also made it clear that some of the employees had

limited experience in using computers in their day-to-day activities. The staff's unfamiliarity with computers presumably did matter, but less so than the application's shortcomings because they failed to benefit from the application, which was not robust or sustainable. The standard application did not reflect the practice, norms and values of Lisbeth and colleagues and can be categorized as 'design from nowhere' (Suchman 2002).

Women as a group are singled out in both Agenda 21 and by WSIS. The meal production in Swedish school kitchens is dominated by women and has low status, and few IT applications have so far been implemented in the municipality's meal production. These circumstances show the importance to pay particular attention to how gender intersect in design (Mörtberg & Elovaara 2007; Jansson et al. 2007) or how gender and technology is a 'mutually constitutive relationship' (Wajcman 2000, p. 460).

In Lisbeth's as well as in the managers' accounts, it became obvious that Lisbeth and her colleagues in this particular municipality neither participated in the design nor in the purchase of the e-commerce solution. It was, however, unclear if others in the municipality had been involved during the development process. The work in the kitchens is mobile. It became obvious that the employees had to leave the kitchen to make the orders, due to a stationary computer. With the manual routines it was possible to remain in the kitchen and still have control of the activities as well as performing some of them. Further, the staff had no additional time to deal with the ordering system. The main reason for the implementation was to rationalize the municipal invoicing process, thus, the activities in the kitchens were not at the heart of the process but were integrated into the e-commerce application. Stationary solutions are probably more suitable to accounting practice rather than to activities conducted in the kitchens and to be sustainable, in the meaning of being integrated into long-term work practices, the system should in fact have supported the mobile practice in the kitchens. This may have strengthened the e-commerce applications role in the school kitchens, and would probably have had a higher potential of being adapted into the daily practices, resulting in more employees accepting it.

As the manager for meal production for schools also highlighted, the weakness of the e-commerce application was, among other things, the systems designers' lack of familiarity with the practice where the application was implemented. The managers had an overview of all kitchens and the activities and this, together with Lisbeth's experiences, show how this design and implementation can be located in the position of 'design from nowhere' (Suchman 2002). The designers seemed to have considered themselves, their knowledge and experiences to be sufficient when they developed an application for a practice like the school restaurants. They seemed not to consider the knowledge of others or that experiences and knowledge are diverse, partial and depend on people's doings and actions in day-to-day activities such as those in the school meal restaurants (Haraway 1991). PD is an approach with the aim to involve all stakeholders in the design in order to gain understanding of practices, to involve others as well in the design process and not to trust only the designers. Bødker et al. (2004) argue that the necessity to understand prospective users work practices is in fact an important part of a sustainable design:

However, in order to develop sustainable visions of new IT usage, the designers need to gain an understanding of the work – which frequently, upon closer examination, turns out to be quite well-organized (Bødker et al. 2004, p. 285)

Bødker et al. (2004) argue how IT design requires knowledge about practices and fundamental traditions in order to design for sustainability. We argue that the experiences of the e-commerce application and the knowledge of traditions, norms and values related to the work practice

in the kitchen shows the necessity of integrating cultural aspects to achieve sustainability in the design of IT/IS. Care and wellbeing by serving tasty dishes to the school children are norms and values associated with the practice in the kitchen (Alander 2007) and are an important part of the knowledge tradition that should be included in cultural sustainability. The analysis shows how the e-commerce application neither renewed nor maintained important values and norms rooted in the practice in the kitchen (Hawkes 2001). In fact, a consequence of the e-commerce application was that new activities were introduced that disturbed the day-to-day practices in the kitchens. The system, however, did not allow the employees to create positive relationships with it and, instead of supporting their work, it created a new set of bugs and errors. This could have been prevented by applying a cultural sustainability approach that focuses, in this case, on the traditions of routines, the knowledge and values that build the rationale of the practices established in the kitchen (Stuedahl 2004).

As we know, green or eco design has for a long time influenced urban planning and architecture with principles built on sustainability. A well-known argument is that IT can support the sustainability of a future society but the time has come to turn the question around and ask how we can design IT systems and services in more sustainable ways. A framework to integrate ecological dimensions as guiding principles in interaction design has been developed by Blevis (2006, 2007). In this paper we have paid particular attention to the social and cultural factors related to design and use of IT. We have used some examples of transformations taking place in Swedish school kitchens as a consequence of the implementation of e-services. Based on our analysis, we argue for the necessity to also integrate the four dimensions of sustainability, social, economic, ecological and cultural, in the design of IT/IS. This, we argue, will extend the ecological guiding principles emerging in interaction design, and might help us to develop new ways of thinking and articulating ideals of sustainable design in the IT/IS field.

ACKNOWLEDGMENT

This paper could not have been written without the helpful people in the school; thank you all! We are very grateful to anonymous referees for helpful comments on earlier drafts of this article, and to Heather Owen for the editing.

REFERENCES

Alander, S. (2007). *Offentliga storkök i det gröna folkhemmet: diffrakterade berättelser om hållbar utveckling* [Institutional kitchens in the green welfare state – diffracted narratives on sustainable development]. Dissertation, Luleå University of Technology, Luleå.

Bjerknes, G., & Bratteteig, T. (1995). User participation and democracy, a discussion of Scandinavian research on system development . *Scandinavian Journal of Information Systems, 7*(1), 73–98.

Blevis, E. (2006). *Advancing Sustainable Interaction Design: Two Perspectives on Material Effects, Design Philosophy Papers: Collection Four* (pp. 52–69). [Online]. Retrieved April 17, 2008 from http://www.desphilosophy.com/dpp/dpp_journal/journal.html

Blevis, E. (2007). Sustainable interaction design: invention and disposal, renewal and reuse. In R. Grinter, T. Rodden, P. Aoki, E. Cutrell, R. Jeffries & G. Olson (Eds.), *Proceedings of the SIGCHI Conference on Human Factors in Computing Systems, CHI 2007* (pp. 503–512). ACM Conference Proceedings Series. New York: ACM Press.

Bødker, K., Kensing, F., & Simonsen, J. (2004). *Participatory IT Design. Designing for Business and Workplace Realities*. Cambridge, MA: MIT Press.

Braa, J., Monteiro, E., & Sahay, S. (2004). Networks of action: sustainable health information systems across developing countries . *Management Information Systems Quarterly, 28*(3), 337–362.

Brandt, E. (2006). Designing exploratory design games: a framework for participation in Participatory Design? In I. Wagner, J. Blomberg, G. Jaccuci & F. Kenising (Eds.), *Proceedings of the Ninth Conference on Participatory Design: Expanding Boundaries in Design, vol. 1* (pp. 105–114). New York: ACM Press.

Bratteteig, T. (2004). Making change. Dealing with relations between design and use, Dr. Philos Dissertation, Department of Informatics, University of Oslo.

Byrne, E. (2005). Using action research in information systems design to address change: a South African health information systems case study. In *Proceedings of the 2005 Annual Research Conference of the South African Institute of Computer Scientists and Information Technologists on IT Research in Developing Countries SAICSIT '05* (pp. 131–141). White River, South Africa.

Byrne, E., & Sahay, S. (2007). Generalizations from an interpretive study: the case of a South African community-based health information system . *South African Computer Journal, 38*, 8–19.

Cheney, H., Nheu, N., & Vecellio, L. (2004). Sustainability as social change: values and power. In H. Cheney, E. Katz & F. Solomon (Eds.), *Sustainability discourse, Sustainability and Social Round Table Proceeding* (pp. 225–246), The Institute for Sustainable Futures, Sydney and CSIRO Minerals, Melbourne [Online]. Retrieved April 17, 2008 from http://www.minerals.csiro.au/sd/pubs/

Eichler, M. (1999). Sustainability from a feminist sociological perspective: a frame- work for disciplinary reorientation . In Becker, E., & Johan, T. (Eds.), *Sustainability and the Social Sciences: A Cross-Disciplinary Approach to Integrating Environmental Considerations into Theoretical Reorientation* (pp. 182–206). London: Zed Books and UNESCO.

Elovaara, P., & Mörtberg, C. (2007). Design of digital democracies – performance of citizenship, gender and IT . *Information Communication and Society, 10*(3), 404–423. doi:10.1080/13691180701410091

Escobar, A. (1995). *Encountering Development: The Making and Unmaking of the Third World.* Princeton, NJ: Princeton University Press.

Gaver, B., Beaver, J., & Benford, S. (2003). Ambiguity as a resource for design. In G. Cockton & P. Korhonen (Eds.), *Proceedings of the SIGCHI conference on Human Factors in Computing Systems* (pp. 233–240). ACM Conference Proceedings Series. New York: ACM Press.

Greenbaum, J. (1993). A design of one's own: towards participatory design in the United States . In Schuler, D., & Namioka, A. (Eds.), *Participatory Design, Principles and Practices* (pp. 27–37). Hillsdale, NJ: Lawrence Erlbaum Associates.

Haraway, D. J. (1991). *Simians, Cyborgs, and Women: The Reinvention of Nature.* New York: Routledge.

Hawkes, J. (2001). *The fourth pillar of sustainability: culture's essential role in public planning, The Cultural Development Network,* Australia, [Online]. Retrieved April 17, 2008 from http://www.cultureandcommunities.ca/downloads/Salons/Salon3-handout.pdf

Jacucci, C., Jacucci, G., Wagner, I., & Psik, T. (2005). A manifesto for the performative development of ubiquitous media. In *Proceedings of The Fourth Decennial Aarhus Conference* (pp. 19–28). Denmark: ACM Press.

Jansson, M., Mörtberg, C., & Berg, E. (2007). Old dreams, new means: an exploration of visions and situated knowledge in information technology. *Gender, Work and Organization, 14*(4), 371–387. doi:10.1111/j.1468-0432.2007.00349.x

Jansson, M., Mörtberg, C., & Mirijamdotter, A. (2008). Participation in e-home healthcare @ North Calotte. In K. Tollmar & B. Jönsson (Eds.), *Proceedings of the 5th Nordic Conference on Human–Computer Interaction: Building Bridges* (pp. 192–200). ACM Conference Proceedings Series. New York: ACM Press.

Kanstrup, A. M., & Christiansen, E. (2006). Selecting and evoking innovators: combining democracy and creativity. In A. Mørch, K. Morgan, T. Bratteteig, G. Ghosh & D. Svanæs (Eds.), *Proceedings of the 4th Nordic Conference on Human–Computer Interaction: Changing Roles* (pp. 321-330). ACM Conference Proceedings Series. New York: ACM Press.

Karasti, H. (2001). *Increasing sensitivity towards everyday work practice in system design.* Dissertation, University of Oulu, Oulu.

Lafferty, W. M., Aall, C., Lindseth, G., & Nordland, I. T. (Eds.). (2006). *Lokal Agenda 21 i Norge: Så mye hadde vi - så mye ga vi bort – så mye har vi igjen* [Local Agenda 21 in Norway], Unipub forlag, Oslo.

Mörtberg, C., & Elovaara, P. (in press). Attaching people and technology: between e and government . In Booth, S., Goodman, S., & Kirkup, G. (Eds.), *Gender Issues in Learning and Working with Information Technology: Social Constructs and Cultural Context.* Hershey, PA: IG Global.

Mörtberg, C., Stuedahl, D., & Elovaara, P. (forthcoming). Designing for sustainable ways of living with technologies . In Wagner, I., Bratteteig, T., & Stuedahl, D. (Eds.), *Exploring Digital Design Multi-disciplinary Design Practices.* Berlin-Heidelberg, DE: Springer Verlag.

Shapiro, D. (2005). Participatory design: the will to succeed. In O. W. Bertelsen, N. O. Bouvin, P. G. Krogh & M. Kyng (Eds.), *Proceedings of the 4th Decennial Conference on Critical Computing: Between Sense and Sensibility* (pp. 29–38). New York: ACM Press.

Stuedahl, D. (2004). Forhandlinger og over-talelser: kunnskapsbygging på tvers av kunnskapstradisjoner i brukermedvirkende design av ny IKT [Negotiations and persuasion. Knowledge building crosses knowledge traditions in participatory design IT design], Series of Dissertations No. 34', The Faculty of Education, University of Oslo.

Suchman, L. (2002). Located accountabilities in technology production. *Scandinavian Journal of Information Systems, 14*(2), 91–105.

Visvanathan, S. (1991). Mrs Brundtland lovely non-magical cosmos, *Lokayan Bulletin, 9*(1). *Alternatives,* 3.

Wackernagel, M., & Rees, W. E. (1996). *Our Ecological Footprint: Reducing Human Impact on the Earth.* Philadelphia, PA: New Society Publishers.

Wajcman, J. (2000). Reflections on gender and technology studies. In what state is the art? *Social Studies of Science, 30*(3), 447–464. doi:10.1177/030631200030003005

WCED (World Commission on Environment Development). (1987). *Our Common Future.* Oxford, UK: Oxford University Press.

WSIS (World Summit on the Information Society). (2003) *Geneva 2003 and Tunis 2005 Declarations of Principles. Building the Information Society: A Global Challenge in the New Millennium,* [Online] Retrieved July 15, 2008 from http://www.itu.int/dms_pub/itu-s/md/03/wsis/doc/S03-WSIS-DOC-0004!!PDF-E.pdf

ENDNOTES

[1] The notion of ecological footprints has its focus on the flows of energy and material that goes to and from a particular entity, e.g., a household, city, or county, – translates the flow to correspond with the land and water needed to maintain the flows. Thus, this approach builds on a method to calculate a certain consumption impact on the ecological system (Wackernagel & Rees 1996).

[2] Sara Alander collected the data for her doctoral thesis (see Alander 2007).

[3] © Taylor & Francis Ltd, *Information Communication & Society, 13*(1), 68-87; Mörtberg, Christina, Stuedahl, Dagny, and Alander, Sara (2010); Why Do The Orders Go Wrong All The Time? Exploring Sustainability in an E-Commerce Application in Swedish Public School Kitchens. Reprinted with permission.

Chapter 35
Information and Communication Technologies for the Good Society

Wolfgang Hofkirchner
Vienna University of Technology, Austria

ABSTRACT

The appearance of notions of a "good society" does not come as a surprise, given the recent crises in the fields of economy, the financial markets, or the climate change. These notions play a decisive role in the context of implementing ICTs. This chapter contends that ICTs – like any technology – make sense in the context of normative visions only that make technology a means to an end. The vision of a good society must nowadays refer to the global challenges confronting the further development of societies. In doing so it identifies ICTs as facilitators of the advent of a Global Sustainable Information Society which makes ICTs meaningful or it classifies them as meaningless gadgets or even as detrimental for designing the future. It is Gunilla Bradley who can take credit for devoting her lifework to raising awareness of the impacts of ICTs on humans and the ethical implications of research in that field.

Gunilla Bradley's lifework has been intrinsically motivated by safeguarding human well-being and the search for societal conditions that enable individual self-fulfillment, given the rapid development and deployment of converging computer, tele- and media technologies. Her scientific perspective is normative. Her vision is "the good ICT society" (2006, 197), "the good society for all (GSA)" (2006, 229). In that she is a pioneer and has been serving as lightfire for the emerging field

of ICTs and society (a term by which I intend to comprise all scientific endeavours to design and assess ICTs in their societal context, whether they originate in Science and Technology Studies, New Media Studies, Computer Science or else).

It's an opportune moment to discuss the "good society". The current financial crisis that brought about the current economic crisis does question the current neoliberal system and its belief in the free market. In doing so, it makes the quest for a "good society" topical. And indeed, the attention that is given to the issue of a "good society" has

DOI: 10.4018/978-1-60960-057-0.ch035

recently been rising. Suffice to mention that, in the political field, ten years after Tony Blair and Gerhard Schröder produced their declaration of the European "third way" in June 1999, British and German Social Democrats invite to a debate on "Building the Good Society" in Europe (Cruddas and Nahles 2009), or that, in the academic field, there is a trend to base good life research issues being investigated in connection with technologies more and more upon considerations of what is the good society – in that vein, e.g., the director of the European division of the International Association of Computing and Philosophy, Philip Brey, had his talk at the Seventh European Conference on Computing and Philosophy 2009 on "The Proper Role of Information Technology in a Good Society".

My own considerations regarding the good society gained tremendous momentum when I became acquainted with a remarkable publication on behalf of the European Union. In April 1997, an EC High-Level Expert Group on Social and Societal Aspects of Information Society, chaired by Luc Soete, and under the participation of well-known scholars like Manuel Castells who ranks today under the most cited authors on information society matters, finalised a report under the title "Building the European information society for us all".

The basic tenet they departed from is the insight that "the information society signals more than a major change in the technological paradigm that underpins our society." The policy challenges ICTs raise "transcend the simplistic notions of rapid adjustment to an externally, technologically determined future in which people have little or no say" and "the sooner these are addressed the better" (63).

The notions "wisdom" and "wise society" were introduced in this context and appeared for the first time and, unfortunately, so far, for the last time in an official document of the European Commission (16): "One of the main effects of the new ICTs has been to speed up and cut the cost of storing and transmitting information a billion-fold, thereby "energising", in the words of the Bangemann report, "every economic sector" ("Europe and the Global Information Society", Brussels, 1994). However, these new technologies have had no such effect on the generation or acquisition of knowledge, still less on wisdom [Which we identify as "distilled" knowledge derived from experience of life, as well as from the natural and social sciences and from ethics and philosophy.] . One would hope, of course, that society would be shifting more and more towards a "wise society", where scientifically supported data, information and knowledge would increasingly be used to make informed decisions to improve the quality of all aspects of life. Such wisdom would help to form a society that is environmentally sustainable, that takes the well-being of all its members into consideration and that values the social and cultural aspects of life as much as the material and economic. Our hope is that the emerging information society will develop in such a way as to advance this vision of wisdom."

The adoption of the competitive Lisbon strategy rendered the vision of this report obsolete. The positive aspect one might be inclined to ascribe to this report is that it anticipated or, at least, accompanied the shift in European Union policy thinking from technological issues exclusively to the inclusion of economic issues testified by the subsequently accorded framework programmes for European research and development. New buzzwords – the "knowledge-based economy" and the "knowledge society" – began to partly complement and partly replace the precedent talk of the "information society". However, the turn, if any, seems to have come to a halt half way. Deep changes that affect the quality of life, environmental sustainability, individual well-being, social and cutural needs as demanded by the report are still waiting for implementation. Neoliberal worshipping seems to have been sacrificing wisdom needed more than ever.

In 2004 I cast the normative vision of the "Global Sustainable Information Society" albeit, for a start, under a similar term when giving an invited lecture with the title "The Great Bifurcation: A Sustainable Global Information Society or Extinction" at the University College Cork, Ireland. Given that contemporary society undergoes a critical phase of evolution – marked by global challenges – which might end up in devolution, I have been conceiving of this phase in system theoretical terms: there is a bifurcation between a breakthrough towards a stable path of societal development that is based upon a novel principle of organisation of society, on the one hand, and a breakdown of the system at all, on the other. This is what I call the Great Bifurcation.

The breakthrough branch is tantamount to what, since my years at the Paris-Lodron University of Salzburg, I am used to calling the development of a "Global Sustainable Information Society" (GSIS) (see Hofkirchner et al. 2007). The purpose of this notion is to guide an integrative assessment and design of ICTs and their social settings which is a step in my activities intended to transcend social sciences and informatics. But this concept is of a more general importance. I argue that it is shaping ICTs that will be of decisive importance to societies that, in turn, are shaped by ICTs. For ICTs provide the means for enhancing the collective intelligence of the information society on different scales – the capability to reach goals by synergetic effects. The continuation of societal evolution becomes less and less probable without a quantum leap in collective intelligence achievable by means of ICTs that are designed for just that purpose. In that perspective, the Internet of today and its follow-up provide the material underpinning for a global consciousness that intervenes in the Great Bifurcation.

To be more to the point, by a GSIS I understand a society that is:

1. capable of making use of knowledge
2. for fighting the dangers of breakdown due to anthropogenic causes
3. on a global scale.

That is, I suggest the most universal value to be met by a good society be sustainability that denotes a society's ability to perpetuate its own development.

I, furthermore, suggest that sustainability be broken down into:

1. a social part, called social compatibility, which is inclusiveness and fairness – to be broken down, in turn, into equality in cultural terms, political freedom and solidarity as to economy –,
2. an ecological part, called environmental compatibility, and
3. a technological part, called technological compatibility, by which I mean a balanced relationship of new with old technologies – to be broken down, again, into usefulness, usability, efficiency, reliability, security, safety and other values.

The main argument is that not only a society that exploits nature (as was found with reduced notions of sustainability) but also a society that does not meet the criterion of social compatibility because of the exclusion of have nots (who are excluded from the usage of commons) or a society that does not abide by technology assessment would in the long run break down and not qualify for being sustainable.

To be more detailed, in the sociosphere social actions are carried out. Tangible and intangible goods are produced and consumed. Every social being is called to co-design the collective in which the supply of the goods is provided. The more actors have access to the supply, the more the sociosphere is well-balanced, fair, just. Thus, justice is the value we can identify at the level of the sociosphere.

In this sphere the actors as social beings construe social relations concerning rules (culture), regularities (polity) and resources (economy) (Hofkirchner and Fuchs 2003).

Culture is about rules in society, including the regularities of political life. It is the field of discourse in which the actors can express themselves as long as they happen to gain influence by sharing the power to define values, ethics, morals (Artigiani 1991). The power of definition legitimises actors to act in a specific way. The ideal of equality would be fulfilled, if all cultural actors shared the same power of definition.

Politics is about power, namely, power of decision. The disposal of means of power means the ability to influence decision-making processes about circumstances of life in general including economic affairs. It represents regularities of how actors pursue interests. By resorting to power, actors are authorised to determine themselves. The more political actors have a determining influence on decisions, the more they are deemed free. Thus freedom is an inherent value of the political sphere.

Economy is about self-preservation of the actors through access to resources. Economy is that sphere of society where the actors carry out work in order to meet their demands. The social relationships that emerge here and channel the self-preservation of the actors are property relations – property being the disposition of resources. According to the power of disposition resources are allocated to the actors, that is, goods are distributed to them. The regulative idea for the allocation is solidarity.

"Ecosphere" is the label for that sphere of society that comprises the flows of matter and energy in support of the physical life of the actors. Contrary to all other forms of life on our planet, humans are able to consciously design their metabolism and to produce their *umwelt* whenever nature itself is not capable of reproducing itself for the sake of humans. Ecological sustainability denotes such a delicate balance between the human nature and the humanised nature. It can only

be reached when the value of respect for nature scores high.

Technology is to augment the actors that take the role of productive forces in that they produce something when they aim at something. The technosphere is the sphere in which the actors of society carry out their instrumental activities. Instrumental activities are the use of technologies as well as the creation of new technologies. The overall aim to which the technological augmentation of productive forces is to contribute is to secure a peaceful development of civilisation.

Thus altogether you find here the same values that have been affirmed in the ecumenical process at the 1983 Vancouver assembly of the World Council Of Churches, albeit in a slightly different wording: "Justice, Peace and the Integrity of Creation" (see Niles 2003).

Exclusion from activities in one of the spheres means that the respective value intrinsic to the sphere in question is not fully realised. Exclusion from activities in the sociosphere produces alienation from fellow humans, that is, the failure of not building equality leads to lacking in influence. The missing implementation of freedom in the political sphere generates powerlessness, and non-compliance with solidarity in the economic sphere is tantamount with expropriation. Exclusion from activities in the ecosphere results in alienation from nature and exclusion from activities in the technosphere yields alienation from technology.

Exclusiveness is a characteristic of societal relations of domination. Exclusion identifies societies in which some actors dominate other actors. The realisation of domination finds its predisposition in possible incongruencies in the interplay of individual and society. As it is in the nature of a GSIS to be inclusive, the interrelation between the individual and the society is to acknowledge their mutual enrichment. Exclusiveness denies a lasting future for society.

ICTs and society as a transdisciplinary research field orients toward the fulfilment of values that are antagonists of the rule of domination. ICTs inhere the potential for that fulfilment. But they can also be used to prolong exclusions and hinder the advent of a GSIS. The inclusion of stakeholders in the genesis of technology makes the design process a participatory one and ensures a discourse that will marginalise exclusions.

Thus the vision of a GSIS as the good society is consequential for the study of ICTs and society. The object of study can be seen as any condition that is crucial for the shaping of ICTs for a GSIS. These conditions cover facilitators of, as well as impediments to, the shaping of technologies for a sustainable development.

If we distinguish between sociosphere, ecosphere and technosphere, there are interrelationships inbetween them and relationships within them that are fostering or are detrimental to societal development at any granularity – from the individual to the world society. The object of study consists in a variety of antagonisms. Since informatisation is rather a catalyst of fundamental societal developments which are given a new appearance than a creator of possibilities *ab novo*, the antagonistic aggravation of tendencies in societal development on the threshold of the global information age is the continuation of lasting antagonisms. Regarding all societal spheres together, the beginning of the information age can be characterised by an antagonism between the information rich and the information poor in which the antagonism between inclusion and exclusion is continued in a different form.

In the cultural sphere the human process of self-expression of actors turned historically, under the premise of domination, into an antagonism between equality and lacking in influence due to false consciousness. This antagonism turns again, in the course of informatisation, into an antagonism between (scientific) rationality and (mass) mediatised manipulation. The information revolution affects the mutual dependence of science, on the one hand, and values, ethics, morals, on the other, by giving more emphasis to the role scientific thoughts play within society.

Science is committed to truth. Will the penetration of everyday life with science help suppress rules of social interaction that are not in compliance with findings that are claimed to be true and, in turn, will it help place an obligation on science to undertake inquiries for the sake of humane purposes only and will it thereby help create a true noosphere as Teilhard de Chardin (1975) and V.I. Vernadsky were envisioning? Or will it contribute by disinfotainment to distorting consciousness and distorting conscience, instead?

In the political sphere self-determination has become antagonistic when there has been domination. The antagonists are freedom and powerlessness which appear as e-democracy and Big Brother to the inside and to the outside when entering the information age. The introduction of ICTs alters the nature of the polity: it becomes the agora of "noopolitik" where governmental and non-governmental actors meet, while bureaucracy turns into "cyberocracy" (Arquilla and Ronfeldt 1999). What is at stake here is: Will the informatised polity empower the political actors? Or will it, instead, extend the control over them, be they interior or foreign (Information Warfare)?

In the economic sphere, there is self-preservation having been exposed to the clash of solidarity with expropriation in dominantly ordered societies and to the clash between the great hypertext which comprises all knowledge of humanity – "cosmopedia" (as Pierre Lévy coined it 1994, see 1997) – and information monopolies under the influence of ICTs. The information age is characterised by knowledge becoming an essential resource itself, becoming a new factor in the economic production process of society (Toffler 1980). "Knowledge mining", however, is confronted with a certain attribute of knowledge which has consequences for the proprietary handling of it. In sharp contrast to other goods, knowledge is a good that, in principle, is not used up after being used, it does not vanish. For that reason, knowledge turns into a seemingly infinite resource while economy is said to deal with scarcity. Thus the basic question of the informatisation of the sphere of economy runs: Will knowledge be made accessible for each economic actor who is in need of it? Or will knowledge be kept in the bounds of private ownership and treated as commodity, instead?

Summarising, as to the sociosphere, there is an underlying antagonism between the human beings and the "Net" (as pointed out by Castells 1996-1998). This antagonism of the information age goes back to the antagonism between justice and alienation from fellow human beings which is the form in which the production of sense appears in the epoch of domination. By the increasing number of ICT applications dislocated throughout the sociosphere the network society arises (Castells 1996). Networking means the increasing interdependence of the actors and the increasing dependence of the actors on access to the means of managing this interdependence which are provided by ICTs. Will networking facilitate the access to the supply and increase justice and, thus, raise social integrity? Or will it contribute to social disparities and increase potential conflicts and raise the digital divide, instead?

As to the ecosphere, the human process of survival has been unfolding under domination into the contradictory tendencies of respect for and alienation from nature that again metamorphose, given the rise of the information society, into the contradiction between human beings and "Gaia" (Lovelock, 1987). Industrialisation multiplied material and energetic fluxes to an extent never seen before on earth. The flows threatened to get out of control. James R. Beniger (1986) calls the information revolution in this respect "control revolution" by which control over the flows can be regained. The question arises: Will the control revolution be used for restoring the balance between human living beings and their umwelt and raise ecological integrity? Or will it further the degradation of environment by means of computer usage, instead?

As to the technosphere, domination has been realising possible incongruities of human instru-

mental activities and making peace and security fight alienation from technology. ICTs intensify this conflict in the form of human beings in opposition to the "Megamachine" (Mumford 1964). The spread of ICTs brings about a change in the very sphere of using and creating technology. Technology itself changes. By coupling with the computer which mechanises certain abilities of the human brain the machine of the industrial age which only mechanised abilities of the human body turns into an automaton. This holds for the whole realm of the infrastructure of society. The ambivalence of informatised technology comes to light: Will automation contribute to augment productive forces and further security and peace and by that raise civilisational integrity? Or will it serve destructive purposes and raise the vulnerability of the information society, instead?

This approach is normative but doing justice to the factual at the same time. For it includes not only an account of the potential that is given with the actual but also an evaluation of the potential which sorts out the desired. Thus ICTs and Society in the perspective of the GSIS vision embraces an ascendence from the potential given now to the actual to be established in the future as well as an ascendence from the less good now to the better then which altogether yields the Not-Yet in critical theorist Ernst Bloch's sense (1967). It identifies facilitators and inhibitors of a good society.

The vision of the GSIS does not orient towards a utopian "nowhere" but searches for real possibilities, that is, possibilities that are anchored in reality. They are concrete and demonstrate that the search for a good society, that is, a better society is not in vain. Those realised possibilities can be envisioned as the foreshadowing of the better society.

It's worth noting that it is only a vision of the good society like the GSIS that gives reason to technological developments that are senseless in themselves unless coupled to humane values which makes them a means to an end. Without such an end they would be meaningless.

Figure 1. ICTs on the levels of things, of living beings, and of individuals in the perspective of a GSIS

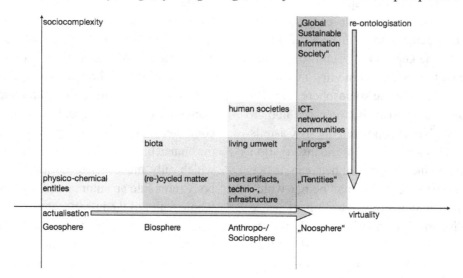

Take the following three developments in which ICTs, computers and Internet might be the driving force behind a convergence with other technologies (NBIC):

1. Pervasive or ubiquitous computing or ambient intelligence: technologists promise to make our human habitat smart, that is, endowed with chips linked to a net to become, in a tailored way, responsive to individual needs;

2. in analogy to this Internet of Things an Internet of living beings, of organisms, that are inhabitants of our *umwelt* as kind of an artificial web of life;

3. and the Internet on the level of the networked individuals of a Facebook society.

All of these developments are devoid of sense like those resulting in gadgets we know from our experiences as participants in the network society as long as there is no safeguard that they serve a humane purpose. Applying a GSIS perspective can set the stage for the development of meaningful technologies in an evolutionary context (see Figure 1).

The x-axis describes the dimension of virtuality and the y-axis the dimension of sociocomplexity. Virtuality means space of possibilities, sociocomplexity the complexity that arises when individual systems form a suprasystem. In the course of evolution, the space of possibilities might rise as well as the level of complexity of the systems. Physico-chemical entities, once exclusively defining the space on Planet Earth as Geosphere, turn, with the rise of biota, into matter that is cycled and recycled by biota and become part of a Biosphere, then turn, with the rise of human societies and the transition from Biosphere to an Anthropo- or Sociosphere, into inert artifacts as which they form the so-called techno- or infrastructure of human societies, and turn finally, with becoming "intelligent", "smart", by means of ubiqutous computing into what Floridi (2007) calls "ITentities". Biota turn, with the rise of human societies into the living *umwelt*, and turn, with becoming connected to the informatised infosphere, into what Floridi calls "inforgs". Human societies turn, with becoming connected to the informatised infosphere, into communities networked by ICTs.

Floridi coined also the term of "re-ontologisation" in that context. By that he means the reworking, reengineering of the infosphere – which according to him is the space of information – such that its ontological nature is transformed. The question is whether or not the technological trends described above and to be found at the respective levels are tantamount to the re-ontologisation of human societies. I contend the position that it is only under the conditions of a GSIS that the actualisation of virtuality through ICTs can be said to be tantamount to a qualitative leap onto a new level that re-ontologises the whole anthropo-/ sociosphere and transforms it into a "noosphere" envisaged by Teilhard de Chardin and Vladimir I. Vernadsky (Hofkirchner 1997). Without the shaping of ICTs in accord with the requirements of a GSIS the technological future will be thumb and dull and, eventually, lead to extermination.

A vision of the good society needs also indicators which allow the measurement of the advancement of society towards its betterment. The GSIS vision longs for the development of combined indicators of informationality (not only the spread of ICTs but also the generation of wisdom), sustainability (not only in ecological terms but also in social terms), and globality (not only regarding economy but also regarding world internal policy as well as the birth of a consciousness comprising all humanity).

So far there have been several attempts on preparing indicators for sustainable development. One attempt resulted in two sets approved by the Commission on Sustainable Development (CSD) in 1995, published in 1996, and after a revision process, again in 2001. 22 countries participated thereafter in pilot-testing these indicators. The latest revision in 2007 identified 50 indicators.

In 1996, at the invitation of the OECD, five working groups worked together to develop a follow-up of the above mentioned sets of indicators at a global level. Originally, the outcome of the working groups was termed "International Development Goals". In 2000 these goals became the "Millennium Development Goals (MDGs)". They can be regarded as intermediate stage to comprehensive sustainable development, as Crowley (2009) points out: "Despite their limitations however, the MDGs constitute the only at present globally focused endeavours by the world community of governments, international organisations and civil society to foster and enhance sustainable development" (77).

They comprise 8 goals (with 18 targets subsumed) addressing the social issues of

* extreme poverty and hunger;
* universal primary education;
* gender equality and the empowerment of women;the health issues of
* child mortality;
* maternal health;
* HIV/AIDS, malaria, and other diseases; the issue of environmental sustainability; and the issue of a global partnership for development.

To conclude, Gunilla Bradley's highlighting of the individual in the network age is not opposed to but, actually, necessitates, and is complementary to, the vision of the good society. The vision I consider necessary is that of a society that is characterised by its informationality, its sustainability and its globality – characteristics that support each other: GSIS. It's not a blueprint of a good society but rather a framework of conditions that have to be met if the development of societies shall enter the sustainable path.

Within this GSIS perspective ICTs can and shall be considered:

* as component of a technosocial system that comprises humans and is, in turn, a subsystem of society;
* as shaping society that shapes, in turn, ICTs;
* as providing a potential for true community-building shining forth as glimpses of a better future, while society provides impeding conditions for the actualisation

of this potential which are, in principle, removable.

REFERENCES

Arquilla, J., & Ronfeldt, D. (1999). *The Emergence of Noopolitik, Toward an American Information Strategy.* Santa Monica, CA: RAND Cooperation.

Artigiani, R. (1991). Social Evolution, A Nonequilibrium Systems Model . In Laszlo, E. (Ed.), *The New Evolutionary Paradigm* (pp. 93–129). New York: Gordon & Breach Science Publishers Ltd.

Beniger, J. R. (1986). *The Control Revolution.* Cambridge, MA: Harvard University Press.

Bloch, E. (1967). *Das Prinzip Hoffnung (3 vols.).* Frankfurt, DE: Suhrkamp.

Bradley, G. (2006). *Social and Community Informatics, Humans on the Net.* London: Routledge.

Castells, M. (1996). *The Rise of the Network Society, The Information Age: Economy, Society and Culture* (*Vol. I*). Cambridge, MA/Oxford: Blackwell Publishers.

Castells, M. (1997). *The Power of Identity, The Information Age: Economy, Society and Culture* (*Vol. II*). Cambridge, MA/Oxford: Blackwell Publishers.

Castells, M. (1998). *The End of Millenium, The Information Age: Economy, Society and Culture* (*Vol. III*). Cambridge, MA/Oxford: Blackwell Publishers.

Crowley, P. (2010). *Information and Communication Technologies Enabling to Create a Self-Organising Civil Society "Knowledge and Service Commons" and "Capability" Capacities to Counteract "Chaos Points".* Dissertation, University of Salzburg, Austria.

Cruddas, J., & Nahles, A. (2009). Building the Good Society, The Project of the Democratic Left. Retrieved from http://www.goodsociety. eu/wp-content/uploads/2009/04/building_the_ good_society.pdf

European Commission. Directorate-General for Employment, Industrial Relations and Social Affairs (ed.) (1997). *Building the European information society for us all, Final Policy Report of the high-level expert group.* Luxembourg, LU: Office for Official Publications of the European Communities.

Floridi, L. (2007). A Look into the Future Impact of ICT on Our Lives. *Journal of the Information Society*, *23*(1), 59–64. doi:10.1080/01972240601059094

Hofkirchner, W. (Ed.). (1997). Vladimir I. Vernadskij, Der Mensch in der Biosphäre, Zur Naturgeschichte der Vernunft. Wien, AU: Peter Lang.

Hofkirchner, W., & Fuchs, C. (2003). The Architecture of the Information Society. In J. Wilby. & J. K. Allen (Eds.), *Proceedings of the 47th Annual Conference*, ISSS (pp. 1-10). The International Society of the Systems Sciences.

Hofkirchner, W., Fuchs, C., Raffl, C., Schafranek, M., Sandoval, M., & Bichler, R. (2007). ICTs and Society – The Salzburg Approach. Towards a Theory for, about, and by means of the Information Society. In ICT&S Center Research Paper Series, 3. Retrieved from http://icts.sbg.ac.at/ media/pdf/pdf1490.pdf

Lévy, P. (1997). *Collective Intelligence, Mankind's Emerging World in Cyberspace.* New York: Plenum Trade.

Lovelock, J. (1987). *Gaia.* Oxford, UK: Oxford University Press.

Mumford, L. (1964). *The Myth of the Machine, The Pentagon of Power*. New York: Harcourt Brace Jovanovich.

Niles, D. P. (2003). Justice, Peace and the Integrity of Creation. In Ecumenical Dictionary. Retrieved from http://www.wcc-coe.org/wcc/who/dictionary-article11.html

Teilhard de Chardin, P. (1975). *The Phenomenon of Man*. New York: Harper & Row.

Toffler, A. (1980). *The Third Wave*. London: Collins.

Section 7
Ethical Aspects on ICT

Chapter 36
Can Computers Decide what is Legal and Illegal?

Jacob Palme
Stockholm University, Sweden.

ABSTRACT

Humans are able to understand that rules must not be adhered to 100% all the time. There are special cases, where the rules should not be adhered to. Computers do not have this ability. A society where computers are judges will not be a nice place to live in. This chapter illustrates with practical examples why computers should not be judges.

INTRODUCTION

The main theme of this chapter is that one should be very careful with programming computers into becoming judges (Figure 1). The reader may react with the question: OK, we should not program computers into becoming judges. But why is this such a big issue? We could program computers to do lots of useful things, even if we don't make them into judges. Why write a chapter on why we should not make computers into judges, why is this such a big issue?

Well, if you think a little more, you will find out that it is extremely common that computers are some kind of judges. Not in the common case

of judges who work in courts and make verdicts. But it is very common that rules about how humans should behave are written into computer programs, and that the programs are written in such a way that their users are forced to adhere to these rules. The people who design and write computer programs will in many cases be rule-makers. By the way they design the programs, they decide which rules are valid among people who use these programs. Computer programs are full of detailed rules about how the world should work.

- Messages may have a limited length.
- It may be illegal to include pictures in certain messages.
- In order to use the software you have bought, you are forced to sign a check-

DOI: 10.4018/978-1-60960-057-0.ch036

Figure 1. Computer as judge, possible or not?

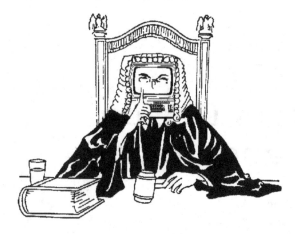

box saying that you agree to long, detailed "conditions of use", which you have no option to negotiate in any way, and which probably are very unreasonable. If you do not check that box, the software you have bought will not work.

- To perform a certain action in the administrative system at your workplace, you have to fill in long detailed forms with information, which makes the systems cumbersome to use, and which are not really necessary.

- Requests for permission do not allow you to specify the reasons for your request in the way you would prefer.

- Etc, etc.

Life is full of these minor or major obstacles posed by computer systems. They are, in fact, rules. They specify what you may do and not do. Often in ways which are cumbersome and unnecessary complex. Because the rule-makers, the designers of the software, want to impose their rules on you. Real life is full of such rules. But when the rules are written on chapter, you have the option of doing things in simpler ways. No one will usually check or require you to adhere to all rules, fully and in every detail.

A well-known method for work-force conflict is that everyone does everything exactly according to rules, making things much more time-consuming so that tasks are not ready in time. In reality, we ignore many rules when we feel they are too complex or unnecessary, if we follow all rules in every detail, work grinds to a halt.

But when the rules are enforced by computer programs, there is no option of making life simpler by not always follow every directive exactly. And these are examples where computers act as judges, forcing you to exactly abide by every rule. And that is why computers often makes life unnecessarily complex.

EXAMPLES OF RULES IN REAL LIFE

Example: A breath analyzer (Swedish: Alkolås) is a tool to prevent drunken driving. The driver breathes in the analyzer. If there is too much alcohol in the breath, the driver is not permitted to start the car. But there can be special cases. Suppose the husband has a heart attack or a stroke. His future survival depends on getting him to the hospital rapidly. His wife has drunken a little. In this case, it might be wise to let her drive him to the hospital in spite of having a little alcohol in her breath.

In fact, one way of installing a breath analyzer is not to let it stop her from driving (*stopper*). Instead, it will report the violation, and a real judge, afterwards, checks if her driving should be permitted in this special case (*reporter*). This may be a better way of implementing the breath analyzer, because the human can understand the need to diverge from the rule in this special case.

Letting the breathalyzer stop her from driving is a case of making a computer into a judge. And letting a human afterwards decide if she was right in driving in this exceptional case may be a better way of implementing such a rule. In fact, breath analyzers have been implemented in both ways, both as *stoppers* and as *reporters* of violation.

Some people may claim that the computer was not a judge. The human who decided that the breath analyzer should work as a *stopper* was the real judge. But in reality the computer, if implemented as a *stopper*, will act as a judge and may cause the husband to die in the special case where his life depends on getting him to the hospital rapidly. There may be cases where it is best to let a computer stop illegal behaviour. But one should consider carefully if a *reporter*-type of implementation may be better than a *stopper*-type of implementation in cases like this.

THE REAL USE OF LAWS AND REGULATIONS

Why do we have laws and rules? One way of understanding this is to say that laws and rules are ways communicating experience and practice. People with a lot of experience with issues will write the rules in order to help people with less experience to act in the best way. Looking at laws and rules in this way makes it easier to understand why rules interpreted by humans are more acceptable than rules interpreted by computers. Sometimes, it is necessary to set up courts and other systems for enforcing the rules. This is not always necessary. And the very hard way of programming adherence into computers may be even less necessary.

An example of a rule in real life is the rule saying that you may not pass a street-crossing against a red light. This may be a good rule to follow in real life. But what if a child is starting to run across the street, in front of a car. Then you may save the life of the child by stepping out and stopping the child. And no one will stop you or prosecute you for this violation. Life is full of such cases where it is sometimes better to not follow every rule exactly. But if the rules are enforced by technical systems, computers, you do not have this option, you have to follow every rule exactly, all the time (Figure 2).

People who create computers, and who build rules into the systems, do not always understand the dangers of always enforcing every rule, all the time, using the computers to enforce every detail of every rule.

DETAILED FORMS

Everyone has encountered situations where you have to fill in a form to get something done. And where you do not have to fill in every detailed field every time. Someone says: "Just sign your name here", and you do, and things gets done, even if you have not filled in every field in the form. But if the filling in of this form is controlled by a computer, you may always have to fill in every detailed field. The every-day rationalization which we do so often is not possible. Sometime, of course, it is important to follow the rules, like point the hose at the base of the fire before pressing the lever to release the fire-extinguishing foam. But sometimes the rules contain details you can skip to get things done faster.

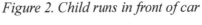

Figure 2. Child runs in front of car

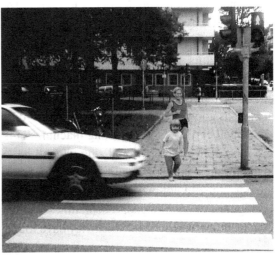

EVERY-DAY RATIONALIZATION

In many workplaces, people will perform tasks more efficient each year than the day before. This is called "every-day rationalisation", the optimization of tasks done by doing things in simpler and more efficient ways. But if tasks are done by the use of computer, the computer will sometimes prevent such every-day improvement in doing things. (Hoare 1975, Palme 1997).

Sometimes, it is important that people do perform every detail and not pass over any step. Air-line pilots have checklists, in order to help them remember to do every check on the list. This is important for safety, to prevent accidents. In such cases, technical means of ensuring that people do perform every step are sometimes used, just because such technical means ensure that you do not skip any step. Night watchmen have special keys they have to put in locks when they walk around the building. These keys ensure that they do not forget, through laziness, from walking around the building. But if the night watchman hears a sound which should not be there, he will of course hurry to the place of the noise, to check if someone is trying to break-in. The technical systems does not prevent him from diverging from the normal route, even if this means that he will not click the keys in the right order that night!

In other cases, it is not really necessary to do every step. And the human ability to rationalize everyday life by skipping certain actions is useful and makes life simpler. I have a baking recipe for baking biscuits, which specifies that you have to add ingredients in a certain order, then mix, then add more ingredients. I have found that the biscuits are just as good when I just throw all the ingredients together and start the baking machine. This is a kind of everyday rationalizing which I have made for the baking of biscuits. And in this case, the machine did not prevent this rationalization.

Figure 3 shows how people sometimes circumvent technical restrictions which they have found not necessary. I am sure you have seen many other examples from your own life.

Sometimes this may be necessary. For example, there is a human tendency to stop performing actions which are necessary only to avoid seldom occurring risks. Example: A pilot forgets an item on the pre-flight check list, or a night watchman forgets to go to a normally empty part of the building. In such cases, it may be necessary to use technical means to ensure that the human follows the rules, for example the night watchman must turn a key to show that he has passed that part of the building. But this does not forbid the night watchman from disobeying the rules in special cases, for example skip the empty corridor if there is a thief in another part of the building. The danger is when the computer does not allow you to do things in other ways than those foreseen when programming it.

People are in fact very clever in circumventing restrictions in order to do what has to be done. See for example Figure 3. I have searched on the internet, and found hundreds of copies of this picture on different web pages.[1] Obviously, many people have felt that this picture shows something important!

Figure 3. Human ingenuity in circumventing mechanical obstacles

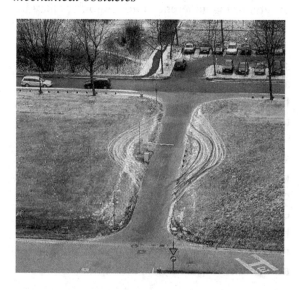

BALANCED COMMUNICATION IS BETTER THAN ONE-SIDED

Power is addictive (Hoare 1975). By this is meant that people who are put in a position of power, will tend to utilize that position to favour their belief in what is the proper way of doing things. There is nothing evil in this, it is just that they believe they have good competence in how things should be done. If they are given the task of designing computer software, they will want to use their competence to design the computer software according to their knowledge about how things should be done. This is a kind of communication process. They are communicating their competence in how things should be done in the design of the computer software just as rule-makers communicte their knowledge of how things should be done in the rules they make. The danger with this is that it is a uni-sided communication process. It is only from the designers, to the users, not bi-directional. It is a communication process promoting a feeling of helplessness, which is known to cause depression and dissatisfaction (Seligman 1975). And uni-directional communication processes are almost always bad. Good communication processes are almost always bi-directional. Only bi-directional communication gives the richness of give-and-take, argument-and-counterargument, my idea-against your idea, which are characteristics of good communication processes. Bi-directional communication processes mostly are characterized by I say you have no say, Listen but not speak which are characteristic of undemocratic, dictatorial mode of communication. Not only will software design per se be one-sided unidirectional communication processes, but the communication processes provided by computer software designed by people in power, tend to be unit-directional.

Now you may say as counter-argument, that "My company has a very democratic process of designing software with committers representing all user groups overseeing and guiding the software design". Or "My company have design groups consisting of representatives of our customers who oversee software development". And if a company have such democratic committees, surely, things are not bad! Wrong! As son as a person is appointed into such a group for overseeing software design, that person becomes a person of power (assuming that you really give influence on software design to these groups, and that these groups are not token groups with no real power) will immediately become a person of power, a person for who all the dangerous thought processes of people in power will crop up as described in the beginning of the previous paragraph. Win-win solution which are characterized of bi-directional communication processes are difficult or impossible with uni-directional processes (Harris 1969, Gordon 1970).

My cable-TV company has a web form for changing my subscriptions. All changes which give them more income are easy and simple to do using the web form. All changes which give them less income (such as unsubscribing from a channel) are impossible in the web form, and force me to write a postal letter to them with my request for a change. If, for example, I want for one month add a channel to my subscriptions, I will have to perform a add channel operation (easy to do using their web form) but if I want to reduce my cost I have to perform a subtract channel operation (can only be done by postal mail) and which is one month delayed. It is of course not by mistake they have designed their system in this way. They hope that I will be lazy and perform only one of these two operations, causing them an income of many months of subscriptions to this channel, when I i reality only wnated to see one particular program.. This way of designing the web dialogue is useful in companies which want to maximize their profit by making all user actions which increas in the costs to the user easy to perform, and all decreases of the cost to the customer difficult and cumbersome to perform.

It is not by chance that this problem occurs with a cable-TV company. Cable-TV compaies

Figure 4.

Human beings have a need to be able to influence their life. They will be more happy and satisfied, and will be able to do a better job, if they can influence their life, and use their abilities to perform their tasks better and better.

⬇ ⬇

Conventional solution: Let the users influence the development of the software system they are going to use.
Corrective action: Users require new features of the software, developers are overloaded with work to adjust the software, there is a huge backlog of tasks, the software gets more and more complex through many haphazard extensions.

Alternative solution: Design the software so that the users can, themselves, modify it according to their present and future needs.
Corrective action: Educate special so-called "local experts", who work locally in the local user groups, and help users with extension of the software to their needs.

are monpolies with lots of power. Such companies have very high capabilities to control free speech, since it is so diffiucult or impossible to switch to a different cable-TV company. They utulize their position in power to increase their revenues.

USER INFLUENCE

See Figure 4.

A TOO DILIGENT PORN STOPPER

A funny example of how misuse of power can occur in a communication system.

A person I know sent a message containing a part of a script to a friend through a messaging software provided by people "who wanted to do good". The script in his message contained the following too lines:

```
#define one 1 /* foo menu */
#define two 2 /* bar baz */
```

And it arrived corrupted in the following way:

```
#define one 1 /* foo me */
# fine two 2 /* bar baz */
```

What had happened was that the "be good"-software in the messaging system censored all messages containing porn, and the word nude was regarded as indicative of porn. If you look carefully, you can see that two last two letters in the first line and the first two letters of the second line makes the word "nude". Porn, cries the friendly software and corrupts this script, which had nothing at all to do with porn.

In general, designing programs which pass through only "good" messages and no "bad" messages (according to your particular idea of what is "good" and "bad"), are very difficult to design. Dictatorial countries like "The People's republic of China" and "Singapore" make attempts. Programs to prevent the word "sex" have difficulty with "Middlesex", a local government in England. And should you stop information about breast cancer because it contains the word "breast"?

IS THE INTERNET ILLEGAL

Usage of the Internet is in fact illegal according to the privacy projection laws in many countries. These laws makes it illegal to send personal information unless in special restricted ways. If I write a letter to my brother saying that our mother is going to try out a new miraculous cancer treatment method, with large success probability, this happy letter was probably illegal according to Swedish law for many years. It contains personal information about an easily identifiable person. And the personal information is medical information, which should only be permitted, according to the privacy protection laws. I ran one of the first BBS-es in Sweden starting in 1978. My BBS was forbidden by the Swedish Data Inspection Board, saying that it was against the Swedish data inspection law. A few years later, an author was forbidden by the Swedish Data Inspection Board, from writing a book. In 1978, I was forbidden from running one of the world's first e-mail systems, because it allowed people to send personal information to each other. Nowadays, through strong acions of lobbying, I and people who understand the dangers with laws on computer usage, have succeeded in changing the Swedish laws, allowing such applicatons like e-mail which was previously forbidden.

Actually, almost all usage of the Internet is illegal according to the privacy protection laws in many countries. In later years, the Data Inspection Boards have become a little more cautious. But it is very difficult to design laws making the internet illegal "by mistake". that is because the privacy protection laws are basically against certain kinds of "free speech", and internet is by design a system for "free speech".

MUST THE COMPUTER STOP ALL UNWANTED BEHAVIOUR

There is a tendency, among designers of computer systems, to believe that the ideal computer system is a system designed so that it guides people into the correct and good behaviour and prevents all unwanted behaviour. The danger with such systems is that they are too controlling. In real life, one often has to step through steps which are incorrect on the way towards a correct solution. Look at the mostly used of all computer applications. These are:

- Word processing software for writing texts, like for example Microsoft Word.
- Spread-sheet software such as Microsoft Excel.
- Web browsers for looking at the world wide web.
- E-mail software for sending messages.

All these software systems are based on giving the user maximum freedom. Microsoft Word is not successful by preventing "incorrect" texts, but in giving freedom to write whatever the user wants. Spread-sheet software are successful by giving maximum freedom in designing different kinds of calculations between cells. E-mail is not successful by forbidding the writing of "incorrect" messages but by permitting any kind of message with any kind of content. Web browsers are successful by the freedom of looking at all information all over the web. Successful designers of software systems are not successful by designing software which prevents illegal usage, but by designing software which gives maximum freedom of usage.

When discussing software design with people doing the design, it sometimes seems as if they are of the opinion that good software must stop all kinds of incorrect usage of the software. The designer's knowledge of the task must be used to prevent all incorrect usage.

A reverse variant of this belief is the belief among some computer crackers that everything which was possible to do must be permitted. "It was your fault", says the cracker, "by making it possible, you made it legal". In fact, lots of things which can be done using a computer are still illegal. Making the software to allow something does *not* make that action permitted or legal.

I have noted this often in discussing regarding the design of the administrative system we use at our university do manage courses, lecture room allocation, student marks, etc. For example, it is not correct for students beginning discussing their thesis writing before they have achieved success in most other courses. The system enforces this, and refuses to provide administrative support for students who want to start their thesis work earlier. However, it is often useful to base a thesis on tasks in earlier courses. This is hampered by the system. This is just one of many examples of how the systems causes unnecessary trouble by enforcing unnecessary rules regarding how to write a thesis. Let the tutor, not the computer, decide when a certain student can beging working on his thesis!

It is not necessary to put all kinds of control of incorrect usage into computer systems. Instead, it is best to let people decide what is correct in their usage. Humans are better at checking what is right and wrong than computer software.

CALENDAR SCHEDULING

One example of a kind of software system which easily becomes unnecessarily restrictive is calendar systems, i.e. software for managing the allocation of times for meetings, etc. Such software can incorporate lots of rules regarding how *good* calendaring should work. It might be better not to put all kinds of rules into such software. And if such systems have to manage certain kinds of issues, it can perhaps better be managed by letting the software *warn* of possible problems rather than forbid them. Human can then decide whether to take action after such warnings, instead of letting the software take action in usually very clumsy ways. For example, certain meetings may be more important than other meetings. It may be necessary to reschedule other, already scheduled meetings, to assign time for other, more important meetings. But it may not be ideal to design the software to handle this. It might be better to have *humans* decide whether to take action because of such rules or not. All rules must not be built into the software. Some rules may not be suitable to put into the software. For example knowledge that meetings with Mr. Jones should never be scheduled on Monday mornings, may not be nice to put into

the software. Calendaring systems are typical of systems where you can put any number of special rules into the software, but where this may not always be suitable or even possible.

CONCLUSION

*   The successes of human society is based on the flexibility of humans and their willingness to adapt their activities to different circumstances.
*   Humans are most happy and productive if they can influence their living environment and contribute to solving problems together.
*   Laws and regulation are a form of communication between humans. They are in reality only guidelines, people have to adapt to varying circumstances and interpret and apply the rules with understanding and human compassion. If everyone had to adhere 100% to all laws and regulations, human societies would not work any more.
*   This is usually no problem when the laws and regulations are written on chapter. But if the laws and regulations are programmed into computers, so that the computers control what is allowed and not allowed, serious problems will often occur. In the best case, people will only be unhappy and unproductive, in the worst case, major catastrophes can occur.
*   Computer software must be designed to allow flexibility and human choice. Laws and regulations should be interpreted by humans, not by machines.
*   Making the software more complex, to include in it more different special handling of special circumstances, will often only make it worse. Instead of complex software, software should be flexible and open-ended.

- There is a human tendency when designing software to want to include in it "proper procedure" and "experience how things should be done". This tendency can easily produce unusable or unsuitable software.
- Possible exception from the above: Certain security rules, where enforcement is necessary to overcome human weaknesses.

REFERENCES

Gordon, T. (1970). *P. E. T. - Parent Effectiveness Training*.

Grip, A. (1974). *ADB-system och kommunikation (Data processing and communication)*. Lund, Sweden: Hermods-studentlitteratur.

Harris, T. A. (1969). *I'm OK - You're OK*. Quill.

Hoare, C. A. R. (1975). Software Design: a Parable. *Software World, 5*(9 & 10), 53–56.

Martin, D. C. (1997). Empowering Educators and Parents: Content Advisories for the Internet. In *Proceedings of the ITiCSE*. ACM.

Palme, J. (1975). *Interactive Software for Humans* (An abbreviated version was published in *Management Informatics, 7*(1976), pp. 4-16).

Palme, J. (1997). *User influence on software design may give less good software*. Computer Mediated Communication.

Palme, J. (2000). *A personal history of CMC* (Honorary publication dedicated to Yvonne Wærn on Her Retirement).

Seligman, M. E. P. (1975). *Helplessness: On depression, development and death*. San Francisco, SF: W.H. Freeman & Company.

Vetandets Värld. (2006). *(In Swedish broadcasting, audio). Den mänskliga faktorn som förklaring till olyckshändelser. Vetandets värld*. Sveriges Radio.

ENDNOTE

[1]   In order to find the original creator of the picture and pay for the usage of the picture in this chapter. I have not been successful in this.

Chapter 37

eHealth and Ethics:
Theory, Teaching, and Practice

Diane Whitehouse
The Castlegate Consultancy, UK

Penny Duquenoy
Middlesex University, UK

ABSTRACT

The use of information and communication technologies (ICT) is increasing rapidly in many spheres of contemporary life in Europe. The ethical use of ICT in all areas of its application is of growing importance. This is especially evident in the field of healthcare. The regional, national, and Europe-wide electronic aspects of health services and systems are related fundamentally to these two developments. This chapter explores the relevance of ethics to eHealth generally. It outlines two main contrasting ideas that have influenced ethical thought: Kantian ethics and consequentialism. It investigates the ways in which teaching and practice for ICT professionals and trainees can be enhanced and extended to increase the awareness of ethical issues in eHealth. It takes as examples two technological applications that are in increasing use in the eHealth field: electronic health records and radio frequency identification devices. The chapter ends with a brief discussion and conclusions about how this ethical awareness can be expanded beyond ICT professionals to other stakeholder groups, and to other eHealth technologies or applications.

INTRODUCTION

eHealth has variously been referred to as medical informatics or medical information systems, clinical informatics or clinical information systems, health informatics or health information systems, or information and communication technologies

(ICT) for health (Duquenoy et al., 2008a). A number of definitions have been outlined in both the academic literature and in policy-related documentation (COM(2004) 356 final; COM(2007) 860 final; Eng (2001); Eysenbach (2001); Oh et al. (2005); Pagliari et al. (2005)). In this paper, we have selected from the text of the eHealth action plan (COM(2004)356, p4) one of the more pragmatic definitions:

DOI: 10.4018/978-1-60960-057-0.ch037

[eHealth] describes the application of information and communications technologies across the whole range of functions that affect the health sector.

This paper is written in the context of health as it affects people's daily lives, enhances the overall well-being of Europe's citizens, and influences the continent's social and economic status. We focus on health supported by electronic means.

The paper describes what eHealth is, what ethics is, and how the two relate to each other particularly within a teaching or training context.

It is directed chiefly towards raising ethical awareness about eHealth applications for ICT professionals and for trainee or prospective professionals. Choosing a comprehensive definition of eHealth enables us to explore ICT applications in their variety and richness. Here, however, we concentrate our analytical efforts on radio frequency identification (RFID) devices and electronic health records.

The paper is completed by asking whether, and in what way, this ethical awareness can be extended to the design, implementation and use of other types of eHealth-related applications, and included in the education and training of other stakeholders. While the proposals outlined here limit themselves to the European scene, they can certainly be extended to a wider, international, perspective.

The paper is particularly intended as a complement to the longstanding work of Professor Gunilla Bradley who focused her ideas so keenly on the importance of human needs in relation to ICT, and has always had a profoundly holistic approach to ICT (cf. Bradley, 2009).

EHEALTH IN EUROPE: GENERAL OVERVIEW

eHealth has been under development in Europe for two decades and, elsewhere, for over four.

In the European Union, the early foundations of eHealth were laid in the late 1980s. Pilot studies were co-financed as early as the second stage of the European Union. From an initial funding of €20 million in 1988, investment in this domain of research and development later expanded tenfold during its Sixth Framework Programme (2002 to 2006). The Commission is now co-financing the Seventh Framework Programme that runs from 2007 to 2013. The amount of financing provided by the Commission dedicated to eHealth in this latest Framework Programme over this time-period is expected to be well over €200 million.

Large amounts of co-financing are now being invested in the deployment of eHealth. The research and development commitment of the Commission has been paralleled by work on the practical aspects of eHealth in the Competitiveness and Innovation Framework Programme (CIP) Information and Communication Technologies (ICT) Policy Support Programme (PSP) (more frequently known simply by its abbreviation as the CIP ICT PSP). This scheme supports the practical advance and integration of ICT use in various public sector domains among the Member States. In eHealth, the ministries of health, eHealth competence centres and industry partners in 12 Member States are focusing on electronic health data (health records/medication records or "patient summaries"), and ePrescribing. The first of these areas is one on which we concentrate in this paper.

eHealth also became an area for strong policy development with the formulation of a plan for policy convergence (COM(2004) 356 final). This plan is soon due to be completed and – presumably – also for some form of renewal or update. Although progress has been steady over the plan's seven-year lifetime, many of its accomplishments started to come to fruition – and have even been reinforced by further policy documentation – over its last three years of operation.

In particular, 2008, 2009 and 2010 have been key years for eHealth in Europe. For example, in the specific contexts of patient mobility, cross-border health services, and eHealth interoperability, a Proposal for a Directive – which has now received even greater support – and a Recommendation were adopted (COM(2008)414 final; COM(2008)3282 final). In 2008, a policy document was also published on telemedicine (COM(2008)489 final).

EHEALTH IN EUROPE: A GROWING COMMITMENT TO DEPLOYMENT

Europe's Member States have committed themselves to collaborate on eHealth[1]. They are currently working together intensively to form a high-level governance framework that will begin to operate formally by the end of 2010. The aim of this governance will be to ensure that health ministries and their high-level leaders and decision-makers cooperate on the key aspects of an eHealth strategy for Europe, working together on eHealth implementation and on monitoring their collective progress[2]. These initiatives are highly likely to incorporate the involvement of a wide range of stakeholders.

There is much current emphasis on the deployment and application of eHealth. eHealth is commonly perceived by policy-makers and decision-makers as a key enabler of good healthcare and as a means of reinforcing the European Union's common values and goals for its health systems. Two-thirds of Europe's Member States believe that their health policy priorities can be supported by eHealth (European Commission, 2007). Every European Member State possesses its own eHealth road map or action plan, and all the States are now building their own initiatives to implement eHealth services, systems, and applications. There are many commonalities among the 27 States. However, there is still considerable disparity among them with regard to their stages of innovation and how they are putting eHealth into practice. This 2007 overview (Ibid) shows that the deployment of the main, common eHealth

services in European countries has been motivated by such concerns as the quality of care and access to care for patients/citizens, which both have ethical aspects. A further review is taking place in 2009-2010[3].

The majority of Member States are now introducing, building, and using three technical domains: infrastructure, electronic health records or cards, and interoperability (Ibid, p13-15). The link between Europe's cited policy directions in eHealth and the actual commitment of the Member States to these particular fields is currently becoming clearer.

The co-financing initiatives of the CIP ICT PSP have increased the extent of collaboration among European Member States. Since 2008, two large-scale undertakings have been established: the first, a European-wide pilot project known as epSOS[4] which focuses on eHealth interoperability; the second, a thematic network which supports comprehensive stakeholder engagement in eHealth called CALLIOPE[5]. Several other similar initiatives also illustrate complementary Europe-wide action. An example here is STORK[6], which focuses on information security and the identification and authentication of users in such settings as eHealth.

European and international organisations are showing a renewed interest in eHealth as a market or business. Many elements of the relevant industries are endeavouring to work together on a number of eHealth-related initiatives: one example is the Continua Health Alliance[7]. In late 2007, the European Commission also launched a platform known as the Lead Market Initiative. This initiative emphasises the notion of the public sector as a driver of technological innovation and potential industrial growth – eHealth is one of the six domains to which attention is directed (COM(2007)860 final).

The health sector has always been a field strongly bound up with ethical questions. Here, we offer a brief overview of some key issues that relate to ethics generally before we apply them in more detail to eHealth.

ETHICS

Ethics is a branch of moral philosophy. It has several schools of thought and action. The consideration of ethics and ethical theory in relation to human behaviour is known as normative ethics. It contrasts with more abstract discussions on morality (i.e. meta-ethics). In the context of this paper, we are interested in normative ethics – the practical application of ethics.

Ethical theories are useful points of departure to enable people to make appropriate choices and to act according to those choices. They provide people with a form of toolkit that can enable them, at any moment in time and in any specific context, to understand the particular moral position taken and the reasoning which underpins a specific moral choice. Each moral choice is complemented by its own criteria and constraints.

In recent years, different ethical theories have been used to assess the ethical implications of ICT. Two of the most common theories used are Kantian ethics and utilitarian ethics.

First, Kantian ethics argues that it is human will that motivates moral action. However, the will can only motivate itself from a rational foundation (Kant, 1981). Rationality implies autonomy (i.e. self-determination); rational argument dictates that all human beings must be equal. Two propositions are the result of this approach. They are, to treat humanity always as an end in itself and never as a means to an end; and, then, in the words of Kant, "Act only on that maxim which you can at the same time will to be a universal law" (Ibid, p421).

Second, utilitarian ethics is located in the field of 'consequentialist' ethics, and is sometimes referred to as consequentialism. Here, the principles of moral actions are considered to be based on their consequences. The principle of utility (the 'utility principle') is that right actions bring the greatest happiness to the greatest number of people. This 'greatest happiness' is determined as being either that which is of the highest value or which does the least harm.

Kantian and utilitarian ethics have led to the taking of two distinct positions. In the first, there is a consideration of human autonomy and respect for others. In the second, a basis is provided for addressing, deciding on, and assessing a specific course of action that is focused on the greatest benefit.

EHEALTH AND ETHICS

High-level, ethical, principles can be brought to bear on specific areas of application. They have been applied to the practice of medicine, the field of health and, more recently, the combined fields of eHealth (i.e., medicine or health and ICT). The more applied the field, the more specific, focused, and contingent are the particular ethical questions. The technologies that are involved in a particular context add yet another layer of complexity.

Codes of ethics often articulate the ethical principles that underpin any given context or setting. These codes provide the ethical foundation for many organisations, and particularly for professional bodies.

The complexity of modern society and communities of work means that the ethics of specific occupations (e.g. their codes of ethics, behaviour, or practice) need to be given careful consideration when two or more such professional or occupational groups collaborate. Challenges might arise: are the professions/occupations similar, do they share the same values, are there any areas of potential conflict among the two (or more) fields, and are there any particular gaps in their thinking/acting?

The ICT industry encompasses a range of disciplines that include electronic engineering, computer science, and information management. The ethical principles of these professions usually fall into different groupings. However, in general, their codes of practice state that they each protect the public interest, uphold the standards of the specific profession, promote knowledge transfer, and require a commitment to personal integrity.

Of direct relevance in the case of this paper are the rules of conduct for Health Informatics Professionals which were drawn up in the United Kingdom under the auspices of the Health Informatics Committee of the British Computer Society. These rules of conduct recognise the role played by ICT in the field of medicine (Kluge, 2003). Several fundamental ethical principles were laid down in this document. They are the: Principle of Autonomy; Principle of Equality and Justice; Principle of Beneficence; Principle of Non-Malfeasance; and the Principle of Impossibility (the last of these principles relates to the assumption that it must be possible to meet the rights and duties that are expressed by the preceding four). These principles are transposed into concrete and practical uses that are aligned with the responsibilities of Health Informatics Professionals.

Here, the ICT professional has "a duty to ensure that appropriate measures are in place that may reasonably be expected to safeguard: The security of electronic records; The integrity of electronic records; The material quality of electronic records; The usability of electronic records; The accessibility of electronic records." (Ibid, p14).

These five characteristics of electronic health records are regarded by Health Informatics Professionals as important to the provision of healthcare. Each characteristic describes an aspect of the data store that could be compromised by technical mediation. In simple terms, these are the possible crisis-points of technically-mediated patient information.

The effective presentation of patient information can be construed as providing "the correct information at the right time, to the right people"; it is the basis for a strong ethical foundation to eHealth (Duquenoy et al, 2008b). This is not an easy task given the increasingly complex organisational and technical interactions implied by eHealth.

TEACHING ETHICS TO ICT PROFESSIONALS

In this section, we highlight the challenges of teaching ethics in the kind of discipline, such as ICT, where ethics has traditionally been an unfamiliar topic. We advocate the benefits of using examples, cases, and analogies. Whereas we concentrate here on teaching ethics to ICT professionals, using eHealth as our specific example, we later expand our discussions to a more holistic approach of interacting with other stakeholders in the eHealth domain.

In some professions, such as medicine and law, the consideration of ethics forms an inherent part of the particular profession's (and professionals') job. Such an approach has a long history and is well understood; ethics is a traditional component of any training offered to the student, and is likely to be treated in each of the various topics taught to the trainee professional.

This is not, however, the case for students of information systems or informatics. In this field of interest, unfortunately, the ethical implications of technologies were not recognised for a long time. Even today, many ICT practitioners find it hard to associate or reconcile the topic of ethics with their training about technologies.

Teaching ethics to technology students is made difficult in several ways. First, ethics tends to offer an abstract, highly conceptual, and even – at times – ambiguous approach to solving problems. Second, technology students tend to be practically-minded, hands-on problem solvers. Third, technology is usually developed with a focus on a specific task that is isolated from a wider context of use. As a result, using the electronic database of patient records as in our example, it can be difficult for technology students to see how building such a database has some form of ethical importance.

Ethics must therefore be made relevant to technology students. They need to be shown the direct connection between technology applications and human beings and the impacts – whether beneficial or detrimental – on people's everyday lives. How best to do this?

Ethics is about promoting benefits and reducing harm. While this is a relatively simple message, it can actually be more difficult to assess what might constitute a benefit and what might constitute a harm. These are fundamental elements of ethical discussion, and it is here that reference to different ethical theories can help. Technology students do not necessarily need to be persuaded by the principles of a particular theory (although many students will lean towards one theory rather than another in their personal preferences). They do, however, need to use the principles as a foundation for discussion in order to draw out the key elements of the subject under debate.

These two elements – the connection between technology and people, and the consideration of ethics – can also be brought together quite simply. First, an introduction to a set of ethical principles is needed. Alongside this, one simple approach can be developed by selecting well-chosen case studies (whether hypothetical or real) or by focusing on concrete examples – what can be called eHealth in practice. A much wider range of technologies with pertinence to eHealth could of course be explored.

Here, we consider two technological applications in further detail: patient electronic health records and RFID devices. We cover in particular the issues of justice and equity. There has generally been a trend to examine justice and equity in the domains of eInclusion and eAccessibility[8] rather than in the eHealth field, however, this is becoming increasingly a pressing field of examination.

ELECTRONIC HEALTH RECORDS AND RADIO FREQUENCY IDENTIFICATION DEVICES

For the sake of simplicity, here we look at only two specific forms of technology that have a relevance to the healthcare field. These two applications were explored in detail at the International Federation for Information Processing summer school on "The Future of Identity in the Information Society – Challenges for Privacy and Security" held in the Czech Republic in 2008[9]. The theoretical and empirical background, especially to the field of RFID, was examined in an earlier paper (Whitehouse and Duquenoy, 2009).

We demonstrate how the application of ethics to specific technologies can be handled in a very practical way. The creation of illustrative templates or charts can encourage the consideration of particular ethical issues. At stake are questions that relate to the impacts of the technology on human beings and on information storage and transmission.

We place our discussion of ethics in the framework of the four issues that were raised earlier in relation to the work of Kluge (2003): non-malfeasance, beneficence, autonomy, and justice/equity. However, rather than covering all four of the potential ethical issues at stake, we choose to focus on the specific matter of *justice/equity*. Our preference for the choice of this field relates to the growing importance in Europe of users' rights in relation to technology use[10] and, in parallel, the rise in awareness of patients' engagement and involvement in their own healthcare[11].

Here, we discuss the usefulness of a specific ethical theory or an ethical approach (cf. Kluge, 2003), and how these underlying principles can provide a tool to tease out, identify, and assess ethical issues.

Electronic Health Records

Patients' health records may be held in a computer database either locally or centrally. Locally-held records may be stored at a doctor's premises or in a group practice shared among several general practitioners. Centrally-held records may be stored in a national database at either an institutional or a governmental level. Generally, locally-held data are less likely to be compromised by security issues than are centrally-held data which are transmitted over a network.

Patient data may also be held in a more distributed manner and/or collated from a range of sources. They could eventually be held by the patient him or herself. It is these options which may be increasingly widely explored, especially given the importance of cloud computing and the possibility of shared services (including health, social, and care services – whether public or private or a mix of the two).

In its widest possible context of use, the development of an electronic health-related database could cause many complex situations to arise that have a bearing on ethics. For example, the sharing of patient data among or between different healthcare professionals, departments, and other information systems could affect the confidentiality of a patient's data or it could compromise the integrity and timeliness of the treatment of the data.

There are at least two concerns that relate to the records application itself, and to the information that it holds. First, a lack of understanding of the particular technologies involved could place certain patients at a disadvantage. Second, the digital format of records could allow for the categorisation of patients according to fields such as age, gender, incidence of ill health (e.g., cancer), the geographic location of their home, or type of lifestyle (such as a person's addiction to cigarettes, leisure drugs, or alcohol). The technical and organisational capabilities for sorting these various data fields could impact on equality and equity generally. Such information can of course

be used in ways that reinforce justice and equity positively e.g., by increasing the understanding of the level of good public health in the community, region, or the country generally or by ensuring equal health treatment whatever the person's socio-economic background. On the other hand, the information could be used negatively to reduce the amount of treatment available to the particular individual and the ways in which such treatment is distributed.

A well-recognised approach to justice/equity would indicate that all patients should be able to have electronic records, so that no person (patient/citizen) is discriminated against[12]. The implication is that all patients should be treated equally. The same rationale and basis for information collection would be used, and non-discriminatory judgements would be made in relation to the basis of the information that is collected. All instances of data collection and transmission should be equal and fair for all patients. All patients should be reassured of the material quality of the record and that the record's content can be interpreted appropriately. If devices or records are designed to be used by patients (for example, for people who may have to read data on-screen or who may have to record and change data for themselves), then devices should be designed with a view to ensuring that all patients should be capable of using them easily. If patients are to have access to records, then all patients should have the same kinds of opportunities to access their own records.

Radio Frequency Identification Devices

RFID is based on small devices that can store data (information) which can be communicated to a receiver for some designated purpose. The device is attached to a host (artefact, human, animal). The ethically interesting – and provocative – characteristics of RFID devices are that they are small (possibly even un-seen) forms of ICT; they can be attached in some way to someone or some object (such as clothing, a piece of equipment, or a badge). They can collect, store, and transmit information using a range of radio frequencies.

To examine the ethical issues that might arise from RFID, we need to consider the fundamentals of the technology and its relationship to the 'ethical entity' which in the case of this paper is a human being. In terms of *the location* of the RFID device, it can matter substantially whether the device is worn externally on a wristband, or is embedded on an internal artefact such as a hip replacement, or is implanted in human tissue. If the device is attached externally, could it cause the patient embarrassment or could it cause them to be discriminated against? If an internal device is deemed to be less discriminating (as well as being beneficial in other important ways), do all comparable patient-cases have the opportunity to benefit from similar technologies? Is there some form of potential interference that could be triggered by a device and cause undue harm to others? Are all patients who carry/use such devices assessed individually in terms of potential harmful effects, i.e., is there an equal interest to assess the needs of each patient? In terms of location, issues arise with regard to complementary or parallel use of other devices and technologies: operationally, is the device likely to interfere with other nearby devices or *vice versa*? Can any radio waves from the device itself, or from one or a combination of nearby devices, affect the patient?

Relating the use of RFID devices to the ethical principles of non-malfeasance, beneficence, autonomy and justice (equity) can help to facilitate ethical decision-making (cf. Kluge, 2003). Thus, very generally, a range of questions would need to be asked when considering the *envisioned use* of the RFID device for a health-related purpose. Specifically, is anyone harmed (such as the patient, or others)? Does the technology promote well-being (does it protect the patient from harm or keep the patient safe)? Is the patient's autonomy respected (i.e. is there respect for the patient's degree of personal choice and independent decision-making)?

Does the use of the device promote justice and equity (or, conversely, does it permit discrimination and inequality)?

Approaching equity/justice in relation to RFID devices might particularly emphasise such issues as: the rationale and basis for use; non-discrimination with regard to the security of the data transmitted; fairness and equality of data collection and transmission; assurances with regard to the data's eventual interpretation; the ease of usability of the devices and equipment; and the access and availability of the devices to all patients on an equitable basis. These kinds of concerns are indeed very similar to those which are also raised in this paper in relation to electronic health records.

RAISING ETHICS AWARENESS IN OTHER AREAS

This paper has focused on raising an awareness of ethics with ICT professionals and trainees. It has used eHealth as a specific example, and has drawn attention to two applications in this domain: electronic health records and RFID devices.

Given the increasing spread of the use of ICT generally, and specifically within the field of eHealth, there are a number of other elements that need to be considered when raising an awareness of ethics.

First, not all ICT professionals enter their profession through the route of higher education – although clearly that entry-point has become more and more the norm. Other levels of education and other professional domains are important.

Second, the debate and discussion strategy used in teaching to bring out the ethical dimensions of technology is equally applicable to other groups, but may need to be conducted in a different context. Forums, or 'spaces for discussion' (Berleur et al. 2000; Berleur et al. 2009) enable participants within a particular domain to explore and gain understanding of different ethical perspectives, and to relate discussions to personal experiences and situations.

Third, formal training programmes are not necessarily going to be either appropriate or helpful with regard to the relevant education of patients, their carers or their families, and they are unlikely to be a feasible option for these groups. What can be achieved, however, would be a general raising of ethical awareness on the part of those who are outside a conventional institutional setting (e.g., a university; a training centre; a hospital; or a clinic), and yet who are nevertheless direct stakeholders in eHealth.

Fourth, in recent times, technologies have begun to provide opportunities to participate in discussions remotely – for example, discussion spaces started from blogs, or facilitated by social networking sites (Whitehouse, 2009). Some of the benefits of face-to-face interaction may be lost using these means, but gains can be made by virtue of the fact that physical presence is not required. This opportunity could be especially relevant to people who experience constraints, in health terms, in terms of physical presence, geographic mobility, or employment conditions.

Fifth, raising ethical awareness is especially important where technologies are used at-a-distance (e.g. telemedicine or telecare), and where the ethical implications may not be so easily or immediately perceived. For example, a diabetes monitoring aid may send information electronically (e.g. *via* wireless connections) to a remote healthcare practitioner. Would either of the users (patient or healthcare professional) understand the potential for compromising data integrity using this means (Duquenoy 2009)?

DISCUSSION

eHealth by its very definition involves the use of ICT in a field which is likely to involve not only a far wider range of professional personnel than simply ICT professionals but also many other people with a wide range of educational and professional competences.

In the eHealth domain, a wide range of different professions and occupations may need to work together alongside ICT professionals, e.g. administrators, clinicians, insurers, nurses, pharmacists, and researchers. These may also interact with other groups of individuals, e.g. patients, carers, and family members.

The ethical aspects of technology are as valid for healthcare professionals as they are for their ICT counterparts. Healthcare professionals would probably not need to be convinced of the role of ethics within their own professional domain, but they should also know how the introduction of technology could impact on their own ethical practices.

Ethical training is therefore increasingly a multi-lane highway rather than simply being a two-way street. The needs involve: an understanding of ethics on the part of the technologists; an understanding of technology on the part of the healthcare (and other) practitioners; and an understanding of both ethics and technology on the part of people who may be neither ICT nor eHealth specialists, but may simply be concerned about their own health, the health of those close to them, or the health of those for whom they care or with whom they work.

Key challenges in this context are likely to be faced by people who have either so far resisted deliberately an introduction to or use of the technologies or whose age and circumstances have caused them to avoid their use.

The complexity of ethical choices does not necessarily have to be simplified. However, it needs to be more easily understood using tools, techniques, and approaches that can aid decision-making. Understanding ethics in a specialist field is in itself challenging, however, understanding it in its more everyday context may be even more provocative. Analytical frameworks are needed to facilitate this, as well as means to apply more theoretical ethical thinking to actual practice.

We anticipate that the framework which we outline in this paper may facilitate a growing clarity of thinking with regard to the possible ethical options at stake in any given practical situation and the various rationales that underpin them.

CONCLUSION

In a larger context, there is a growing convergence among the various domains, services, technologies and applications that are under development and use in modern society. This trend is as relevant to eHealth as it is to other social and organisational domains. Indeed, it may be even more so, given the considerable challenges – social, organisational, demographic, and economic – to Europe's healthcare.

The range of technologies that can be used contemporarily is already impressive. This list is likely to be increased still more comprehensively in the future: this ever-widening range of possibilities is explored, for example, in work by the Institute for Prospective Technology Studies (IPTS) assisted by empirica[13] and projects such as The Senior Project[14]. The IPTS study explains that eHealth is helping to move healthcare from a more institutionally-based model to a patient-centred one (increasingly, there is also a portrayal citizen-driven healthcare). The technologies to be used are being operated close to the patient, whether e.g., on the skin of or even within a patient, or are located in a patient's more intimate, domestic sphere e.g. in her or his home. As these trends develop, an understanding of technologies and their ethical concerns will become increasingly relevant to patients themselves, their carers, and families.

There may indeed be trade-offs or compromises that need to be made among these various challenges. One potential polarity may be the ethics of computing use and the economics of technology use. On the other hand, these dilemmas may also share common ground. Today's focus on the sustainability of society provides a larger context in which such issues can be resolved and it may even encourage their resolution.

We can look forward to a greater in-depth investigation of ethical issues and ICT. Important examinations of applied ethics are already being undertaken in relation to a wide range of technological applications, whether contemporary or future-oriented. These occur in current European co-financed projects such as ETICA and EGAIS.[15] More specifically, in relation to eHealth, various ethical dilemmas are being explored in European projects such as ETHICAL.[16]

ACKNOWLEDGMENT

We wish to acknowledge that this paper builds on earlier work relating to eHealth and ethics (Whitehouse and Duquenoy, 2009) although this text enhances and expands considerably that first set of ideas.

REFERENCES

Berleur, J., Burmeister, O., Duquenoy, P., Gotterbarn, D., Goujon, P., Kaipainen, K., et al. (Eds.). (2008). *Ethics of Computing Committees. Suggestions for Functions, Form, and Structure*: IFIP-SIG9.2.2. IFIP Framework for Ethics of Computing (pp. 1-35), Laxenburg, AU: IFIP Press.

Berleur, J., Duquenoy, P., d'Udekem-Gevers, M., Ewbank de Wespin, T., Jones, M., & Whitehouse, D. (2000). Self-regulation instruments – Classification – A preliminary inventory. HCC5, Geneva 1998; SIG9.2.2 January 2000; SIG9.2.2. June 2000; IFIP – WCC-SEC 2000.

Bradley, G. (2009). The Convergence Theory and the Good ICT Society - Trends and Visions . In Schlick, C. M. (Ed.), *Industrial Engineering and Ergonomics* (pp. 43–55). Aachen, DE: Springer Berlin Heidelberg. doi:10.1007/978-3-642-01293-8_4

COM 3282 final (2008, July 2). *Commission recommendation of 2nd July 2008 on cross-border interoperability of electronic health record systems.*

COM 356 final (2004, April 30). *e-Health – making healthcare better for European citizens: An action plan for a European e-Health area.* Luxembourg: European Commission

COM 414 final (2008, July 2). *Proposal for a Directive on the application of patients' rights in cross-border healthcare.*

COM 489 final (2008, November 2). *Telemedicine for the benefit of patients, healthcare systems and society.*

COM 860 final (2007, December 21). *A lead market initiative for Europe.*

Duquenoy, P. (2009). Taking a holistic approach to exchanging health information over a global network. In Mordini, E., & Permanand, G. (Eds.), *Ethics and health in the Global Village: Bioethics, globalization and human rights* (pp. 287–304). Rome: CIC Edizioni Internazionali.

Duquenoy, P., George, C., & Solomonides, A. (2008b). Considering Something ELSE: Ethical, Legal and Socio-Economic Factors in Medical Imaging and Medical Informatics In H. Muller, G. Xiaohong, L. Shuqian (Eds.), *Special Issue of the International Conference MIMI2007 on 'Medical Imaging and Medical Informatics'* (pp.227-237), Beijing, China. Computer Methods and Programs in Biomedicine, *92* (2008), 2(3). Ireland, Elsevier.

Duquenoy, P., George, G., & Kimppa, K. (Eds.). (2008a). *Ethical, Legal, and Social Issues in Medical Informatics.* IGI Global: Medical Information Science Reference.

Eng, T. R. (2001). *The eHealth Landscape: A Terrain Mapping of Emerging Information and Communication Technologies in Health and Health Care.* The Robert Wood Johnson Foundation.

European Commission. (2007). *eHealth priorities and strategies in European countries.* Luxembourg: Office for Official Publications of the European Communities.

Eysenbach, G. (2001). What is e-health? *Journal of Medical Internet Research, 3*(2), e20. doi:10.2196/jmir.3.2.e20

Kant, I. (1981). *Grounding for the Metaphysics of Morals* (Ellington, J. W., Trans.). Indianapolis: Hackett Publishing Company.

Kluge, E.-H. (2003). *A Handbook of Ethics for Health Informatics Professionals.* London: Health Informatics Committee, British Computer Society.

Oh, H., Rizo, C., Enkin, M., & Jadad, A. (2005). What is eHealth? (3): A Systematic Review of Published Definitions. *Journal of Medical Internet Research, 7*(1), e1. doi:10.2196/jmir.7.1.e1

Pagliari, C., Sloan, D., Gregor, P., Sullivan, F., Detmer, D., & Kahan, JP. (2005). What is eHealth? (4): A Scoping Exercise to Map the Field. *Journal of Medical Internet Research, 7*(1), e.

Whitehouse, D. (2009) Book review. The Medicalization of Cyberspace. In *Journal of Information, Communication and Ethics.* February 2009. 7 (2/3), 211-213.

Whitehouse, D., & Duquenoy, P. (2009). Applied Ethics and eHealth: Principles, Identity, and RFID. In V. Matyáš et al. (Eds.) *IFIP AICT 298* (pp. 43-55). Laxenburg, AU: IFIP Press.

ENDNOTES

[1]   See the conference declarations of at least three high-level (Ministerial) conferences in 2007 and, 2008, and 2009: http://ec.europa.eu/health-eu/news/ehealth/ehealth2007_en.htm ; and http://www.ehealth2008.si/ ; and http://www.epractice.eu/en/library/281916 Accessed 5 January 2010

2   See the Council Conclusions of 1 December 2009: http://eur-lex.europa.eu/LexUriServ/LexUriServ.do?uri=OJ:C:2009:302:0012:0014:EN:PDF Accessed 6 January 2010

3   "eHealth strategies" http://www.empirica.com/themen/telemedizin/projekte_en.php Accessed 10 January 2010

4   http://www.epsos.eu/ Accessed 6 January 2010.

5   http://www.calliope-network.eu/ Accessed 6 January 2010.

6   https://www.eid-stork.eu/index.php?option=com_frontpage&Itemid=1/ Accessed 6 January 2010.

7   http://www.continuaalliance.org/ Accessed 5 January 2010.

8   Examples of relevant studies include ICT and ageing http://www.ict-ageing.eu/ Accessed 10 January 2010.

9   http://www.buslab.org/SummerSchool2008/schedule.html/ Accessed 7 January 2010.

10   One example is the possible future focii of a European Commission Directorate-General on justice, fundamental rights, and citizenship. A second is the increasing perception that the European Union's post-i2010 and EU2020 initiatives may concentrate, at least in part, on user rights in relation to the Internet.

11   A two-year project called Value+ (which ended in February 2010) developed a policy statement on patients' meaningful involvement in health-related projects, and produced a toolkit and handbook for patients' associations as well as project leaders. See http://www.eu-patient.eu/Initatives-Policy/Projects/ValuePlus/ Accessed 20 July 2010.

12   On the other hand, there may be individuals who for various reasons prefer not to have such an electronic health record held on their health data.

13   http://www.empirica.com/themen/telemedizin/projekte_en.php/ Accessed 10 January 2010.

14   http://www.seniorproject.eu/ Accessed 11 January 2010

15   ETICA http://moriarty.tech.dmu.ac.uk:8080/pebble/default/2009/05/28/1243516800000.html/ and EGAIS http://www.egais-project.eu/?q=node/3/ Accessed 10 January 2010.

16   http://www.ethical-fp7.eu/ Accessed 10 January 2010.

Chapter 38
Ethical and Social Issues of the Internet Governance Regulations

Jacques Berleur
Facultés Universitaires Notre-Dame de la Paix, Belgium

ABSTRACT

In this paper we debate some fundamental normative issues of the Internet governance. This is addressed in terms of technical regulations, self-regulations, and the legal regulations; this debate gives rise to a set of social and ethical questions whose answers may impact our lives.

IN HONOUR OF GUNILLA BRADLEY

Before all, I am very pleased to repeat here the terms of the IFIP-WG9.2 Namur Award that honoured Gunilla Bradley in 1998:

"Gunilla Bradley, professor in Technology and Social Change at the Royal Institute of Technology in Stockholm, Sweden, and now professor in Informatics at the University of Umeå and at Mid Sweden University, is a pioneer within interdisciplinary research concerning IT and its impacts and the interrelations between techniques, organisations and humans. In her work, she has always refrained from fractionalising to keep a holistic perspective and she has never tired in her mission

to put forward human needs and possibilities in relation to IT structures. Her internationally successful text book Computers and the Psychosocial Work Environment presents the essence of her continuous research: work places and environments that are psycho-socially sound produce viable and profitable services and products. This was first outlined in her Ph.D. thesis in 1972 and has been pursued nationally and internationally since in enterprises and government organisations. Her work has influenced lawmakers to include in laws the need for psychological and social adaptation of work to human factors, and she has influenced scholars all over the world through lectures, conferences and textbooks. Today, her work remains cross-disciplinary by comparing and analysing societal and psychosocial challenges in modern IT domains, such as

DOI: 10.4018/978-1-60960-057-0.ch038

rural versus suburban communities and various interactive creative learning environments. Her dedication enlightens us all concerning the need for true human qualities in the IT era.

Gunilla Bradley also stands out as a role-model for women in IT, encouraging researchers of many disciplines to follow their own minds, even though it is not always the fashion of the day. She has persistently underlined the needs and possibilities of all those women who historically, in batch systems, in on-line systems with display terminals and micro-computers, made up the basic work force required for the developments that led to today's and tomorrow's IT systems - in this way empowering humans on all levels with the knowledge of what is needed to carry out human-oriented, viable but also economically feasible developments.

In the opinion of WG9.2, the work of Professor Gunilla Bradley firmly supports the work and spirit of WG9.2 now and into the future. By offering this award to Professor Bradley, a women is honoured who symbolises the persistence required to create better awareness of the social implications of information technology."[1]

Let me now contribute to what I think has been in accordance with one of Gunilla Bradley's own preoccupations.

ETHICAL AND SOCIAL ISSUES OF THE INTERNET GOVERNANCE REGULATIONS

If Vinton Cerf, one of the fathers of the Internet and the founder of the Internet Society (ISOC) is to be believed, then "As we move into a new century marked by the Internet's ubiquitous presence, we must dedicate ourselves to keeping the network

unrestricted, unfettered, and unregulated." [Cerf, 1999][2]

Ten years later, after the subprimes crisis and its consequences at the worldwide level, many countries have insisted for setting up regulations, mainly of the financial but also of the activities that have global consequences.

It is naïve to say that the Internet is unregulated. Lawrence Lessig and Joël Reidenberg have pointed out three levels of regulations: 1) technical, code, infrastructure; 2) market, commerce, business, self-regulatory, and 3) legal.[3] Pierre Trudel of the University of Montreal, distinguished seven levels which constitutes a continuum: the common law, the ruling of the States, the contractual techniques, the self-regulation, the soft law, the standardization, and the technical normalisation.[4]

We shall restrict ourselves to three levels: the technical regulations, the self-regulations, and the legal regulations, trying to raise the social and ethical questions that are linked to those levels.

THE TECHNICAL REGULATIONS

It is usual to mention three organisations, which regulate the Internet from a technical point of view: the Internet Engineering Task Force (IETF), the Word Wide Web Consortium (WWWC) and the Internet Corporation for Assigned Names and Numbers (ICANN). Let us briefly describe their role before raising the social and ethical issues.

Internet Engineering Task Force (IETF)

Its main roles are schematically, and among others:

Promotion of standards and norms which assure the full interoperability of the Networks

Areas: transport, routing, security to the users, the Internet Protocol. The IETF is "the protocol engineering and development arm of the Internet"

Approximately more then 130 working groups in 8 areas with more or less 2000 technician volunteers (http://www.ietf.org/dyn/wg/charter/ipv6-charter.html)

Working groups in 8 areas, +/- 2000 technicians-volunteers

Since March-April 1966 until October 2009: 5734 RfC (Request for comments), i.e. norms

Independent organisation, supported by the Internet Society (ISOC), **without juridical status.**

It is said it has functioned along a "consensus method under the auspices of "benevolent dictators".[5]

Let us take an example, coming from the IPv6 Working Group:

The IPv6 working group is responsible for the specification and standardization of the Internet Protocol version 6 (IPv6). IPv6 provides a much larger global addresses space than its predecessor IPv4. This enables global end-to-end communication and restores valuable properties of the IP architecture that have been lost in the IPv4 Internet. The core IPv6 standards are widely implemented and are starting to see global deployment.

The IPv6 working group was originally chartered by the IESG as the IP Next Generation (IPng) working group to implement the recommendations of the IPng Area Directors as outlined at the July 1994 IETF meeting and in "The Recommendation for the IP Next Generation Protocol," RFC1752, January 1995.

The primary focus of the IPv6 w.g. is to complete the standardization of the IPv6 protocols, and to review and update the IPv6 specifications based on implementation and deployment experience, and advancing them on the standardization track as appropriate.[6]

Of course, any expert can participate in the process, but I have doubts that considerations other than technical are taken into consideration. For example, what to do socially useful and to decide the appropriateness of the norms with so many addresses: a trillion of trillion of trillion of trillion (4 times) addresses?

The World Wide Web Consortium (W3C)

Briefly described:

*   Recommendations about WWW infrastructure in domains such as web architecture and its related technologies, the formatting of documents (html, xml, …), enhancing interaction or developing the accessibility for all,… Also responsible for the Platform for Internet Content Selection (PICS).
*   An "open" organisation **without juridical status**, hosted alternatively by INRIA(Fr) [today (January 1st, 2003) replaced by ERCIM, European Research Consortium for Informatics and Mathematics], MIT (USA) or KEIO University(Japan)
*   "Open": but annual full membership = US$ 50000;

Some of its recent initiatives:

*   The platform for Privacy Preference 1.0 (P3P1.0) Specification;
*   The Web accessibility Guidelines (WGAG)2.0;
*   The Mobile Web initiative, without forgetting its Platform for Internet Content Selection, standard for filtering notably illicit or harmful content on the Internet (PICS).

What can be said here is that the decision process is far from democratic. The W3C comprises 500 member organisations, product vendors and technological services, content suppliers, utility companies, research laboratories, standardization organizations, governmental representatives, and so on. But it is said that no decision is taken without the approval of the charismatic Tim Berners-Lee.

The Internet Corporation for Assigned Names and Numbers (ICANN)

The third regulator has surely been the focus of the opponents to a system of Internet regulation. It was not, as the two previous one, the fruit of individuals' charisma, but rather the fruit of the liberal ideology of technicians and Internet Engineers. Moreover, the Department of Commerce of the United States wanted to keep the hand on the attribution of TCP/IP addresses and of domain names and on the overall coordination of the critical functions of the Internet, which was the main role of ICANN. All the UN Fora, like the WSIS (World Summit on Information Society, 2003 and 2005) and its subsequent IGF (Internet Governance Fora (annual meetings since 2006) were poisoned by the ICANN question directly linked to the Internet Governance issues. Whilst all the other instances were, in the spirit of a multistakeholder approach, the US Department of Commerce wanted to keep the control of ICANN.

Things have recently evolved., through a document that is called "Affirmation of Commitment by the United States Department of Commerce (DOC) and the Internet Corporation for Assigned Names and Numbers".[7]

Many people rejoiced about this "affirmation", most probably because it put an end to the US monopoly. But I am afraid that they just read between the lines and not the text itself. Let me say first, positively, it is surely a step forward. But it doesn't forbid a critical regard.

ICANN, created in 1998, has known many updates: the JPA (Joint Project Agreement) was the 7th amendment of the original MOU (Memorandum of Understanding)! Now (September 30, 2009) the DOC declares ICANN is independent and is not controlled anymore by any one entity. But when reading carefully, "DOC affirms its commitment "to a multistakeholder, *private sector led*" (We underline) adding that "ICANN commits to perform and publish analyses of the positive and negative effects on its decision on the public …", and add that ICANN remains "a not profit organisation headquartered in the United States of America." When it is said that ICANN is "a multistakeholder private sector led", any people are wondering where is the role of the civil society and of the Governments. The civil society seems satisfied by the agreement they reached between ICANN and the "Non Commercial Users Constituency" (NCUC) during the recent Seoul meeting.[8] We cannot forget that other structure within ICANN must still find their place: the Governmental Advisory Committee (GAC) and the At Large Advisory committee (ALAC). A new story to be open!

Moreover, an even more important step for the management of the Internet will be in September 2010 or in September 2011, for the termination or renewal of the contract for the IANA functions between the DOC and ICANN.[9]

Social and Ethical Issues about Technical Regulations

Without emphasis let us list some of the social and ethical issues that we see as emerging from the technical regulations:

- An Internet's root server system of 13 main routers in the world: 10 in the USA, 2 in Europe, 1 in Asia (ICANN coordination)!!!
- What kind of democratic control for the decision process of Internet Governance and of ICANN, as regards, for example, competition law (abuse of dominant position and monopolies, prohibition of cartel, collusion and related practices), consumers rights, and of internal public and private law.
- The rules for attributing ".org" to Public Interest Registry (PIR) by ICANN to ISOC, and other TLD: unknown procedure;
- Issues at stake with IPv6, for example. 3,4 10^{38} addresses (340 trillions of trillions of

trillions of trillions, vs. 4 10^9 for IPv4). To do what? For which kind of society? To the advantage and benefit of whom? We must also assess the resistance: again migration costs from IPv4 to IPv6.[10] Who will decide?

- Does Internet technical regulation reinforce "public resource" / "common good" aspects?
- There are *many public policy concerns:* competition, consumers' protection, IPR, privacy, freedom of access,... In the hands of whom?
- DNS issues: they are identifiers for social identity, commerce,...
- Respect of the countries *diversity*, regarding its own Internet (legislative) policy; GAC in ICANN is an "advisory committee";
- Private organisation taking important decisions shaping the future of society, our ways of living and accessing and sharing information without clear participation and consensus on strategic decisions. This is a major issue in our modern world where democracy and ethics are merging;
- ICANN: how to resolve disputes of the vested interests as represented in the organisation?
- Where are the developing countries in ICANN, in GAC? (see *Digital Freedom Network*: "ICANN through its actions and inactions has succeeded in sidelining the interests of developing countries", May 19, 2003, http://dfn.org)
- Where are developing countries, and a.o. China in this negotiation of standards? Several countries are threatening to have their own system;
- The possible architectures of Cyberspace are many, "the values that these architectures embed are different, and one type of difference is *regulability* – a difference in the ability to control behaviour within a

particular cyberspace. Some architectures make behaviour more regulable; other architectures make behaviour less regulable. *These architectures are displacing architectures of liberty*.[11]

- Limits and validity of technical norms?
- How should the ar. 6000 technical norms (RfC) decided by 2000 people and few organizations without recognized status become universal norms?
- ...

THE SELF-REGULATION

Two definitions to frame our reflection: « Self-regulation is a resort to norms voluntarily developed and accepted by those who take part in an activity ».[12] « A legal technique according to which the rule of law is created by the persons to which that rule of law is aimed to be applied - those rules being elaborated by the persons themselves or their representatives ».[13]

It is sure that in the recent years there has been a proliferation of codes, guidelines, charters...: 'The Ten Commandments of Computer Ethics' [CEI, 1992][14], 'One planet, One Net: Principles for the Internet Era [CPSR, 1997][15], The User Guidelines and Netiquette [Rinaldi, 1999][16], The Wartburg Online Magna Charta [Magna Charta, 1997][17], The EuroISPA Codes/Guidelines of Conduct [EuroISPA, 1997-1999][18],... IFIP-SIG9.2.2 has analysed 40 such documents, and established a classification of the Inventory of self-regulation Instruments.[19]

When you look, for instance at the codes of the Internet Service Providers, you are astonished by their content:

- Concern about 'illegal material' (child pornography, racism propaganda,...), youth protection; commitment to cooperate with hotlines...;
- Data protection, confidentiality and e-mail secrecy;

- Need for decency: no violence, no hatred, no cruelty, no incitement to commit crimes;
- Fair trading, acting decently with the customers, giving them clear information, including about pricing, etc., but they decline any responsibility.

When looking at the sectoral codes, you are confronted with more and more contractual clauses, and a stress on practices in accordance with professional standards, as for instance: Health: candour and trustworthiness, quality of information, products, services, the best *commercial* practices (our emphasis), the highest standards by Health Care Professionals [IHCC, 2000][20].

The Global Business Dialogue on Electronic Commerce (GBD-e). This case is interesting. They have Summits of CEO and their "sherpas" (Tokyo 2001, Brussels 2002, New York 2003, Kuala Lumpur 2004, Brussels 2005, Taipei 2006, Tokyo 2007, San Francisco 2008, München 2009). They stated recommendations about: consumer confidence, Internet payments, convergence, cybersecurity, digital bridges, eGovernment, new business models, IPR, SPAM, taxation, and Trade/WTO. They had also a *Cyber Ethics Statement* but without any reference to their real "business".[21]

Social and Ethical Issues about Self-Regulation

Selfregulation: General Questions

- Self-regulation: its place in the normative order?
- Content: who decides what is to be considered as a policy or a social or ethical issue?
- How should private actors have a normative role *for all*?
- The role of the regulators to protect citizen and customers?
- The signs of real *participation* in drafting the codes of the actors are rare: where is democracy?

- Is self-regulation making the economic actors more responsible?
- Very often the slogans of self-regulation are:
  - 'The least State possible is the best',
  - 'Let us avoid a greater degree of statutory regulation',
  - 'Let business self-regulate the Net'

These slogans belong to the "knee-jerk antigovernment rhetoric of our past", and cannot persist without damage for a democratic society.[22]

"Between the strong and the weak, it is the freedom which oppresses and the law which frees."
(Lacordaire, quoted by M. Vivant)

Self-regulation, and/or "co-regulation" (See "Paris 1999 Summit of the Regulators"), or "multiregulation" (M. Vivant, University of Montpellier)

Self-Regulation: Its Relationship to Ethics and Deontology

- The impression is that when we leave the general principles of the deontological approach for more specific principles expressed in contractual terms, social aspects and ethics are more and more absent.
- Difference between professional deontology and self-regulation: ethics can find its place - more easily - in the first, because the « boundaries » of the profession are better delineated, and then members participation and public democracy are possible.
- Sectoral self-regulation: same situation as in the profession? Difficult to argue, since the clauses are nearly purely contractual.
- General principles codes are not the same as the sectoral ones. But in any case the *titles and preambles should make explicit the status* of those documents, and they

should all be *negotiated* in a *participatory* manner.

- Our deep conviction: those documents are *more self-protecting than self-regulating*, which is the opposite of giving the public the capacity of knowing and evaluating our behaviour in society. Do they protect all the parties, or aren't they protecting only their authors?

- The dimension of multistakeholderism is far from being present!

Social and Ethical Issues, Shortly

We should:

- Request more professionalism from professional bodies, i.e. clearer statements on issues in specialised fields where they develop their competence;

- Anticipate threats and dangers (Early warning function);

- Increase international exchange between professional societies and institutional groups, respecting the cultural, social, and legal differences;

- Reflect on the "shift from deontology for informaticians to a deontology of informatics under the control of the law" (Herbert Maisl);

LEGAL REGULATIONS

To believe that Internet is not legally regulated is also a utopia. The law creates confidence and is necessary for many Internet transactions. It creates a clear frame of reference, subjugates players to stipulations that guarantee security, fairness, and a good outcome. Moreover, it gives the public power for complaints. Doubtless, its territorial limits are questioned at a time of the global network, and the construction of supranational spaces like the European Union and the increasingly discussions at the level of organizations such as OECD,

WIPO, WTO, the Council of Europe, and so on, allow the progressive establishment of adequate international regulatory consensus.[23]

Considering only the European Regulatory Framework, we are faced with numerous Directives and Recommendations:

"In response to the conclusions of the special European Council of Lisbon of 23 - 24 March 2000, and building on the Communication on the results of the public consultation on the 1999 Review of the Electronic Communications Sector and the principles and orientations for the new Regulatory Framework, the Commission proposed in July 2000 a package of measures for a new regulatory framework for electronic communications networks and services. The package consists of five proposed European Parliament and Council directives under Article 95, one Commission directive to be adopted under Article 86 and one proposed Commission Decision on a regulatory framework for radio spectrum.

In addition, the Commission proposed a European Parliament and Council Regulation for unbundled access to the local loop, which was adopted in December 2000 and entered into force on 2 January 2001 [Regulation (EC) No 2887/2000 of 18 December 2000]. The Commission proposal for a Regulation for unbundled access to the local loop was adopted by the European Parliament and Council in December 2000 and has been in force since 2 January 2001.

Before submitting these proposals, the Commission had examined the impact of convergence on this sector and had conducted an examination of the use in the Community of radio spectrum by Member States and by non-governmental bodies.

The new regulatory framework is intended to provide a coherent, reliable and flexible approach to the regulation of electronic communication networks and services in fast moving markets. The directives provide a lighter regulatory touch where markets have become more competitive yet ensure that a minimum of services are available to all users at an affordable price and that the basic rights of consumers continue to be protected. "[24]

Those European documents cover: Framework Directive, Access and Interconnection Directive, Authorisation Directive, Universal service Directive, Data protection Directive, Consolidated Directive on Competition in the market for communications services, Regulation on unbundled access to the local loop, Commission Guidelines on market analysis and assessment of significant market power under the Community regulatory framework for electronic communications networks and services, Commission Recommendation on Relevant Product and Service Markets within the electronic communications sector susceptible to ex ante regulation, and List of standards and/or specifications for electronic communications networks, services and associated facilities and services.

On the USA side, there is perhaps less legislative work, but this does not mean "no policy". One should refer to[25]:

- US IT policy documents, website of the US General Services Administration http://www.gsa.gov: http://www.gsa.gov/Portal/content/policies_content.jsp?contentOID=117087&contentType=1006&PMES=1
- and http://policyworks.gov/policydocs/policy_list.htm,
- Role of PITAC (President's Information Technology Advisory Committee) mainly under Clinton-Gore administration: http://www.ccic.gov)
- Digital Millennium Copyright Act of 1998,

- Children's Online Protection Act of 1998 (COPA, Commission on Online Child Protection),
- Children's Online Privacy Protection Act of 1998 (COPPA)
- USA-UE Safe Harbor Principles (Opinion of the « Commission art. 29 », 4/2000 of 16 May 2000
- USA Patriot Act 2001: http://www.epic.org/privacy/terrorism/hr3162.html
- New US Draft of Internet and Broadband Legislation Proposal (November 2005)

It is obvious that one of the most litigious issues between Europe and USA has been the question of privacy. Finally, the discussion produces the "Safe Harbour Principles, but as soon as signed, the Bush Administration wanted to cancel the agreement. But it is still in use, if not really applied! The best – a must – book on *Computer Ethics*, as seen from the US point of view, and larger, is the bestseller Handbook of Deborah Johnson.[26]

We must finally mention the *Convention n° 185 on Cybercrime* of the Council of Europe. It has been signed by the members of the Council, but also unusually by USA, Canada, Japan, and South Africa. The domain of its content are: Illegal access, Illegal Interception, Data interference, System Interference, Misuse of devices, Computer-related forgery, Computer-related fraud, Offences related to child pornography, Offences related to infringements of copyrights and related rights, and Attempt and aiding or abetting.

Social and Ethical Issues in the Logic Development of Legal Regulations

The following logic may be read through the legal regulations with their own controversies:

It started with the Protection of the content and of the investments in the information society: for instance, about the intellectual property and related rights, ... but in Europe, with some "draw-backs" in the traditional legislation about copyright. In the United States, the 1998 *Digital Millennium Copyright Act* is protecting even technical measures that will restrict the access. When the content was guaranteed, it was to *the transaction to be protected* (B2B and B2C): identification of the parties, authentication of the messages, confidentiality, ... See on both sides of the Atlantic, legal regulation about the electronic signature, and in Europe, the directive on eCommerce, June 2000. Finally, it was needed to *protect the content and the transaction*, and then, detect and sue the illegal or the illicit. See the convention n° 185 on Cybercrime. Increasing Cybersurveillance hurting the freedom of expression and the privacy protection. Nobody can deny that this process has been developed not to protect first the citizen but the business. Let us mention, for instance, about the IPR, the reaction of the "Pirate Party":

"The Pirate Party wants to fundamentally reform copyright law, get rid of the patent system, and ensure that citizens' rights to privacy are respected. With this agenda, and only this, we are making a bid for representation in the European and Swedish parliaments. (...) The official aim of the copyright system has always been to find a balance in order to promote culture being created and spread. Today that balance has been completely lost, to a point where the copyright laws severely restrict the very thing they are supposed to promote. The Pirate Party wants to restore the balance in the copyright legislation. All non-commercial copying and use should be completely free".[27]

PROVISIONAL QUESTIONS

- The process of regulation is everywhere.
- At each level – technical, self-regulatory, and legal – it is difficult to really identify the actors. There is a nebula of actors. Who is finally regulating? Lack of transparency. Predominance of hidden (or vested?) interests – not always the same.
- The question "Who is regulating?" is a democratic question and "then" an ethical question, or at least a social question.
- Where are the challenges treated ?
  - At a political level, an agenda and an action plan have been fixed (WSIS, phase Geneva [December 2003] and Tunis Tunis Tunis Tunis [November 2005])[28]: which follow up of the 10 "action lines"?
  - At a research agenda level: scientists should help to prepare the parties to the Internet Governance Forum - especially in countries where the level of expertise is lacking of resources.
- Some main issues?
  - Before building "An Internet for All", let us question which and where are the people's needs!
  - Respect for humankind's diversity;
  - Respect for cultural diversity, multilingualism;
  - Equality of access, including education to the "Information/Knowledge Society"
  - Social justice and "digital divide";
  - Respect of the dignity of the person - protection of the youth and especially of minors;
  - Racism, hatred, denegation of crimes against humanity, incitation to crime, drugs traffic, violence... A "real" censorship not opposed to the freedom of expression
  - Anchor the virtual in the real.
  - ...
- Pending proposals:
  - Internet Governance Forum: A Bill of Rights;
  - Council of Europe: A Charter of rights and duties for the Internet users;

- ◦ There are more and more people advocating that the question of rights is becoming more and more central;
- ◦ But which legal tradition? Jurisprudential or more "normative"?
- ◦ And: how to reach a reconciliation of cultural diversities?
- ◦ ...

As a final word, we should remember the definition of the Internet Governance as expressed during the Tunis WSIS meeting, the fruit of difficult discussion within the Working Group on Internet Governance: *"Internet governance is the development and application by Governments, the private sector and civil society, in their respective roles, of shared principles, norms, rules, decision-making procedures, and programmes that shape the evolution and use of the Internet."*[29] This definition could be a signpost for further elaboration of any Internet regulation! We are still far from satisfying that ideal of multistakeholderism and having a democratic, social and ethical Internet Governance!

ENDNOTES

[1] http://www.info.fundp.ac.be/~jbl/IFIP/cadresIFIP.html (January 1998)

[2] Vinton CERF, *On the Internet*, July-August, 1999.

[3] Lawrence LESSIG, *Code and other laws of Cyberspace*, New York, Basic Books, 1999. Joel R. REIDENBERG in «Governing Networks and Cyberspace Rule Making», *Emory Law Journal*, 1996, p. 911ff.., and in «Lex Informatica: The Formulation of Information Policy Rules through Technology», *Texas Law Review*, vol. 76, 1988, p. 553-584

[4] P. TRUDEL, F. ABRAN, K. BENYEKHLEF and H. SOPHIE, *Droit du cyberespace*, Montréal, Thémis, 1997; P. TRUDEL, «Les effets juridiques de l'autoréglementation», *Revue de droit de l'université de Sherbrooke*, vol. 19, no 2, 1989.

[5] *The Economist*, June 10, 2000

[6] http://www.ietf.org/mail-archive/web/ietf-announce/current/msg00107.html (May 2004)

[7] http://www.icann.org/en/announcements/announcement-30sep09-en.htm (30 September 2009)

[8] Civil Society reps, ICANN Board bridge differences at Seoul Meeting, Internet Governance Project, http://blog.intergovernance.org/blog/_archives/2009/10/25/4361022.html

[9] http://www.icann.org/en/general/iana-contract-14aug06.pdf

[10] *Computer*, IEEE-CS, August 2001

[11] Lawrence LESSIG, *Code and other laws of Cyberspace*, op.cit.

[12] Pierre TRUDEL, Les effets juridiques de l'autoréglementation, in: *Revue de Droit de l'Université de Sherbrooke*, 1989, vol. 19, nr. 2, p. 251

[13] Pierre VAN OMMESLAGHE, L'autorégulation. Rapport de synthèse. In: *L'autorégulation*, Bruxelles, Ed. Bruylant, 1995, pp. 233-274

[14] Computer Ethics Institute (CEI), Washington (D. C.), The Ten Commandments of Computer Ethics, 1992, www.brook.edu/ its/cei/cei_hp.htm;

[15] CPSR (Computer Professionals for Social Responsibility), The Civil Society Democracy Project, http://www.cpsr.org/internet-democracy/

[16] *The Net: User Guidelines and Netiquette, by Arlene H. Rinaldi*http://www.fau.edu/netiquette/net/

[17] *Online Magna Charta, Charta of Freedom for Information and Communication, 'The Wartburg Charta', 1997*, http://sem.lipsia.de/charta/gb/chartagb.htm

[18] EuroIspa, http://www.euroispa.org/

[19] IFIP-SIG9.2.2
International Federation for Information Processing Special Interest Group " IFIP Framework on Ethics of Computing *Self-Regulation Instruments – Classification – A Preliminary Inventory*, http://www.info.fundp.ac.be/~jbl/IFIP/sig922/selfreg.html (June 2000)

[20] *Internet Health Care Coalition, eHealth Code of Ethics*http://www.ihealthcoalition.org/ethics/draftcode.html (2004-2010)

[21] Global Business Dialogue on electronic commerce: GBDe, http:///www.gbd-e.org

[22] Lawrence LESSIG, *Code and other laws of Cyberspace*, op.cit.

[23] Pierre TRUDEL (ed.), *Le droit du Cyberespace*, Thémis, 1995.

[24] Telecoms, Regulatory Framework, Introduction and Presentation http://ec.europa.eu/information_society/topics/telecoms/regulatory/new_rf/index_en.htm#Introduction (2000-2002)

[25] That information was provided to us by □ Rob KLING himself, from the Rob Kling Center for Social Informatics, http://rkcsi.indiana.edu/

[26] Deborah G. JOHNSON, *Computer Ethics*, 4th edition, Prentice Hall, 2009.

[27] The Pirate Party, http://www.piratpartiet.se/international/english

[28] World Summit on the Information Society, http://www.itu.int/wsis/index.html

[29] WSIS, Tunis Agenda for the Information Society, § 34)

Chapter 39

Moral Considerations for the Development of Information and Communication Technology

Darek M. Haftor
Stockholm University, Sweden & Linnaeus University, Sweden

ABSTRACT

This text reports findings from an inquiry into the normativity inherent within the developmental work of Information and communication Technologies (IT). While IT has arrived to human affairs to stay, and may be used both for good and bad, it has an unparalleled potential to impact our world! There exists a considerable set of research contributions that address the normative aspects of IT-usage – which is important! However, the process of IT-development is also important as it may be regarded as foundational for the IT-usage – it is during the development that important normative decisions are made that will open and close possible kinds of IT-usage. Unfortunately, there are few research contributions that inquire the ethical considerations inherent in the developmental work of an IT-artefact. Further, the few contributions that exist seem to assume a particular moral stance and are typically articulated in terms of a moral code of conduct. Unlike such contributions, the present text advances a conceptual framework for the guidance of IT-professionals' ethical considerations during the development of IT-artefacts. This framework offers a set of conceptual categories that support a formulation of specific questions, to help to unearth inherent moral norms. The proposed framework distinguishes between the typical kind of working phases when an IT-artefact is developed and the kind of stakeholders that both can make moral decisions and those that can be impacted buy such decisions.

PROLOGUE

I first met Professor Gunilla Bradley in 1997 when I was a graduate student. From the very beginning,

DOI: 10.4018/978-1-60960-057-0.ch039

and increasingly thereafter, Professor Bradley has been a source of inspiration to me and a role model for my own research – not in substance but in form. I have perceived Professor Bradley as an unorthodox scholar, not afraid of posing questions that no one has asked before, of crossing intellectual disciplines in a way they have never been crossed before, and of integrating sound explorative and descriptive theory building with normative guidelines aimed at human wellbeing.

Professor Bradley was one of the first researchers in the world to address the social and socio-psychological consequences of Information Technologies deployed in a human environment such as in the workplace. This was at a time when all attention was concentrated on developing this technology and on its performance. Today we see this kind of inquiry as given; then it was considered at best odd, sometimes even hostile. As my relationship with Professor Bradley developed over the years into friendship, I have realised that the greatness of a scholar is not defined by her intellect but by the heart that guides it, and motivates facing up to challenges and difficulties in the quest for truth relevant for human wellbeing!

In my aspiration to link to the Bradley spirit of human concern, I propose to present a modest contribution for reflections upon the moral conditions unconditionally inherent in the very development of Information Technology artefacts.

INTRODUCTION

Assume a situation where a computerised information system is developed and, in the course of this development, subjected to various functional tests in order to assure desired system quality. The following normative question may emerge: Should the anticipated users test the new system, or not? Assume further that there are various types of anticipated users, e.g. those well acquainted with using systems and those who are not. In such an instance: should representatives from both groups be used to conduct tests, or not? – And why?

This is the type of practical situation addressed in this text as we present some of the preliminary findings from an ongoing inquiry into the normative considerations of Information and Communication Technology (IT) and its profes-

sionals. While no final answers to these questions will be provided here, a conceptual framework will be introduced, aimed to guide normative considerations and decisions in the course of the development of IT-artefacts. The remaining part of this Introduction provides a context to this inquiry and then presents a structure for the text as a whole.

Information and communication technologies are embedded in most human and social affairs, and this embedding is most likely to continue. The assumption here is that as with any technology, IT may be both good and bad, depending on how it is utilised. Unlike any other technology, however, IT possesses the unique ability to affect our world, which requires careful normative and particularly moral consideration. While most such moral inquiries today seem to address the question of how to use an IT-artefact that has been constructed and deployed, the present inquiry focuses on the moral conditions of the actual development of an IT-artefact and its master: the IT-professional!

This text presents two interrelated discussions. First, an elaboration of some of the central moral characteristics of technology in general and specifically IT. This provides the context for the second elaboration which addresses the structures of norms embedded in the development process of an IT-artefact, including its key stakeholders. The outcome of elaboration is a *proposed conceptual framework aimed to guide moral reflections of IT-professionals during their development of IT-artefacts*.

Unlike other contributions to this area, this elaboration does not attempt to provide another code of moral conduct for IT-professionals, which must inevitably be based upon a selection of ethical values.[1] Rather, the framework proposed here aims to guide the moral reflections of the IT-professional independently of moral convictions, be they utilitarian, deontological, Christian, or other. Figure 1 illustrates the positioning of this inquiry. As the conceptual framework presented here is in the midst of its development, the final

Figure 1. Illustration of the position of this inquiry, namely to provide guidance for moral reflections upon the development of an IT-artefact, as conducted by IT-professionals

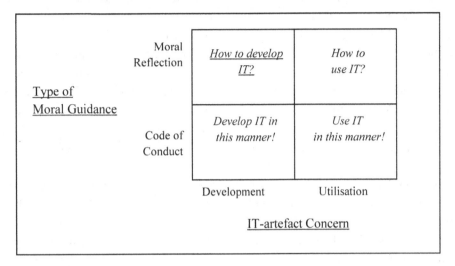

part of this text offers some suggestions for its further development.

NORMATIVITY OF INFORMATION AND COMMUNICATION TECHNOLOGY

The first part of this section presents some reflections upon the normativity inherent in technology as such, with the aim of manifesting the need for dedicated ethical reflection while the second part elaborates on the embedded normativity that is peculiar to IT – all this to establish a foundation for the following elaboration of a conceptual framework

Central Characteristics of Technology

We may recall that the term *technology* as such is etymologically derived from the Greek "*techne*", meaning craft, and "*logia*", previously denoting "*saying*" and now the "*logic of*". Together these terms provide us with "*technologia*" or the "*logic of craft*". Technology may for example be

contrasted with knowledge (Greek "*episteme*"), characterising our world as it is while "*techne*" is the craft that intervenes into our world. In this way, we may regard technology as man's knowledge, skills and usage of tools and crafts to affect the world he lives in.

A further important distinction lies in the technology itself, as it refers to both the material objects being used, such as a hammer, a medicine, a computer etc., and to systems with methods, procedures, organisations and techniques (Franklin, 1999; Strijbos & Basden 2006). For example, in the case of a carpenter, the term technology can both be used for the hammer itself and for the way in which it is used to achieve a predefined aim of intervention in the world, here to hang a painting on the wall!

Given this understanding of technology, we can now articulate one crucial characteristic of all technology: that our utilisation of technology to impact the world generates an *instrumentalisation of human actions*! In other words, technology is used to support and/or enable us to conduct certain activities, for example a spade supports us in more efficiently digging a ditch in the ground; a telephone enables us to talk to other fellow humans far away from us. While the first example instrumentalises our actions in a supporting manner, meaning that we would probably be able to dig the ditch without the spade, albeit not as efficiently; the latter example instrumentalises our action in an enabling manner, meaning that standing in Amsterdam we would not be able to speak to our colleague in Stockholm without this technology: the telephone system!

An important implication of these intervening features of technology is its inherent dual normativity. One kind of normativity comes from the fact that all technology – whether an ultrasound machine for medical cancer diagnosis or the actual procedures that are designed so the machine can make the diagnosis – comprises embedded norms, or is based upon a set of (value based) norms. This is the case as technology, and for example its artefacts, are the result of a deliberate design process, which assumes the mode of how things *ought to be*, rather than how things *are* in the world, and as such is selective. This selectivity is unconditionally normative.[2]

The second normativity inherent in all technology comes from the way it is actually used; in a person's instrumentalisation of his/her actions. For example, nuclear power technology, in itself, embeds a set of norms from its development process. However the actual use of nuclear power also has a second distinct set of norms embedded into it. *We may thus conceive norms inherent in the process of technology development and then norms inherent in the utilisation of technology, after it has been developed.*[3] The first category is the concern of the inquiry presented here.

Key Characteristics of Information and Communication Technologies

Moving the attention to the main theme of interest in this discussion, one can ask the question: what are the peculiar characteristics of Information and Communication Technologies? To be sure, IT does inherit the above-mentioned characteristics of technology as such, those which are inherent in all technology irrespective of whether it is IT, nuclear technology, bio technology or any other type of technology.

Instances of IT may include book printing technology, radio, television, telephones, monitoring and controlling systems in nuclear power plants or surgery rooms, a bank's automatic teller machine, the Internet – with its various offerings such as electronic journals, e-books and e-shopping – car dashboards comprising systems providing information, video games, automatic customer payment systems in the supermarkets ... among thousands of other instances! It seems that IT is immersed everywhere in our human and social affairs, whether in a private, public, social, or professional context. In total, all these artefacts and procedures, in one way or another, support and enable us to conduct certain activities. If we ask ourselves: *Would I like to live in a world where none of this IT exists?* We assume that most of us would say: *No!* Yet any technology, including IT, comprises benefits and disadvantages. We will return to this later on.

If we assume a structural elaboration, we can start with the characterisation of IT as a sort of Information Processing System (IPS), after Newell and Simon (1972), which stipulates that all kinds of IPS, whether natural or artificial, have the following four fundamental functions: to generate information, to transform information, to store information, and to transfer information. We refer here to artificial IPS or IT and are ignoring the existence of natural IPS such as human neural systems or genes. Given this functional specification of IT, its purpose can be questioned! In this context, we understand that IT has two inherent generic benefits that may be defined as generic purposes: one is to inform and the second is to automate (Zuboff, 1988). Hence, IT may enable communication by transferring information[4] over a long distance; as with telephones, radio, television, and the Internet. However, IT also enables us to automate activities, such as simple arithmetical calculations, automatic mechanisms to lock or unlock an office door, or advanced automation of a production line in the automotive industry, etc.[5]

While discussing the central characteristics of technology as such, we formed the conclusion that technology instrumentalises human activities. Transferring our attention to this particular type of technology, IT, we can further qualify this characteristic as being peculiar to IT as it is able to instrumentalise a certain area of human action, namely human reason! Hence, while other technologies may instrumentalise human physical activities, such as digging a ditch, IT instrumentalises human mental[6] activities, such as arithmetical calculations. This is a unique characteristic of IT: no other technology is able to instrumentalise human reason! This unique characteristic has profound implications in terms of IT's capability to change our world! The examples of IT-systems described above manifest the vast benefits that IT can offer mankind, whether by eliminating dangerous acts for man, conducting lifesaving activities, or providing pleasure. On the other hand, IT may cause damage. Stanley Kubrick's seminal movie '*2001: A Space Odyssey*' is an icon illustrating the damage that can result from instrumentalisation of human reason! The spaceship's all-controlling main computer, HAL 9000, is sufficiently intelligent to mimic a kind of unenlightened self-interest that is all too human!

The ability of IT to instrumentalise human reason provides the generic abilities described above – automation and communication – which in turn expose man to two generic threats. The first is automation enabling control, which in turn threatens human integrity, while the second is the communication which enables mediated human communication, which in turn threatens the authenticity of human communication.

Control may prove to be valuable for man, one example is the health monitoring systems that continuously monitor key health variables of a person and forward them to a physician for diagnosis. On the other hand, unsolicited control

of our shopping behaviour, as conducted by a major supermarket chain, is something to which many of us are unwilling to be subjected, as it violates our integrity!

Likewise, IT-mediated communication such as e-mailing has enabled communication opportunities between people and organisations as never before. On the other hand, the ever increasing amount of so-called SPAM (i.e. unsolicited commercial and other mailings) exposes us to false information, such as banking proposals which attempt to deceive us financially.

Neither of the problems control vs. integrity and communication vs. authenticity are generated by IT – these problems have been around for a long time. What is new here is the IT context; the speed, magnitude and scope assumed by the two problems: integrity and authenticity can now be violated in a way hitherto unknown to us! We shall now move on to the two IT contexts that generate these threats.

So far we have attempted to establish that IT is a unique technology in that it possesses the ability to instrumentalise human reason, which in turn can generate benefits and cause damage to human and social affairs. This opens the quest for normative reflections as to how we ought to utilise IT to create benefits and not damage. In this regard we wish to articulate a further distinction that differentiates on the one hand between IT as implemented in human affairs to serve ends and utilised as such, and on the other hand the working process of IT development and implementation in human affairs, the latter is a precondition that generates the former, and the main concern of this document. Ethical reflections upon the utilisation of IT, such as means of utilising Internet to create benefit rather than harm is crucial for the wellbeing of human affairs, and a significant amount of reflections on this have been published. However ethical reflections on the development of IT are also crucial as they open and close the functional and normative space of IT utilisation, and can thus be perceived as more fundamental than the ethical reflections on how to IT should be utilised. Unfortunately, ethical reflections upon the IT development process have generated only a limited amount of attention within the research community; and where so, of a particular type only; this is the concern of this elaboration and proposal.

These reflections have typically been made in terms of proposals for a code of ethics aimed at IT professionals, such as the *"ACM Code of Ethics and Professional Conduct"*.[7,8] An example of such a moral imperative is: *"Contribute to society and human well-being."* While we welcome this particular moral statement, such an approach to ethical meditation does have its limitations. Firstly, it is very generic in its nature, in other words it is applicable to everything - most people would probably subscribe to its intention on an intuitive basis - yet it does not say a great deal about how it could be fulfilled, or the significance of fulfilling it in a particular real-life situation. Secondly, and more importantly, such imperatives are selective in their preference to a particular type of moral position and its value sets – yet this is also necessary (e.g. Moor, 1985; Berleur & Brunnstein, 1996; Johnson 2001). Not everyone submits to a particular moral imperative position and its specific value set, for a variety of reasons. Therefore, the present elaboration focuses on a meta-level of such professional ethical norms without subscribing to a particular ethical preference – whether it be utilitarianism or other type of consequentialism, some deontological position, any type of virtue ethics, or the Christian ethics. The focus here is rather to provide structural guidance for conducting moral reflections and considerations for IT professionals in their professional IT development.[9] For this reason, the structure of the IT development process will be characterised in the next section in order to create a foundation for the forthcoming proposal for a framework to guide such reflections.

CHARACTERISATION OF IT-PROFESSIONALS

This section provides a characterisation of the core tasks of IT-professionals, to act as a basis for deriving a framework for ethical reflection of professional conduct. The method of this derivation comprises two steps: first, the establishment of the key activities of an IT-professional and secondly, identification of the normativity structures inherent in these identified activities.

The starting assumption here is that the central subject matter of an IT-professional is the IT-artefact.[10,11] Therefore the key question here is: how is an IT-artefact developed? Fortunately, the so-called Information Systems discipline, since its inception after World War II, has been extensively occupied with the formulation of numerous methods for the development and management of IT-artefacts (Friedman & Dominic, 1991). While there are numerous so-called methodologies and processes governing the development and management of IT-artefacts (Avison & Fitzgerald, 2002), this context presents a generalised structure, meaning the general activity types that seem to be included in most of the current methodologies for the development of IT-artefacts (Avison & Fitzgerald, 2002; Weaver, et al 2002). This general view states that the development and management of an IT-artefact may be understood in terms of seven types of activities typically conducted by the IT-professional. These types of activities are: inception, analysis, design, construction and testing, deployment, maintenance, and finally abolishment[12] – see Figure 2 for an illustration. The following sections provide a brief characterisation of each of these activity types, or working phases, together with some central ethical considerations.

Inception

The Inception phase denotes the initiation of the development of an IT-artefact; it is here that the need or opportunity for a new, or changed, IT-

Figure 2. Illustrates a process for the development of IT-artefacts, as assumed for the present elaboration

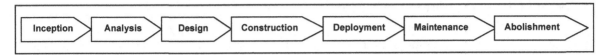

artefact emerges. This the least understood and researched activity type while at the same time being one of the most important for the whole development of such an artefact. Inception connotes here the often subtle change of mental state, within one or several human minds, from a state of no mental or conscious notion of the development of an IT-artefact into a mental state where such a notion does exist. Such emergence of an idea for a new IT-artefact may take place in a formal organisational meeting but also when a customer complains or when an employee is on vacation. This is then followed by various communicative, argumentative and dialogic activities which often lead to some type of formalisation of the emerged situation, frequently in terms of a project being set up and necessary resources being allocated. The next step may then be to conduct a pre-analysis (constituted by an opportunity and feasibility investigation which may also include a business case diagnosis) resulting in some kind of recommendation for the next step: to continue with the development initiative, how to do so, or to bring it to an end.

It is important to recognise that this emergence of the awareness of a need or an opportunity takes place in a pre-given context. This pre-given context is constituted by existing determinative and normative structures that open and close the opportunities for further development. They may include the physical situation – people, buildings, factories, machines – the mental situation – previous experiences, education and training – the cultural situation – differences and similarities in the opinions, suggestions and political structures involved – and also aesthetical preferences, legal

stipulations, or ethical positions of what is right or not.

In this Inception phase of the development of an IT-artefact some key moral questions emerge: what is the content of the initial proposal itself, who is to approve whether the pre-analysis is to be conducted or not, who is to be defined as responsible for conducting such a pre-analysis, and who should be involved in this pre-analysis; what kind of knowledge should be included in this pre-analysis and what kind of preferences (values) should be assumed (e.g. economic aiming at business benefit of the proposal, political aiming at power re-distribution as may be the case with the unions). Other considerations regard the actual content of the recommendation as a result of the pre-study: whether it is positive, i.e. can we go ahead with the next phase or it is negative, i.e. do we stop: the decision is a normative standpoint as to what should or should not be done!

Analysis

The term Analysis is used here to denote working activities with the aim of providing a concise definition of the desired IT-artefact, often in terms of the functionality and information the systems should offer the users, be they human or machine. This what-definition may vary in scope, from hardware and software characteristics to organisational workflows, roles and competencies, as well as other aspects, such as financial or vendor considerations.

The work-tasks of the analysis expose IT-professionals to various normative and thus ethical considerations, such as: who should conduct this analysis and who should be responsible for it, and further who should be involved and who should be considered in this analysis, what type of knowledge should be utilised and what set of values should be assumed, and how much resources – time or money - should be allocated for this phase. Once these questions have been dealt with another type of questions will arise regarding the actual content of the formulation of *the what*. For example, will the introduction of a new check-out system in the supermarket imply that cashiers will lose their jobs and that older customers will have to learn how to handle fully automated check-outs? If so; who is to decide this, why and on what grounds?

As with the Inception phase, the Analysis phase determines the space of options of the forthcoming working phases, particularly Design. For example, if the scope of an Analysis is limited to a particular department of an organisation, then the Design work will most likely also be concerned with the selected department and not much more.

Design

The next phase is the Design phase. Typically, this is aimed at the production of a specification for how the desired IT-artefact should be realised. Hence, while the work during the Analysis phase is concerned with *the what* of an IT-artefact, the Design work is concerned with *the how*. A simple example will illustrate this distinction: the Analysis may specify that a desired IT-device will be able to store text documents while the Design may then specify that this storage is to be achieved using binary code or ASCII code, or both.

For the IT-professional, Design work contains numerous moral considerations. Firstly, the questions of who should conduct the design and who should be responsible for it, and then who should be involved and who should be considered in this work, what type of knowledge should be utilised and what set of values should be assumed, and how much resources should be allocated for this phase – i.e. time and money?

Construction

In the present conception, the Construction work for the proposed IT-artefact is conceived in terms of two sub-phases of work. Firstly, the formulation of a plan for the construction and testing of the system and secondly the actual execution of this construction and testing. As with the previous working phases, a set of decisions need to be made here. The planning of the construction and testing phase requires decisions regarding who should conduct this design and who should be responsible for it, thereafter who should be involved and who should be considered in this work, what type of knowledge should be utilised and what set of values should be assumed, and how much resources should be allocated for this phase – i.e. time and money? As was the case with the Design phase of the IT-artefact, the planning should include sub-phase decisions with regard to *the ought to* of the construction plan and its content. The plan needs to specify the order of the construction work and the tests, the people involved in the construction and tests with details of their skills, experiences and preferences. For example, crucial differences may emerge depending on whether a specification is formulated in India or in the Netherlands.

Deployment

Given that an IT-artefact has been constructed it needs to be Deployed within its desired context. This typically requires that two types of work be done by the IT-professionals: to plan the deployment and to execute it! As with the Design and Construction phases discussed above, there are a number of normative considerations: the IT-professionals must justify who should conduct the planning and execution of the deployment and who should be responsible for it, and then who should be involved and who should be considered in this work, what type of knowledge should be utilised and what set of values should be assumed, and how much resources should be allocated for this phase – i.e. time and money? Again, the planning sub-phase of the deployment plan will specify the people involved in the construction with their skills, experiences and preferences – for example, should the deployment be according to the all-at-once manner or should it be done step-wise? Who will justify this? Yet another type of normative consideration that frequently emerges during construction and deployment work is that the plans defined to specify the execution are not feasible, in one way or another. Sometimes central items may have been omitted while in other cases the given specification cannot be executed due to faulty thinking. In whatever case, the question is: what to do? Should the specification work be re-iterated or not, who is to decide this and what will the consequences be?

Maintenance

The Maintenance of an IT-artefact may involve a set of various activities, which is partly dependent on the situation at hand. One central sub-phase is the evaluation of the IT-artefact in relation to performance criteria, whether they are defined in advance or have emerged during the evaluation process. A second central type of activities to be conducted are those that require that the current IT-artefact can maintain its operation and perfor-mance as it is – for example, a database typically requires regular de-fragmentation in order to maintain its data access performance. Further, if the software includes errors then adjustments need to be made, which is a type of problem fix-ing. Comprehensive adjustments may result in the work being instead classified as development work requiring its own analysis, design, construction and deployment. This would clearly require that someone make and justify a normative decision.

As is the case with the previous phases, all types of Maintenance work mentioned here and elsewhere in this document, may include a plan-ning phase and an execution phase. This brings us

back to the normative type of questions mentioned before, regarding the set-up of the work to be conducted and the actual content of the outcome of this work.

Abolishment

While very few researchers seem to address the question of the abolishment of an IT-artefact, it is a crucial and sometimes very challenging work-stream for the IT-professional! Examples of challenges include: what happens with the data in the database system? What should be done with the physical artefacts after the system is closed down? Who should decide whether or not the sys-tem should be closed down? As with the previous phases, detailed planning needs to be done prior to the execution of an abolishment. This exposes the IT-professional for the two types of normative considerations, the set-up of the planning work and the content of the outcome of the planning and execution tasks![13]

The Two Types of Developmental Norms

The notion of the development process of an IT-artefact as the core task of an IT-professional enables an identification of two types of norms inherent in such developmental work.

This first type of normativity emerges from the empirical insight that as soon as a develop-mental task is to be conducted, someone has to conduct it, and the questions then are the *who, why, how, when*, etc. These types of norms may be understood to be initial or fundamental as they constitute the very pre-condition for carrying out necessary developmental tasks.

The second type of normativity emerges from the empirical insight that each of the working phases described above – e.g. analysis, design, or construction – is selective in some manner. For example, someone must make the decisions regarding what functionality an IT-artefact should or should not have! These types of norms may be understood as terminal or directly forming the outcome of each working phase and thus eventually the final outcome: the IT-artefact!

This implies that both types of norms identified here; the foundational and the forming, derive from the fact that IT-professionals, when conducting their profession, are forced to be selective: there is unconditional selectivity inherent in the development process of any IT-artefact! The term 'unconditional selectivity' is used here to denote that a professional participating in the development of an IT-artefact is *thrown into a situation*[14], and cannot avoid making normative decisions – e.g.: 'should user group two participate in the user tests, or not?'

While this elaboration has so far been centred on the IT-artefact, the next step is to identify the key stakeholders involved in these working phases.

Stakeholders of the IT-Development

Given the work-process of an IT-professional as presented here, the second central area of elaboration here is the kind of stakeholders typically involved in the presented process to develop development an IT-artefact.[15] While the above characterisation of the typical activities for the development of an IT-artefact articulates the type of ethical questions that are imposed by such a process, the following articulation of the stakeholders aims to identify and to answer these questions and to analyse the impact of the answers. In other words, the stakeholders contextualised within this developmental process provide a certain space of moral considerations.

The first stakeholder of the development process of an IT-artefact is the actual IT-professional and the fellow-colleague IT-professional.[16] As characterised above, IT-professionals are the actors developing the IT-artefacts. An assignment to develop an IT-artefact is typically conditioned by various local norms, for example a given financial budget and a limited time-frame, and is justified by a strong financial cost and benefit motivation. An IT-professional, and his/her fellow-colleagues, gives rise to a certain relationship of fellowship as both share the same assignment-interests; however there may also emerge another type of interest caused by an eventual interdependency between two or more IT-professionals, for example when a certain task conducted by one IT-professional will determine the work of another IT-professional at a later stage in the process of the IT-artefact development. This type of dependence creates a need for responsible actions and considerations between the IT-professionals.

The second stakeholder of the development process is the Owner of the IT-artefact being developed by the IT-professionals. The owner is here understood to be someone, a person or an organisation, with the power to initiate and terminate an IT-artefact initiative. Frequently, the owner may be a company that has assigned another company to develop an IT-artefact. In this sense the owner has a particular interest in the IT-artefact, typically motivated by a desire to use it in a certain manner to a certain end, such as automating certain business processes in its organisation. The relationship between the Owner and the Professional seems to have a reversed symmetry. While the Owner approves the overall purpose of the IT-artefact and allocates and controls the needed resources for its development, the professionals have the capability to produce such an artefact within the given conditions. In this sense, these two stakeholders seem to have most influence over the development process of an IT-artefact – these stakeholders are also the moral power-holders of such a process.

A third central stakeholder is the Employer of the IT-Professional. Frequently, the IT-professional is employed by a company and assigned tasks or an area of tasks. The interest of the Employer is therefore to ensure that the IT-professional conducts his or her tasks with proper quality and in an efficient manner. In this sense there emerges a relationship between the IT-professional and the

Employer where the latter dominates the former in terms of having the power of assigning him or her to a certain project and/or area of tasks, and also setting certain expectations as to the quality and efficiency of the IT-professional's work. On the other hand, the Employer is dependent upon the work of the IT-professional, in order to be able to generate the outcome committed, typically by the owner – hence there seems to be a reversed asymmetry between these two stakeholders as well.

The fourth central stakeholder to be articulated here is the forthcoming *User* of the IT-artefact[17] – i.e. those actors that will use the system. This role may be in an organisational setting (e.g. a secretary using an invoice management system) or in a social context (e.g. a friend connecting up with a friend on Facebook). One of the challenges of the user role emerges from the empirical observation that the *actual* user can be the *intended user* but also an *unintended user*. A further challenge is that an actual user may *actually use* the developed IT-artefact as intended or otherwise – it is reasonable to assume here that the original developers of the Internet never conceptualised the possibility of financial transactions and related crime! While theses challenges must be important in terms of the functionality of an IT-artifact, they also pose a central ethical challenge: should we develop IT-artefacts that can be misused and thereby hurt other people? Therefore the IT-professional both opens and closes opportunities for the user's usage of the IT-artefact, which is a position with responsibility. For example, while an invoice management system may create a lot of challenges for a secretary if it requires new types of tasks to be conducted; it may also represent the opposite: it may eliminate part of the administrative burden from a secretary's daily work-load.

We have now reviewed the key stakeholders we assume to play a key role in the development of an IT-artefact. This identification may never be assumed to be final, and other kinds of stakeholders may be included where and when needed – such as the Public Stakeholder or the User's Client, or the Educator of the IT-professional. However, for the proposal put forward in the present elaboration, the listed stakeholders will suffice.

A GUIDE FOR THE NORMATIVE CONSIDERATIONS OF IT-PROFESSIONALS

The elaboration here has so far produced two conceptual structures: first a characterisation of the IT-development process, as a means to understand the kind of activities and thus decisions typically taken when an IT-artefact is developed, and thereafter a characterisation of the typical stakeholders of such a development; these stakeholders are both those who make normative decisions during the developmental work and those who take the consequences of such decisions.

The next step, in the present elaboration, is to combine these two structures into one two-dimensional conceptual framework – see Table 1 for an illustration. Starting with the process for the development of an IT-artefact, constituted here by seven distinct working phases each with its own subject-matter specific normative questions; this process provides two kinds of generic normative questions: the initial and the terminal, which govern all the constituting phases. The consequence of this is that for each working phase, the involved and affected stakeholders can be asked to reflect critically upon the normative content of the specific questions pertinent to each of the two kinds of generic norms. Secondly, for each development phase and for each kind of generic norm, one or more stakeholders may constitute one or two of the following roles: the decision-maker and the consequence-taker. The decision-maker may ask him- or herself: what normative decision should I make and what may the consequences of this decision be for me and for others? The framework proposed here enables the derivation of a set of operational questions to facilitate such a self-critical normative reflection. Examples of

Table 1. Illustrates the proposed framework for normative reflection of IT development

Stake-holders	Kind of Norms	Kind of working activities of the development and handling of an IT-artefact						
		Inception	Analysis	Design	Construction	Deployment	Maintenance	Abolishment
IT Pro-fessional	Initial	Decision-taker	Decision-taker	Decision-taker	Decision-taker	Decision-taker	Decision-taker	Decision-taker
		Conse-quence-takers	Conse-quence-takers	Conse-quence-takers	Conse-quence-takers	Conse-quence-takers	Conse-quence-takers	Conse-quence-takers
	Terminal	Decision-taker	Decision-taker	Decision-taker	Decision-taker	Decision-taker	Decision-taker	Decision-taker
		Conse-quence-takers	Conse-quence-takers	Conse-quence-takers	Conse-quence-takers	Conse-quence-takers	Conse-quence-takers	Conse-quence-takers
Owner	Terminal	Decision-taker	Decision-taker	Decision-taker	Decision-taker	Decision-taker	Decision-taker	Decision-taker
		Conse-quence-takers	Conse-quence-takers	Conse-quence-takers	Conse-quence-takers	Conse-quence-takers	Conse-quence-takers	Conse-quence-takers
	Initial	Decision-taker	Decision-taker	Decision-taker	Decision-taker	Decision-taker	Decision-taker	Decision-taker
		Conse-quence-takers	Conse-quence-takers	Conse-quence-takers	Conse-quence-takers	Conse-quence-takers	Conse-quence-takers	Conse-quence-takers
Employer	Terminal	Decision-taker	Decision-taker	Decision-taker	Decision-taker	Decision-taker	Decision-taker	Decision-taker
		Conse-quence-takers	Conse-quence-takers	Conse-quence-takers	Conse-quence-takers	Conse-quence-takers	Conse-quence-takers	Conse-quence-takers
	Initial	Decision-taker	Decision-taker	Decision-taker	Decision-taker	Decision-taker	Decision-taker	Decision-taker
		Conse-quence-takers	Conse-quence-takers	Conse-quence-takers	Conse-quence-takers	Conse-quence-takers	Conse-quence-takers	Conse-quence-takers
User	Terminal	Decision-taker	Decision-taker	Decision-taker	Decision-taker	Decision-taker	Decision-taker	Decision-taker
		Conse-quence-takers	Conse-quence-takers	Conse-quence-takers	Conse-quence-takers	Conse-quence-takers	Conse-quence-takers	Conse-quence-takers
	Initial	Decision-taker	Decision-taker	Decision-taker	Decision-taker	Decision-taker	Decision-taker	Decision-taker
		Conse-quence-takers	Conse-quence-takers	Conse-quence-takers	Conse-quence-takers	Conse-quence-takers	Conse-quence-takers	Conse-quence-takers

such questions for the Initial or Foundational normativity include:

a. Who is initiating this initiative, or working phase, and why?

b. Who could initiate this initiative, or working phase instead?

c. Who is involved in carrying out this working phase, and why?

d. Who could be involved in carrying out this working phase instead?

e. Who has selected the actors for this working phase, and on what grounds?

f. Who could select the actors for this working phase instead?

g. What directions are given for doing the work in this working phase, and why?

h. What directions could be given for carrying out this working phase instead?

i. What knowledge and experience base is introduced into this working phase, and why?

j. What knowledge and experience base could be introduced into this working phase instead?

Secondly, examples of questions for triggering self-critical normative reflections for Terminal or Formative normativity include:

a. What is proposed in the proposals generated in this working phase, and why?

b. Who will be influenced by these proposals, and how?

c. What could be proposed instead?

d. Who could be influenced instead?

e. How could the influence be different?

f. What worldview guides the formulated proposals, and why?

g. What worldview could provide guidance instead?

The operative questions set out here are only suggestions to illustrate how the framework proposed here can be translated into the concrete work of an IT-professional. These questions are built on the Churchman-Ulrich approach of polarisation between the is-situation and the ought-to-situation, here articulated as 'could-be', thus facilitating the unearthing of the inherent normativity in human affairs.

Normative Considerations Form a Particular Normative Standpoint

The framework for the guidance of normative considerations of IT-professionals as proposed here is a guide for *the kind of reflections* that could be made in order to self-critically oversee the inherent normativity of such development. This means that this proposal should not be regarded as a set of direct recommendations for the decision to be made in a particular professional situation. The actual decisions, as to what should or should not be done, are largely determined by the values assumed by the decision-maker(s). In the text below we will provide an example of this by contrasting a situation and its key decision with two distinct normative positions: the utilitarian[18] approach and a deontological[19] approach.

We shall assume as an example the need for test-groups for a new IT-artefact: a new inventory management system. One of the IT-professionals involved observes that the selected testers are younger women only and suggests to the test leader that the group also include older people who may have less experience of IT-systems but more experience of inventory management. However, such an expansion of the testing scope may threaten the budget and delivery schedule, two matters of great relevance to the employer and the owner.

The utilitarian position would be to investigate the positive and negative consequences, compare them and choose those that are the most significant. Assume thus that the negative consequences of expanding the tests as suggested would be budget and delivery schedule overrun, which would in turn trigger a penalty for the IT company producing the IT-artefact, implying a decrease in payment of 10%. This in turn would imply that the IT-professionals would not be paid bonuses for timely delivery within budget. Further, this could also endanger the relationship between the IT company and its client, as far as future business opportunities are concerned. Assume further that the only positive argument would be the fact that a wider segment of the targeted users of the IT-artefact would be given the opportunity to evaluate the IT-system and provide input for possible adjustments relevant to this segment of users. In such a case the utilitarian decision would clearly go for not expanding the tests.

On the other hand, a deontological position, such as the Kantian, would motivate the opposite decision. This is so as the categorical imperative stipulates that no human being should be utilised merely as a means (or instrument) toward a higher goal; rather humans should be the end in themselves.

SUMMARY

The introduction of contemporary information and communication technologies in human and social affairs opens opportunities and challenges. Unlike any other technology conceived by humankind, this technology can instrumentalise human rationality and thereby possesses a unique ability to change our world. This unique ability bears with it the need for careful responsibility and normative considerations both in the use of this technology and during its very development – as discussed in this investigation.

A conceptual framework is proposed here to guide normative, and particularly moral, reflections that the IT-professionals may make while developing any IT-artefact. This framework has two dimensions, one that characterises the lifecycle of an IT-artefact while the other that articulates a set of key stakeholders of the artefact. In each phase of the lifecycle of the artefact, a set of normative questions may be defined followed by a search for answers. Unlike other normative guidelines, this proposal does not assume a particular moral standpoint in a specific question; it rather points explicitly and critically to the kind of normative considerations to be made. In this sense, an IT-professional, whatever his or her moral conviction,

may be guided in his or her reflections, within a set of particular values.

The conceptual framework proposed here is still in its early phases and requires further development. One example is the assessment of whether the two dimensions of the framework do sufficient justice to the empirical situations of IT-artefact development. Secondly, a set of specific guiding questions for each phases of the lifecycle and each stakeholder, would facilitate and further govern the IT-professional's reflections.

REFERENCES

Alter, S. (2002). *Information Systems, Foundation of E-Business* (4th ed.). Upper Saddle River: Prentice Hall.

Avison, D., & Fitzgerald, G. (2002). *Information Systems Development: Methodologies, Techniques and Tools* (3rd ed.). Berkshire, UK: McGraw-Hill.

Bateson, G. (1972). *Steps to an ecology of mind*. New York, NY: Ballentine Book.

Berleur, J., & Brunnstein, K. (1996). *Ethics of Computing, Codes, spaces for discussion and law*. London, UK: Chapman & Hall.

Churchman, C. W. (1968). *The Systems Approach*. New York, NY: Delacorte Press.

Franklin, U. M. (1999). *Real World Technology* (Rev.edition). Concord, ON: House of Anansi Press.

Friedman, A. L., & Dominic, S. C. (1991). *Computer Systems Development: History, Organisation and Implementation*. New York, NY: John Wiley.

Heidegger, M. (1962). *Being and Time*. (translated by J. Macquarrie). New York, NY: Harper & Row: New York.

Johnson, D. G. (2004). *Computer Ethics* (3rd ed.). New Jersey, NJ: Prentice Hall.

Ladd, J. (1991). Collective and Individual Moral Responsibility in Engineering: Some Questions . In Johnson, D. (Ed.), *Ethical Issues in Engineering*. New Jersey, NJ: Prentice Hall.

Moor, J. H. (1985). What is Computer Ethics? *Metaphilosophy*, 4(16), 266–275. doi:10.1111/j.1467-9973.1985.tb00173.x

Newell, A., & Simon, H. A. (1972). *Human problem solving*. Englewood Cliffs, NJ: Prentice-Hall, Inc.

Peirce, C. S. (1891). The architecture of Theories. *The Monist*, 1(2), 161–176.

Shannon, C. E., & Weaver, W. (1949). *A Mathematical Theory of Communication*. Eleventh edition, 1967. Urbana, IL: University of Illinois Press.

Simon, H. A. (1960). *The New Science of Management Decision*. New York, NY: Harper & Row Pub.

Strijbos, S., & Basden, A. (2006). *In Search of an Integrative Vision for Technology*. New York, NY: Springer. doi:10.1007/0-387-32162-4

Ulrich, W. (1994). *Critical Heuristic of Social Planning: A New Approach to Practical Philosophy, (First published 1983)*. Chichester, UK: Wiley.

Weaver, P., Lambrou, N., & Walkley, M. (2002). *Practical Business Systems Development using SSADM: A complete tutorial guide* (3rd ed.). Pearson Education Ltd., Edinburgh Gate.

Weizenbaum, J. (1976). *Computer Power and Human Reasoning: From Judgement to Calculation*. San Francisco, SF: W.H. Freeman.

Zuboff, S. (1988). *In the Age of the Smart Machine. The Future of Work and Power*. Oxford, UK: Heineman.

ENDNOTES

[1] The empirical insight that guides this inquiry is that all IT-professionals unconditionally make moral decisions when doing their work. Secondly, the moral position assumed here is that IT-professionals ought to make their professional-moral decisions consciously and explicitly, thus motivating this inquiry.

[2] Since David Hume (1711-1776) we have been aware that it is not logically or rationally possible to derive *what ought to* be from *what is*, hence the need for a normative preference and decision about the desired situation.

[3] We do recognise that there is a logical circularity between the two types of technology normativity when technology artefacts as such are utilised to enable the development of technology – however this circularity is not temporal and can therefore be disregarded in this discussion.

[4] Information & Communication Technologies process *information*, which is not of key concern for our investigation here; however bearing in mind that there exist two competing notions of information – the physical or engineering one, that regards information merely as symbols or signals (after Shannon and Weaver 1949)), and the hermeneutic-semiotic or social one, that regards information as symbols with significance or meaning to its observers (e.g. Peirce, 1891; Bateson 1972)) – we wish to clearly state that this investigation assumes the latter.

[5] In this context, we are aligned with Alter's (2002:6) notion of an information system that is regarded as a work system supporting other work systems by processing data.

[6] This elaboration does not address the classic question of artificial intelligence; whether or not an information processing system can duplicate human or natural intelligence. In this context, we simply maintain that IT

enables duplication of certain human mental activities, such as manipulation of symbols (c.f. Weizenbaum 1976).

7　Association of Computing Machinery – see http://www.acm.org/about/code-of-ethics

8　Other similar propositions may be found at IEEE: http://www.ieee.org/portal/cms_docs/about/CoE_poster.pdf

9　This kind of focus on the developmental process of an artefact, in contrast to the focus on its use, has been suggested for the engineering community in general, see: Ladd (1991).

10　In very general terms, the term IT-artefact refers to man's creation of information processing technology, where technology includes both physical artefacts, with software and hardware, and working procedures and organisations.

11　We do acknowledge that IT-professionals may be engaged in other working tasks than those related to IT-artefacts, such as recruitment, management of people or budgeting, yet these are regarded here as complementary and not core subject matter tasks, and are thus disregarded in the present elaboration.

12　The mentioned order is a logical, not necessarily temporal, meaning that each consequent phase presupposes the outcome of the previous phase, to be successful, however temporally regarded, in the various tasks within the different phases may be conducted in parallel or other order.

13　All the types of working tasks for IT-professionals as described here suggest that there may emerge subspecialisations of the IT-profession; this is indeed frequently the case. For example: System Analyst, System Designer, Database Manager, System Tester, Maintenance Engineer, etc. In the present elaboration, all these are regarded as subclasses of the general category of IT-professional.

14　This is in the sense of Heidegger's '*thrownness*'; (Being and Time, 1962).

15　The stakeholder approach to normative situations has been advanced by a set of independent schools of thoughts, where one advanced school of management ethics, within the so-called Systems Approach, is the Churchman-Ulrich critical heuristics approach, offering a set of specific stakeholders (c.f. Churchman 1968; Ulrich, 1994).

16　A sub-set of the IT-Professional that may be conceived here is the vendor/supplier category, which is assumed to be included in the former and more general category.

17　The IT-user role may also be further decomposed into such roles as primary end-users, the user-support providers, and other – this is however not relevant for the current elaboration.

18　We understand Utilitarian Approach to be the moral imperative that everyone ought to adopt so as to bring about the greatest amount of happiness for the greatest number of people.

19　We understand Deontological Approach to be the moral imperative to never treat another human being merely as a means but always as an end.

Chapter 40

Critical Systems Thinking and Information Technology:
Some Summary Reflections, Doubts, and Hopes through Critical Thinking Critically Considered, and Through Hypersystems[1]

Kristo Ivanov
Umeå University, Sweden

ABSTRACT

This chapter presents a summary of some features of soft systems methodology—SSM, and of critical systems thinking—CST as they have been experienced from the point of view of the field of applications of information technology. It highlights the manner in which CST completes SSM in the context of the design of computer support in the form of HYPERSYSTEMS, and evidences some problematic aspects of the two approaches which push the practitioner into philosophical issues. One concluding hypothesis is that further developments of systems practice must be sought at the interface between formal science, political ethics, analytic psychology, and religious thought. For tutorial purposes, a great amount of literature is related to these issues.

SOFT SYSTEMS METHODOLOGY

SSM has been comprehensively presented in an extensive work (Checkland, 1981) but the following will be edited out of a more recent, and therefore presumably more developed, presentation of SSM that is related to informations systems (Checkland, 1988). It will sometimes be completed and followed by my comments.

Information systems can be seen as an organized attempt at meaning—creation—from—data by a social institution. The creation of meaning is seen as requiring a "semantic information theory" that may be grounded on the welcomed theory of "speech acts" in modern philosophy. An SSM idea that is considered crucial is that a set of activities be linked as to form a purposeful whole that could itself be regarded as a kind of system, a "human activity system". Such systems can be adequately clearly described only in relation to a particular world view, or *Weltanschauung*. Methods—models—systems that are relevant to debate real-world activity are developed (in a logic—driven stream of analysis), and compared with real-world ac-

DOI: 10.4018/978-1-60960-057-0.ch040

tion in a problem situation, in order to structure a debate about change. The problem situation itself is simultaneously explored (in a social stream of analysis) as a culture, with social and political characteristics. It feeds both the former choice (design) of relevant systems and the debate about change among participants/designers/users/end users/(ever-changing)-organizational members. This view of social reality is that of an ever changing outcome of a social process in which human beings continually negotiate and renegotiate, and so construct with others their perceptions and interpretations of the world and the rules for coping with it, rules that are never fixed once for all.

Future computer projects need to be complemented with such a technical—social—political *process* for continuous thinking and rethinking of organizations tasks and processes [activities], together with the rethinking of the enabling information flows. When iterations of the process produce models which are *widely agreed* to be relevant in a company [problem] situation, then such *consensus* activity models can be converted into information flow models, and the more traditional methods of information system design can be initiated. Lately there have been attempts, ideas and projects to design multimedia computer support of similar processes and their iterations (Forsgren, 1989; Lundquist and Huston, 1990). The activity models can be transformed into traditional information flow models (Checkland, 1970), as known in the field of information systems analysis (Langefors and Sundgren, 1975), by asking of each activity: (a) what information is required in principle to do this activity, in what form, with what frequency, from what source?, and (b) what information is generated by doing the activity? Even if prototyping as related to continuously learning systems apparently makes the idea of stable information flows obsolete, it is still true that some provisionally stable structure of the information system must be available in order to be periodically revised. Co-constructiveness

requires constructiveness. Learning systems are in the best case expected to increase the frequency of revisions or updatings, or then, to create structured databases of continuous opinion polls.

SSM CRITICALLY REVISITED

It is now time to reflect on the SSM approach summarized above. Lately there has been an articulated criticism of SSM at the interface with critical systems thinking. It will be covered later but for the time being we can note a kind of summary of this criticism that was presented in a recent paper (Gregory, 1989). It is stated there that the soft systems approaches were unable to deal with the fundamentally conflictual nature of social systems. Influential students of the method of social science in the context of analysis of radical, antiorganization approaches noted that the home of the twentieth century's critical theorists was the so called Frankfurt school. As alternatives or complements to SSM are in fact mentioned the "critical systems heuristics" that is directed at practical action of a critically normative nature, and the "theory of communicative competence" that provides a clear and pure theory of social interaction and of the means of societal reproduction, a rational reconstruction of the formal conditions required for communicative competence, i.e. the ideal speech situation. It is noted that the term "critique" has a long history. It was first used to describe the art of informed judgement appropriate to the study of ancient texts, whether the Classics or the Bible. The appeal to critique gradually displaced the criterion of truth, from revelation towards clear and rational, or critical, thought. The critical approach proposed by the critical heuristics of social planning is seen to remediate the failure of the critical theory of communicative competence in bridging the gap between *theoretical justification* and *political or strategic action.* It seeks to bridge this gap between theory and praxis by introducing the notion that any theory of society must be critically normative, and hence practically oriented. This means treating the model of communicative competence as an ideal which cannot be practically achieved, but can be striven for. This means striving not at an objective solution but merely at a *critical* solution. Critically normative reflection, however, must not remain extrinsic to systems thinking and system practice, or simply "added on" to instrumental-strategic reasoning.

It is not easy to follow this rather abstract criticism of an approach like SSM which has the intrinsic merit of being quite empirical. It will be therefore fruitful to meet SSM's problems first on its own grounds. SSM already in its early programmatic declarations was quite sensitive to its political interpretations. It was therefore stated (Checkland, 1981, pp. 281ff.) that the social systems theory implicit in SSM covers the area in which influential surveyors of socio-logical paradigms had located the critical theory of the so called Frankfurt school as represented by Jürgen Habermas. It was claimed that the differences between the two approaches stem from critical theory's *more overtly political stance.* SSM had not yet any *theory of how the structure of society, especially its stratification, might limit fundamentally the range of debate about change.* To critical theory's "communicative competence" corresponded SSM's consensual debate that has as criteria of success its *usefulness to the actors (instead of its validity for the analyst).*

One trouble with this position is that the choice of actors, and especially customers or problem owners, must certainly be "ethically valid" for the analyst who will espouse SSM. An analog point could be made for SSM's easy going admission that stages 5 and 6 of the methodology (comparing conceptual models with reality, and implementing "feasible and desirable" changes) will be inhibited by society's structure. It is further admitted that there are limitations on our creative freedom and on our powers of rational criticism since we and our values are products of existing institutions

and past traditions, "but this does *not* mean that the use of SSM methodology *cannot* in fact be emancipatory for the actors concerned".

Even disregarding for the time being the questionable WHY-NOT?-flavor of the double-negation above, that I will address later, it should be noted that the position taken by SSM with regard to institutions and traditions displays a "Lockean" bias in the tradition of British empiri-cism, in that ethical man is assumed to be born as a blank tablet to be written on by institutions and traditions. In other words, we are far from "categorical imperatives". The issue is also the choice of *which* institutions and traditions are to be fostered, since some of them may be assumed to be better than others in certain ignored respects.

All this, eventually, undermines the trustwor-thiness of an ethics that tends to get reduced to a communicative competence that, in turn, gets easily reduced further to a kind of politics of negotiations and re-negotiations of perceptions and interpretations of the outer world.

One most conspicuous claim by SSM, in spite of all emphasis on the unlimited negotiability of social (as opposed to natural) reality, is that the negotiations about the *method* (SSM) are explicitly constrained: "But *the way* one finds out about [so-cial reality] may in principle be reasonably stable: hence the importance of methodology rather than findings, of *process* rather than *content*....The unquestioned prime value embodied in 'a systems approach' is that continuous, never ending learn-ing is *a good thing*" (Checkland, 1981, p. 285, my emphasis). What is conspicuously missing in the context of the claim is a discussion of what is to be meant by a *good learning* as opposed to the statement that *learning is good.* It is therefore symptomatic that both the words knowledge and learning, not to mention ethics, are missing in the subject index of the SSM basic textbook (ibid.). To the extent that at least *meaning* is considered, it is selfassuredly observed that the social scientist will be reduced to studying not exactly social reality but only the *logic of situations,* producing findings of the kind "in situation A, a likely outcome is B", without any guarantee that this will hold in any particular situation: "And over the years, with the growth of human knowledge, the 'logic of situations'—which will involve actors' attribution of meaning—will gradually change" (ibid., p. 71). Ethical relativism in SSM is thereby enhanced by the missing dimension of purposes, in spite of the avowed standpoint against "determinists, dictators, or demagogues" (not to mention dogmatists) (ibid., p. 285). It could be instructive to compare the ethical relativism of this unproblematic reference to the logic of situations with other qualified attempts at the origins of moderns social systems theory (Churchman, 1961, p. 183ff.).

SSM authors have recently criticized the idea of purposeful systems, and have substituted (e.g. work process) activities for purposes (Checkland, 1988) while paradoxically referring to *purposeful* activities of work processes. Our suggestion (Docherty & Ivanov, 1990) is that the attempt to bypass the assumedly old-fashioned question of purposes, as also evident in later developments of soft systems methodology (Checkland, 1988; Checkland & Casar, 1986), is rather a symptom of the inadequacy of available theories in accounting for the political and ethical dimensions. It leads to paradoxical appeals to concepts such as purposeful activities, effective/efficacious/efficient systems or activities (Atkinson and Checkland, 1988, p. 714), culturally feasible or politically acceptable solutions, or agreed-accomodated purposeful activity systems.

SSM's criticism of systems teleology (Checkland, 1988) has been formulated in terms of assuming that this teleology implies depictive mirroring views of systems *out there in the world*, instead of implying a constructive process of model building that captures possible *perceptions of* the world. This charge against SSM appears to be related to other charges which have been made against dialectical systems theory for allegedly implying that an independent observer (analyst) is able to arrive at an "objective" knowledge of

the clients' *Weltanschauungen* (Oliga, 1989, p. 53). This criticism unfortunately, seems to be a straw-man argument. It may have been motivated by a misunderstanding that arises out of the SSM's unconscious unintended empirical-realistic bias in the dichotomies of idealism-empiricism (Churchman, 1979, p. 41, and chap. 12] or idealism-realism (Churchman, 1968, chap. 14) that are well recognized in the dialectical-pragmatist systems approach, particularly in the context of "Hegelian inquiring systems" (Churchman, 1971). This may be the reason why the critics themselves so often refer unproblematically to the "real world" without detailing the issue of perception as related to teleology. The dialectics between purposes and activities appears in fact to have been well acknowledged in the context of the criticized social systems teleology, even if the ultimate import of this dialectics could not be ascertained (Churchman, 1971, pp. 249ff.).

It may be the case that SSM looks for a new balance between political negotiation and ethics. But the whole ethical context may in fact be too complex to allow us to get away with its renaming and formal reduction to "enacting a social process in which humans seek to maintain or modify relationships according to applied standards which are themselves the product of the previous history of the relationship maintaining/modifying activity" (Checkland, 1988, p. 382). An equally problematic earlier version was the conception of social reality as being "the ever-changing outcome of the social process in which human beings, the product of their genetic inheritance and previous experiences, continuously negotiate and re-negotiate with others their perceptions and interpretations of the world outside themselves" (Checkland, 1981, pp. 283f.). Earlier analogous approaches admitted at least the challenging connection to the field of (natural) law (Ivanov, 1972, pp. 4.45f., 5.26f., 5.34, A11.10).

Under the label of apparently a-theoretical and non-purposeful multimedia structured discourses, opinion polls, negotiations, or decision support we will then find an unconscious revival of the sociologistic schools of undemanding conversational "interpersonal relations" (Lasch, 1977, pp. 135-138). that will be difficult to distinguish from misunderstandings and abuses of an "experiencing of relations...[that] is or is expected to be satisfying in itself" (Atkinson & Checkland, 1988, p. 13, quoting Geoffrey Vickers]. This recalls what elsewhere has been addressed as the "Don Juán syndrome" (Ivanov, 1986, pp. 135ff). Negotiations with co-workers on the basis of shared information space (Bannon & Schmidt, 1989, p.365f) and effective communication that allows both ambiguity and clarity (Robinson, 1989) then will not entail purposeful organization of actions under the legitimate constraints of institutions and traditions (Ivanov, 1986). They will rather express the fact that "the administration of justice gives way, in a therapeutic society, to a complicated process of negotiation....Justice is fixed by means of ...bargains among interested parties" (Lasch, 1977, p. 174). Such bargains could include certain kinds of negotiations between labor and capital (Bischofberger and Zaremba, 1985, cf. Ivanov, 1986, pp. 143ff.) that constitute the pride of influential Scandinavian approaches to systems development (Ehn, 1988).

SSM appears ultimately to be impaired theoretically by what may be important shortcomings besides the question of teleology versus activities considered above. SSM does not consider that activities consume resources. Resources, without theoretical support, are stretched to include even *information* resources. Activities, however, co-produce in an environment that cannot be defined except in terms of social actors like decision makers. Activities may then be correlates of *subsystems* in that they must be related to other subsystems in face of the problem of design separability. Because of this the above mentioned SSM information flow models must probably be structured in terms of morphological—functional—teleological classes (Churchman, 1971, chap. 3) that require an explicit relating of Weltanschauung to activities, and may

destroy the possibilities of the flow metaphor itself, and of the semantic information theory in terms of the theory of "speech acts" that was welcomed by SSM. Fundamental concepts like methods—models—systems are not penetrated in that they are often used as synonyms. Comparisons are made with so called real—world action (in a problem situation) in spite of the disclaimer that the real world can only be controversially perceived and negotiated but not described. Fundamental categories of social actors that are correlates of purposes, e.g. participants—designers—users—end users—(ever changing) organizational members, are used sometimes (Checkland, 1988) in an unclear intermingled way in the context of loosely structured negotiations. On other occasions the richness and nuances of social-political roles have been overtly recognized (Checkland, 1981, p. 294; Checkland, 1986) but it is this looseness of the structure of practical negotiations through an "open, participative debate" that may be at the heart of the SSM-problems. This is not to say that SSM cannot be or has not been helpful in many practical non controversial consultancy situations where political and ethical evaluations are not paramount, if one only knows how to determine what is not controversial. This is rather a challenge for its evaluation and improvement with a particular focus on basic concepts and primitives or categories.

CRITICAL SYSTEMS THINKING

It is at this point that recent critical systems thinking—CST related to early seminal work (Ulrich, 1983), may contribute by means of sharpened critical categories that attempt to counter the basic paradox of the ideal models of practical discourse that correspond roughly to SSM's negotiation towards wide agreement and consensus. It is a kind of attempt that has some features in common with the hypersystems approach mentioned below.

Before we go into CST let's remark that it seems to rely heavily on a "Kantian twist" of the influential critical tradition in philosophy. The formulations of CST-LST variants, however, have often been programmatic and somewhat lofty. It is, for instance, asserted (Midgley, 1989), that critical systems—CS— are emancipatory in the context of the researcher's ideology and praxis, and that the explicit focus is on the ideology of the individual researcher in determining method-ology and outcomes, implying also an extended understanding of praxis. It is a systemic idea of the relationship between theory and praxis in which the two are inseparable [as in pragmatism?]. It uses working methods derived from either the positivist of interpretive camps. *Positivist* techniques will reflect a *perception of agreement* on problematic areas, between all those who are perceived as being involved or affected. Ownership of the perception lies with the researcher. *Interpretive* techniques of interpersonal exploration will reflect a *percep-tion of disagreement* between people who are also perceived to have power relationships with each other, that will not obstruct this exploration. CS' conceptualization of situations as a series of questions with different contexts, results in "methodological partitioning" taking center stage in the debate, and providing a far richer source of information than if he had been working with just *one* methodological approach. CS represent the *second epistemological break* in systems science — the first having occurred when SSM moved away from positivist approaches toward interpretive ideas.

In the context of liberating systems theory— LST— (Flood, 1989, presents a bibliography], it has been proposed (Schechter, 1989) that LST developers must answer the question of (1) For whom? Consultants-customers-users-owners-clients, (2) To do what? Goals-activities, efficiency and effectiveness, viability and adaptation, learn-ing and development, all leading to liberation and social justice. The activities will be to support problem owners in their efforts to address their own problematic situations, i.e. in "management" activities that include creating fundamental social change, e.g. destroying oppressive social systems. It is remarked that there is a "serious gap" towards dimensions such as beauty, the aesthetic, the erotic, the spiritual, but this is surprisingly stated to be "worthy of a separate project". (Stolterman, 1989, instead, suggests that the aesthetic project should not be separate.)

In the context of "interpretive systemology" (Fuénmayor, 1989), it is remarked that the open-ing of possibilities brought up by interpretive discussion should be translated into a process of enlightenment which is rich in political con-sequences, depending upon the institutional preconditions for practical discourse among the general public. The striving is to gain a pluralist dialectical understanding of social phenomena, the unconcealment of that which normally is taken for granted. Surprisingly and paradoxically, however, this will be done without any disturbing pragmatic intention of the research, since that would be very likely to coincide with e.g. the interests of those in power, having the ultimate effect of stopping the unconcealing drive.

Let us now go back to a recent presentation of CST itself. In a summarizing account (Ulrich, 1987) it is remarked that ideal models of practi-cal discourse paradoxically presuppose what they are supposed to produce, namely, cogent rational argumentation—the ability and will of all participants to argue in a compelling way and to rely on nothing but the force of better argument. This paradoxical "utopia" seems to be a typical Kantian heritage as represented by the late developments of the tradition of critical social theory. It has certainly been the object of criticism that per se could have been devastating (Ottmann, 1982, is a valuable example]. It has, however, the merit of stimulating, as in CST, the design of conversation-negotiation systems, and the dealing with argumentation-negotiation break-offs. They are akin to what sometimes has also been called "conversation killing" (Levén

& Nordström, 1989) even if conversation killing may be conceptualized in vastly diverse terms (Churchman, 1971, pp. 104f, 119, 172f).

In order to support the identification of justification break-offs and the challenging of boundary judgments or normative presuppositions in systems design, CST groups twelve boundary questions in four classes, each comprising three kinds of categories: social roles, role-specific concerns, and key problems. The four classes ask for the normative OUGHT of (a) the sources of motivation: client, purpose—measure of performance, (b) sources of control: decision maker, components, environment, (c) sources of expertise: designer, expertise, guarantor, and (d) sources of legitimation: the affected people's witnesses, their emancipation, and their world views—Weltanschauung. The twelve OUGHT questions above are then to be contrasted with the pertaining answer to the corresponding IS question, laying open the normative basis of the planning system and its evaluation.

A paradoxically recursive question appears at this point in that the identified or postulated boundary OUGHT judgements remain dependent for their justification on a discursive process of consensus formation—a rational discourse—among the involved and the affected by the system. The normative content can be justified only through the voluntary [informed!] consent of all those who might be affected by the consequences. In order to foster reflection and the discursive dialogue process about the normative implications of systems designs, CST proposes that Kantian "polemical" employment of alternative boundary judgements be used to challenge the expert's own normative presuppositions. Affected citizens can secure for themselves an advantage of argumentation by imposing the burden of proof upon the involved expert who may then be embarrassed for being unable to prove the superiority of his assumed normative judgement. Such an approach will hopefully mediate the conflicting demands of democratic participation of all affected citizens,

and those of rational compelling argumentation on the part of the involved planners and experts.

It is then seen that CST attempts to "push" further the struggle for conversation-negotiation by fostering the rational conditions and presuppositions of this process. This is done in the same spirit as early critical-constructive approaches to development of computer applications which aimed at "allowing a gradual learning, self improvement of the information system" (Ivanov, 1972, pp. 5.37ff.)

It may be instructive to compare the above presentation of CST with the latest program for LST as formulated by the same author (Ulrich, 1989) on the basis of his earlier "critical heuristics". A critical solution to the problem of the antinomies of *pure reason* as envisaged by Kant is to seek to lay open the conditions that are presuppositions for our knowledge and understanding, reflecting on the fact that such conditions are never totally given to us through experience and logic. Critical heuristics attempts something analog in the domain of *practical (ethical) reason*. Rather than concentrating on the theoretical goal of demonstrating the in-principle possibility of "objective" generalizable justification of normative validity claims, it will focus on the task of helping practitioners achieve at least a critical solution. This is done by developing *methodological tools and models of rational argumentations,* and helping us in the everyday task of dealing critically with situations of *imperfect rationality.* Churchman's process of "unfolding" in the dialectical pragmatism of his systems approach fosters certainly an ethical discourse but it requires support in its "justification". Dialectical pragmatism is namely strong in driving the process of critical self-reflection but relatively weak in justifying its standard of critique, while the opposite happens in scientism. We need an alternative paradigm of rational criticism, one that would truly free itself from the unreflected presuppositions of scientism and thus might guide us toward a nonscientistic model of critical systems science. The key to such an alternative paradigm lies (for the espoused critical social theory of Habermas) in the *language-pragmatic* or *communication-theoretic* turn of practical philosophy. Its implications are a program of *communicative rationalization* of society. Functional rationalization by empirical-analytic science is then complemented and controlled by the dimension of communicative rationalization that is attained by the institutionalization of practical discourses. [Complementing, however, in this case may not imply integration but rather eclectic juxtaposition]. Such discourses seek to secure value transparency and consensus regarding disputed normative assumptions. This is done by testing the generalizability of the implied norms of action or, at least, the degree to which the propositions in question depend on non generalizable normative assumptions that benefit specific interests. The underlying utopia is the emancipatory idea of a *community of free and self-responsible citizens coming together and seeking to achieve consensus on matters of public (nonprivate) concern by means of argumentative, oppression-free will-formation and democratic majority vote.* [Pragmatism, however, denies the sharp separation of public and private]. The key strategies toward LST share a common inspiration by Kant's critical philosophy. The underlying concept of critique is one of emancipatory self-reflection with respect to the conditioned nature of our knowledge and understanding. The built-in emancipatory utopia of a community of free, communicatively competent and self-responsible citizens does not preclude a critically handled *methodological pluralism*, but it is supposed to preclude mere methodological eclecticism and ethical relativism. It gives a systematic place to moral judgement, as well as to the practice of democracy. So long one of the latest presentations of CST.

CST CRITICALLY REVISITED

Before going into details it may be noted that some of those who have criticized SSM's short-comings from a critical point of view (Jackson, 1989) tend to make altogether too unproblematic claims for the rescuing capability of the critical approach. It is, for instance, stated that the only possible justification for implementing the results of a soft systems study must be that results and implementation have been agreed upon after *a process of full and genuine participatory debate* among all the stakeholders involved or affected. Soft systems thinkers should therefore be critical of all social arrangements which prevent the kind of *open, participative debate* which is essential for the success of their approach, and which is the only justification for the results obtained. As for Stafford Beer's viable systems model—VSM—what is required is a *democratic milieu* in which to operate properly: the philosophy of SSM demands *communicative competence* as the foundation of the process it orchestrates. The goal is man's emancipation from slavery.

This is obviously all right, but the satisfactoriness of CST in these same respects is not clear and accountable unless one happens to subscribe already to Marxism and to Habermas. The tone of the "shoulds" is strongly ethical, not to say moralistic, but the ethical content of Marxism and of Marx-influenced schools of thought is, to say the least, problematic for many people (Carpi, 1989, pp. 60-62; Riley, 1983; Thompson and Held, 1982).

If we leave for the moment these more encompassing issues we may revert to the detailed text of the CST-presentation above. One initial problem that may be observed in the CST approach above is that the idea of "burden of proof" has a political power component that may be also an ethical one. What if those powerful agents who organize the negotiations and who ought to feel embarassed by polemical questions do *not* feel embarassed? What if they, instead, state for example that "We find that it is too expensive to bear the burden of proof that you want to impose on us" or "It is too expensive to elicit the voluntary consent by all those who might be affected by the system and its consequences", etc. This was recently acknowledged by CST (Flood and Ulrich, 1990, p. 24), but the proposed answers run into serious difficulties like the following one.

One aspect of this issue is what has been elsewhere called the problem of the "WHY—NOT?" strategy, or the strategy of easy questions and difficult answers (Ivanov, 1989). The more difficult the answers become because of easily formulated questions, and the lesser the number of knowledgeable potential answerers becomes, the easier will be to disrupt the possible wisdom that has been accumulated in history and tradition. This turns out to be *a fundamental debated shortcoming of Kant's thought in what concerns the ability to integrate religion with ethics, to integrate history and tradition with the Enlightenment ideal of an "invisible Church" that along an endless approximation converges at the infinity into a moral society or ethical community* (Ferretti, 1989, p. 49ff.; Scheler, 1988, p. 69f.). That may be one reason why CST refers to *logically* compelling polemical arguments (Ulrich, 1987, p. 281) but not to historically or *psychologically-emotionally* compelling complementary components such as amply considered, for example, in the pragmatist tradition (William James) or in the rhetorical tradition of antiquity. On the contrary, we may hear that a rational discourse or an ideal speech situation is the one that has the best chance to liberate us from the "historical compulsions" of the past, or to correct "false consciousness" and deliberately distorted forms of communication, or simply "psychological distortions" due to "individual bias", even if unfortunately it may fail to correct psychological (but not logical!), social and physical constraints that have been inherited (Bernstein, 1976, pp. 216f, as quoted by Gregory, 1989, p. 279; Hirschheim & Klein, 1989, pp. 1209ff.; Gregory 1989).

This appears to be the Kantian background of the ideal discourse situation where on the one hand certain kinds of WHY—NOT? are deemed necessary for the development of the invisible Church while the questions so posed undermine the legitimacy of the "expert" visible-Church positions that happen to have been conquered in the historical process of sweep-in and endless approximation. It all bears a flavour of "Singerian inquiring systems" in the context of the social systems theory that inspired CST (Churchman, 1971, pp. 194ff). It may also be the background for why teology, and in particular ecumenical efforts and so called natural teology (Mondin, 1988, pp. 435ff), may have something to teach us about the conditions for dialogue as well as for ideal and practical discourse where deep emotions and values beyond the cogency of logic are taken into account. All this may be relevant to the effort to oppose the Kantian attempt to dissociate knowing from the reality of the intelligible world, and to subordinate teology to ethics (ibid., p. 189, 191). It may also help to understand why the "social construction of reality" implied in the ideal discourse and possibly implemented in constructive computer applications may occasionally recall the charge that Kantian Protestant Puritan reason is a "system of external espionage" constrained by the laws of an external *logic* as opposed to an internal *psychology*. "The external technicism of production in Anglo-Saxon countries — as first programmatically conceptualized by Francis Bacon — stands in the most intimate spiritual continuity with this internal technicism of the ruling of impulses" (Scheler, 1957; Scheler, 1988, pp. 84f). It would be not surprising, then, to see the external technicism of the social construction of reality being promptly implemented in computer applications that put forth claims of having an ethical potentiality. They would be embodyments of an external technical logic that apparently revives prestige words like democracy and participation but works in practice mainly as systems of external espionage. Constructiveness, then, would be trying to obviate the shortcomings of our ethical conceptions, whether Kantian-Protestant or not.

This motivational background of the social construction of reality as appearing in CST ideal models of practical discourse and in the constructive design of computer applications may also illuminate the difficulty that these approaches have in grasping the meaning of the conflict-creating gaps between logic and emotions, between reason and power, and in bridging them. It will be recalled that Kant's critical conception of ethics may be regarded as having contributed to the split of its content on the one hand in logic, and on the other in psychology, akin to the split between law/duty/justice, and love (Niebuhr, 1986, p. 144; Wojtyla, 1980, p. 81f). It is therefore a little late, in the modern context of computer science conceptualized as an embodiment of logic, to reinstate ethics in logic by means of Kantian approaches. A superficial sense of togetherness—cooperation offered by ethical constructive communities may have mainly the effect of alleviating the tragic loneliness of the systems hero that has been conditioned by Kantian suicidal misunderstandings of the relations between "logic, ethics, and the ego" (Weininger, 1903, chap. 7), and has not been consoled by Marxian or Freudian theoretical complements.

The inability to face emotional, and therefore also political, conflict is evidenced by liberating consultants' often recurrent claim that "so many as possible" involved or affected people be swept participatorily into the constructive ideal discourse. At the same time, however, there is a certain resistance in sweeping in and accounting for the participation of any real "deadly opponent", as it has been recommended in early approaches to constructive quality-design of information systems (Ivanov, 1972, chaps. 4-5; Ivanov, 1957). In other words, "so many as possible" harmless dialogue partners or supporters, yes; but "deadly opponents", no. Deadly opponents, if not downright malevolent, are at least odd, illogical or crazy. In principle they should participate, especially in

jobs far away from the consultants' home-base, but that would be too dangerous or expensive in time and emotional efforts, considering the higher purposes of the assumedly noble endeavour: worldwide democracy through progressive marketing of profitable ideas. So goes often the argument, even in constructive quarters, when the matter boils down to concrete daily development work. The question here is whether CST, seen as a qualification of SSM, can do anything about it.

Participation risks to get reduced to constructive multimedia information technology that is supposed to streamline continuously structured opinion polls in organizations. It is to be hoped that they will profit at least of the lessons from survey techniques, interviewing and psychological testing techniques, or economic and social statistics: validity, reliability, and all the rest (Bauer, 1966; Morgenstern, 1963].

There are other ambitious currents of critical systems thinking which, in the Marxist-Frankfurt tradition, address some of the above issues. They tend, however, to reduce the ethical dimension to the social and political one. The power-ideology —PI— thinking (Oliga, 1990), for example, attempts to address the question of *origins* of the conflicts that SSM and constructive approaches seem to take for granted. These approaches are insightfully envisaged as mainly attempting to fix conflicts or differences in perceptions by means of so called continuous learning that is grounded on relatively simple means-ends schema. It does not even incorporate the pragmatist lessons on morphological-functional-teleological classes in the study of purposeful activities. The emergence of interests is seen as a function of discursive constructive processes aimed at reaching decisions and means of acting on the basis of such decisions (Mitroff, 1988). The PI-thinking notes that in so doing one forgets that those processes themselves, the ensuing decisions and possible actions, are all circumscribed by an initial set of unequal and differential conditions of the dominant social system: "Indeed, one wonders what, in the first place, the social struggles are all about in such uncritical conceptions of power" (Oliga, 1990, p. 38). The constructive-relativistic answer is, of course: "Well, let's then have an additional learning dialogue about *that*".

PI-thinking, however, is soon confronted with the question of the lack of a concept of truth (not of good). Critique presupposes criteria for distinguishing falsity from truth, where provisional truth cannot be equated to the result of constructive negotiations. If true interests cannot be distinguished from expressed preferences, prevailing power relations become the ultimate arbiters of true interests and truth.

It is interesting to note that this kind of problems enables an understanding of why critical theory needed to recur to psychoanalysis. "Related to this is the view that a theory of truth must somehow provide a conception of *reason* and *rational* action in terms of which certain *forms of consciousness* can be said to be ideological and judged to be *irrational*" (ibid., p. 39). Because critique seeks the true meaning of an ideology in relation to a historical context, it lacks the grounds on which to assert a priori criteria of its own truth, that must be considered as historically conditioned. "Because critique cannot develop formal a priori criteria of what counts as ideology, its strength lies not in a body of theoretical statements from which empirical states of affairs might be inferred but in a theory-dependent method that guides research into the *meaning of a form of consciousness by relating it to its contexts of interests and realities*. The philosophical implications are that for critical theory not to undermine its own claim to a *relative rationality* it must criticize a form of consciousness 'immanently'. That is, 'criticism gains its right to impute ideological meaning to a text insofar the text is irrational with regard to its own criteria of adequacy'" (Oliga, 1990, p. 40, my emphasis, quoting M. Warren about "Nietzsche's concept of ideology").

That was not clear. CST claims that the implications for systems theory are that these insights

can be read as an attempt to broaden the inquiry beyond the "structural" aspects of systems control. This is done by focusing on the *process* of organizational power relations and the functioning of ideologies, including the *significance of forms of subjective consciousness* or the *ideological formation of human subjectivities* (ibid., p. 46). To me this seems to be rather vague, but it is certainly akin to the spirit of the so called human action theory and action control theory, based on Soviet psychology, that have lately been adduced in the context of interactive computer systems and can be seen as an attempt to qualify constructiveness of computer applications (Nilsson, 1989).

In summary, it will be noted that PI-thinking senses some important limitations of SSM regarding the consideration of the nature of social control imposed upon a social system, seen as the "product of conscious actions of human beings as makers or victims of history". Nevertheless, the frequent reference to consciousness, forms of consciousness, reason, criteria of truth, rationality, relative rationality, and irrationality, points at psychological issues that once upon a time required the leaning of the Marxian-Kantian heritage on psychoanalysis. It will, in fact, be noted that the psychology of Marx's historical time was either hypertext-like associationistic-connectivistic, or mainly a Hegelian socialization or politization of the science and psychology of Kant, the first master of "forms of subjective consciousness" who still related to ethics and religion.

Today we need no more to keep ourselves circumscribed to this heritage. There is the option of Jungian analytical psychology, conditioned by Kant's phenomenology or phenomenalism, Nietzsche's cultural criticism, William James' pragmatism and by psychoanalysis itself. It is true that such conception of human (ir)rationality may be accused of implying that ideology is a "naturalistic", instead of being a "historical" phenomenon (Oliga, 1989, pp. 4ff.). By naturalistic it is then meant that it is essentially rooted in unhistorical forms or in the universal character or essence of

503

human nature, in the psychical structure of the individual, in the innate predispositions of the human mind, in the non-logical preconceptions or prenotions inherent in the human intellect, or in the unconscious impulses, instincts, and human passions and desires. By contrast, the historical conception views ideology as produced and re-produced through human practice, reflecting the historical development of men's social relations.

Disregarding the embarassing fact that PI itself apparently regards reason and rationality as rather "naturalistic", and has serious troubles with its so called criterion of truth, it must be noted that analytic psychology's conception of prenotions allows for both a historical-political dimension *and* an ethical-religious one (Odajnyk, 1976; Progoff, 1973), even if these aspects have not yet been studied as much as for psychoanalysis. If, under such premises, ideology is still to be regarded as naturalistic, so much worse for ideology.

There is a growing evidence that the answer to these questions must be conquered at the interface between philosophy and religion, in particular Christianity. The striving for progressive amplification of the ethical discursive community and the construction of growing social relations, family—nation—humanity, may well be conceptualized for instance in Christian terms in the context of studies of human action that bridge the Kantian disjunction between theoretical and practical reason (Blondel, 1973; Ferretti, 1989, p. 230f).

KANTIAN ETHICS REVISITED

It will be noted that at least of couple of systems theorists who have been very concerned with systems ethics (Churchman, 1979; Ulrich, 1983) have relied very heavily on a Kantian philosophical basis. SSM is phenomenologically influenced, and critical social theory was originally influenced by the Kantian revolution developed further through Hegel and Marx, and supported by psychoanalysis. It will also be noted that a recurrent persistent

theme in most, if not all attempts to develop a social systems approach has been the reliance on the basically *social* idea of "so many as possible", "communication", "emancipation", etc.

These key words relate mainly to Jürgen Habermas' critical social theory. It has been remarked (Ladmiral, 1984, p. 1130, my trans.) that there is undoubtedly a persistent deficit in the anthropology constructed by Habermas, which can be related to his moralism of Protestant inspiration. It marks a deviation in comparison with the first generation of the Frankfurt school in what concerns its treatment of the emotional sensory world, even if the theory of communicative action would make place for the idea of "bodily attraction". For the rest, Habermas seems to relativize progressively the psychoanalytic model, and to turn more and more towards the idea of "reconstruction". It indicates an ex-planation [mise à plat] of what is implicit, i.e. a systematic explanation of a pre-theoretical knowledge that is mastered only at the level of practice. The emancipatory interest and the utopic-prophetic dimensions of neo-marxism inherited from earlier critical theorists have come to be played down. Instead, Habermas seems to approximate further a rationalism that is inspired mainly by the tradition of Enlightenment, and a "realism" that emphasizes the growing convergence with Max Weber. In effect the exigence for emancipation has been confirmed to be of a rational nature, and to be conveniently rooted in the "structure of language". Above all, Habermas emprehends the reconstruction of the materialistic and historical genesis of reason, whose "procedural" nature is engendered by language itself, since "with the first pronounced phrase, a will of universal and unconstrained consensus expresses itself without ambiguity".

It seems to me that it is less attractive to subscribe to this account of Habermas' development that, for once, is less loaded with prestige words. In any case it is possible to reflect on the fact that critical social theory tends more towards abstract reason and towards language (as an obvious ethical tool?) than towards ethics itself which, as a concept, does not appear to have a central place in the discourse. The message has a somewhat prophetic tone, revealing a new participatory dialogue-prophecy that has not yet been implemented within the university itself, not even in the limited "laboratory" conditions of its own institutional setting. Habermas, in fact, apparently ridicularizes the "old mandarins" or at least questions the nineteenth century's belief in the totalizing power that the inner dynamics of research work would have (Habermas, 1990). The new mandarins of the participatory prophecy, however, apparently do not realize that the university, on the basis of reason as substitute for religion, can be seen as one of the most extensive and intensive historical attempts to start implementing an ideal discourse in society as a whole. The inner dynamics of research corresponded to the inner dynamics of reason. In all its social complexity the university would serve as a forerunner and model of a progressively "democratic" society based on reason. (Betz, 1971, pp. 123f.; Simpson 1951).

Prophecies recall the concern for the ethical dimension. Nevertheless it has been difficult to clarify its theoretical status, and whether it was subsumed under the social-political dimension, and if so, on what grounds.

Let's recall possible questions about Kantian ethical thinking. I am not a professional philosopher, even if philosophical pragmatism hints at the necessity of everybody attempting to be one. In any case the following lines will be pragmatically oriented towards supporting one main intuition, in spite of Kantian reason having been "canonized" by the philosophical community. It is the hypothesis that both SSM and CST share some basic assumptions about the problematic subsumption of ethics under politics. It is also the hypothesis that this is not good, and that it leads us into a kind of vicious circle, in that it tempts systems scientists to develop themselves and their trade by pulling up themselves, as it were, by the hair.

Since Kant's work is extremely complex it would be prohibitive, especially for non professional philosophers, to risk to get caught up and seduced by plunging into it. To search for possible shortcomings in Kantian thinking by following the threads of Kant's own original work (Kant, 1989) implies a temptation to espouse his own concealed presuppositions incurring furthermore in the WHY-NOT?-problem mentioned above. It implies also a superficial non-hermeneutical view of "what Kant actually meant". Because of this it seems convenient to complete occasional readings of and about Kant, as his thought has been considered relevant in the systems context (Churchman, 1971, chap. 6; Churchman, 1979, chap. 6; Ulrich 1983], with an outline of the criticism that historically has been directed against Kant's work.

It may be particularly informative to choose a summary of this criticism as it has been surveyed by somebody who nevertheless *defends* Kant's ethical positions (Carpi, 1989). The opposition to Kant, the launcher of modern critical philosophy, came from several diverse quarters as represented by the key schools of idealism (G.W.F. Hegel, Karl Marx, Benedetto Croce), phenomenology (Georg Simmel, Max Scheler), empiricism and neopositivism (Betrand Russell, Hans Kelsen), realism (Jacques Maritain), and others (J.G. Hamann, J.G. Herder, F.W.J. Schelling). In spite of much emphasis on critical philosophy and much reliance on Kant we have heard very little about this criticism of critique, with the possible exception of the wholesale acceptance of Marxist criticism and wholesale dismissal of the ignored but conjectured positivist-empiricist criticism.

A study of the opposition to Kant is, however, strongly recommended to all of us who wish to advance systems thinking in the political-ethical aspects, and in close contact with the formal sciences that are embodied in the ongoing so called computer revolution. Now, back to the announced questions.

1) Kant formulates many fundamental and sharp distinctions that are very controversial, and have very definite consequences in defining "gaps" that consequently are hopefully to be bridged by (paradoxically Kantian?) systems approaches. But: "distinctions are the weapons of the elite"? (Churchman, 1971, p. 270). Or, is it lack of religiosity that is the main weapon? (Buber, 1958, p. 93). Some such distinctions that have become "classical" and are apparently implied in CST are, for instance: theoretical-pure and practical-ethical reason, ethics and religion, gnoseology and ontology, reason and will, noumenon-spontaneity-freedom and phenomenon-causality-necessity, virtue and happiness. Do we understand why we are willing to accept these distinctions?

2) Kantian thought emphasizes the notion of *science* seen as universal and necessary knowledge (of "nature"). By so doing it may have unintendedly favored misunderstandings leading to prestige-inflation of natural and formal science, such as in scientism, not the least in the context of systems thinking. Which should be the place of "lesser sciences" like psychology and anthropology, compared with logic and mathematics, in critical thinking? What place would CST grant to "a metaphysical psychology to un-Locke our ailing world" that develops the meaning of all those perceptions that allegedly contribute to false consciousness? (Griffin, 1989).

3) In opposition to Hegelian thought which tends to believe that all political institutions have a moral value, fostering a reduction of ethics to politics, Kantian thought finds that both law and politics must be judged by ethics. Such an ethics, however, was conceived in terms of a concept of freedom (cf. liberation) that is metaphysical and relates to the person independently upon social-political institutions. This is what differentiates Kantian thought and original revisionistic social-democratic thought from so called liberation philosophies (Hegel, Marx, Storicism). Such liberation philosophies have been accused to deny transcendence. They "divinize" man and, in spite of all emphasis on communicative competence, close definitively the door to discussions about theology and religion. In fact I have not seen these words being mentioned in the CST literature, and CST has still to develop the meaning of liberation.

4) Kantian ethics calls for an appreciation of moral imperatives that could enable an *ethical conversation*, when other imperatives as contained in holy books have been "explained away". It is, for instance, possible to conceive of a computer program that not only works along the Kantian categories of systems definitions, but also counters every fundamental proposal for action in an "activity system" with the question of whether one would like to see the maxim of his action enpowered to become an universal law. Or rather: "Would you act as if the maxim of your proposed action had to be erected by your will to a universal law of nature [in its broadest sense of "form"]?" Furthermore it will be observed that Kantian thought considers several duties that may also be seen as enabling ethical conversation, i.e. fostering both "future generations" and "conversation pushing" as opposed to conversation killing. These duties are dintinguished as being duties *towards oneself,* (e.g. concerning suicide and lies), and *towards others* (like charity, gratitude, and sympathy). Should such important aspects of an ideal speech situation be considered in future computerized CST-models of hypersystems? Or will this suggestion be accused of Kantian liberalism, or for attempting a reversal towards early critical theory's reliance on psychoanalysis and naturalistic thought? What about C.G.

Jung's analytical psychology instead of Freudian psychoanalysis for taking care of feeling and perception? (Griffin, 1989). Does Kantian "empiricization" of psychology and anthropology, as contrasted to the universalization of reason and logic, contribute to CST's and to the computer revolution's emphasis on the latter to the detriment of the former, as well as contribute to SSM's poverty in the treatment of "perceptions" of the world? Why are such words as charity, gratitude, love seldom if ever mentioned? And finally:

5) Does the (unavoidable?) failure to implement (self-doomed?) Kantian wishful thinking on "transcendence" of ethics into religion throw us into the arms of political ethics, an ethics in the form of constructive-ideal speech situation, akin to a vague concept of "divinized" Democracy that exposes us to demagogical technicalities and Faustian bargains in the computer-network revolution?

In summary: while CST refers unproblematically to "an untenable pre-Kantian understanding of rationality" (Flood and Ulrich, 1990, p. 8), others (Greif, 1988, in the introduction, p. 6f, 13) recall that thinkers like A. N. Whitehead sought to return to pre-Kantian modes of thought, circumventing the Kantian critique by correcting some errors in pre-Kantian philosophy: both Whitehead and Jung are postmodern in that they both reject tenets of the modern worldview (Weltanschauung), yet without returning to a premodern approach. They retain the formal commitment of modernity to rational empiricism, but they reject some of the substantive presuppositions of modernity.

INFORMATION TECHNOLOGY AND HYPERSYSTEMS

In the search for promising development of the ideas above one way could be to explore computer implementation of the systems concept that has been proposed in terms of the idea of co-constructive hypersystem (Forsgren & Ivanov, 1989). The core of the hypersystem idea would be to keep track, by means of adequate "pointers" or links between simple or composite nodes of hypertext computer software, of the relationships between various affected social actors' instantiations of the "primitives" (basic social systems concepts) during the process of solution or learning. The question about which social actors or agents will be thus swept-in, and in what kind of communication or self-reflection, may be discussed in terms of error-accuracy (Ivanov, 1972; Ivanov, 1987), of the classical issue of "power and ideology" (Oliga, 1990), or "metaphysical psychology" (Griffin, 1989), but also in terms of ethics and religion.

The primitives mentioned above could be the categories of the original dialectical social systems approach (Churchman, 1979, pp. 79ff.): (1) Clients, purposes, measures of performance, (2) Decision makers, components, environment, (3) Planners, implementation, guarantor, and (4) System philosophers, enemies of the systems approach, significance. They could be also CST's categories reviewed above, or SSM's so called CATWOE-categories: (1) Customers, (2) Actors, (3) Transformation processes, (4) Weltanschauung, (5) Ownership of the system, (6) Environment. At an apparent level of meta-systems it has also been suggested that various paradigms of information systems development be described and interpreted in terms of the categories: (1) Key actors (the "who" part of the story), (2) Narrative (the "what", or the key activities), (3) Plot ("why" did the action take place, akin to causes and purposes), (4) Assumptions (the fundamental beliefs or Weltanschauung, or epistemological-ontological assumptions) (Hirschheim & Klein, 1989). Several authors have recently liked to create their own variants of the original categories, without affording to ground their categorizations in basic considerations of controversies in philosophy and in scientific method. The difference, of course, is that certain sets of systems categories (notably Churchman's) establish demanding and commiting *relations* between categories, fostering ethical disciplined thinking. So, for instance, one would not talk, as in SSM, about "environment" without a commitment about who is/should be the decision-maker, and which are the clients' purposes.

Reference is often made to a learning process. Such a process is rather a dynamic continuous learning-follow-up of the particular systems problem. There will be communication, opinion polls, dialogue-negotiation, conversation or discussion, but they will be mainly or initially about certain primitives (primitive concepts) and their relations, a certain model or structure, with particular functions or goals, and they will strive to involve at least certain particular actors or role bearers whose absence would hide the problems of power and of emotions (Ivanov, 1972; Ivanov, 1986).

The question is whether the hypersystem idea in the outlines of its particular computer implementation in terms of co-constructive computer applications (Forsgren, 1988; Forsgren, 1989; Forsgren & Ivanov, 1989) or other similar approaches (Mitroff, 1990) will be able to meet social-political and ethical realities that have been exemplified in other comparable contexts (Docherty & Ivanov 1990; Flood, 1989; Gibson & Ludl, 1988; Ivanovm 1986; Ivanov, 1986; Ivanov, 1987; Oliga, 1990). The so called learning process that is based on the dogma that learning is good, but where neither the meaning of (good) learning nor purposes or constraints are discussed in order to build the ground for some political-ethical evaluation, opens the doors for endless expensive consulting, negotiating, innovating, and purchasing of computer equipment that works as a communication-negotiation "shell" (Bond & Gasser, 1988; Greif, 1988). If we welcome this new technology, what about the old knowledge? (Ivanov, 1988). The consultant may be akin to "the analyst as facilitator" in the paradigm of social relativism (Hirschheim & Klein, 1989). Working

for the clients or problem owners may be just an unintended contribution to make our world more frenetically commercial as one grinds out a vast array of products and services to assuage the hungry appetites of world citizens, wherever they may live in the new global democratic economy (Böhler, 1970). The social construction of reality may eventually run into the SSM negotiation process mentioned above, into a search for wide agreements and consensual activity models. Such constructiveness can easily turn out to be the expression of a basically *technical* idea, a generalization of the very idea of technology which, either supported by constructive computer applications or not, claims to incorporate the human sciences (Dahlbom, 1990, p. 25). It may therefore easily appeal to social engineers who believe that they will build up revolutionary social ideas into technical equipment. Therefore the challenge may be to turn the analyst-as-facilitator in the spirit of social relativism either into the analyst-as-labor-partisan in the paradigm of radical structuralism or, (preferably?), in into the analyst-as-emancipator or the analyst-as-social-therapist in the paradigm of neohumanism (Hirschheim and Klein, 1989). That might be all right, if one only knew a good meaning of these terms, and no other alternatives were available.

The success of any computer implementations will then probably depend to a great extent upon the soundness and the implementability of the proposed categories. They, in turn, rely on the soundness of the Kantian, neomarxist and pragmatist political-ethical conceptions, which have been objects of an extensive criticism that is apparently ignored in our contexts and in recent developments of constructive social systems theory. In this context one may wonder whether the forms of poetry or of dramatic dialogue have any relation to categories, and whether particular categories in a Kantian sense, including logic, place any fundamental restrictions on the human power of expression in its dependence upon content. The rhetoric tradition of argumentation (Fisher, 1987) may inspire some alternative approaches (Hahn and Jarke, 1988, is just an attempt). Compare, about song: "The dimension disclosed by the tones can certainly be called 'inner life', but it is not the inner life of the subject as opposed to the object; it is not the inner world of the self but of the world, the inner life of things. This is precisely why the singer experiences inner life as something he shares with the world, not as something that sets him apart from it....Music prevents the world from being entirely transformed into language, from becoming nothing but object, and prevents man from being nothing but subject." (Göranzon et al., 1988, quoting the musicologist and philosopher Victor Zuckerkandl).

In the best case it may be found out that the importance of our technical implementation efforts in hypersystems is akin to the importance of Robert Pirsig's motorcycle in fostering critical reflection on philosophical issues, like the purpose or meaning of a trip, that per se may improve future system thinking (Pirsig, 1974). In the worst case it may be found out that the importance of the efforts "has less to do with their direct usefulness to organizational decision making and more to do with their symbolic value", promoting an image of leading-edge consultancy and facilitating the marketing of other products (Gibson & Ludl, 1988, p. 282f.). Even in this latter case there are possibilities for legitimate meaningful research in regarding the computer as an image in a psychological Rorschach-projective test (Turkle, 1980) or as a mathematical-psychological construct (Ivanov, 1989).

CONCLUSION

My growing conviction is that provisional answers to many of the above questions must be sought along the developments of dialectical pragmatism and dialectical systems theory (Churchman, 1971; Churchman, 1979). Critical systems thinking (Ulrich, 1983) may help us to sharpen the political and ethical dimensions of systems thinking, but only if pushed to the interface between philosophical ethics, analytical psychology, and reconquered reinterpreted religions. I am thinking, in particular to the religion closest at home, i.e. Christianity, not because it should be the most "attractive" but because it most likely conceals our deepest presuppositions and has been the most studied in the context of science (Blumenberg, 1985; Buckley, 1987; Ferré, 1987; Lewis, 1988; Riley, 1986).

Computer applications actualize the basic shortcomings of Kantian-Marxian normative thought regarding the gaps between formal science, human science, ethics, and religious thought. Such applications might in the future try to incorporate some of the suggestions in this chapter by "imposing" interactively to the computer users ethically loaded questions that, if possible, should also be aesthetically, e.g. poetically, attractive. Such questions, to be interactively related to each other and to various agents' answers, could deal, for instance, with systems primitives or categories, boundary judgements, categorical imperatives. Instead of working mainly as systems for external espionage, for consensus and negotiation, or for marketing, the system of questions would be especially designed to awaken the constructive ethical concerns of those who succeed in getting involved in the technical equipment. We would, at the same time, be on guard against the "technological imperative" at least as much as we do against ethical imperatives. It may be the case that anything that is worth doing in these respects must be done without any technical equipment.

REFERENCES

Atkinson, C. J., & Checkland, P. B. (1988). Extending the metaphor 'system'. *Human Relations*, *41*(10), 709–725. doi:10.1177/001872678804101001

Bannon, L., & Schmidt, K. (1989, January). *CSCW: Four characters in search of a context.* In First European Conference on Computer-Supported Cooperative Work (pp. 358-372), Gatwick, London.

Bauer, R. A. (Ed.). (1966). *Social indicators.* Cambridge, MA: The MIT Press.

Bernstein, R. J. (1976). *The restructuring of social and political theory.* Oxford, UK: Basil Blackwell.

Betz, F. (1971). On the management of inquiry. *Management Science.* 18(4, Dec., part 1), B-117-B-133.

Bischofberger, E., & Zaremba, M. (1985). *Arbete före kapital.* Stockholm, SE: Brevskolan.

Blondel, M. (1973). *L'action: Essai d'une critique de la vie et d'une science de la pratique* (Orig. published 1893). Paris, FR: Presses Universitaires de France.

Blumenberg, H. (1985). *The legitimacy of the modern age (Originally published as Die legitimität der Neuzeit. Frankfurt: Suhrkamp Verlag, 1966, 1976).* Cambridge, MA: MIT Press.

Böhler, E. (1970). Conscience in economic life . In Zbinden, H. (Eds.), *Conscience* (pp. 43–77). Evanston, IL: Northwestern University Press.

Bond, A. H., & Gasser, L. (Eds.). (1988). *Distributed artificial intelligence.* San Mateo, CA: Morgan Kaufman.

Buber, M. (1958). *Ich und Du* (Special ed., first ed. 1923. Swedish trans. Jag och Du, Stockholm: Bonniers, 1962. Page refs. to Sw. trans.), Stockholm, SE: Bonniers.

Buckley, M. J. (1987). *At the origins of modern atheism.* New Haven/London, CT/UK: Yale University Press.

Carpi, O. (1989). *Kant: L'etica della ragione.* Rimini, IT: Panozzo.

Checkland, P. B. (1981). *Systems thinking, systems practice.* New York, NY: Wiley.

Checkland, P. B. (1986). *The politics of practice. Paper for the IIASA Int. Roundtable The Art and Science of Systems Practice.* Laxenburg, Austria: International Institute of Applied Systems Analysis.

Checkland, P. B. (1988). Churchman's "anatomy of system teleology" revisited. *Systems Practice,* 1(4), 377–384. doi:10.1007/BF01066580

Checkland, P. B. (1988). Information systems and systems thinking: Time to unite? *International Journal of Information Management,* 8(4), 239–248. doi:10.1016/0268-4012(88)90031-X

Checkland, P. B., & Casar, A. (1986). Vicker's concept of an appreciative system: A systemic account. *Journal of Applied Systems Analysis,* 13, 3–17.

Checkland, P. B., & Griffin, R. (1970). Information systems: A systems view. *Journal of Systems Engineering,* 1(2), 29–42.

Churchman, C. W. (1961). *Prediction and optimal decision: Philosophical issues of a science of values.* Englewood Cliffs, NJ: Prentice-Hall.

Churchman, C. W. (1968). *Challenge to reason.* New York, NY: MacGraw-Hill.

Churchman, C. W. (1968). *The systems approach* (References are to pages of the 2nd ed., 1979). New York, NY: Delta

Churchman, C. W. (1971). *The design of inquiring systems: Basic principles of systems and organization.* New York, NY: Basic Books.

Churchman, C. W. (1979). *The systems approach and its enemies.* New York, NY: Basic Books.

Dahlbom, B. (1990). *The idea that reality is socially constructed (Manuscript, 12 Jan. 1990.).* University of Gothenburg, Dept. of Philosophy.

Docherty, P., & Ivanov, K. (1990, 18-21 June). Computer support of decisions in a social-political environment: A case study." Prepared for the IFIP TC 8.3 *Conference on Environments for Supporting Decision Processes*, Budapest, Hungary. Page refs to rev. edition as report UMADP-WPIPCS 26.90, Univ. of Umeå, Institute of Information Processing.

Ehn, P. (1988). *Work-oriented design of computer artifacts*. (Doctoral dissertation). University of Umeå, Arbetslivscentrum and Almqvist & Wiksell International. Umeå-Stockholm.

Ferré, F. (1987). *Language, logic, and God* (Reprint of the 1961 ed.). Chicago/London: IL/UK: University of Chicago Press.

Ferretti, G. (1989). La filosofia verso la religione: Itinerari dello spiritualismo e del neotomismo. In Ciancio, Ferretti, Pastore & Perone (Eds.), *lotta con l'angelo*: *La filosofia degli ultimi due secoli di fronte al Cristianesimo*. Torino, IT: Società Editrice Internazionale SEI.

Ferretti, G. (1989). La ragione ai confini della trascendenza cristiana. In Ciancio, Ferretti, Pastore & Perone (Eds.), *lotta con l'angelo*: *La filosofia degli ultimi due secoli di fronte al Cristianesimo*. Torino, IT: Società Editrice Internazionale SEI.

Fisher, W. R. (1987). Technical logic, rhetorical logic, and narrative rationality. Argumentation: *An International*. [Dordrecht]. *Journal. on Reasoning*, *1*(1), 3–21.

Flood, R. L. (1989). Liberating systems theory: A summary and literature review. Proceedings of the ISSS Int. Society for the Systems Sciences, *33rd Annual Conference*: *Vol.2,* Edinburgh, Scotland (With a bibliography of 34 entries.)

Flood, R. L., & Ulrich, W. (1990). Testament to conversations on critical systems: Thinking between two systems practitioners. *Systems Practice*, *3*(1), 7–29. doi:10.1007/BF01062819

Forsgren, O. (1988). *Samskapande datortillämpningar [Constructive computer applications]* (Doctoral diss., Report UMADP-RRIPCS-3.88.). University of Umeå, Inst. of Information Processing.

Forsgren, O. (1989). The first "co": A prototype of a learning co-constructor." Proceedings of the ISSS Int. Society for the Systems Sciences, *33rd Annual Conference, Vol.1*, Edinburgh, Scotland.

Forsgren, O., & Ivanov, K. (1989, April). *From hypertext to hypersystem*. Prepared for the EMCSR 90, Tenth European Meeting on Cybernetics and Systems Research, Vienna, Austria. 1990. Umeå University, Inst. of Information Processing.

Fuénmayor, R. (1989). Interpretive systemology: A critical approach to interpretive systems thinking. Proceedings of the ISSS Int. Society for the Systems Sciences, *33rd Annual Conference*: *Vol.2,* Edinburgh, Scotland.

Gibson, D. V., & Ludl, E. J. (1988). Group decision support systems and organizational context. In R.M. Lee, A.M. Cosh & P. Migliarese (Eds.), *Organizational decision support systems*. Amsterdam, NL: North-Holland.

Göranzon, B., Florin, M., & Sällström, P. (1988). Dialogue. *AI & Society*, *2*(4), 279–286. doi:10.1007/BF01891362

Gregory, W. J. (1989). Critical theory and critical systems heuristics: The history and development of an emancipatory systems approach to social change. Proceedings of the ISSS Int. Society for the Systems Sciences, *33rd Annual Conference*: *Vol.2,* Edinburgh, Scotland.

Greif, I. (Ed.). (1988). *Computer supported cooperative work: A book of readings*. San Mateo, CA: Morgan Kaufman.

Griffin, D. R. (Ed.). (1989). *Archetypal process: Self and divine in Whitehead, Jung, and Hillman*. Evanston, Ill: Northwestern University Press.

Griffin, D. R. (1989). A metaphysical psychology to un-Locke our ailing world . In David, D. R. (Ed.), *Archetypal process: Self and divine in Whitehead, Jung, and Hillman* (pp. 239–250). Evanston, Ill: Northwestern University Press.

Habermas, J. (1990). *Die Idee der Universität-Lernprozesse. Eine Art Schadensabwicklung. 1987 Suhrkamp. Frankfurt a.M. Swedish trans.* Umeå, Sweden: K. Nilsson, Umeå University, Inst. of Information Processing.

Hahn, U., & Jarke, M. (1988). A multi-agent reasoning model for negotiation support. Organizational decision support systems. In R.M. Lee, A.M. Cosh & P. Migliarese (Eds.), *Organizational decision support systems.* Amsterdam, NL: North-Holland.

Hirschheim, R., & Klein, H. K. (1989). Four paradigms of information systems development. *CACM, 32*(10), 1199–1216.

Ivanov, K. (1972). *Quality-control of information: On the concept of accuracy of information in data banks and in management information systems* (Doctoral thesis.) The University of Stockholm and The Royal Institute of Technology, Stockholm, Sweden.

Ivanov, K. (1986). *Systemutveckling och rättssäkerhet: Om statsförvaltningens datorisering och de långsiktiga konsekvenserna för enskilda och företag [Systems development and rule of law].* Stockholm, SE: SAF:s Förlag.

Ivanov, K. (1987). Public records and trade-offs. Legal Informatics . In Tuominen, P. (Ed.), *The Inst. for Nordic Law at the University of Lapland. Lapland, FI: Rovaniemi.*

Ivanov, K. (1987). Rule of law in information systems research: The role of ethics in knowledge-building procedures, especially in the updating of inference networks. In P. Järvinen (Ed.), *Proceedings of the Tenth Information Systems Research Seminar in Scandinavia,* Tampere-Vaskivesi, FI: University of Tampere.

Ivanov, K. (1988). Expert-support systems: The new technology and the old knowledge. *Systems Research, 5*(2), 293–100.

Ivanov, K. (1989). Computer applications and organizational disease. The well-being of organizations . In Churchman, C. W. (Ed.), *The well-being of organizations* (pp. 283–312). Salinas, CA: Intersystems.

Ivanov, K. (1989). Is the AI society a symptom of a cultural crisis? Proceedings of the ISSS Int. Society for the Systems Sciences, *33rd Annual Conference, Vol. 3.* Edinburgh, Scotland.

Jackson, M. C. (1989). The critical kernel in modern systems thinking. Proceedings of the ISSS Int. Society for the Systems Sciences, *33rd Annual Conference, Vol. 2.* Edinburgh, Scotland.

Kant, I. (1989). *Scritti di filosofia della religione* (Trans. essays from the German, by G. Riconda). Milan, IT: Mursia.

Ladmiral, J. R. (1984). J. Habermas. In D. Huisman (Ed.), *Dictionnaire des philosophes.* Paris, FR: Presses Universitaires de France.

Langefors, B., & Sundgren, B. (1975). *Information systems architecture.* New York, NY: Petrocelli/Charter.

Lasch, C. (1977). *Haven in a heartless world: The family besieged.* New York, NY: Basic Books.

Levén, P., & Nordström, T. (1989, March). Socially responsive systems. Presented at the conference Support, society and culture: Mutual uses of cybernetics and science, *The Int. Federation for Cybernetics*, Amsterdam. Report UMADP-WPIPCS 22.89, Umeå university, Inst. of Information Processing, Umeå, Sweden.

Lewis, C. S. (1988). *Christian reflections* (Walter Hooper, Ed. First published in 1967). Glasgow, UK: Collins.

Lundquist, T., & Huston, M. M. (1990). Information rich environments for continuous organic development—CODE. *Manuscript. Submitted to the J. of Applied Systems Analysis.* Luleå Institute of Technology and Texas Women's University.

Midgley, G. (1989). Critical systems: The theory and practice of partitioning methodologies. Proceedings of the ISSS Int. Society for the Systems Sciences, *33rd Annual Conference, Vol.2,* Edinburgh, Scotland.

Mitroff, I. I. (1988, Winter). Crisis management: Cutting through the confusion. *Sloan Management Review,* 15–20.

Mitroff, I. I. (1990). *Can appropriate technology help in the battle against crises? Computer software for crisis management. Submitted for publication to Security Management Review.* University of Southern California, Graduate School of Business, Center for Crisis Management.

Mondin, B. (1988). *Scienze umane e teologia.* Roma, IT: Urbaniana University Press.

Morgenstern, O. (1963). *On the accuracy of economic observations.* Princeton, NJ: Princeton University Press.

Niebuhr, R. (1986). *The essential Reinhold Niebuhr: Selected essays and addresses* (Ed. and intr. by R. McAfee Brown). New Haven/London, CI/UK: Yale University Press.

Nilsson, K. (1989). Designing for creativity: Toward a theoretical basis for the design of interactive information systems. *Proceedings of the 12th IRIS Conference - Information Systems Research in Scandinavia,* Skagen, Denmark. Aalborg University, Inst. of Electronic Systems. Aalborg. Report UMADP—WPIPCS 20:89, Umeå university, Inst. of Information Processing. Also as report UMADP-RRIPCS-8.89, University of Umeå, Inst. of Information Processing.

Odajnyk, V. W. (1976). *Jung and politics: The political and social ideas of C.G. Jung.* New York, NY: Harper & Row.

Oliga, J. C. (1989). Ideology and systems emancipation. School of Accountancy and Commerce, Nanyang Technological Institute, Singapore. ISSS Int. Society for the Systems Sciences, *33rd Annual Conference,* Edinburgh, Scotland, 2-7 July 1989.

Oliga, J. C. (1990). Power-ideology matrix in social systems control. *Systems Practice, 3*(1), 31–49. doi:10.1007/BF01062820

Ottmann, H. (1982). Cognitive interests and self-reflection . In Thompson, J. B., & Held, D. (Eds.), *Habermas: Critical debates* (pp. 79–97). London, UK: Macmillan.

Pirsig, R. (1974). *Zen and the art of motorcycle maintenance.* New York, NY: Bantam Books.

Progoff, I. (1973). *Jung's psychology and its social meaning* (Original ed., 1953), Garden City, NY: Anchor Press/Doubleday.

Riley, P. (1983). Marx and morality: A reply to Richard Miller . In Pennock, J. R., & Chapman, J. W. (Eds.), *Marxism* (pp. 33–53). New York/London, NY/UK: New York University Press.

Riley, P. (1986). *The general will before Rousseau: The transformation of the divine into the civic.* Princeton, NJ: Princeton University Press.

Robinson, M. (1989, March). Double level languages and cooperative working. Support, society and culture: Mutual uses of cybernetics and science. *The International Federation for Cybernetics*. Amsterdam, The Netherlands.

Schechter, D. (1989). For whom and to do what? Questions for a liberating systems theory. Proceedings of the ISSS Int. Society for the Systems Sciences, *33rd Annual Conference, Vol.2*, Edinburgh, Scotland.

Scheler, M. (1957). *Der Bourgeois und die religiöse Mächte* (*Vol. 3*). Bern-München, DE: Gesammelte Werke.

Scheler, M. (1988). *Lo spirito del capitalismo; e altri saggi* (Trans. collection of essays from German orig.). Guida, IT: Napoli.

Simpson, G. (1951). Science as morality. *Philosophy of Science*, *18*(2), 132–143. doi:10.1086/287139

Stolterman, E. (1989, August). System design methods as creativity "killers". *Proceedings of the 12th IRIS Conference - Information Systems Research in Scandinavia*, Skagen, Denmark. Aalborg University, Inst. of Electronic Systems. Aalborg. Report UMADP—WPIPCS 20:89, Umeå university, Inst. of Information Processing.

Thompson, J. B., & Held, D. (Eds.). (1982). *Habermas: Critical debates*. London, UK: Macmillan.

Turkle, S. (1980). Computers as Rorschah. *Society*, *17*(2), 15–24. doi:10.1007/BF02700055

Ulrich, W. (1983). *Critical heuristic of social planning*. Bern, CH: Paul Haupt.

Ulrich, W. (1987). Critical heuristics of social systems design. *European Journal of Operational Research*, *31*(3), 276–283. doi:10.1016/0377-2217(87)90036-1

Ulrich, W. (1989). Liberating systems theory: Four key strategies. Proceedings of the ISSS Int. Society for the Systems Sciences, *33rd Annual Conference, Vol. 2*, Edinburgh, Scotland.

Weininger, O. (1903). *Geschlecht und Character: Eine prinzipielle Untersuchung* ((Page refs. to Ital. trans. *Sesso e carattere*. Milano: Feltrinelli/Bocca, 1978). Wien/Leipzig, AU: Braumüller.

Wojtyla, K. (1980). *I fondamenti dell'ordine etico*. Città del Vaticano, IT: Libreria Editrice Vaticana.

NOTE

This article is a revised version. The original article was first published in 1991 in the *Journal of Applied Systems Analysis*.

Section 8
Trans-Disciplinary Studies

Chapter 41

Engaged Scholars, Thoughtful Practitioners:
The Interdependence of Academics and Practitioners in User-Centered Design and Usability

Susan M. Dray
Usability Professionals' Association & Dray & Associates, Inc., USA

ABSTRACT

The current schism between academia and practice exists for many understandable reasons, mostly to do with the very different incentives and life realities that each face. However, it represents a dangerous threat to the legitimacy of the field of user-centered design. This article first discusses the fundamental differences between academics and practitioners, and then suggests a variety of ways that we each can work to break down the barriers so that together we can advance the field.

INTRODUCTION

Our field faces threats to its legitimacy which we will have trouble dealing with if we allow there to continue to be a split between academia and practice. Many academics face obstacles in the way of more "relevant" research that would be more meaningful to practitioners, and practitioners tend to see academic research as not relevant to them in reinforcing their professional identity, skills, and legitimacy as the organizational experts in user research. Meanwhile, many practitioners feel they are threatened by a perceived commoditization and co-opting of user-centered design (UCD) and

user experience (UX) work. These two trends or tendencies are rarely mentioned together. How, they are related, and how we address these issues will have a significant bearing on whether our field will continue to advance or whether it will wither.

In this essay I first explore the different dynamics of the worlds of academia and product development and how these differences affect the nature of the work we do. Then, I show why the world of practice needs an infusion of academic rigor that can only come from changes in the nature of academic research and the adoption of a more academic style of critical thinking in the world of practice.

In fairness, I fully acknowledge that the following analysis makes generalizations for which

DOI: 10.4018/978-1-60960-057-0.ch041

there are many exceptions. There are certainly academics who have made major contributions to practice and are committed to relevance and there are practitioners who are thoughtful and rigorous in their thinking. There are also people in academia whose roles are structured so that they have some similarities to practitioner roles, and conversely people in industry who do function more like academics (such as people in industrial R & D groups). But one way or another, I maintain that even most exceptional people have to contend somehow with the problematic dynamics I describe below.

ACADEMIA VERSUS PRACTICE

As an applied field, we are not alone in experiencing a tension between academia and the world of applied practice. For example, in medicine, doctors need the fundamental knowledge that comes from research such as that on, say, evolving anti-biotic resistance in microbes due to over-prescription of antibiotics. However that research may provide little guidance for them on how to deal with the things like anxious patients who are demanding antibiotics, the pressures toward "productivity" and the fact it takes less time to write the prescription than to explain to the patient why that is not a good idea, the concerns about having to respond to a complaint filed with customer services by a dissatisfied patient, fear of liability if they do not provide an active treatment, etc. How they actually act will depend on a complex combination of rewards and incentives, past history, social dynamics of the clinic, and experience.

In our own field of usability and UCD, the tension or gap between academia and practice has a long history. The challenge of the relationship between academics and practitioners is a perennial issue at our sister organization, SIGCHI, where there have major effort to ensure that the CHI conference meets the needs of academics and practitioners, but it is still difficult to bring the

academic communities together collaboratively. Indeed, UPA emerged partly from a community of professionals who felt the need for a practitioner conference distinct from CHI.

As Avi Parush (2006) points out, many practitioners engaged in design, evaluation and/or implementation of technology feel that academic research is not useful to their day-to-day life in companies. He quotes an unnamed practitioner as saying:

"There are very few, if any, research articles published in scientific and academic journals that can be utilized effectively in the practice of HCI design" (p. 61)

In this journal, Caroline Jarrett (2007) has described how to write research papers that appeal to practitioners. In general, practitioners look for and need research when they encounter a knotty problem that they need to solve or when they are approaching a new situation and are looking for guidance. As Jarrett points out, for practitioners, "research reading generally has to have a business purpose." (p.1) . She gives a number of excellent suggestions to researchers to help them to explain their research in more practitioner-friendly ways, and this is certainly a good start, but for many practitioners, research in general is still rarely "relevant" to them. This suggests that the problem is not only with how research is written, but also in what they say and whether the pre-occupations of researchers are helpful to practitioners.

INCENTIVES AND PRESSURES IN THE ACADEMIC CONTEXT

Why is it so hard for so many academics to do research that practitioners will consider "relevant"? The answers come from understanding the incentives and dynamics that influence the career paths of academics.

In academia, the most basic measures of success are typically scholarly publishing and obtaining grants. It is a truism that faculty must "publish or perish." Anything that increases success in obtaining grants and producing publications in refereed publications increases career success. The quickest and easiest types of papers to write tend also to be the most narrow – and unfortunately, these are also the least likely to be considered "relevant" and "useful" by practitioners. Operationalizing sticky real-world problems is difficult and messy. Conducting rigorous research in the real world is extremely challenging logistically. It is also much easier to get funding and to be productive if you buy into an existing research tradition and extend it through a modest variation on what has been done before. These are the social pressures towards "normal science" that Thomas Kuhn discussed in his classic, *The Structure of Scientific Revolutions* (1996)

When academic research takes the form of experimentation, academics are likely to focus on isolating variables to discover the abstract relationships among them, using artificial simulations. Research that involves proof of concept for new forms of human-computer interaction usually is also carried out in an artificial context and with a very narrow focus. A noted researcher acknowledges the pressures toward a narrow and artificial focus in his blog, writing that:

"The reviewers [for the CHI conference which is considered by academics to be among the most prestigious venues for publication] simply do not value the difficulty of building real systems and how hard controlled studies are to run on real systems for real tasks. This is in contrast with how easy it is to build new interaction techniques and then to run tight, controlled studies on these new techniques with small, artificial tasks." (Landay, 2009)

The goal of tenure adds to the pressures that skew the choice of research topics. The emphasis on volume of publications is especially true for young faculty who, in order to achieve tenure, must churn out papers and get grants. Therefore, the pressure to do research that is tightly focused and relatively easier to publish can push young faculty to do less "relevant" research. This becomes a habit over the 7 years leading to tenure decision, and as we all know, longstanding habits are very hard to break. This same dynamic influences graduate students who may be interested in academic careers, since there is also increasing competition for academic posts in our field. Also, graduate student research must be circumscribed so it is feasible for the student to graduate in a reasonable time.

Most academics will spend much of their careers investigating a particular problem area, with increasing depth and focus – and some would say narrowness – over time. In addition, one's colleagues at other universities reinforce this specialization by partnering on publications, presentations at conferences, and grant proposals. It is almost unheard of for an academic to switch to an entirely different field – e.g., to move into Humanities from Computer Science – and such a switch would require significant re-tooling, additional education and an excellent rationale to be taken seriously.

In none of the above do I mean that academics are lazy or avoiding complex problems. Rather, they are simply following the natural incentives and shared interests of their community. Work driven by theoretical interest in the nature and influence of particular variables naturally pushes for narrowness of focus, isolation of variables through controlling confounds. Operationalizations of independent and dependent variables can only capture particular manifestations, and in the choice of operationalization the emphasis is on ease of measurement.

However, increasingly, students are finding that jobs in academia are scarce. Many academic programs now have terminal Masters Degrees or industry-focused programs that are intended to prepare students for life as practitioners. While some of these include teaching by practitioners, most do not, although many include internships or other industry experience as part of the program.

While academic research may not be seen as "relevant", it is usually rigorous. Academics deepen their understanding by applying rigorous analysis and thought to decoding underlying principles and developing theories to explain their findings. This focus on rigor is a hallmark of the best academics. They know their research will be exposed to criticism by specialists from their own discipline. While this may promote caution in the topics taken on, it has the virtue of incentivizing methodological soundness and critique.

INCENTIVES AND PRESSURES IN THE WORLD OF PRACTICE

The messy world of practice is replete with interesting, "relevant," and knotty problems and challenges. In contrast to isolating variables to study them for their own sake, every product development decision reflects the intersection of and tradeoffs among huge numbers of variables. The challenges of product development in the business world are thus inherently extremely difficult to address rigorously. Furthermore, research in the business world takes place in a culture where there are unfortunately many disincentives to the rigorous and critical thinking at which our academic colleagues excel.

Rather than "publish or perish" as the guiding principle, practitioners live by the mantra "produce or perish." The goal of their work is the integration of user-centered information into the development of products or services so these will be useful and usable. Therefore, the information practitioners seek about users, context and usability are all intended to support those products or services, rather than to satisfy an intellectual interest. Personal career success depends on the perception that you make a valuable contribution

to helping products progress through the pipeline, and that your contribution increases the chance of commercial success—preferably that you are indispensable to this. Deepening knowledge of the relationships among abstract variables is of little use in itself, and does not increase your standing. Focusing on these without tying the dialogue back to concrete product-development decisions can interfere with career success by making you seem too "academic" which is an epithet in many corporate settings.

The context of product development has a tendency to suppress skepticism and critical thinking. This is not to say that product ideas can't be questioned, but there are always issues that the team feels it has already made and moved on from. Questioning these can lead to be seen as obstructionistic. When the consensus begins to move in a certain direction, there can be intense pressure on practitioners to be silent about their qualms. Practitioners often must demonstrate enthusiasm at least about the basic product concept. Cognitive dissonance that inhibits questioning grows the more that has already been invested in the product.

There are many examples of products where everyone other than the people on that team wonder how on earth the product has gotten so far down the pipeline, because of "obvious" flaws. For example, we once did ethnographic research on consumer behavior for a team working on a battery-powered machine to take care of odors in the refrigerator. It was extremely obvious early on that this concept made no sense to consumers because it was solving a "problem" that consumers did not perceive that they had. Either they did not perceive odors in their fridge (even when we did), or they had other, cheaper solutions (e.g., a box of baking soda) that worked fine for them. They saw no reason to buy a costly machine requiring batteries to do the job that the baking soda did just fine. The team, however, was passionate that this product WAS terrific and maintained that we had simply chosen the wrong people to visit. It was only a year and many millions of dollars later that the product was finally cancelled, due, it would seem, to "lack of a market" – something we had told them a year earlier.

Practitioners live in highly pressurized settings where decisions have to be made quickly, often without as much information, time for planning methodology, or for analysis as would be ideal. The time to think deeply about findings and interpretation is greatly compressed. In fact, taking time in this way is a negative because the focus is on speed, not deep understanding. As a colleague of ours at a large company quipped, "Close enough is close enough." Time is measured in hours or days, sometimes in weeks, rarely in months or quarters, and almost never in years. In these circumstances, practitioners must find ways to gather, analyze, and present data quickly, efficiently, cogently, and compellingly in ways that "work" in their organization.

One manifestation of the time pressure is the need to present "topline" findings before doing a full analysis of data, often within one or two days of completing the data collection. This is a symptom of an environment where the audience is also under tremendous time pressure and cannot take the time to wrestle with nuances. Someone has to take responsibility to be prescriptive and make strong recommendations, and putting too much emphasis on describing nuances can seem like hedging.

The implications of the fact that the audience for practitioners is NOT composed of specialists in UX and UCD cannot be over-emphasized. UCD professionals in companies work in a highly cross-disciplinary environment. This has many benefits, such as fostering cross-disciplinary learning, but it also presents many challenges. Colleagues in other, related disciplines are also trying to have influence with decision makers, and experience the same pressures toward prescriptive simplification. Success can be determined not by who has the "best" methodology or analysis, but by who best understands the concerns of the decision

makers and communicates in the most concise, compelling, memorable, and simple prescriptive ways. People talk of the "PowerPoint culture" that focuses on form and brevity rather than content and rationale. Career success is heavily influenced by the judgment of people outside of the profession. UCD practitioners cannot assume that these people know of or are interested in the fine points of methodology that allow well-trained UCD people to make a contribution that is distinct from that of other people who bring in data about users and customers or recommend aspects of product strategy based on beliefs or information about people (marketing, sales people and field representatives, customer support people, etc.).

Another implication of working in a cross-functional environment is that it is important to maintain collegial relationships and choose one's battles. This means that there is a tendency to defer to others rather than confronting underlying paradigm differences or critique each other's methods.

Another factor that comes into play is the relative fluidity of the UX practitioner's career. Rarely does someone stay in the same job or even the same specialty for an entire career the way an academic typically does. People often move around – both within a company, between companies. and to new areas of specialty. For instance, in the 9 years of my own career prior to becoming a consultant, I worked in 2 different companies and did Human Factors research for the military, analyzed user manuals, conducted ethnographic research in a variety of settings, worked in the corporate IT department, developed ergonomic guidelines, created a cross-functional methodology to incorporate organizational factors in the design and implementation of internal IT systems, developed user interfaces of thermostats, control systems and other products (consumer products, industrial controls, forms, online applications, etc), did user testing, ran focus groups, managed a systems training group, created and ran a usability lab, did organizational development consulting and finally, directed an integrated UX team. In addition, some of these were individual contributor roles while others were management roles at a variety of levels from first-line supervisor, to middle manager, to executive. There was a thread there, of course, but each new job was radically different from the last and almost every transition was with a new group and required that I learn new skills. This is hardly unusual in our field. As a result, practitioners often are in roles for which they lack formal training, and must rely instead on learning on-the-job.

WHY DOES THIS MATTER?

I am not articulating the differences between academia and industry because I believe mutual understanding is a good thing (although it is). Rather, it is because I think that bridging the gulf is crucial to the future of our field, because it will strengthen the quality of both academic and applied work, and help us deal with trends in the market that can dilute our contribution.

For example, just as UX practitioners are moving around in their careers, so too are people moving into UX and UCD roles from many other areas. Sometimes they have had at least some formal preparation in the form of a course or seminar, but often, they have not. Instead, just like the moving UX pro, they learn by doing. This means that, while there is the benefit of new perspectives being infused into UX, there is also the risk that the field will lose its distinct identity.

Related to this is the commoditization and co-opting of UX by other disciplines. In the past, usability could lay claim to a professional identity based on a particular set of practices or methodology—usability testing. Of course we have more to offer than just critiquing of other people's designs, including applying our research skills to deeper levels of product definition. However, as usability has moved out of the usability lab and the usability profession has expanded its mandate to look not just at usability (narrowly

defined as the ease of accomplishing a defined goal) but also at defining what those user goals are, understanding the context of use, looking at perceived value and emotion, its overlap with other disciplines has increased.

For instance, marketing people in companies and in agencies are increasingly selling usability and other user experience research services, or sometimes co-opting them under other names, but with a not-surprising tendency for them to resemble the methods that come out of the intellectual culture of marketing research, with its heavy reliance on self report. Marketing groups typically have larger budgets, and hold management's ear in a way that HCI people often don't. This creates the risk of decreasing the perceived value and distinctiveness of the usability profession. Competition for the turf of introducing understanding of users into product development means that professions and vendors are under pressure to differentiate themselves. This leads to proliferation of branded research methods being sold on the basis of their intuitive appeal to decision makers who may well not have the knowledge or inclination to carefully weigh their validity. This environment promotes a proliferation of methodological fads, and of pundits fighting for visibility by making provocative, memorable, and simplistic pronouncements that undermine disciplined and nuanced thinking. These trends raise the question of what is our profession's intellectual core. What defines usability and UX as a body of knowledge and a profession at all? If we do not have a strong and constantly updated conceptual base, why is our opinion any more valid than anyone else's? How do we justify our particular approaches to observation, collection of data, analysis, or understanding of users a basis grounded in research?

Part of the answer is an infusion into industry of the type of critical thinking associated with academia, and of practice that is backed up by sound research. By critical thinking I mean being willing to ask things like the following and being prepared to evaluate the answers:

- Course of action X implies assumptions Y and Z. How do we know them to be true, and what are the risks if we are wrong?
- Is this a data-based decision or a philosophy-based decision? Is there data that could help?
- What is the nature of the data? How was it collected? Was the methodology sound?
- Whether the data is qualitative or quantitative, was it analyzed rigorously or merely impressionistically and taken at face value?
- Does the data really support this interpretation or allow us to draw this conclusion? Have we ruled out other reasonable and important alternative interpretations? What other research would do so?

For academic work in our field to play this role of supporting practice, it needs to focus on things that matter to practitioners, but it is not only the practitioners who will benefit. Such "engaged scholars" will find a wealth of extremely interesting, perplexing, and complex problems to research – great grist for those who want to make a difference in the world. Researchers who get too locked into "normal science" elaboration of existing research paradigms will miss out on new research questions of interest that will be raised by the evolution of new technologies. Here are some other areas that come to mind:

- Studies of methodological validity under realistic conditions
- Empirical assessments of common product development practices and approaches
- A paradigm for case studies that lets us draw generalizable lessons from rich experiences in the trenches
- Once we have this, we need to test some of these generalizations

- Longitudinal studies of the process and dynamics of product adoption and the behavior change that goes with it, since many business decisions are based on "intuitive" psychological theories of how masses of people change behavior to adopt technology

Academics benefit in practical ways from closer connections with the commercial world as well. In some companies, there are opportunities for academics to partner with practitioners to do research that would not be possible by either side alone but that can answer real needs for information. Practitioners can sometimes help provide access to key populations of interest, and can help leverage corporate resources to provide funding for certain types of research activities. In addition, deeper understanding within academia of the world of practice can help academics do a better job of preparing their students to function as professionals in the face of the pressures they will encounter as they increasingly go into jobs in industry rather than in academia. Alliances can help provide students with real-life experience that makes them more marketable in tough economic times, and can also provide industry with thoughtful practitioners who understand both the rigor of academia and the pace of industry. In short, both academics and practitioners stand to benefit from strengthening the bridge between academia and practice.

THE ROLE OF PROFESSIONAL ASSOCIATIONS

The challenge of the relationship between academics and practitioners is a perennial issue and there are no easy answers to the friction between us. However, given the importance of the issue, it is critical that we find ways to work collaboratively together. How can we accomplish this? Just as professional associations bring together people from a variety of disciplines and geographic locales, I believe that professional associations also have an opportunity to demonstrate how academics and practitioners can work together to create the kinds of win-win situations that provide us all with the benefits that our differences can bring. In professional groups, we can find a forum to discuss potential approaches – both for individuals and for our larger profession – and can debate, tweak, challenge, and find ways to integrate solutions so they can really work. Professional associations also can draw upon their memberships across the world for different approaches that work in different places, to give ideas and share wisdom.

The more we truly are engaged scholars and thoughtful practitioners, the larger the positive impact our field can have. I think that is worth aiming for.

REFERENCES

Jarrett, C. (2007). Problems and Joys of Reading Research Papers for Practitioner Purposes. *Journal of Usability Studies*, *3*(1), 1–6.

Kuhn, T. (1996). *The Structure of Scientific Revolutions*. Chicago, IL: University of Chicago Press.

Landay, J. (2009). I Give Up on CHI/UIST. Blog entry, November 7, 2009. Available at: http://dubfuture.blogspot.com/2009/11/i-give-up-on-chiuist.html (checked November 10, 2009)

Parush, A. (2006). Practice and Research in Human Computer Interaction: Towards a common ground. *Interaction*, *13*(6), 61–62. doi:10.1145/1167948.1167994

NOTE

©UPA, *Journal of Usability Studies*, Volume 5, Issue 1, pp. 1-7; Dray, Susan M. (2009); "Engaged Scholars, Thoughtful Practitioners: The Interdependence of Academics and Practitioners in User-Centered Design and Usability. Reprinted with permission.

Chapter 42
Habits of the Mind:
Challenges for Multidisciplinary Engagement

Myra H. Strober
Stanford University, USA

ABSTRACT

The extraordinary complexity of knowledge in today's world creates a paradox. On the one hand, its sheer volume and intricacy demand disciplinary specialization, even sub-specialization; innovative research or scholarship increasingly requires immersion in the details of one's disciplinary dialogue. On the other hand, that very immersion can limit innovation. Disciplinary specialization inhibits faculty from broadening their intellectual horizons - considering questions of importance outside their discipline, learning other methods for answering these questions and pondering the possible significance of other disciplines' findings for their own work. This article seeks to understand more fully the factors that enhance and impede cross-disciplinary conversations and the possible longer-term effects of those conversations. Based on 46 interviews with a sample of seminar participants, it examines the experiences of faculty members who ventured (voluntarily) into multidisciplinary waters and its implications for the organization of disciplines and universities.

INTRODUCTION

The complexity of knowledge in the contemporary world creates a paradox. On the one hand its sheer volume and intricacy demand disciplinary specialization, even subspecialization, because innovative research or scholarship increasingly requires immersion in the details of disciplinary dialogue. On the other hand that very immersion can limit innovation. Disciplinary specialization inhibits faculty from broadening their intellectual horizons: for example, by considering questions of importance outside their discipline, learning other methods for answering these questions, and pondering the possible significance of other disciplines' findings for their own work.

To push the frontiers of knowledge forward and create knowledge that helps to solve the problems

DOI: 10.4018/978-1-60960-057-0.ch042

of the world, we need not only discovery within disciplines, but also integration across them (Boyer 1990; Weingart 2000). Yet few faculties engage in research or teaching outside of their own field. The academic reward structure for hiring, promotion, salary, grants, and prizes provides powerful incentives to specialize narrowly and few opportunities to integrate knowledge from other fields of study (National Academy of Sciences, National Academy of Engineering, and Institute of Medicine 2005). Also, the jargon and shorthand in which members of disciplines often speak and write, and the profound difference in cultures across disciplines, make cross-disciplinary forays arduous. While faculty say they see the value in multidisciplinary scholarship (Boyer 1990) organizational, economic, and cultural barriers keep most from pursuing cross- disciplinary work. Most faculty also discourage cross-disciplinarity in graduate education, ensuring that the next generation of scholars will also find it difficult to break out of disciplinary confines.

Foundations are particularly interested in fostering interdisciplinarity. For example, in a recent issue of the Chronicle of Higher Education, Vartan Gregorian (2004), the President of the Carnegie Foundation and former President of Brown University and the New York Public Library, wrote:

We must reform higher education to reconstruct the unity and value of knowledge... The complexity of the world requires us to have a better understanding of the relationships and connections between all fields that intersect and overlap—economics and sociology, law and psychology, business and history, physics and medicine, anthropology and political science. (Gregorian 2004 B12)

A recent report by the National Institute of Medicine on the National Institutes of Health (NIH) argues for more integration within the sciences and between the sciences and behavioral and social sciences: "[S]ome parts of the scientific frontier require... the mobilization of interdisciplinary research teams... Increasingly, investigators will need to integrate knowledge... And greater prominence must be given to research in the behavioral and social sciences" (National Institute of Medicine 2003: 51–52).

Similarly, the Keck Foundation, in creating the Futures Initiative in 2003, argued: "Training individuals who are conversant in ideas and languages of other fields is central to the continued march of scientific progress in the 21st century" (National Academy of Sciences, National Academy of Engineering, and Institute of Medicine 2005: x).

One of the reasons why foundations, government agencies, and leaders of institutions of higher education would like to see faculty move in the direction of more multi- disciplinary work is that they believe there are more opportunities for creativity and breakthroughs at the intersections of disciplines.

In 2000, Atlantic Philanthropic Services (now Atlantic Philanthropies) provided two-year grants to three leading American research universities (to maintain their anonymity, I call them Washington, Adams, and Jefferson) to create broad (not problem-specific) seminars for the purpose of encouraging dialogue across disciplines. The decision to concentrate the grants in research universities was made because multi- disciplinary dialogue among faculty members is perhaps most difficult to achieve at research universities, where there is considerable pressure to publish in one's own discipline, where cross-disciplinary teaching is seldom valued, and where the sheer size of the institution prevents faculty from easily meeting colleagues in other fields.

There were six seminars in all, each meeting once a week for one academic year. In 2002 I received a grant from the Ford Foundation to study those seminars in order to understand more fully the factors that enhance and impede cross-disciplinary conversations and the possible longer-term effects of those conversations. Based on 46 inter- views with a sample of seminar participants, this article examines the experiences of faculty members who ventured, voluntarily, into multidisciplinary waters.

Given the importance now being placed on creating the conditions that foster cross- disciplinary exchange, my study focuses upon the following questions: What were the difficulties and successes in the scholarly discussions? How did faculty use knowledge from other disciplines? How did barriers to cross-disciplinary integration of knowledge operate? What kinds of intellectual and affective connections did participants make in their own minds and in relationships with colleagues? Also, with respect to these seminars potentially serving as models for other institutions, I considered the following: What can other institutions interested in developing more cross-disciplinary exchange on their campuses learn from the seminars at Washington, Adams, and Jefferson?

DEFINING TERMS

Before proceeding to an overview of the results of this work (the full study will be published as a book), it is important to define the terms used. The dictionary defines a discipline as a branch of knowledge or learning (from the Latin disciplus, a learner). However, for the purpose of distinguishing between disciplinarity and interdisciplinarity, this definition is too ecumenical; interdisciplinary fields are also branches of knowledge or learning.

Using knowledge criteria alone (e.g., the existence of a distinctive theory, paradigm, body of information, methodology, or scholarly journal) to decide whether a branch of knowledge is a discipline, subdiscipline, or multidiscipline is a hopeless task. Based on such criteria, would clinical psychology be deemed a discipline or subdiscipline? Is statistics a discipline, or a branch of mathematics? Is women's studies a discipline? Knowledge criteria alone do not result in agreement among academics on these matters, in part

because knowledge changes even while particular debates rage and in part because participants in the debate are not impartial spectators.

Having a field or subfield declared a discipline has numerous advantages; branches of knowledge that are deemed disciplines are rewarded by being made departments at academic institutions. As such, they receive protection for both their disciples and their knowledge base—theories, methods, content, and procedures for ascertaining "truth" (Lohmann 2003). They obtain financial resources and are permitted to hire, promote, and give tenure to faculty based on their own collective scholarly preferences. They are permitted to develop curricula and offer courses, train undergraduates, and certify them as majors—and, most importantly for the perpetuation of their field, select, train, examine, and certify doctoral students.

Using departmental status as a proxy for discipline is akin to using revealed preference theory in economics. Economists point out that in studying the behavior of consumers, it is difficult to know, a priori, their underlying tastes and preferences. However, once consumers make a purchase, their behavior reveals those underlying tastes and preferences. Similarly, although academics cannot agree in the abstract which branches of knowledge are disciplines, by observing their collective behavior in making what they think are disciplines into departments, the definition of disciplines is revealed.

Using revealed preference theory in this way makes it obvious that the definition of a discipline has political as well as epistemological dimensions. The history of women's studies, for example, indicates that because of its low status, and perhaps because of gender discrimination, its practitioners have had a difficult time convincing academic authorities to give it departmental status (Boxer 1998, 2000). Moreover, the political and epistemological dimensions of achieving disciplinary status are not independent. Rather, it is likely that the vast majority of academic institutions' refusal to create women's studies departments, which forced women's studies scholars to achieve tenure and promotion within the disciplines in which they were trained and hired, had a negative effect on the development of cross-disciplinary or interdisciplinary theories in women's studies (Messer-Davidow 2002).

It is important for disciplinary status that there are many departments with the same designation. Having departmental status in only a few institutions (as is the case for women's studies now) is insufficient for disciplinary status, because new doctorates have an insufficient number of institutions at which to seek jobs. In other words, for a field to be a discipline there must be both "identity and exchange" (Turner 2000: 51). The identity comes from achieving departmental status. The exchange comes from a market for new doctorates. Indeed, Turner defines disciplines as "cartels that organize markets for the production and employment of students by excluding those job- seekers who are not products of the cartel" (Turner 2000: 51).

Although in some respects this definition of disciplinarity is unsatisfactory, because it relies so heavily on political as opposed to purely epistemological considerations, it is in fact useful for understanding interdisciplinarity. One of the hallmarks of interdisciplinarity is the difficulty that scholars or researchers who have been trained and socialized in one field experience when they attempt to talk to or work with scholars trained and socialized in other fields. By defining disciplines as synonymous with departments, we ensure that faculty or other doctorates who wear a particular disciplinary label have all been socialized in pretty much the same way. This is not to say, necessarily, that the socialization "took" equally well for all, but to be assured that their initiations and on-going customs and culture are simultaneously quite different from those of other scholars and quite similar to those with the same disciplinary label.

The terms cross-disciplinary, multidisciplinary, interdisciplinary, and transdisciplinary are often used interchangeably, but they have different meanings. To confuse the matter further, different authors use the terms differently (e.g., Gibbons et al. 1994: 4–6).

I define cross-disciplinary and multidisciplinary synonymously; both mean that two or more disciplines are being used, but that they are not integrated. I use the term inter- disciplinary when there is an integration of some aspects of the disciplines (method, theory, content, perspectives), but where, despite the integration, the separate disciplinary perspectives are still discernible. I use the term transdisciplinary where there has been such a degree of integration of disciplines that tracing distinct disciplinary traits is difficult.

HABITS OF THE MIND

Each of the three institutions I studied took the cross-disciplinary seminars in a different direction. Washington confined the seminar to the social sciences. In the first year, discussions began with Open the Social Sciences, the Gulbenkian Commission's plea for greater integration across the social sciences (1996). In the second year, they narrowed their focus further and selected a group of social scientists to examine the concept of inequality. Adams University sought to bridge the two cultures defined by C. P. Snow (1959/1998) and selected a group of humanists and scientists to discuss science studies in the first year and ethics in the second. Jefferson had the most varied faculty mix of all—social scientists, scientists, humanists, and artists (including a composer, a painter, and an actress/director). In both years, the discussions began with a consideration of Edward O. Wilson's book, Consilience: The Unity of Knowledge (1999).

The structure and leadership of the seminars also varied. At Washington, each seminar was run by a (different) prestigious senior faculty member (one a political scientist and one an economist) and the university's top administrators participated actively in both years. At Adams, the seminars were run in both years by a non-tenure-line humanities faculty member who had had experience with interdisciplinary programs at another university. No administrators participated in Adams' seminars. At Jefferson, the first year seminar was run by a senior faculty member in the humanities who had been a dean; a prestigious emeritus faculty member, also in the humanities, led the second year seminar. In both years, both former and current administrators participated.

Each seminar was to have a participant-observer, who was to take notes and circulate them periodically to participants and, in abbreviated form, to Atlantic. At Washington and Jefferson, the same faculty member served as participant-observer for both years. However, at Adams, faculty decided they did not want their proceedings recorded and so there was no note-taker and the only person who participated in the seminars for both years was the leader.

At Washington and Adams, administrators at both the university and departmental levels were intent upon improving their institutions' positions in various national prestige rankings. They viewed the seminars as opportunities not only to promote cross-disciplinary dialogue, but to fulfill other purposes as well: to provide "perks" for key faculty who were considering relocating, as a means for employing a new faculty member's significant other, as a means for developing specific new interdisciplinary programs, and as a venue for discussing departmental reorganizations. Jefferson, on the other hand, while less prestigious than Washington or Adams, was more relaxed about its national ranking and saw the seminars as primarily an intellectual activity, an opportunity to get its intellectual "stars" better acquainted with one another, and a venue for incubating new cross-disciplinary courses. As a result, the participants, leaders, and topics of the Washington and Adams seminars were chosen to fulfill multiple goals. Jefferson, on the other hand, chose seminar participants, leaders, and topics solely for the purpose of creating intel-

lectual excitement and cross-fertilization. These two different models had a profound influence on the proceedings of the seminars and the seminars' effects on participants.

What I seek to do here is to show some of the difficulties seminar participants experienced in overcoming their habits of mind in order to engage in cross-disciplinary dialogues. As will become evident, habits of mind include not only disciplinary content, but also styles of thinking, styles of presenting, and styles of questioning. It is important to recognize from the outset, however, that the snippets I provide here present a very incomplete accounting of these three seminars. The reader should not conclude from this material that the seminars were unsuccessful. On the contrary, there were numerous positive outcomes and almost all of the participants said they would sign up again. I am merely trying here to highlight some of the difficult issues for this special edition.

PERSPECTIVES AND EXPERIENCES

Adams

The seminars at Adams were more contentious than those at either Washington or Jefferson. Some of this was due to the absence of any administrators, who, at the other universities, tended to foster a decided atmosphere of civility; some was due to the fact that the woman who led the seminars for both years was not a tenure-line faculty member. She had been chosen in part because she had a background in interdisciplinarity (indeed she was more knowledgeable about interdisciplinarity as a subject of study than any leader or participant in any of the six seminars) and in part because the university needed to find a position for her in order to be able to hire her partner, whom they were actively courting. She had no say in the topics of the seminar or in the selection of seminar participants; these were chosen by a dean and a senior central administrator.

In the seminar leader's words, in the first year the participants fought the science wars, and in the second year, the culture wars. The seminar "blew up" in the first year, when an economist was critiquing readings and a presentation in what he reported to me was his "usual style"; a young woman of color (a post-doctoral fellow in religion) called him insensitive and chastised him. The economist's response was to leave the seminar and refuse to return, despite some modest efforts by the seminar leader to change his mind. Here is an account of the "fight" from a psychologist in the seminar:

[The economist] did a very serious critique of game theory, straight on... And then, the post-doc... thought it was too harsh or too mean or not communal... not the kind of thing a Quaker would have done or something. I don't know... But... [the economist] was claiming that his... style... that's what [economists] were trained to do... And this person from religion, where you wouldn't do that, was appalled, shocked that someone would say, "That's a stupid idea." I don't think... [the economist] ever said, "That's a stupid idea."... He said, "That argument doesn't flow," or something like that, and then he pursued it. And that's the game... [But] that wasn't the game for this woman, and she laid into him for doing it in a very, I felt, a very aggressive way... I think it came out of her views of the world. I think it was her religious background of having to build a community of people who work together... I don't think she was a Quaker, but [she] kind of [thought] we should come to consensus.

In the second year, nobody left the seminar, but the two key antagonists in the culture wars, a senior white man in analytic philosophy and a young woman of color in English, battled all year. Here is the philosopher's reply to my question about the meaning that the seminar had for him:

Well, I had thought that the culture wars were over and that everybody had seen that the emperor of postmodernism was naked, but I was completely mistaken. My colleagues in English and cultural studies and literature, who participated in the seminar, cast me into despair about the level of intellectual seriousness and willingness to be intelligible. Their concern with mere fashionability, and sheer ignorance of these disciplines... I was just appalled.

"Sheer ignorance of other people with different views?" I asked:

Of their own disciplines, of the theories and ideologies that they were trying to help themselves to, of the subject matter with which they are traditionally supposed to be concerned, and about the meaning of the word "ethics". I thought this was a word in ordinary English use, but they didn't know what it was.

I asked for clarification: "I'm still not clear how the fault lines worked here, where people divided":

Well, the fault lines were thus: when [three people in the seminar] presented our material, it was intelligible to the others and resulted in give-and-take, a debate, a discussion about the substance of the theses we were defending or attacking... When they [the postmodernists] talked, we couldn't understand what they were saying and we kept asking them to explain, to translate, and they were completely incapable of doing so.

When I interviewed a younger woman from English and asked her about her experiences in the seminar, she acknowledged the repeated unpleasant encounters with the philosopher and said that, primarily, what she had taken away from the seminar was an appreciation of her own discipline:

I think that the seminar has in some ways made me more attached to my own disciplinary bias... It has sharpened my own attachment to a form of literary reading... I mean, of course, every discipline has their various methodologies of interpretation, and I suppose I began to value and refine my own sense of what mine is in this seminar.

In both seminars there was inadequate a priori appreciation by the key antagonists, the seminar leader, and the other seminar participants of the vast disciplinary gulfs that needed to be navigated in order for productive dialogue to take place. The need to define terms carefully in all discussions and to negotiate styles of presentation and questioning was never made clear. Despite the seminar leader's experience in the first year, she was unable or unwilling to raise these issues early enough in the second year to encourage more fruitful discussion.

Nevertheless, when I interviewed the historian in this seminar, he expressed great satisfaction with it, telling me he thought that he was "the happiest person in the seminar", that he would never have been able to read Derrida on his own, and that post- colonial theory had given him some tools that he could use in his own work. He thought the problem with the seminar had been that the junior and senior faculty had not shown the necessary respect for one another. Interestingly, the young female English professor, when asked whether she would have participated in the seminar again, responded that she would have, but that she would have "demanded respect".

When I talked with the senior central administrator at Adams, who had been involved in choosing the seminar participants and topics, she commented that she thought that successful interdisciplinary dialogue requires rigor, but that it also requires "a willful suspension of one's own concept of what rigor means". More mutual respect and more willful suspension of participants' own concepts of rigor would have gone a long way toward improving the climate of the seminars at Adams.

Jefferson

The seminars at Jefferson were far more amicable than those at Adams, but my interviews with two participants in the second seminar—a mathematician and a dramatist—provided additional examples of the cultural divides across disciplines and the difficulties in bridging them. The second Jefferson seminar was led by a distinguished professor emeritus of English, who had much experience of leading cross-disciplinary seminars over the years and had also been a participant in the first year's seminar. However, despite his status, he, like the non-tenure-track leader of the Adams seminars, had no say in the choice of seminar participants. He did, however, shape the seminar topic, which he defined as "representation in each of the disciplines".

In all of my interviews with participants in the second Jefferson seminar, respondents told me that the mathematician in the seminar "had not participated". He came regularly, but never spoke. My interviewees were perplexed by this. Below is my discussion with the mathematician about his participation in the seminar:

Me: I was much less an active participant than I had hoped, [than I] would have liked to have been.

Him: Any particular reason?

Him: [Pause] I think it wasn't really my medium, my natural habitat, to be in a situation like that. I hadn't gotten used to that kind of interaction. It is quite different from the way mathematicians interact.

Me: Could you explain that to me? What did you see as the differences?

Him: Mathematicians interact much more... one-on-one, or in small groups... In the context of a seminar, where one person is presenting something that they are working on or know well, there's really not much discussion, as such... Most of the discussion happens on a one-on-one basis, at some other time outside of that seminar... It really takes time... for most mathematicians to absorb ideas and to under- stand what it's all about... like my conversation habits... I want a lot of time to think and to formulate precisely. I think that's part of what made me a less active participant, because in the seminar, people were, you know, talking all the time... I wanted to take a little time to think about what I'm going to say, and then the discussion's been done. It really wasn't for me.

Despite the fact that the mathematician had a very clear understanding of why he didn't speak in the seminar (except when he presented), nobody else in the seminar did, as evidenced by their perplexity about it. Nobody had ever asked him the reasons for his non-participation and so nobody could help him to bridge the enormous gap between his style of thinking, presenting, and questioning and the dominant style in the seminar, which was set by the English background of the seminar leader.

Still, although he did not participate in the discussions, the mathematician felt he had got a great deal out of the seminar:

Me: If you had it to do all over again, would you participate or would you take a pass?

Him: I'd participate.

Me: Why?

Him: Because it was so interesting. Because I learned so much... Before, I really had very little sense of what, for example, a sociologist really works on and how they go about their work... If I did it again, now I have a sense of that... so I might appreciate it more and participate more, be a more active participant.

The dramatist had a different cross-cultural issue with the same seminar. She objected to the critical stance that English professors, in particular, took to texts. She preferred to withhold judgement and "try on" ideas. I asked her: "What did you see as the most important issues that took place in the seminar, intellectual issues, themes, ideas?":

How we responded to work... We read Consilience as our first book... I thought it was exciting to be taken on a journey, sort of follow the thread, you know, and to try on his ideas. That's sort of my way of analysis. I was initially quite shocked at how some of the more, I guess, traditional aca- demics responded, not only to Consilience, but to the work in general, by being extremely criti- cal, which, initially, I saw as destructive. I came to under- stand over time that it was their true process of ascertaining the value of the ideas in the book; whereas, to me, I start with a positive attitude and I try the ideas on and see what I can find as an artist. You know, I'm given a script, I dive in, I see what's there, rather than going, it's bad, because I could never then connect to the work and do it justice.... I would say that isolated me in the seminar in a rather extreme way. I did come to terms with the fact that this was not of cruel or evil intent, though it would never be my way of approaching the analysis... My training has been... to engage in it and try to go with it rather than to withdraw and judge it... You know, they saw things I didn't see, [but] I think I had more fun than they did.

The most important connection the dramatist made in the seminar was with a chemistry professor. Both were considering offering a new course together on theatre and science that would include such plays as "Proof", "Arcadia", "In the Matter of J. Robert Oppenheimer", and "Copenhagen".

ENTERING MULTIDISCIPLINARY WATERS

The purpose of the seminars at Washington, Adams, and Jefferson was to foster conversations across disciplines. Those who wrote the grant proposals hoped that such conversations might lead to team-taught courses and/or joint research proposals. It would have been highly unrealistic to expect that one-year's worth of weekly conversations or any possible tangible outcomes of those conversations would result in truly integrated courses or research proposals.

As Steven Brint has argued, for many faculty, disciplines are comforting and venturing outside them is scary: "Every academic knows the experience of reading something from outside his or her discipline and knows the unsettling feeling it induces. Disciplines in fact provide a core element of the identity of most intellectuals in Modern America" (2000: 210).

Yet some academics do in fact venture out of their disciplines and appear to delight in doing so. Several faculty I interviewed were not only interested in cross-disciplinary work, but were the sole authors of books that were truly interdisciplinary. Faculty seem to span a spectrum with respect to multidisciplinarity. Some are allergic to it, in part because they don't feel they have criteria to assess its quality (Mansilla and Gardner). Others say they like it, but don't act that way. Still others revel in it.

Drawing on Archilochus (a seventh-century-BC Greek soldier-poet), Erasmus of Rotterdam, and Isaiah Berlin, Steven Jay Gould (2003) argues that some scholars, like hedgehogs, stick to a single effective strategy throughout their academic careers, while others, like foxes, devise many strat-

egies. Needless to say, the foxes in the seminars got more out of the readings and discussions than the hedgehogs. Interestingly, for some faculty the main benefit of the seminar was the development of self-awareness; they discovered that they were foxes (or more frequently, hedgehogs), although they didn't phrase their new self-knowledge in those terms.

In many ways the fox/hedgehog distinction is misleading when applied to multidisciplinary work at research universities. In the first place, it is not the case that successful academics in research universities can choose whether to be a fox or a hedgehog. They must all be certified hedgehogs before they can be foxes. All candidates for faculty promotion and tenure at research universities, even those who show fox-like tendencies early on, must gain their reputations in a relatively narrow specialty. Moreover, even those who seek to be foxes must retain a deep connection to their specialty. Other- wise, it is unlikely that they will be sought out as collaborators. So although one may be a pure hedgehog, one cannot be a fox without also being a hedgehog.

Taking all of this into account, one of the students in my graduate seminar came up with a more fruitful way of distinguishing between those who prefer to dig deeply into a single discipline and those who prefer to roam more widely across disciplines. He labels those who stay close to home "I" and those who roam "T", arguing that a "T" can be "broad" only if it stands upon an "I" (Landes 2005).

Although it is useful to note the differences between pure hedgehogs and fox/hedge- hogs or between "I" and "T" faculty, the distinctions don't do much to explain why certain faculty seem more open to multidisciplinarity or interdisciplinarity than others. While it is possible to seek personality characteristics to explain the differences, I don't take my work in that direction, in part because I am skeptical of the notion of personality differences for explanatory purposes and also because I have very little evidence on faculty members' personality characteristics. Instead, I use social and anthropological perspectives to explain both the propensity to engage in cross-disciplinary dialogue and the difficulties of doing so.

An anthropological perspective leads toward an understanding of disciplines as distinct cultures (Becher 1989; Geertz 1983) that initiate their faculty into particular ways of thinking and behaving. Moreover, disciplines continually reinforce those styles of thinking and behaving. Certain disciplines (e.g., history) teach their doctoral students to be rather open-minded about paradigms, theories, and research methods (Bromme 2000; Klein 1990). Other disciplines (e.g., economics) teach their doctoral candidates to be relatively closed-minded about alternative ways of viewing human behavior or using alternative research methods. As a result, many historians are like sponges in multidisciplinary situations, eager to soak up what their colleagues have to say, while economists tend to "communicate" mainly by telling others that they would make more progress on whatever problem is on the table if they simply viewed it from an economic perspective.

This is not to say that all historians are interested in being foxes and all economists are hedgehogs. In fact, many economists are neither foxes nor hedgehogs. They often venture out of economics, but not for the purpose of learning new strategies through dialogues with other disciplines. Rather, they seek, often quite successfully, to apply their own disciplinary theories and methods to other social sciences on subjects previously considered out of the economist's sphere, such as the family, politics, and education.

When discussing the effect of discipline on propensity toward cross-disciplinarity, it is important to distinguish between science and non-science and between cross- disciplinarity within science and cross-disciplinarity between science and non-science. Scientists appear to navigate cross-disciplinarity within science far more successfully than humanists do within the humanities, and certainly more successfully than social scientists

do within the social sciences. Part of this may be because of the similarity of scientists' training and the easy transferability of the scientific method across particular science disciplines. Part of it is also because scientists view the disciplinary boundaries among the sciences as rather fluid; they seem much more instrumental about their work than others in the academy. If there is an important technique, machine, or theory that seems applicable to their work, they have little interest in its disciplinary origins and much greater interest in learning, or having their post-docs learn, whatever it is from the other disciplines that will propel their own projects forward.

In many instances, openness to other sciences also makes scientists open to learning about disciplines outside of the sciences. They may be avid readers of history or fiction or they may remember fondly their undergraduate reading in the humanities and wish to hear more about them, although, since their exposure to the humanities was generally pre-post-modern, they can be baffled by some of the more recent analyses. Scientists are also often open-minded with respect to the social sciences, recognizing in particular the importance of economics and politics to science and often eagerly seeking to understand more about economic and political forces in society. Of course, this openness and interest does not always translate into a desire to team-teach or create joint research projects with humanists or social scientists, but sometimes it does.

I am certainly not arguing that disciplinary affiliation by itself predicts interest or effectiveness in multidisciplinary endeavors. Several other characteristics matter—for example, gender and age, as well as the current productiveness of one's research program and developments in one's field. Gender sometimes makes a difference because so many women in the humanities and social sciences have been involved with women's studies, which has given them an early and often positive experience of multi- disciplinary work. They are often already familiar with colleagues and their work in other disciplines at their university and elsewhere and understand some of the language and research methods of disciplines other than their own.

Age, on the other hand, all other things being constant, may well be negatively related to a propensity toward interdisciplinarity. For most scholars, the longer one has been in a discipline, the more one's habits of mind become fixed. Theories, research methods, ways of reasoning, colleagues, and networks all become familiar sources of success and reward. Moreover, the longer one has been in a discipline, the more investment one has made in these habits of mind; seeking new intellectual territory has increasing opportunity costs.

Conversely, age gives one the opportunity to take more risks. Having already achieved success as a hedgehog, one can afford to become more fox-like. In academia, becoming a fox is inherently more risky than remaining a hedgehog. It requires a high up-front investment in new learning, the development of new networks, movement into uncharted territory, and the possibility that there will be little or no payoff. Yet on the other hand, the payoff may be quite large, perhaps larger than anything to be gained through straight disciplinary endeavors. Faculty who have already been successful are in a better position to assume the risk of multidisciplinary work.

The decision to become more multidisciplinary depends also on where one's research is at. If there are clearly more gains to be made by continuing on a pure disciplinary path, perhaps with some added tools or methods from another field, then the impetus to seek multidisciplinary paths will be small. If, on the other hand, one's line of research has come to a natural halt, or one has become bored with one's project, then looking for new problems or ideas in other disciplines may become quite attractive. Also, if the field is moving in a more multidisciplinary direction, individual scholars may be motivated to follow suit. For example, many political scientists have

begun to learn more about economic maximizing models and game theory as these have taken hold in their own discipline.

Cross-disciplinary work is formidable not only because of language problems—the extreme difficulties in communicating across the specific languages, jargon, and short-hands of the various disciplines. Equally important are the cultural differences across disciplines—the amount of text material normally read, the manner of seminar presentations, the style of thinking and talking in groups, and the degree and style of critique normally given. Even in the seminars that were restricted to social scientists, the cultural differences among the disciplines played a major role for some seminar participants.

The seminar leaders, without being aware of it, each brought to the table a distinct disciplinary style of seminar organization and leadership. Rules with regard to a wide variety of subjects including level of civility, degree of democratic decision-making, style of presentations, style of discussion of texts, and style of leadership were instituted without group discussion by seminar leaders, based on their own disciplinary cultures. These leaders either did not recognize, or did not care, that other members of the seminar came from disciplines with quite different disciplinary styles. Not surprisingly, participants whose disciplinary cultures were closest to that of the seminar leader tended to report that they felt comfortable in the seminar and got more out of it. At the same time, participants whose disciplinary cultures were quite different from that of the seminar leader reported that they were uncomfortable and that that discomfort often interfered with their learning.

None of the leaders or administrators thought about the likely interpersonal inter- actions of seminar participants. Rather, the questions asked in the selection process concerned individual intellectual qualities and political issues in the university. For example, administrators and those seminar leaders who had input into the selection process asked not only about whose work was "really interesting", but also about who might change their mind about taking a job in another university in response to an outside offer if they were given this extra "bennie" of two courses off to participate in the seminar. They also asked about who could help them improve relations with the central administration in a department that had had its resources cut.

In those cases where group interactions were considered, the questions raised were about intellectual or political matters, not about potential interpersonal interactions. With regard to the intellectual dimensions of the seminars, there was no consideration given to the question of which disciplinary perspectives might most fruitfully interact, and which might lead to out-and-out warfare. The most salient kinds of group-related question asked by those choosing participants were: Who can bring a particular intellectual perspective to the table? How can we make sure that all of our "stars" get to know one another better?

Economic analysis of risk is useful with regard to understanding the effects of the seminar on faculty teaching and research, and the role of institutions in encouraging or impeding changes in faculty teaching and research (Tilghman 2005). To understand the economic approach to interdisciplinarity and risk, we need to ask first what it is that faculty and their institutions are seeking to maximize. The answer that is increasingly given by economists and sociologists who study higher education is that both faculty and their institutions seek to maximize prestige (Breneman 1970; Garvin 1980; Massy and Zemsky 1994; Melguizo and Strober 2005; Stinchcombe 1990).

For faculty, this single-minded utility function is far too simplistic a depiction of reality. Faculty also seek to satisfy their curiosity and to enjoy their work. Many also wish to make a contribution to the betterment of their fellow human beings. However, for most faculty, and perhaps especially those at research universities, maximization of prestige is at least one factor to

be considered when they decide which research projects to pursue.

An economic framework assumes that in the pursuit of prestige, and perhaps also in the pursuit of other goals, both faculty and institutions weigh the likely benefits and costs of various courses of action. In seeking to determine how much of their research and teaching should be disciplinary and how much, if any, should be multi- disciplinary, they look at the probable payoffs and costs of each type of work. In many ways, investing time in disciplinary activities is like investing in bonds. The returns are relatively predictable, but unlikely to be spectacular. Investing in stocks, on the other hand, or spending time in multidisciplinary or interdisciplinary activities, is riskier. That is, in both cases, there is greater possible harm and greater variability in returns. Both stocks and fox-like research have the potential for very high payoffs, but also the potential for disaster. In much the same way that investors combine stocks and bonds in an investment portfolio, in accordance with their risk tolerance, we can envision faculty and institutions of higher education seeking to create optimal disciplinary/multidisciplinary teaching and research "portfolios" to spread their risk.

All other things being equal, the longer one's time horizon, the more risk tolerance one has. This is why, for example, as workers approach retirement age they are counseled to increase the portion of their portfolio in bonds and decrease the proportion in stocks. Those with a shorter time horizon can much less easily weather a decline in their portfolio. By the same token, universities, with a much longer time horizon than individual faculty, have greater risk tolerance for interdisciplinary activities. To induce faculty to increase their multidisciplinary and interdisciplinary activities, so as to maximize institutional prestige, universities must put certain structures and incentives into place that will reduce risk for faculty.

Similarly, junior faculty and post-docs (and, by extension, doctoral students) who need to work toward tenure (or an acceptable dissertation) have an even shorter time horizon than other faculty, and thereby face even greater risk if they engage in multi- disciplinary or interdisciplinary activities. Yet it is in the institution's interest to expose junior faculty, post-docs, and doctoral students to multidisciplinary and interdisciplinary projects early in their careers, before they become set in their intellectual ways. To do this, institutions need to help younger scholars to reduce the risk of engaging in such work by changing job and tenure criteria and procedures.

An article by James March (1991) entitled "Exploration and Exploitation in Organizational Learning" examines the optimal mix for an organization of two strategies-- exploitation of known technologies versus exploration of new ones. If we think of exploitation as disciplinary work and exploration as multidisciplinary or interdisciplinary work, we can make use of March's analyses when looking at institutional optimization of disciplinary versus interdisciplinary activities. By extension, we can also apply March's insights to individual faculty decisions.

March lays out some fundamental differences between exploitation and exploration:

The essence of exploitation is the refinement and extension of existing competences, technologies, and paradigms. Its returns are positive, proximate, and predictable. The essence of exploration is experimentation with new alternatives. Its returns are uncertain, distant, and often negative... Such features... lead to a tendency to substitute exploitation of known alternatives for the exploration of unknown ones, to increase the reliability of performance more than its mean. (1999: 85)

Because of this tendency, March argues, organizations need to take positive steps to encourage exploration. They need to "work to sustain ... exploration in the face of adaptive processes that tend to inhibit it" (1999: 85).

March's article is theoretical and does not deal with the question of the optimum distribution of disciplinary versus multidisciplinary or interdisciplinary work at universities in the real world. However, it is interesting that at least two university presidents have suggested that, in their view, in an optimal world, multidisciplinary research would constitute about one-fifth of all research at their university. Since the current percentage of multidisciplinary work at most universities is probably not this high, analyzing multidisciplinarity from a risk perspective suggests that administrators who wish to move more faculty in the direction of greater multidisciplinarity will need to build new structures and procedures that reduce their risk of doing so.

SUMMARY: LESSONS LEARNED

The cross-disciplinary seminars at Washington, Adams, and Jefferson created difficult dialogues. Yet, overwhelmingly, seminar participants said the seminars were important to their intellectual growth. When asked, "If you had it to do over again, would you?" almost all said yes, although many hedged their assent with phrases like, "Only if certain things were different". Given the widespread interest in fostering conversations across disciplinary lines, it is instructive to examine these wishes for change in the seminars. Although they didn't always point in the same direction, certain lessons are clear.

First, seminar participants, and particularly the seminar leader, need to understand explicitly, from the outset, that they are engaged in a difficult cross-cultural activity, that habits of mind are deeply engrained, and that they represent a significant challenge for multidisciplinary conversation. Second, if there are wide differences in age and status among participants, these need to be recognized explicitly and discussed as part of the seminar proceedings. It is counterproductive to discuss only intellectual matters and ignore matters of process. Third, seminar participants generally needed more clarity about the purpose of the seminars and the criteria for success than was provided. Fourth, while diversity of perspectives and willingness to engage in debate were critical to the success of the seminars, so was civility and a respect for others' ideas and styles of thinking and presenting. Fifth, leading multidisciplinary seminars is exceedingly challenging. Leaders should be given training prior to the seminars and opportunities to talk with administrators about the progress of the discussions over the course of the year. Problems should not be permitted to fester.

Sixth, after multidisciplinary seminars have been completed, a member of the administration should interview participants about their experiences. I found many opportunities for follow-up that were squandered because no-one from the university learned about them. Moreover, several participants told me that it was only through talking to me that they themselves became clear about what they had learned in the seminars and what they wished to follow up. Seventh, if university administrators want seminar participants to teach new courses or develop new research projects as a result of their seminar experiences, they have to provide resources to seed these activities and they have to remove existing impediments to team-teaching and grant proposals that cross administrative boundaries. Multidisciplinary work is costly and risky. To encourage such work, the costs and risks need to be addressed and transformed.

REFERENCES

Becher, T. (1989). *Academic tribes and territories: Intellectual enquiry and the cultures of disciplines.* Milton Keynes: Society for Research into Higher Education and Open University Press.

Boxer, M. (1998). *When women ask the questions: Creating women's studies in America.* Baltimore, MD: Johns Hopkins University Press.

Boxer, M. (2000). Unruly knowledge: Women's studies and the problem of disciplinarity. *NWSA Journal, 12*(2), 119–129. doi:10.2979/NWS.2000.12.2.119

Boyer, E. L. (1990). *Scholarship reconsidered: Priorities of the professoriate.* Princeton: The Carnegie Foundation for the Advancement of Teaching.

Breneman, D. (1970). *The Ph.D. production function: The case of Berkeley (Paper P-8).* New York: Ford Foundation Program for Research in University Administration.

Brint, S. (Ed.). (2000). *The city of intellect.* Stanford, CA: Stanford University Press.

Bromme, R. (2000). Beyond one's own perspective: The psychology of cognitive interdisciplinarity. In Weingart, P., & Stehr, N. (Eds.), *Practicing interdisciplinarity.* Toronto, CA: University of Toronto Press, Inc.

Frost, S. H., & Paul, M. J. (2003). Bridging the disciplines: Interdisciplinary discourse and faculty scholarship. *The Journal of Higher Education, 74,* 119–143. doi:10.1353/jhe.2003.0013

Garvin, D. A. (1980). *The economics of university behavior.* New York, NY: Academic Press.

Geertz, C. (1983). The way we think now: Toward an ethnography of modern thought . In *Local knowledge: Further essays in interpretive anthropology.* New York, NY: Basic Books.

Gibbons, M., Limoges, C., Nowotny, H., Schwartzman, S., Scott, P., & Trow, M. (1994). *The new production of knowledge: The dynamics of science and research in contemporary societies.* London: Sage Publications.

Gould, S. J. (2003). *The hedgehog, the fox, and the magister's pox.* New York, NY: Harmony Books.

Gregorian, V. (2004). Colleges must reconstruct the unity of knowledge. *The Chronicle of Higher Education, 4*(June), B12.

Gulbenkian Commission on the Restructuring of the Social Sciences. (1996). *Open the social sciences*. Stanford, CA: Stanford University Press.

Klein, J. Th. (1980). *Interdisciplinarity: History, theory and practice*. Detroit, MI: Wayne State University Press.

Landes, M. (2005). *A case in interdisciplinarity: The product design program at Stanford. Unpublished seminar paper prepared for Education 357X*. Interdisciplinarity in Higher Education.

Lohmann, S. (2003). *How universities think. Unpublished manuscript*. Department of Political Science, University of California.

Mansilla, V. B., & Gardner, H. Assessing interdisciplinary work at the frontier. An empirical exploration of "symptoms of quality". Available from http://www.interdisciplines.org/ interdisciplinarity/papers/6; INTERNET.

March, J. G. (1991). *Exploration and exploitation in organizational learning*. Organization Science [Special Issue: Organizational Learning Papers in Honor of (and by) James G. March] 2, 71–87.

Massy, W. F., & Robert, Z. (1994). Faculty discretionary time: Departments and the academic ratchet. *The Journal of Higher Education, 65*, 1–22. doi:10.2307/2943874

Melguizo, T., & Myra, H. S. (2005). *A prestige model of the determinants of full-time faculty salaries at four-year institutions in the U.S.* Unpublished manuscript.

Messer-Davidow, E. (2002). *Disciplining feminism: From social activism to academic discourse*. Durham, NC: Duke University Press.

National Academy of Sciences, National Academy of Engineering, and Institute of Medicine. (2005). *Facilitating interdisciplinary research*. Washington, DC: The National Academies Press.

National Institute of Medicine. (2003). *Enhancing the vitality of the National Institutes of Health: Organizational change to meet new challenges*. Washington, DC: National Academies Press.

Snow, C. P. (1998). *The two cultures*. Cambridge, UK: Cambridge University Press. (Original work published 1959)

Stinchcombe, A. L. (1990). *Information and organizations*. Berkeley, CA: University of California Press.

Tilghman, Ch. (2005). *Considering interdisciplinarity. Unpublished seminar paper prepared for Education 357X*. Interdisciplinarity in Higher Education.

Turner, S. (2000). What are disciplines? And how is interdisciplinarity different? In Weingart, P., & Stehr, N. (Eds.), *Practicing Interdisciplinarity*. Toronto, CA: University of Toronto Press Inc.

Weingart, P. (2000). Interdisciplinarity: The paradoxical discourse . In Weingart, P., & Stehr, N. (Eds.), *Practicing interdisciplinarity*. Toronto, CA: University of Toronto Press Inc.

Wilson, E. O. (1999). *Consilience: The unity of knowledge*. New York, NY: Vintage Books.

NOTE

© Taylor & Francis Ltd, *Social Epistemology, 20*(3&4), 315-331; Strober, Myra H. (2006); Habits of the Mind: Challenges for Multidisciplinary Engagement. Reprinted with permission.

Section 9
The Emerging Message

Chapter 43

In Search for Unity within the Diversity of Information Societies

Darek M. Haftor
Stockholm University, Sweden & Linnaeus University, Sweden

Anita Mirijamdotter
Linnaeus University, Sweden

Miranda Kajtazi
Linnaeus University, Sweden

INTRODUCTION

"We have now a wholly new chance to explore the human side of societal change and take advantage of the technology to shape a good and balanced life. Let us use this opportunity for redesigning society towards peace, democracy and welfare for all...those who will develop, introduce and use technology that promotes peace, a deepening of democracy, welfare and quality of life for all will be the winners" G. Bradley, *"Humans on the Net"*, 2001 p. 21

This final Chapter represents the responsibility, the privilege but also the aspiration of the two editors of this *Gunilla Bradley Festschrift*. The aspiration here is no less than to identify a key message that emerges out of the contributions in this volume considered as a whole. In other words, the question here is: *what do all this research and reasoning say to us?* Of course, each reader of this Volume will derive her or his own interpretation and thus also a key message, which we only see as the richness offered by this Festschrift. Therefore, the key message presented here must be regarded only as one possible message that is formed by the two editors' own predispositions: intellectual, cultural, motivational, and other.

DOI: 10.4018/978-1-60960-057-0.ch043

In presenting the key message proposed, we will not attempt to reproduce all the arguments present in each of the chapters of this Volume. Rather the method employed is more like a cherry picking where various components are selected from each of the contributions, and configured so that the proposed message is advanced yet with the attempt to recognise each of the contributions, in one way or another. Finally, the message presented is made in a manner to facilitate its adoption by non specialists, students from various disciplines, avoiding the use of jargon and extensive conceptualisations. This implies a reduction of the reasoning, risking oversimplification. This risk is assumed for the opportunity to convey the key message to as many readers as possible.

In summary, the key message of this Festschrift, as provided here, is that human beings' use of the various kinds of information and communication technologies (ICT) gives rise to new kinds of societies. These so-called Information Societies expose us for several paradoxes of dialectical character. One such central is that Information Societies provide us with unique opportunities to realise human and social well-being; and this Volume presents a set of important guidelines to reach that end. However, the emerging Information Societies also manifest unparalleled threats to humanity, to societies themselves, and ultimately to humankind as such. At the end, there are no safeguards! Therefore, the need for normative considerations is greater than was the case before the advent of Information Societies and, paradoxically, the advent of the mediated-life shows that the function of truly human values is more important than ever.

CONVERGENCE: THE PRODUCT AND THE PRODUCER

Gunilla Bradley's more than four decade long inquiry into the human condition and well-being, took early focus on the post WWII introduction of ICT into professional, industrial, and then private and social affairs. One way of summarizing and presenting Gunilla Bradley's research, yet not the only one, is through her so-called *Convergence Model*.

This model may be understood as an articulation of a set of ongoing convergences that interact in our societies. The merge of the various kinds of information and communication technologies, such as computing, communication, and media, enables humans to both do current things differently, e.g. write faster a book, and to do new things that were not possible before the advent of ICT, e.g.: to control a spaceship on its journey to the moon or to find a husband in a country far away from own home without ever having visited that distanced place. This technological convergence is the most tangible one yet, in a certain sense, also the most trivial that the Convergence Model articulates. However, one central importance of this technological convergence is that it is simultaneously both *a product* and *a producer*; in the latter it acts as an enabler for and co-producer of the more complex and subtle convergences ongoing in our societies. These are reconfigurations and convergences of our life environments – i.e. work, home, public – and life roles – i.e. professional, private, citizen – and thereby societies as a whole – i.e. values, behaviours, cultures, economies, organisations. These convergences of human and societal functioning both produce and become a product of a particular kind of transformation of our societies, which would not be possible without the ICT. Bradley emphasizes the main change drivers being the interaction between ICT and the process of Globalization where economy and value systems dominate. The central question underlying here, and articulated by Gunilla Bradley, is: *how these ICT-powered societal transformations may lead to human and social well-being?*

AN EMERGENCE OF A NEW SOCIAL ORDER

Contemporary media reports more frequently about societal phenomena that could not be found only two or three decades ago. One example of these are the so-called e-wars, that include hidden attacks on Internet-servers aimed to disable these and as a consequence parallelise million of organisations and people, whether in the context of businesses, public services or private lives. Another example are the people of similar mindsets, engaged in a particular societal question – e.g. freeing a prisoner or forbidding the killing of an endangered species – that in a very short time can identify and communicate with each other, organise plans and guide the conduct of concrete actions toward particular ends, all enabled by Internet, mobile communication, and other advanced technological solutions.

These and many other phenomena not experienced before, suggest that the conditions of social order are transforming, or in other words, the question of how societies are being produced and re-produced is receiving a new answer. Indeed, the question of social order, its characteristics and conditions, have been and is inquired by numerous thinkers, yet without founding *the* *answer*. While Plato (c. 380 BCE) elaborated in his *Republic* how societies should be governed by philosopher-kings, it was probably Thomas Hobbes (1588-1679) who articulated the central question of the Social, namely: *how is social order really possible?* In more concrete terms, the question is about *how can social and fairly predictable order emerge out of actions of large numbers of discrete individuals*, very few of whom know each other personally, and of whom only a very small number are at any one time or place in a position to coordinate their actions by means of explicit agreements?

Hobbes answer then assumed a mono-centric model of governance, where order is produced by means of the law and authority, of an all-powerful ruler – then a King – and backed up by the use of force and the credible threat of punishment. However, the problem of this is that from a point of view of an individual it is sometimes better to break the law than to comply with it. Sometimes the perceived benefit of breaking laws and violating norms – punishment – will be much less than the perceived benefit of getting away with it; in such case it will be rational to break the law rather than to obey it. Hence, conceptions and theories that purport to show that obedience to the established laws somehow benefit each individual, do not guard against the so-called 'free-rider' problem. Since then, numerous of thinkers have attempted to provide an answer to this fundamental question. To be sure, our aim here is not to attempt such an answer; however, the question of the social and its order anticipate a great challenge from the Information Societies, with its emerging polycentric governance modes.

A SOCIETAL SELF-PRODUCTION

One way of conceptualising and understanding the societal complexities, yet far from the only one, is as a network of particular categories of empirical phenomena that interact both with themselves and with each other. These categories are: the Nature, the Human Beings, and the ICT; the latter as a particular subset of the artificial. The constituting content of their interactions may be understood as "*a contribution to the production and re-production of*" a particular category of phenomena; Figure 1 illustrates this interacting network understood here as a Societal Self-Production.

In this conception of a Societal Self-Production, the Nature is contributing to the production and re-production of itself but also the Human Beings and the ICT. Likewise, Human Beings and the ICT, respectively, contribute to the production and re-production of themselves and the other two empirical categories articulated; (the spe-

Figure 1. Societal Self-Production: illustrates the here assumed conceptualisation of the emerging Information Societies. In this Human Beings contribute to the production and reproduction of themselves, including the emergence of the Social, but also of Nature and of the particular kind of artefacts understood as Information and Communication Technologies (ICT). Likewise, Nature is contributing to the production and re-production of itself but also of Human Beings and the ICT. Lastly but not least, ICT is contributing to the production and re-production of itself and also of Human Beings and the Nature. The key message of this conception of the Societal Self-production is the circular manner of co-production where everything seams to interact with everything.

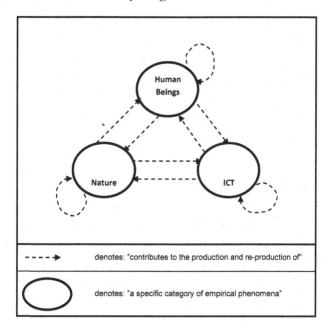

cific character of each kind of the productions is different, these differences though are not important for the message here and therefore not accounted). Further, the origin of this cosmological order is not of concern here, rather the key proposition is that every thing seems to contribute to the production and re-production of everything.

Assuming a human-oriented position here, this co-producing network is to satisfy the various human needs, physical, mental and social. Beside food and shelter and other physical needs, which include safety and security, privacy and yet belonging is central to human beings' well-being, as is physical, intellectual and emotional stimulation, but also visionary experiences and self-fulfilment as driven by human intentionality. In this, the human being is a *collective being by*

nature – unlike some other beings – human being's being together with another human being satisfies central human needs.

The emerging Information Societies give rise to new social structures and cultures in a manner that has not been possible before. People, that live in the same local communities as well as those separated by thousands of miles and many clock hours, can now identify each other, express and share freely their meanings and opinions, argue for their point of view, and accept or not the other fellow citizen's arguments. This freedom of the *human being* produces and re-produces new social structures that in turn enable taking actions that were not possible otherwise, and thereby transforming the central tension of any social system: the individual versus its environment, cultural and natural. The emergence of ICT-enabled social spaces gives rise to new shared meanings that could not be shared before and thereby the creation, re-creation and re-configuration of social fabric and its ethos that would not be created otherwise. It enables the coordination and collaboration of people that are committed to conduct successfully complex tasks – such as brain surgery or inspections of nuclear power stations – yet being physically and temporally separated, but not intentionally! All this, and much more, is the democratic ideal, still not realized everywhere, yet worth striving for in order to contribute to human and social wellbeing!

To this end, the emerging Information Societies bring their instrumentalisation, or mediation, of inter-human communication, in the semantic sense. This is achieved through the forwarding of various signals and symbols that trigger human meaning formulation, sense-making, aimed at an inter-human sharing of meanings, and then of the emergence of understanding, which contributes to learning and potentially human development. However, similarly to the case with the non-ICT-mediated Social, the ICT-mediated Social has inherent inter-human power structures, both formal and informal: some people have and also explore the opportunity to influence other people. This political dimension influences the shaping, production and re-production of social structures, its culture and the very social fabric and ethos of our societies and thereby the ability to provide with unity, and human and social well-being.

SOME GUIDELINES TOWARD WELLBEING

Research on *ICT, Human Beings and Society* provides us all with a large amount of empirical experiences that may be transformed into normative guidelines regarding how to positively enable, yet not necessary secure, the realisation of human and societal wellbeing in a democratic context.

These guidelines give directions for how to design, develop and utilize ICT toward that end.

Examples of this include enabling *free and equal access* to ICT and its networks and information therein. However, as access as such does not guarantee free expression and communication, there is also a need to enable free and *active creation of the content*: the information. This in turn makes it important to secure the *integrity of information*, its accuracy – safeguarded for misrepresentations and manipulations. There is also a need to secure that the access to the 'neural system' – to use a biological analogy – of Information Societies is not limited by the various ergonomic qualities by striving to provide *human-oriented ICT-devices*. The latter may mean *active adaptations to each individual* human being, to hers or his physical and mental *deficiencies*, to the various *cognitive and affective profiles* and styles, and also providing required social and cultural *metaphors* for the interaction and navigation, among many others.

However, it is not only the characteristics of information or the very ICT-artefacts that influence the success, or otherwise, of human beings' interaction with the ICT and therefore with other human beings. Various contextual aspects also need to be accounted for. This may include both *organisations* and *communities* that act as the context in a given situation of human being's information interaction. These contexts include formal and informal decision-making and *power-structures*, its subtle *cultural patterns*, the actual *working-routines*, job designs or operating procedures, and the existence or the absence of *educational and communicational* routines; all aimed to enable successful ICT-access, utilization and therefore mediation of inter-human interaction. Central to this is the prevention and also reduction of *physical and mental stress* and the enabled establishment of *human being's influencing and even control of him or her self* or own destiny. Securing these and other related measures should be the mission for our societies contributing to the production of human and social wellbeing in a democratic context.

Beside this central social re-production function, Information Societies have yet another important opportunity that may become crucial for its wellbeing. It may contribute to the realisation of a *de-materialisation* of human and social activities – for example, the conduct of a telesurgery for a patient far away, instead of flying in him or her. The importance of this opportunity of de-materialisation is manifested frequently in the various debates and demonstrations, and also their failures, aimed to handle the sustainability of the natural resources and the associated global warming. Failure to handle successfully these challenges to our Nature – such as illustrated in the recent 2009 Copenhagen-meeting – may produce social unrest in a manner that may challenge any democracy!

THE SEARCH FOR UNITY IN THE SOCIAL DIVERSITY OF THE INFORMATION AGE

ICT in social contexts co-produces the Information Societies that offer human beings new and unparalleled opportunities to create novel social networks, new cultural configurations with innovative ideas, commitments and aspirations, and also new political structures. In this, human beings distanced geographically, temporally, and also socially – gender, age, profession, social class – can spontaneously configure new social spaces with its peculiar social fabric and ethos – all this in a way that was not possible prior to the advent of ICT in human and social contexts. In this, an active inclusion and co-creation is imperative to enable the realisation of social compatibility aimed at social sustainability and the avoidance of societal break-downs.

However, this production and re-reproduction of Information Societies also manifest a greater threat than ever. The configuration of social structures and processes aimed at domination, manipulation and oppression of fellow human

beings may now be realized in an unparalleled manner! Small groups of people, spread globally and with advanced knowhow of complex ICT-systems, guided by unfair intentions, may implement disasters that whole armies of soldiers were unable to do prior the advent of the Information Society. Imagine what happens if the ICT-systems of all hospitals, all banks, and all nuclear power stations, are taken over by someone who has unpleasant intentions…?

Plato inquired extensively, in his *Republic,* for safeguards to human and social wellbeing, and found the democratic solution unreliable. One of the reasons is that whatever societies are produced and self-reproduced, this constitution never happens in a vacuum; there are, unconditionally, some normative foundations pre-existing the evolution of a society that influence and govern the course of such reproduction and development. Human and social future is partly a function of its present and its past; fortunately not completely. Even the Habermasian notion of the *ideal speech situation*, where every citizen is given the opportunity to freely express and argue for her or his position, and where any manipulative measures are eliminated, there is the possibility of a mass-psychosis, as history manifest too often, where collective evil is advanced, ultimately in a self-destructive manner, as is evidenced daily by extended suicidal incidents.

In this we may recall that ICT as such is not a value-neutral artefact! Like all technology, ICT is a human invention produced by the idea and aspiration of human's mastery and control over her or his environment! To this end, it seems that we, Human Beings, have produced our own paradox, and prison. On the one hand we live by and aspire for *human freedom*, which is a central ideal of a democratic society, on the other hand though our lives are governed and advanced by human being's supremacy and *control of its environment* – as manifested by scientism and its icon: ICT. The paradox in this is: how can we human beings realise *freedom* in a world, natural and social, that is subjected to this *control*?

To this ambivalent position toward the dialectical reproduction of the physical and cultural spheres we bring the *compass needle* to contribute to a development toward human and social well-being: this guidance and governance must come from all of us, by seeking a unity within the ever transforming social diversity. Gunilla Bradley has provided us with an answer: *Let us use this opportunity for redesigning society towards peace, democracy and welfare for all... those who will develop, introduce and use technology that promotes peace, a deepening of democracy, welfare and quality of life for all will be the winners.*" (*Humans on the Net*; 2001 p. 21)

Compilation of References

(Ed.). (2009). Texting to Death (Editorial). *New York Times*. Retrieved 15 September 2009 from, http://www.nytimes.com/2009/09/15/opinion/15tue3.html

Abbott, A. (1995). Sequence analysis: New methods for old ideas. *Annual Review of Sociology*, *21*(4), 93–113. doi:10.1146/annurev.so.21.080195.000521

Abercrombie, N., Turner, B. S., & Hill, S. (2000). *The Penguin Dictionary of Sociology*. London: Penguin.

Åborg, C. (2002). *How does IT feel @ work? And how to make IT better: Computer use, stress and health in office work*. Ph D Thesis, Department of Information technology, Uppsala University.

Abowd, G., & Mynatt, E. D. (2000). Charting Past, Present, and Future Research in Ubiquitous Computing. *ACM Transactions on Computer-Human Interaction*, *7*(1), 29–58. doi:10.1145/344949.344988

Abu Dhabi Future Energy Company (Masdar). (2009). The Masdar Initiative. http://www.masdar.ae/en/Menu/index.aspx?&MenuID=42&CatID=12&mnu=Cat

Adamczyk, A., & Bailey, B. P. (2004). If Not Now, When? The Effects of Interruption at Different Moments within Task Execution. *CHI 2004*, Vienna, Austria.

Adams, R. J., & Khoo, S.-T. (1996). *QUEST: The interactive test analysis system* (*Vol. 1*). Melbourne: Australian Council for Educational Research.

Administration on Aging. (2009). Aging statistics. Retrieved April 24, 2009, from http://www.aoa.gov/AoARoot/Aging_Statistics/index.aspx

Agar, J. (1998). Introduction: History of computing: Approaches, new directions and the possibility of informatic history. *History and Technology*, *15*(2), 1–5. doi:10.1080/07341519808581938

Ahrentzen, S. (1990). Managing conflict by managing boundaries: how professional home workers cope with multiple roles at home. *Environment and Behavior*, *22*(6), 723–752. doi:10.1177/0013916590226001

Aiken, L. H., Sochalski, J., & Anderson, G. F. (1996). Downsizing the hospital nursing workforce. *Health Affairs*, *15*(4), 88–92. doi:10.1377/hlthaff.15.4.88

Åkerstedt, T., Kecklund, & G., Axelsson, J. (2007). Impaired sleep after bedtime and worries. *Biological Psychology*, *76*, 170–173. doi:10.1016/j.biopsycho.2007.07.010

Alander, S. (2007). *Offentliga storkök i det gröna folkhemmet: diffrakterade berättelser om hållbar utveckling* [Institutional kitchens in the green welfare state – diffracted narratives on sustainable development]. Dissertation, Luleå University of Technology, Luleå.

Alexander, J. K. (2006). Efficiency and Pathology Mechanical Discipline and Efficient Worker Seating in Germany, 1929–1932. *Technology and Culture*, *47*, 286–310. doi:10.1353/tech.2006.0109

Allvin, M., & Wiklund, P. Härenstam, & A., Aronsson, G. (1999). *Frikopplad eller frånkopplad [Disconnected or out of touch]*. National Institute for Working Life, Stockholm, Sweden.

Allvin, M., Aronsson, G., Hagström, T., Johnasson, G., Lundberg, U., & Skärstrand, E. (1998). *Gränslöst arbete eller arbetets nya gränser.* Stockholm: National Institute for Working Life, Arbete och hälsa 21.

Alter, S. (2002). *Information Systems, Foundation of E-Business* (4th ed.). Upper Saddle River: Prentice Hall.

Alty, J. L. (2003). Cognitive workload and adaptive systems . In Hollnagel, E. (Ed.), *Handbook of cognitive task design* (pp. 129–146). New Jersey: Lawrence Erlbaum Associates.

Alvesson, M. (2002). *Understanding Organizational Culture.* London: Sage Publications.

Anders, S., Patterson, E. S., Woods, D. D., & Ebright, P. (2007). Projecting Trajectories for a New Technology Based on Cognitive Task Analysis and Archetypal Patterns: The Electronic ICU. *8th Annual Naturalist Decision Making Conference.* Asilomar, CA.

Anders, S., Patterson, E. S., Woods, D. D., & Schweikhart, S. (2008). Shifts in Functions of a New Technology Over Time: An Analysis of Logged Electronic Intensive Care Unit Interventions. *Human Factors and Ergonomics Society 52nd Annual Meeting.* New York, Human Factors and Ergonomics Society.

Anderson, C. (2006). *The long tail: why the future of business is selling less of more.* New York: Hyperion.

Andersson, C., Camenisch, J., & Crane, S. Fischer-Hübner, S., Leenes, R., Pearson, S., Pettersson, J.S., & Sommer, D. (2005). Trust in PRIME. In *Proceedings of the 5th IEEE Int. Symposium on Signal Processing and IT*, December 18-21, 2005, Athens, Greece.

Andriessen, J. (2003). *Working with Groupware: understanding and evaluating collaboration technology.* New York: Springer.

Angus, D. C., Linde-Zwirble, W. T., Sirio, C. A., Rotondi, A. J., Chelluri, L., & Newbold, R. C. III (1996). The effect of managed care on ICU length of stay: implications for medicare. *Journal of the American Medical Association, 276*(13), 1075–1082. doi:10.1001/jama.276.13.1075

Annett, J. (2003). Hierarchical Task Analysis . In Hollnagel, E. (Ed.), *Handbook of cognitive task design* (pp. 17–35). New Jersey: Lawrence Erlbaum Associates.

Apted, T., Kay, J., & Quigley, A. (2006). Tabletop sharing of digital photographs for the elderly. In *Proceedings of the 2006 SIGCHI conference on Human Factors in computing systems.* Canada.

Armour, P. G. (2000). The five orders of ignorance: Viewing software development as knowledge acquisition and ignorance reduction . *Communications of the ACM, 43*(10), 17–20. doi:10.1145/352183.352194

Armstrong, T. J., Buckle, P., Fine, L. J., Hagberg, M., Jonsson, B., & Kilborn, A. (1993). A conceptual model for work-related neck and upper limb musculoskeletal disorders. *Scandinavian Journal of Work, Environment & Health, 19*, 73–84.

Arnetz, B. B. (1997). Technological stress: psychophysiological aspects of working with modern information technology. *Scandinavian Journal of Work, Environment & Health, 23*(3), 97–103.

Arning, K., & Ziefle, M. (2008). Development and validation of a computer expertise questionnaire for older adults. *Behaviour & Information Technology, 27*(4), 325–329. doi:10.1080/01449290802127153

Arquilla, J., & Ronfeldt, D. (1999). *The Emergence of Noopolitik, Toward an American Information Strategy.* Santa Monica, CA: RAND Cooperation.

Article 29 Data Protection Working Party. (2004). Opinion on More Harmonised Information provisions. 11987/04/EN WP 100, November 25 2004.

Artigiani, R. (1991). Social Evolution, A Nonequilibrium Systems Model . In Laszlo, E. (Ed.), *The New Evolutionary Paradigm* (pp. 93–129). New York: Gordon & Breach Science Publishers Ltd.

Astor, M., Koch, C., Klose, G., Reimann, F., Rochhold, S., & Stemann, M. (2006). *Zu alt, um Neues zu lernen? Chancen und Grenzen des gemeinsamen Lernens von älteren und jüngeren Mitarbeitern. QUEM-Materialien der Arbeitsgemeinschaft Betriebliche Weiterbildungsforschung e* (pp. 1–165). V. AWBF.

Atkins, D., Boyer, D., Handel, M., Herbsleb, J., Mockus, A., & Wills, G. (2002). *Achieving speed in globally distributed project work.* Winterpark, CO: Human Computer Interaction Consortium.

Atkinson, D., & Walmsley, J. (2003). Time to make up your mind: Why choosing is difficult. *British Journal of Learning Disabilities, 31*(1), 3–8. doi:10.1046/j.1468-3156.2003.00181.x

Atkinson, C. J., & Checkland, P. B. (1988). Extending the metaphor 'system'. *Human Relations, 41*(10), 709–725. doi:10.1177/001872678804101001

Aubert, B. A., & Kelsey, B. L. (2003). Further understanding of trust and performance in virtual teams. *Small Group Research, 34*(5), 575–618. doi:10.1177/1046496403256011

Austin, J. L. (1962). *How to Do Things with Words.* Cambridge, MA: Harvard University Press.

Avgerou, C. (2002). *Information Systems and Global Diversity.* Oxford: Oxford University Press.

Avison, D., & Fitzgerald, G. (2002). *Information Systems Development: Methodologies, Techniques and Tools* (3rd ed.). Berkshire, UK: McGraw-Hill.

Axmann, M. (2002). An online mentorship programme for the online educator: Patterning for success. In *Proceedings of the Australian Society for Educational Technology International and Technology Conference (ASET 2002): Untangling the Web-Establishing Learning Links.* Melbourne, Australia.

Axmann, M. (2004). *Human capital development in an online mentoring system.* MA Thesis, University of Pretoria.

Axmann, M., McKay, E., Banjanin, N., & Howat, A. (2006). Towards web-mediated learning reinforcement: Promoting effective human-computer interaction. In *Proceedings of Web-Based Education (WBE 2007), International Association of Science and Technology for Development (IASTED)* (pp.210-215), Chamonix, France.

Aziz, M. (2004). Role stress among women in the Indian information technology sector. *Women in Management Review, 19*(7), 356–363. doi:10.1108/09649420410563412

Bailey, B. P., & Iqbal, S. T. (2008). Understanding Changes in Mental Workload during Execution of Goal-directed Tasks and its Application for Interruption Management. *ACM Transactions on Computer-Human Interaction, 14*(4), 21. Retrieved from http://doi.acm.org/10.1145/1314683.1314689. doi:10.1145/1314683.1314689

Bailey, R. W. (1996). *Human Performance Engineering: Using human factors / ergonomics to achieve computer system usability* (3rd ed.). Englewood Cliffs, NJ: Prentice Hall.

Baldwin, C. L. (2009). Individual differences in navigational strategy: implications for display design. *Theoretical Issues in Ergonomics Science, 10*(5), 443–458. doi:10.1080/14639220903106379

Ballon, P., Pierson, J., & Delaere, S. (2005). Open Innovation Platforms for Broadband Services: Benchmarking European Practices. In *16th European Regional Conference, Porto, Portugal.*

Bannon, L., & Schmidt, K. (1989, January). *CSCW: Four characters in search of a context.* In First European Conference on Computer-Supported Cooperative Work (pp. 358-372), Gatwick, London.

Bardram, J. E. (2009). Activity-Based Computing for Medical Work in Hospitals. *ACM Transactions on Computer-Human Interaction, 16*(2), 1001–1036. doi:10.1145/1534903.1534907

Bariff, M. L., & Lusk, E. J. (1977). Cognitive and Personality Tests for the Design of Management Information Systems. *Management Science, 23*(4), 820–829. doi:10.1287/mnsc.23.8.820

Barrantes, R. (2005). Analysis of ICT demand: what is digital poverty and how to measure it? In Galperin, H., & Mariscal, J. (Eds.), *Digital poverty: Latin American and Caribbean perspectives* (pp. 29–53). Lima, PE: Practical Action Publishing.

Barthelmess, P., & Anderson, K. M. (2000). A View of Software Development Environments Based on Activity Theory. Retrieved 21 September 2009 from, http://www.ics.uci.edu/~redmiles/activity/final-issue/Anderson/Anderson.pdf

Bartlett, F. (1932). Remembering: A Study in Experimental and Social Psychology. Cambridge University Press. Retrieved December 2009 from http://www.ppsis.cam.ac.uk/bartlett/RememberingBook.htm

Baskerville, R. L., & Wood-Harper, A. T. (1998). Diversity in Information Systems Action Research Methods. *European Journal of Information Systems, 7*, 90–107. doi:10.1057/palgrave.ejis.3000298

Baskerville, R. L., & Wood-Harper, T. A. T. (1996). A Critical Perspective on Action Research as a Method for Information Systems Research. *Journal of Information Technology, 11*, 235–246. doi:10.1080/026839696345289

Bateson, G. (1972). *Steps to an ecology of mind*. New York, NY: Ballentine Book.

Bauer, R. A. (Ed.). (1966). *Social indicators*. Cambridge, MA: The MIT Press.

Bauer, W., & Kern, P. (1994). Human Factors in office design - employee expectations and future trends. In G.E. Bradley & H. W. Hendrick (Eds.), *Human Factors in organizational design and management* (pp.67-72). Amsterdam, NL: North-Holland

Bauman, R. (1986). *Story, Performance, and Event: Contextual Studies of Oral Narrative*. New York: Cambridge University Press.

Baumann, A., Giovannetti, P., O'Brien-Pallas, L., Mallette, C., Deber, R., & Blythe, J. (2001). Healthcare restructuring: the impact of job change. *Canadian Journal of Nursing Leadership, 14*(1), 14–20.

Becher, T. (1989). *Academic tribes and territories: Intellectual enquiry and the cultures of disciplines*. Milton Keynes: Society for Research into Higher Education and Open University Press.

Beck, U. (2009). *World at Risk*. Cambridge, UK: Polity Press.

Bedeian, A. G., & Zammuto, R. F. (1991). *Organizations: Theory and Design*. Chicago, IL: Dryden Press.

Bekker, M., & Long, J. (2000). User Involvement in the Design of Human-Computer Interactions: Some Similarities and Differences between Design Approaches. In McDonald, S. & Cockton, G. (Eds.), *People and Computers XiV: Proceedings of the HCI 2000* (pp. 135-147). New York: Springer.

Bell, D. (1968). *The coming of post-industrial society: A venture in social forecasting*. New York: Basic Books Inc. Publishers.

Benevolo, L. (1980). *The History of the City* (Culverwell, G., Trans.). Cambridge, MA: The MIT Press.

Beniger, J. R. (1986). *The Control Revolution*. Cambridge, MA: Harvard University Press.

Benkler, Y. (2006). *The Wealth of Networks: How Social Production Transforms Markets and Freedom*. New Haven, CT: Yale University Press.

Berger, P. L., & Luckmann, T. (1966). *The Social Construction of Reality; a Treatise in the Sociology of Knowledge*. Garden City, NY: Doubleday.

Bergman, M. (1999). *På jakt efter högstadieelevers Internetanvändning* [A study of high school students' use of the Internet]. Licentiate of Philosophy. Uppsala: Uppsala University, Sweden.

Bergmann, M. (2009). User Friendly Policy Management and Presentation. In Fischer-Hübner et al.

Bergmann, M., Rost, M., & Pettersson, J. S. (2006). Exploring the Feasibility of a Spatial User Interface Paradigm for Privacy-Enhancing Technology. In *Proceedings of the Fourteenth International Conference on Information Systems Development (ISD'2005)* (pp. 437-448), Karlstad, August 2005. Published in Advances in Information Systems Development, Springer-Verlag, Germany.

Bergvall-Kåreborn, B., Ihlström Eriksson, C., Rudström, Å., Svensson, J., Ståhlbröst, A., & Åkesson, M. (2009a). *Clarifying the Living Lab Concept.* Luleå, Sweden: Luleå University of Technology.

Bergvall-Kåreborn, B., Holst, M., & Ståhlbröst, A. (2008). Creating a New Leverage Point for Information Systems Development . In Avital, M., Boland, R., & Cooperrider, D. (Eds.), *Designing Information and Organizations with a Positive Lens* (pp. 75–95). Oxford, UK: Elsevier Science /JAI Press.

Bergvall-Kåreborn, B., Ihlström Eriksson, C., Ståhlbröst, A., & Svensson, J. (2009b). A Milieu for Open Innovation - Defining Living Lab. In Huizingh, Conn, K. R. E., Torkkeli, S., & Bitran, M (Eds.). *Proceedings of the 2nd ISPIM Innovation Symposium*, New York.

Berkenkotter, C. (1995). Theoretical issues surrounding interdisciplinary interpretation. *Social Epistemology, 9*(2), 175–187. doi:10.1080/02691729508578784

Berleur, J., & Brunnstein, K. (1996). *Ethics of Computing, Codes, spaces for discussion and law*. London, UK: Chapman & Hall.

Berleur, J., Burmeister, O., Duquenoy, P., Gotterbarn, D., Goujon, P., Kaipainen, K., et al. (Eds.). (2008). *Ethics of Computing Committees. Suggestions for Functions, Form, and Structure*: IFIP-SIG9.2.2. IFIP Framework for Ethics of Computing (pp. 1-35), Laxenburg, AU: IFIP Press.

Berleur, J., Duquenoy, P., d'Udekem-Gevers, M., Ewbank de Wespin, T., Jones, M., & Whitehouse, D. (2000). Self-regulation instruments – Classification – A preliminary inventory. HCC5, Geneva 1998; SIG9.2.2 January 2000; SIG9.2.2. June 2000; IFIP – WCC-SEC 2000.

Bernstein, N. A. (1966). *Essays in the Physiology of Movement and Activity*. Moscow: Medicine Publishers. (in Russian)

Bernstein, R. J. (1976). *The restructuring of social and political theory*. Oxford, UK: Basil Blackwell.

Bessenyei, I. (2008). Learning and teaching in the information society. *Elearning 2.0 and connectivism. Revista de Informatica Sociala*, 9. Retrieved August 8, 2009 from http://www.ris.uvt.ro/wp-content/uploads/2009/01/ibesseneyi.pdf

Betz, F. (1971). On the management of inquiry. *Management Science.* 18(4, Dec., part 1), B-117-B-133.

Bhattacharyya, J. (1995). Solidarity and Agency: Rethinking Community Development. *Human Organization, 54*(1), 60–68.

Bichler, R. M., Bradley, G., & Hofkirchner, W. (2010). Editorial Comment. Sustainable Development and ICTs. *Information Communication and Society, 13*(1).

Bichler, R. M., Bradley, G., & Hofkirchner, W. (2010). Editorial Comment. Sustainable Development and ICTs. *Information Communication and Society, 13*(1).

Bigley, G. A., & Pearce, J. L. (1998). Straining for shared meaning in organization science: Problems of trust and distrust. *Academy of Management Review, 23*(3), 16. doi:10.2307/259286

Birren, J. E., & Schaie, K. W. (2006). *Handbook of the Psychology of Aging*. London: Academic Press.

Bischofberger, E., & Zaremba, M. (1985). *Arbete före kapital*. Stockholm, SE: Brevskolan.

Bjerknes, G., & Bratteteig, T. (1995). User participation and democracy, a discussion of Scandinavian research on system development. *Scandinavian Journal of Information Systems, 7*(1), 73–98.

Blakeslee, S. (2001). Car Calls May Leave Brain Short-Handed. *New York Times*, 31 July 2001. Retrieved 17 September 2009 from, http://www.nytimes.com/2001/07/31/science/car-calls-may-leave-brain-short-handed.html

Blatt, M. (1971). The Effects of Classroom Discussion Upon Children's Moral Judgment . In Kohlberg, L., & Turiel, E. (Eds.), *Moral Research: The Cognitive-Developmental Approach*. New York: Holt, Rinehart and Winston.

Blavasky, H. P. (1889). *The Voice of Silence*. New York: J.W.Bouton. Centenary Edition of the book is published in 1992 by Quest Books Publishers.

Blevis, E. (2006). *Advancing Sustainable Interaction Design: Two Perspectives on Material Effects, Design Philosophy Papers: Collection Four* (pp. 52–69). [Online]. Retrieved April 17, 2008 from http://www.desphilosophy.com/dpp/dpp_journal/journal.html

Blevis, E. (2007). Sustainable interaction design: invention and disposal, renewal and reuse. In R. Grinter, T. Rodden, P. Aoki, E. Cutrell, R. Jeffries & G. Olson (Eds.), *Proceedings of the SIGCHI Conference on Human Factors in Computing Systems, CHI 2007* (pp. 503–512). ACM Conference Proceedings Series. New York: ACM Press.

Bloch, E. (1967). *Das Prinzip Hoffnung (3 vols.)*. Frankfurt, DE: Suhrkamp.

Blondel, M. (1973). *L'action: Essai d'une critique de la vie et d'une science de la pratique* (Orig. published 1893). Paris, FR: Presses Universitaires de France.

Blumenberg, H. (1985). *The legitimacy of the modern age (Originally published as Die legitimität der Neuzeit. Frankfurt: Suhrkamp Verlag, 1966, 1976)*. Cambridge, MA: MIT Press.

Bodker, S., & Sundblad, Y. (2008). Usability and interaction design-new challenges for the Scandinavian tradition. *Behaviour & Information Technology*, *27*(4), 293–300. doi:10.1080/01449290701760682

Bødker, K., Kensing, F., & Simonsen, J. (2004). *Participatory IT Design. Designing for Business and Workplace Realities*. Cambridge, MA: MIT Press.

Böhler, E. (1970). Conscience in economic life . In Zbinden, H. (Eds.), *Conscience* (pp. 43–77). Evanston, IL: Northwestern University Press.

Bond, A. H., & Gasser, L. (Eds.). (1988). *Distributed artificial intelligence*. San Mateo, CA: Morgan Kaufman.

Borgmann, A. (1999). *Holding On to Reality: The Nature of Information at the Turn of the Millennium*. Chicago, IL: University of Chicago Press.

Borja, G., & Björn-Sören, G. (2005). The concept of information poverty and how to measure it in the Latin American context . In Galperin, H., & Mariscal, J. (Eds.), *Digital poverty: Latin American and Caribbean perspectives* (pp. 11–28). Lima, PE: Practical Action Publishing.

Bottorff, W. W. (n.d.). What Was The First Car? A Quick History of the Automobile for Young People. Retrieved December 2009 from http://www.ausbcomp.com/~bbott/cars/carhist.htm

Boumans, N. P. G., & Landeweerd, J. A. (1994). Working in an intensive or non-intensive care unit: does it make any difference? *Heart & Lung*, *23*, 71–79.

Bourdieu, P. (1977). *Outline of a Theory of Practice* (pp. 143–158). New York: Cambridge University Press.

Bourdieu, P. (1993). *The Field of Cultural Production: Essays on Art and Literature*. New York: Columbia University Press.

Boxer, M. (1998). *When women ask the questions: Creating women's studies in America*. Baltimore, MD: Johns Hopkins University Press.

Boxer, M. (2000). Unruly knowledge: Women's studies and the problem of disciplinarity. *NWSA Journal*, *12*(2), 119–129. doi:10.2979/NWS.2000.12.2.119

Boyer, E. L. (1990). *Scholarship reconsidered: Priorities of the professoriate*. Princeton: The Carnegie Foundation for the Advancement of Teaching.

Braa, J., Monteiro, E., & Sahay, S. (2004). Networks of action: sustainable health information systems across developing countries. *Management Information Systems Quarterly*, *28*(3), 337–362.

Bradley, G. (2006). *Social and Community Informatics: Humans on the Net*. London: Routledge.

Bradley, G. (1989). *Computers and the Psychosocial Work Environment. Translated from the Swedish by Struan Robertson.* London: Taylor & Francis.

Bradley, G. (2000). The Information and Communication Society: How People Will Live and Work in the New Millennium. *Ergonomics, 43*(7), 844–857. doi:10.1080/001401300409053

Bradley, G., Holm, P., Steere, M., & Strömquist, G. (1993). Psychosocial Communication and Computerization . *Computers in Human Behavior, 9*(2-3), 157–169. doi:10.1016/0747-5632(93)90004-C

Bradley, G. (2001). Information and Communication Technology (ICT) and Humans - How we will live, learn and work . In Bradley, G. (Ed.), *Humans on the Net: Information and Communication Technology (ICT), Work Organization and Human Beings* (pp. 22–44). Stockholm: Prevent.

Bradley, G. (1989). Knowledge based systems and Work Design . In Haslegrave, C. M., Wilson, J. R., Corlett, E. N., & Manenica, I. (Eds.), *Work Design in Practice*. London: Taylor & Francis.

Bradley, G. (2009). The Convergence Theory and the Good ICT Society - Trends and Visions . In Schlick, C. M. (Ed.), *Industrial Engineering and Ergonomics* (pp. 43–55). Aachen, DE: Springer Berlin Heidelberg. doi:10.1007/978-3-642-01293-8_4

Bradley, L., & Bradley, G. (2001). The Home as a Virtual and Physical Space – Experiences from USA and South- East Asia . In Smith, M., & Salvendy, G. (Eds.), *Systems, Social and Internationalization Design Aspects of Human-Computer Interaction* (pp. 81–85). Mahwah, NJ: Lawrence Erlbaum Associates.

Bradley, G. (1977). *Datateknik, Arbetsliv och Kommunikation. (Computer Technology, Work Life, and Communication).* The Swedish delegation for long term research. FRN. Stockholm, SE: Liber (in Swedish).

Bradley, G. (1979). Computerization and some Psychosocial Factors in the Work Environment. In *Proceedings of the conference Reducing Occupational Stress* (pp. 30-40). New York, 1977. U.S. Department of Health, Education, and Welfare, NIOSH Publication No. 78-140.

Bradley, G. (1993). What Happens to the Work Organization? In W.S., Marras, W., Karwowski, J.L., Smith, & L. Pacholski (Eds.), *Proceedings of the International Ergonomics Association World Conference on the Ergonomics of Manual Work*, June 14-17, 1993, Warsaw, Poland. Washington/London, DC/UK: Taylor & Francis.

Bradley, G. (2001). *Humans on the Net*. Stockholm, SE: Prevent.

Bradley, G. (2003). Humans on the net: psychosocial life environment and e-society. In *Proceedings of the international Conference Risk and Safety Management in Industry, Logistics, Transport and Military Service: New Solutions for the 21st Century*, (pp.27- 36),Tallinn Technical University, Tallinn, Estonia.

Bradley, G. (2003). ICT for deepening human and societal qualities. In *Proceedings of WITFOR 2003. Humans on the Net*. London, UK: Routledge.

Bradley, G. (2005). The Convergence Theory on Information and Communication Technology (ICT) and the Psychosocial Life Environment – The Connected Home. In Salvendy, G. (Ed.). *Proceedings of the HCI International 2005 conference*, 22-27 July 2005, Las Vegas, USA. (CD). Mahwah, NJ: Lawrence Erlbaum Associates.

Bradley, G. (2006). Social Informatics: From Theory to Actions for the Good ICT Society. In J Berleur, M.I. Nurminen, & J. Impagliazzo (Eds.), *Social Informatics: An Information Society for All? Proceedings of the Seventh International Conference on Human Choice and Computers (HCC7)* (pp. 183-194), IFIP TC 9. New York: Springer.

Bradley, G. (2007). ICT, Work Organisations, and Society. In Anttiroiko, A-V. & Mälkiä, M. (Eds,) *Encyclopedia of Digital Government*. Hershey, PA: Idea Group Inc.

Bradley, G. (Ed.). (2001). *Humans on the Net. Information and Communication Technology (ICT) Work Organization and Human Beings.* Stockholm, SE: Prevent.

Bradley, G. E., & Hendrick, H. W. (Eds.). (1994). Human Factors in organizational design and management - IV. Development, introduction and use of new technology - challenges for human organization and human resource development in a changing world. In *Proceedings of the 4th International symposium on Human Factors in Organizational Design and Management.* Amsterdam, NL: North-Holland

Bradley, G., & Bradley, W. (1996). Computers in the Bakery - From Theory to Action. In O. Brown & H. W. Hendrick (Eds.), *Human Factors in Organizational Design and Management-V.* Amsterdam, NL: Elsevier Science. Proceedings from ODAM V, Breckenridge, Colorado, July 31- August 3, 1996.

Bradley, G., & Robertson, M. (1991). *Computers, Psychosocial Work Environment, and Stress. A comparative theoretical analyses or organizations and action strategies.* Plenary presentation at the 11th Congress International Ergonomics Association. Paris 15-20 July, 1991.

Bradley, G., Börjesson, K., & Lundgren, M. (1974). Arbetsmiljö och tjänstemän (Work Environment and Salaried Employees). Report to the Swedish Central Federation of Salaried Employees. Stockholm, SE: TCO.

Bradley, L. (2005). *Home of the Future Japan – Information and Communication Technology (ICT) and Changes in Society and Human Patterns of Behavior in the Network Era.* KTH Research report ISBN 91-7178-052-1. Stockholm: Royal Institute of Technology (KTH).

Brandel, M. (2008). CROWD SOURCING: Are You Ready to Ask the World for Answers? *Computerworld, 42*(10), 24–26.

Brandt, E. (2006). Designing exploratory design games: a framework for participation in Participatory Design? In I. Wagner, J. Blomberg, G. Jaccuci & F. Kenising (Eds.), *Proceedings of the Ninth Conference on Participatory Design: Expanding Boundaries in Design, vol. 1* (pp. 105–114). New York: ACM Press.

Bransford, J. D., Nitsch, K., & Franks, J. J. (1977). Schooling and the facilitation of knowing . In Anderson, R. C., Spiro, R., & Montague, W. (Eds.), *Schooling and the acquisition of knowledge.* New Jersey: Erlbaum.

Bratteteig, T. (2004). Making change. Dealing with relations between design and use, Dr. Philos Dissertation, Department of Informatics, University of Oslo.

Braverman, H. (1975). *Labor and Monopoly Capital; the Degradation of Work in the Twentieth Century.* New York: Monthly Review Press.

Breneman, D. (1970). *The Ph.D. production function: The case of Berkeley (Paper P-8).* New York: Ford Foundation Program for Research in University Administration.

Brennan, P. F., Moore, S. M., Bjornsdottir, G., Jones, J., Visovsky, C., & Rogers, M. (2001). HeartCare: an Internet-based information and support system for patient home recovery after coronary artery bypass graft (CABG) surgery. *Journal of Advanced Nursing, 35*(5), 699–708. doi:10.1046/j.1365-2648.2001.01902.x

Brennan, P. F., Moore, S. M., & Smyth, K. A. (1995). The Effects of a Special Computer Network on Caregivers of Persons with Alzheimer's Disease. *Nursing Research, 44*(3), 166–172. doi:10.1097/00006199-199505000-00007

Breslow, M. J., Rosenfeld, B. A., Doerfler, M., Burke, G., Yates, G., & Stone, D. J. (2004). Effect of a multiple-site intensive care unit telemedicine program on clinical and economic outcomes: An alternative paradigm for intensivist staffing. *Critical Care Medicine, 32*(1), 31–38. doi:10.1097/01.CCM.0000104204.61296.41

Brey, P. (2006). Evaluating The Social And Cultural Implications Of The Internet. *Computers & Society, 36*(3), 41–48. doi:10.1145/1195716.1195721

Brint, S. (Ed.). (2000). *The city of intellect.* Stanford, CA: Stanford University Press.

Bromme, R. (2000). Beyond one's own perspective: The psychology of cognitive interdisciplinarity . In Weingart, P., & Stehr, N. (Eds.), *Practicing interdisciplinarity.* Toronto, CA: University of Toronto Press, Inc.

Brown, J. J., & Sullivan, G. (1989). Effect on ICU mortality of a full-time critical care specialist. *Chest, 96*(1), 127–129. doi:10.1378/chest.96.1.127

Bryant, C. G. A., & Jary, D. (1991). *Giddens' Theory of Structuration: A Critical Appreciation*. London: Routledge.

Brynjolfsson, E., & Hitt, L. (1998). Beyond the Productivity Paradox. *Communications of the ACM, 41*(8), 49–55. doi:10.1145/280324.280332

Buber, M. (1958). *Ich und Du* (Special ed., first ed. 1923. Swedish trans. Jag och Du, Stockholm: Bonniers, 1962. Page refs. to Sw. trans.), Stockholm, SE: Bonniers.

Buchman, J. M. (1985). *Liberty, Market and State: Political Economy in the 1980 New York*. New York: New York University Press.

Buckley, M. J. (1987). *At the origins of modern atheism*. New Haven/London, CT/UK: Yale University Press.

Bughin, J. (2008). The rise of enterprise 2.0. *In Direct . Data and Digital Marketing Practice, 9*(3), 251–259. doi:10.1057/palgrave.dddmp.4350100

Bull, C. Hoose, & J., Weed, M. (2003). *Leisure studies*. London: Pearson Education.

Bullen, C. (1990b). *Bennett. J* (pp. 291–302). Learning from User Experience with Groupware. CSCW.

Bullen, C., & Bennett. J. (1990a, March). *Groupware in Practice: An Interpretation of Work Experience. Center for Information Systems Research Report*, no. 205. Cambridge, MA.

Burgess, P. W., Veitch, E., de Lacy Costello, A., & Shallice, T. (2000). The Cognitive and Neuroanatomical Correlates of Multitasking. *Neuropsychologia, 38*(6), 848–863. doi:10.1016/S0028-3932(99)00134-7

Burjor, A. (2007). *India: The Ancient Past*. London: Routledge.

Butler, B. S., & Gray, P. H. (2006). Reliability, Mindfulness, and Information Systems. *Management Information Systems Quarterly, 30*(2), 211–224.

Buxton, W., Hill, R., & Rowley, P. (1985). Issues and Techniques in Touch-Sensitive Tablet Input. *Computer Graphics, 19*(3), 215–224. doi:10.1145/325165.325239

Bynum, T., & Rogerson, S. (Eds.). (1996). *Global Information Ethics*. Opragon Press.

Bynum, T., & Schubert, P. (1997). In van den Hover, J. (Ed.), *How To Do Computer Ethics- A Case Study* (pp. 85–95). Erasmus University Press.

Byrne, E., & Sahay, S. (2007). Generalizations from an interpretive study: the case of a South African community-based health information system. *South African Computer Journal, 38*, 8–19.

Byrne, E. (2005). Using action research in information systems design to address change: a South African health information systems case study. In *Proceedings of the 2005 Annual Research Conference of the South African Institute of Computer Scientists and Information Technologists on IT Research in Developing Countries SAICSIT '05* (pp. 131–141). White River, South Africa.

Caldwell, B. S. (1990). Development of Models for Park Rangers' Perceived Isolation of National Park Service Areas. *Environment and Behavior, 22*(5), 636–649. doi:10.1177/0013916590225004

Caldwell, B. S. (1994). Developing Robust Mathematical Models of Information Technology Use in Organizations Human Factors in Organizational Design and Management – IV: In *Proceedings of the Fourth International Symposium on Human Factors in Organizational Design and Management* held in Stockholm, Sweden (pp. 526–530). Amsterdam, NL: North-Holland. Caldwell, B. S., & Paradkar, P. V. (1995). Factors Affecting User Tolerance for Voice Mail Message Transmission Delays. *International Journal of Human-Computer Interaction, 7*(3), 235–248. doi:10.1080/10447319509526123

Caldwell, B. S., Uang, S.-T., & Taha, L. H. (1995). Appropriateness of communications media use in organizations: Situation requirements and media characteristics. *Behaviour & Information Technology, 14*(4), 199–207. doi:10.1080/01449299508914633

Camenisch, J., & Lysyanskaya, A. (2001). Efficient non-transferable anonymous multi-show credential system with optional anonymity revocation. In *Advances in Cryptology - Eurocrypt 2001* (pp. 92-118), 2045.

Camenisch, J., Shelat, A., Sommer, D., & Zimmermann, R. (2006). Securing user inputs for the web. In *Proceedings of the Second ACM Workshop on Digital Identity Management* (pp. 33-44). Alexandria, Virginia, USA, November 03 - 03, 2006. DIM '06. New York: ACM.

Campanella, Th. J. (2004). *Webcameras and the Telepresent Landscape. The Cybercities Reader* (pp. 57–63). London, UK: Routledge.

Cannon, W. B. (1928). The mechanism of emotional disturbance of bodily functions. *The New England Journal of Medicine*, *198*, 877–884. doi:10.1056/NEJM192806141981701

Caplan, J. (2008, June 30). The Citizen Watchdogs of Web 2.0. *Time*. Retrieved

Carayon, P., & Gurses, A. P. (2008). *Nursing workload and patient safety - A human factors engineering perspective. Patient safety and quality: An evidence-based handbook for nurses*. Rockville: Agency for Healthcare Research and Quality.

Carayon, P., Hundt, A. S., Karsh, B.-T., Gurses, A. P., Alvarado, C. J., Smith, M., & Flatley, B. P. (2006). Work system design for patient safety: The SEIPS model. *Quality & Safety in Health Care*, *15*(Suppl I), i50–i58. doi:10.1136/qshc.2005.015842

Carayon-Sainfort, P. (1992). The use of computer in offices: Impact on task characteristics and worker stress. *International Journal of Human-Computer Interaction*, *4*(3), 245–261. doi:10.1080/10447319209526041

Carilli, A. M., Coyne, C. J., & Leeson, P. T. (2008). Government intervention and the structure of social capital. *The Review of Austrian Economics*, *21*, 209–218. doi:10.1007/s11138-007-0035-z

Carlson, R. W., Weiland, D. E., & Srivthsan, K. (1996). Does a full-time, 24-hour intensivist improve care and efficiency? *Critical Care Clinics*, *12*(3), 525–552. doi:10.1016/S0749-0704(05)70260-8

Carlsson, I., Collberg, D., Månsson, E., Greiff, M., Starverski, H., Wigerfelt, B., et al. Klapp Lekholm, & A., Persson, A. (2004) *Nära gränsen? Perspektiv på skolans arbetsliv [Close to the edge? Perspectives of the working life in schools]*. National Institute for Working Life, Stockholm, Sweden.

Carpenter, S. R. (1998). Sustainability and common-pool resources: Alternatives to tragedy. *Philosophy and Technology*, *3*(4), 36–57.

Carpi, O. (1989). *Kant: L'etica della ragione*. Rimini, IT: Panozzo.

Carr, A. C., Woods, R. T., & Moore, B. J. (1986). Automated Cognitive Assessment of Elderly Patients: A Comparison of Two Types of Response Device. *The British Journal of Clinical Psychology*, *25*, 305–306.

Carr, N. (2008). *The Big Switch: Rewiring the World, from Edison to Google*. New York: WW Norton & Company.

Carson, R. (1962). *Silent Spring*. Boston, MA: Houghton Mifflin.

Castells, M. (2001). *The Internet galaxy*. Oxford, UK: Oxford University Press.

Castells, M. (Ed.). (2004). *The network society*. Northampton, MA: Edward Elgar.

Castells, M. (1998). *The Rise of the Network Society: The Information Age: economy, society and culture*. Malden, MA: Blackwell.

Castells, M. (1996). *The Rise of the Network Society, The Information Age: Economy, Society and Culture (Vol. I)*. Cambridge, MA/Oxford: Blackwell Publishers.

Castells, M. (1997). *The Power of Identity, The Information Age: Economy, Society and Culture (Vol. II)*. Cambridge, MA/Oxford: Blackwell Publishers.

Castells, M. (1998). *The End of Millenium, The Information Age: Economy, Society and Culture (Vol. III)*. Cambridge, MA/Oxford: Blackwell Publishers.

Castells, M. (2004a). Informationalism, networks, and the network society: a theoretical blueprint . In Castells, M. (Ed.), *The network society* (pp. 3–45). Northampton, MA: Edward Elgar.

Castells, M. (2004). Space of Flows, Space of Places: Materials for a Theory of Urbanism in the Information Age . In Stephen, G. (Ed.), *The Cybercities Reader* (pp. 82–93). London: Routledge.

Castells, M. (2000). Trilogy on *The Information Age. Economy, Society and Culture*. 1996-97 in English. Daidalos Publisher 2000 (in Swedish).

CBC News. (2008, February 1). Federal department's BlackBerry blackout gets mixed reviews. http://www.cbc.ca/news/yourview/2008/02/federal_departments_blackberry.html

Centre for Civil Society. (2009). *What is Civil Society?* Retrieved June 11, 2009 from http://www.lse.ac.uk/collections/CCS/introduction/what_is_civil_society.htm

Centre of Regional Science. Vienna UT. (2007, October). Smart cities – Ranking of European medium-sized cities. Retrieved from http://www.smart-cities.eu

Ceruzzi, P. E. (2005). Moore's Law and Technological Determinism. Reflections on the History of Technology. *Technology and Culture*, *46*, 584–593. doi:10.1353/tech.2005.0116

Chai, K. (2007). A Survey of Revenue Sharing Social Software's Systems. In *Proceedings of International, Workshop on Social Interaction and Mundane Technologies (Simtech)*, Melbourne. Retrieved August 8, 2009 from http://kevinchai.net/images/resources/survey-of-revenue-sharing-social-software-systems.pdf

Chan, W.-S., Stevenson, M., & McGlade, K. (2008). Do General Practitioners Change How They Use the Computer During Consultations with Significant Psychological Component? *International Journal of Medical Informatics*, *77*(8), 534–538. doi:10.1016/j.ijmedinf.2007.10.005

Chan, S. (2007, August 14). U.S. Offers New York $354 Million for Congestion Pricing. *New York Times*. Retrieved from http://cityroom.blogs.nytimes.com/2007/08/14/us-will-give-new-york-354-million-for-congestion-pricing/

Chaparro, A., Bohan, M., Fernandez, J., Choi, S., & Kattel, B. (1999a). The impact of age on computer input devices use: psychophysical and physiological measures. *International Journal of Industrial Ergonomics*, *24*, 503–513. doi:10.1016/S0169-8141(98)00077-8

Chaparro, A., Bohan, M., Fernandez, J., Kattel, B., & Choi, S. (1999b). Is the trackball a better input device for the middle-age computer user? *Journal of Occupational Rehabilitation*, *9*, 33–43. doi:10.1023/A:1021341415404

Charness, N., Holley, P., Feddon, J., & Jastrzembski, T. (2004). Light pen use and practice minimize age and hand performance differences in pointing tasks. *Human Factors*, *46*(3), 373–384. doi:10.1518/hfes.46.3.373.50396

Charness, N., Bosmann, E. A., & Elliot, R. G. (1995). Senior-Friendly Input Devices: Is the Pen Mighter than the Mouse? *103rd Annual Convention of the American Psychological Association Meeting*, New York.

Chateerji, M. M. (1932). *Viveka Chudamani or Jewel of Wisdom of Sri Shankaracharya*. Whitefish, MT: Kessinger Publishing Company.

Checkland, P. B. (1981). *Systems Thinking, Systems Practice*. Chichester, UK: John Wiley & Sons.

Checkland, P. B., Forbes, P., & Martin, S. (1990). Techniques in Soft Systems Practice Part 3: Monitoring and Control in Conceptual Models and in Evaluation Studies. *Journal of Applied Systems Analysis*, *17*, 29–37.

Checkland, P. B., & Holwell, S. (1998). Action Research: Its Nature and Validity. *Systemic Practice and Action Research*, *11*(1), 9–21. doi:10.1023/A:1022908820784

Checkland, P. B. (1981). *Systems thinking, systems practice*. New York, NY: Wiley.

Checkland, P. B. (1986). *The politics of practice. Paper for the IIASA Int. Roundtable The Art and Science of Systems Practice*. Laxenburg, Austria: International Institute of Applied Systems Analysis.

Checkland, P. B. (1988). Churchman's "anatomy of system teleology" revisited. *Systems Practice, 1*(4), 377–384. doi:10.1007/BF01066580

Checkland, P. B. (1988). Information systems and systems thinking: Time to unite? *International Journal of Information Management, 8*(4), 239–248. doi:10.1016/0268-4012(88)90031-X

Checkland, P. B., & Casar, A. (1986). Vicker's concept of an appreciative system: A systemic account. *Journal of Applied Systems Analysis, 13*, 3–17.

Checkland, P. B., & Griffin, R. (1970). Information systems: A systems view. *Journal of Systems Engineering, 1*(2), 29–42.

Chen, C., & Rada, R. (1996). Interacting with hypertext: A meta-analysis of experimental studies. *Human-Computer Interaction, 11*(2), 125–156. doi:10.1207/s15327051hci1102_2

Chen, P. W. (2009). How Mindfulness Can Make for Better Doctors, *New York Times*. Retrieved 13 October 2009 from, http://www.nytimes.com/2009/10/15/health/15chen.html

Cheney, H., Nheu, N., & Vecellio, L. (2004). Sustainability as social change: values and power. In H. Cheney, E. Katz & F. Solomon (Eds.), *Sustainability discourse, Sustainability and Social Round Table Proceeding* (pp. 225–246), The Institute for Sustainable Futures, Sydney and CSIRO Minerals, Melbourne [Online]. Retrieved April 17, 2008 from http://www.minerals.csiro.au/sd/pubs/

Chesbrough, H. (2003). *Open Innovation: The New Imperative for Creating and Profiting from Technology*. Cambridge, MA: Harvard Business School Press.

Chesbrough, H., & Appleyard, M. (2007). Open Innovation and Strategy . *California Management Review, 50*(1), 57–76.

Christensen, H., & Lundberg, U. (2002). Musculoskeletal problems as a result of work organization, work tasks and stress during computer work. *Work and Stress, 16*(2), 89–90. doi:10.1080/02678370213265

Churchman, C. W. (1968). *The Systems Approach*. New York, NY: Delacorte Press.

Churchman, C. W. (1961). *Prediction and optimal decision: Philosophical issues of a science of values*. Englewood Cliffs, NJ: Prentice-Hall.

Churchman, C. W. (1968). *Challenge to reason*. New York, NY: MacGraw-Hill.

Churchman, C. W. (1971). *The design of inquiring systems: Basic principles of systems and organization*. New York, NY: Basic Books.

Churchman, C. W. (1979). *The systems approach and its enemies*. New York, NY: Basic Books.

Churchman, C. W. (1968). *The systems approach* (References are to pages of the 2nd ed., 1979). New York, NY: Delta

Clifford, S. (2009). Doubts about Scare Tactics on Drivers Who Text, *New York Times*. Retrieved 1 September 2009 from, http://www.nytimes.com/2009/09/01/technology/01distracted.html

Cohen, M. H. (2008). Professional communication and teamwork. *Creative Nursing, 14*(1), 17–23. doi:10.1891/1078-4535.14.1.17

Cohen, D., & Prusak, L. (2001). *In Good Company: How Social Capital Makes Organizations Work*. Cambridge, MA: Harvard Business School Press.

Coiera, E. W., Jayasuriya, R. A., Hardy, J., Bannan, A., & Thorpe, M. E. C. (2002). Communication loads on clinical staff in the emergency department. *MJA, 176*, 415–418.

Colero, L. (2007). *A Framework for Universal Principles of Ethics*. UBC Center for Applied Ethics. Retrieved from www.ethics.ubc.ca

COM 3282 final (2008, July 2). *Commission recommendation of 2nd July 2008 on cross-border interoperability of electronic health record systems.*

COM 356 final (2004, April 30). *e-Health – making healthcare better for European citizens: An action plan for a European e-Health area.* Luxembourg: European Commission

COM 414 final (2008, July 2). *Proposal for a Directive on the application of patients' rights in cross-border healthcare.*

COM 489 final (2008, November 2). *Telemedicine for the benefit of patients, healthcare systems and society.*

COM 860 final (2007, December 21). *A lead market initiative for Europe.*

Conchie, S. M., Donald, I. J., & Taylor, P. J. (2006). Trust: Missing piece(s) in the safety puzzle. *Risk Analysis, 26*(5), 1097–1104. doi:10.1111/j.1539-6924.2006.00818.x

Constantinides, E., & Fountain, S. (2008). Web 2.0: Conceptual Foundations and Marketing Issues. *Journal of Direct . Data and Digital Marketing Practice, 9*(3), 231–244. doi:10.1057/palgrave.dddmp.4350098

Cook, J. R., & Salvendy, G. (1999). Job enrichment and mental workload in computer-based work: Implications for adaptive job design. *International Journal of Industrial Ergonomics, 24*, 13–23. doi:10.1016/S0169-8141(98)00084-5

Cooper, C. L., & Marshall, J. (1976). Occupational sources of stress: A review of the literature relating to coronary heart disease and mental ill health. *Journal of Occupational Psychology, 49*, 11–28.

Cooper, C. L. (Ed.). (1998). *Theories of organizational stress.* Oxford: Oxford University Press.

Cooperrider, D. L., & Avital, M. (Eds.). (2004). *Advances in Appreciative Inquiry, Constructive Discourse and Human Organisation.* Oxford, UK: Elsevier.

Cooperrider, D. L., & Whitney, D. (2005). *Appreciative Inquiry - A Positive Revolution in Change.* San Francisco: Berrett-Koehler Publishers.

Cooperrider, D. L., Whitney, D., & Stavros, J. M. (2005). *Appreciative Inquiry Handbook,* San Francisco, SF: Berrett-Koehler Publishers.

CoreLabs. (2007). *Living Labs Roadmap 2007-2010: Recommendations on Networked Systems for Open User-Driven Research, Development and Innovation* (pp. 1–61). Open Document. Luleå, Luleå University of Technology, Centrum for Distance Spanning Technology.

Cox, T. (1985). Repetitive work: Occupational stress and health . In Cooper, C. L., & Smith, M. J. (Eds.), *Job Stress and Blue-Collar Work* (pp. 85–112). New York: John Wiley & Sons.

Craik, F. I. M., & Salthouse, T. A. (2008). *The Handbook of Aging and Cognition.* London: Psychology Press.

Cronbach, L. J. (1957). The two disciplines of scientific psychology. *The American Psychologist, 12*(11), 671–684. doi:10.1037/h0043943

Crook, C., & Barrowclif, D. (2001). Ubiquitous Computing on Campus: Patterns of Engagement by University Students. *International Journal of Human-Computer Interaction, 31*(2), 234–256.

Croon Fors, A. (2006). *Being-with Information Technology: Critical explorations beyond use and design.* PhD Thesis. Umeå University. Sweden: Department of Informatics: Umeå.

Cross, D. G., & Fallon, A. (1985). A stressor comparison of four speciality areas. *The Australian Journal of Advanced Nursing, 2*, 24–36.

Crowley, P. (2010). *Information and Communication Technologies Enabling to Create a Self-Organising Civil Society 'Knowledge and Service Commons' and 'Capability' Capacities to Counteract 'Chaos Points.* Ph.D. University of Salzburg.

Crowley, P. (2010). *Information and Communication Technologies Enabling to Create a Self-Organising Civil Society "Knowledge and Service Commons" and "Capability" Capacities to Counteract "Chaos Points".* Dissertation, University of Salzburg, Austria.

Cruddas, J., & Nahles, A. (2009). Building the Good Society, The Project of the Democratic Left. Retrieved from http://www.goodsociety.eu/wp-content/uploads/2009/04/building_the_good_society.pdf

Csikszentmihalyi, M. (1990). *Flow: The Psychology of Optimal Experience*. New York: Harper and Row.

Cummings, J., Krsek, C., Vermoch, K., & Matuszewski, K. (2007). Intensive care unit telemedicine: Review and consensus recommendations. *American Journal of Medical Quality, 22*(4), 239–250. doi:10.1177/1062860607302777

Czaja, S., & Lee, C. C. (2002). *Designing Computer Systems for older Adults*. New Jersey: Lawrence Erlbaum Associates.

Czaja, S. J. (1997). Computer technology and the older adult . In Helander, M., & Landauer, T. (Eds.), *Handbook of human - computer interaction* (pp. 797–812). Amsterdam: North-Holland.

Czaja, S. J., Rogers, W. A., Fisk, A. D., & Walker, N. (1996). Aging and acquisition of Computer skills. *Aging and Skilled Performance: Advances in Theory and Applications* (pp. 202-221).

Czaja, S., & Lee, C. C. (2008). Information technology and older adults. In M.G. Hollander, T.K. Landauer, & P.V. Prabhu (Eds.), (pp. 777-792), *Handbook of Human Computer Interaction*.

Czerwinski, M., Horvitz, E., & Wilhite, S. (2004). A Diary Study of Task Switching and Interruptions. In *Proceedings of CHI 2004* (pp. 175-182), April 24-29, 2004, Vienna, Austria.

Daft, R. L., & Lengel, R. H. (1986). Organizational Information Requirements, Media Richness and Structural Design. *Management Science, 32*(5), 554–571. doi:10.1287/mnsc.32.5.554

Dahlbom, B. (2003). *Makten över framtiden* [Control over the future]. Sweden: Liber Ekonomi.

Dahlbom, B. (1990). *The idea that reality is socially constructed (Manuscript, 12 Jan. 1990.)*. University of Gothenburg, Dept. of Philosophy.

Dahlgren, A. (2006). *Work stress an overtime work – effects on cortisol, sleep, sleepiness and health*. Thesis: Department of psychology. Stockholm University, Sweden.

Damasio, A. R. (1995). *Descartes' error: emotion, reason, and the human brain*. New York: Harper Collins.

Danielsson, K., & Wiberg, C. (2006). Participatory Design of learning media: designing educational computer games with and for teenagers, in ITSE special issue . *Computer Game-based Learning, 3*(4), 4–20.

Danielsson, C. (2005). *Office environment, health and job satisfaction: an explorative study of office design's influence*. Licentiate Thesis: Royal Institute of Technology, Stockholm, Sweden

Danielsson, U. (1999). Learning in Networks. *Proceedings of the Human Computer Interaction International* (pp. 407-411). Munich, Germany.

Danielsson, U. (2002). *Unga IT- Människor i storstad [Young urban knowledge workers]*. Fiber Science Communication Network, R-02-34, Sweden.

Danielsson, U. (2003). Young urban knowledge workers – The relationship between ICT and the psychosocial life environment. In *Proceedings of Human Computer Interaction International* (pp. 941-945). Crete, Greece.

Danielsson, U. (2007). *Relationships Between Information Communication Technology and Psychosocial Life Environment. Students and Young Urban Knowledge Workers in the ICT-Era*. Sundsvall: Mid Sweden University. Doctoral Thesis no 41, 2007.

Danielsson, U. (2007a). High school students – Relationship between ICT and psychosocial life environment. In *Proceedings of IRIS Information system Research seminar in Scandinavia 30*, Tampere, Finland.

Danielsson, U. (2007b). *Relationships between Information Communication Technology and Psychosocial Life Environment – Students and Young Urban Knowledge Workers in the ICT-Era*. PhD Thesis. Mid Sweden University. Sundsvall, Sweden: Department of Information technology and media.

Danielsson, U., & Danielsson, K. (2008). Boundaries between work and leisure within psychosocial life environment - an interdisciplinary literature review. In *Proceedings of IRIS Information System Research Seminar 31 - Nordic Conference in Informatics*. Åre, Sweden. E-publication

Data Protection in the European Union. Citizens' perceptions (2008, February). *Flash Eurobarometer*. Retrieved from http://ec.europa.eu/public_opinion/flash/fl_225_en.pdf

Davis, F. D., Bagozzi, R. P., & Warshaw, P. R. (1989). User acceptance of computer technology: A comparison of two theoretical models. *Management Science, 35*(8), 983–1003. doi:10.1287/mnsc.35.8.982

Davis, K. (1966). Some Correlates of Responses to the "This I Believe Test". In Harvey, O. J. (Ed.), *Experience, Structure, and Adaptability*. New York: Springer.

Day, P. (1999). Information Policy and Promoting Active Communities in the Information Society. Retrieved from http://www.scn.org/tech/the_network/Proj/ws99/day-pp.html

De Angelis, M. (2006, November 1*). On the "tragedy of the commons* (that is, the tragedy of commons without communities). The Commoner. Retrieved December 4, 2006, from http://www.commoner.org.uk/blog/?p=79

Delgadillo, K., Ricardo, G., & Klaus, S. (2005) Telecentros… ¿para qué? *Lecciones sobre telecentros comunitarios en América Latina y el Caribe*. Quito: Somos@ telecentros.

Delphi Method. Techniques and Applications. Retrieved from http://is.njit.edu/pubs/delphibook/delphibook.pdf

Denzin, N. K. (2001). *Interpretive Interactionism: Applied Social Research Methods*. Thousand Oaks, CA: SAGE Publications.

Dervin, B. (1983, May). *An overview of Sense-Making research: Concepts, methods, and results to date*. Paper presented at the meeting of the International Communication Association, Dallas, TX.

Dhamija, R., & Dusseault, L. (2008). The Seven Flaws of Identity Management: Usability and Security Challenges. *IEEE Security and Privacy, 6*(2), 24–29. doi:10.1109/MSP.2008.49

Dhamija, R., Tygar, J. D., & Hearst, M. (2006). Why Phishing Works. *CHI 2006 Proceedings. ACM Conference Proceedings Series*. ACM Press.

Dhond, G., Ridley, S., & Palmer, M. (1998). The impact of a high-dependency unit on the workload of an intensive care unit. *Anaesthesia, 53*, 841–847. doi:10.1046/j.1365-2044.1998.00522.x

Dietz, P., & Leigh, D. (2001). Diamondtouch: a multi-user touch technology. In *Proceedings of the ACM Symposium on User interface Software and Technology*, USA.

Dijkstra, E. W. (n.d). The next fifty years. Retrieved April 12, 2008 from http://www.cs.utexas.edu/~EWD/ewd12xx/EWD1243.PDF

Dimick, J. B., Pronovost, P. J., Heitmiller, R. F., & Lipsett, P. A. (2001). Intensive care unit physician staffing is associated with decreased length of stay, hospital cost, and complication after esophagal resection. *Critical Care Medicine, 29*(4), 753–758. doi:10.1097/00003246-200104000-00012

Directive 2002/58/EC of the European Parliament and of the Council of 12 July 2002 concerning the processing of personal data and the protection of privacy in the electronic communications sector, Official Journal L No. 201, 31.07.2002.

Directive 95/46/EC of the European Parliament and of the Council of 24 October 1995 on the protection of individuals with regard to the processing of personal data and on the free movement of such data, Official Journal L No. 281, 23.11.1995.

Docherty, P., & Ivanov, K. (1990, 18-21 June). Computer support of decisions in a social-political environment: A case study." Prepared for the IFIP TC 8.3 *Conference on Environments for Supporting Decision Processes*, Budapest, Hungary. Page refs to rev. edition as report UMADP-WPIPCS 26.90, Univ. of Umeå, Institute of Information Processing.

Donabedian, A. (1966). Evaluating the quality of medical care. *The Milbank Memorial Fund Quarterly, 40*, 166–206. doi:10.2307/3348969

Doncaster, C. P., & Davey, J. H. (2007). *Analysis of Variance and Covariance*. Cambridge: Cambridge University Press. doi:10.1017/CBO9780511611377

Donchin, Y., Gopher, D., Olin, M., Badihi, Y., Biesky, M., & Sprung, C. L. (1995). A look into the nature and causes of human errors in the intensive care unit. *Critical Care Medicine, 23*, 294–300. doi:10.1097/00003246-199502000-00015

Dourish, P. (2006). *Implications for Design. CHI: Conference on Human Factors in Computing Systems*. Montréal, Québec, Canada.

Doxiadis, C. A. (1968). *Ekistics: An introduction to the science of human settlements*. New York: Oxford University Press.

Doxiadis, C. A., & Papaioannou, J. G. (1974). *Ecumenopolis: The Inevitable City of the Future*. London: W.W. Norton & Company, Inc.

Draper, E., Wagner, D., Russo, M., Bergner, M., Shortell, S., & Rousseau, D. (1989). Study design - data collection. *Critical Care Medicine, 17*(12), S186–S193. doi:10.1097/00003246-198912000-00007

Driskell, J. E., Radtke, P. H., & Salas, E. (2003). Virtual teams: Effects of technological mediation on team performance. *Group Dynamics, 7*(4), 297–323. doi:10.1037/1089-2699.7.4.297

Droege, P. (Ed.). (1997). *Intelligent Environments - Spatial Aspect of the Information Revolution*. Elsevier. Retrieved from http://books.google.ca/books?id=zo-iwzll0dIC&dq=Intelligent+Environments+-+Spatial+Aspect+of+the+Information+Revolution&printsec=frontcover&source=bl&ots=M8CGS8IO2Y&sig=yK6q4XIZfcA1ShHScyh7eJ5wdBM&hl=en&ei=Vk9aSuLcNom4M72SsEM&sa=X&oi=book_result&ct=result&resnum=1

Drucker, P. F. (1969). *The age of discontinuity: Guidelines to our changing society*. New York: HarperCollins Publishers.

Drucker, P. (1954). *The Practice of Management*. New York: Harper Business Reissue.

Druin, A. (2009). Mobile technologies for the world's children, talk at *Women in ICT lecture series*, Iowa State University, USA, October 9, 2009. Retrieved March 9, 2010 from http://vimeo.com/6990499

Drury, C. G., Holness, K., Ghylin, K. M., & Green, B. D. (2009). Using individual differences to build a common core dataset for aviation security studies. *Theoretical Issues in Ergonomics Science, 10*(5), 459–479. doi:10.1080/14639220802609887

Duquenoy, P. (2009). Taking a holistic approach to exchanging health information over a global network . In Mordini, E., & Permanand, G. (Eds.), *Ethics and health in the Global Village: Bioethics, globalization and human rights* (pp. 287–304). Rome: CIC Edizioni Internazionali.

Duquenoy, P., George, C., & Solomonides, A. (2008b). Considering Something ELSE: Ethical, Legal and Socio-Economic Factors in Medical Imaging and Medical Informatics In H. Muller, G. Xiaohong, L. Shuqian (Eds.), *Special Issue of the International Conference MIMI2007 on 'Medical Imaging and Medical Informatics'* (pp.227-237), Beijing, China. Computer Methods and Programs in Biomedicine, *92* (2008), 2(3). Ireland, Elsevier.

Duquenoy, P., George, G., & Kimppa, K. (Eds.). (2008a). *Ethical, Legal, and Social Issues in Medical Informatics*. IGI Global: Medical Information Science Reference.

Dutton, W. H. (1987). *Wired Cities: Shaping the Future of Communications*. Boston, MA: G. K. Hall & Co.

Eaton, J. J., & Bawden, D. (1991). What kind of resource is information? *International Journal of Information Management*, *11*(2), 156–165. doi:10.1016/0268-4012(91)90006-X

Eccleston, D., & Griseri, L. (2008). How does Web2.0 stretch traditional influencing patterns? *International Journal of Market Research*, *50*(5), 591–616. doi:10.2501/S1470785308200055

Edström, R., & Riis, U. (1997). *Informationsteknik i skolan [Information technology at school.* En fråga om ekonomi och pedagogik. Uppsala Universitet, Uppsala: Pedagogiska Institutionen: Fisch, S. M. (2005). Making Educational Computer Games "Educational." In *Proceedings of the 2005 conference on Interaction Design and Children* (pp. 56-61). Boulder, Colorado. Frankenhauser, M., & Ödman, M. (1983). *Stress: en del av livet [Stress: a part of life].* Brombergs Bokförlag, Stockholm, Sweden.

Egan, T. (2009, June 24). The Self-Service City. *The New York Times, Outposts* (Timothy Egan Blog). Retrieved from http://egan.blogs.nytimes.com/2009/06/24/the-self-service-city/

Egelman, S., Cranor, L., & Hong, J. (2008). You've Been Warned: An Empirical Study of the Effectiveness of Web browser Phishing Warnings. *CH 2008 Proceedings*, Florence/Italy, April 5-10.

Ehn, P. (1988). *Work-oriented design of computer artifacts*. (Doctoral dissertation). University of Umeå, Arbetslivscentrum and Almqvist & Wiksell International. Umeå-Stockholm.

Eichler, M. (1999). Sustainability from a feminist sociological perspective: a frame- work for disciplinary reorientation . In Becker, E., & Johan, T. (Eds.), *Sustainability and the Social Sciences: A Cross-Disciplinary Approach to Integrating Environmental Considerations into Theoretical Reorientation* (pp. 182–206). London: Zed Books and UNESCO.

Eikel, C., & Delbanco, S. (2003). John M. Eisenberg Patient Safety Awards. The Leapfrog Group for Patient Safety: rewarding higher standards. *Joint Commission Journal on Quality and Safety*, *29*(12), 634–639.

Eikelmann, S., Peterson, M., Hasbani, G., & Hajj, J. (2007). The Urgent Need for Companies To Adapt to the Web 2.0 – New Models of Online Consumer Behaviour Demand Changes in Corporate Strategy. *Booz Allen Hamilton.* Retrieved May 8, 2009 from http://www.boozallen.co.uk/media/file/The_Urgent_Need_for_Companies_to_Adapt_to_Web_2.0.pdf

Elovaara, P., & Mörtberg, C. (2007). Design of digital democracies – performance of citizenship, gender and IT. *Information Communication and Society*, *10*(3), 404–423. doi:.doi:10.1080/13691180701410091

Enders, A., Hungenberg, H., Denker, H.-P., & Mauch, S. (2008). The Long Tail of Social Networking - Revenue Models in Social Networking Site. *European Management Journal*, *26*(3), 199–211. doi:10.1016/j.emj.2008.02.002

Eng, T. R. (2001). *The eHealth Landscape: A Terrain Mapping of Emerging Information and Communication Technologies in Health and Health Care*. The Robert Wood Johnson Foundation.

English curriculum and standards framework II. (2000). 375.0009945.

Engstrom, M., Ljunggren, B., Lindqvist, R., & Carlsson, M. (2005). Staff perceptions of job satisfaction and life situation before and 6 and 12 months after increased information technology support in dementia care. *Journal of Telemedicine and Telecare*, *11*(6), 304–309. doi:10.1258/1357633054893292

Epps, J., Lichman, S., & Wu, M. (2006). A study of hand shape use in tabletop gesture interaction. In *Proceedings of the Computer/Human Interaction CHI*, Canada.

Erdmann, L., & Hilty, L. M. (2010). (accepted for publication). Scenario Analysis: Exploring the Macroeconomic Impacts of Information and Communication Technologies on Greenhouse Gas Emissions. *Journal of Industrial Ecology*.

Erdmann, L., Hilty, L. M., Goodman, J., & Arnfalk, P. (2004). *The future impact of ICT on environmental sustainability. Synthesis report. Institute for Prospective Technology Studies*. Sevilla, Spain: IPTS.

Ericson, S. (2001). *A Field Notebook for Oral History* (4th ed.). Idaho Oral History Center. Boise, Idaho: Idaho State Historical Society.

Eriksson, M., Niitamo, V. P., & Kulkki, S. (2005). *State-of-the-art in Utilizing Living Labs Approach to User-centric ICT innovation - a European approach*. Finland: Centre of Distance Spanning Technology at Luleå University of Technology, Sweden, Nokia Oy, Centre for Knowledge and Innovation Research at Helsinki School of Economics.

Escobar, A. (1995). *Encountering Development: The Making and Unmaking of the Third World*. Princeton, NJ: Princeton University Press.

Esenther, A. (2007). *DiamondTouch Mouse Users Manual (Technical Report)*. Cambridge, MA: Mitsubishi Electric Research Laboratories.

Ethics and Human Rights in IT organized by French Commission for UNESCO. Retrieved from portal.unesco.org/ci/en/ev.php-URL

European Commission. (2007). *eHealth priorities and strategies in European countries*. Luxembourg: Office for Official Publications of the European Communities.

European Commission. Directorate-General for Employment, Industrial Relations and Social Affairs (ed.) (1997). *Building the European information society for us all, Final Policy Report of the high-level expert group*. Luxembourg, LU: Office for Official Publications of the European Communities.

Evans, S. A., & Carlson, R. (1992). Nurse-physican collaboration: Solving the nursing shortage crisis. *Journal of the American College of Cardiology, 20*(7), 1669–1673. doi:10.1016/0735-1097(92)90464-X

Evans, C. (1979). *The Mighty Micro: The Impact of the Computer Revolution*. London: Victor Gollancz Ltd.

Ewing, T. (2008). Participation Cycles and Emergent Cultures in an Online Community. *International Journal of Market Research, 50*(5), 575–590. doi:10.2501/S1470785308200043

Eysenbach, G. (2001). What is e-health? *Journal of Medical Internet Research, 3*(2), e20. doi:10.2196/jmir.3.2.e20

Ezoe, S., Araki, S., Ono, Y., Kawakami, N., & Murata, K. (1993). Work stress in Japanese computer engineers: Effects of computer work or bioeducational factors? *Environmental Research, 63*(1), 148–156. doi:10.1006/enrs.1993.1136

Fadel, K. J., & Tanniru, M. (2005). A Knowledge-centric framework for process redesign [Atlanta, Georgia.]. *SIGMIS-CPR, 05*(April), 14–16.

Fairweather, N. B., & Rogerson, S. (2003). The Problems of Global Cultural Homogenisation in a Technologically Dependant World. *Information . Communication & Ethics in Society, 1*(1), 7–12. doi:10.1108/14779960380000221

Ferrari, G. F. F. (2000). *Plato: The Republic.* (T. Griffith, Translation - Original work published 380 BC. New York: Cambridge University Press.

Ferré, F. (1987). *Language, logic, and God* (Reprint of the 1961 ed.). Chicago/London: IL/UK: University of Chicago Press.

Ferretti, G. (1989). La filosofia verso la religione: Itinerari dello spiritualismo e del neotomismo. In Ciancio, Ferretti, Pastore & Perone (Eds.), *lotta con l'angelo: La filosofia degli ultimi due secoli di fronte al Cristianesimo*. Torino, IT: Società Editrice Internazionale SEI.

Ferretti, G. (1989). La ragione ai confini della trascendenza cristiana. In Ciancio, Ferretti, Pastore & Perone (Eds.), *lotta con l'angelo: La filosofia degli ultimi due secoli di fronte al Cristianesimo*. Torino, IT: Società Editrice Internazionale SEI.

Feurstein, K., Hesmer, A., Hribernik, K. A., Thoben, K. D., & Schumacher, J. (2008). Living Labs: A New Development Strategy . In Schumacher, J., & Niitamo, V. P. (Eds.), *European Living Labs - A New Approach for Human Centric Regional Innovation* (pp. 1–14). Berlin, DE: Wissenschaftlicher Verlag.

Field, A. (2005). *Discovering Statistic using SPSS*. London: Sage Publications.

Field, M. J. (Ed.). (1996). *Telemedicine: A Guide to Assessing Telecommunications in Health Care*. Washington, DC: National Academy Press.

Fielding, R. T., & Taylor, R. N. (2000). Principled Design of the Modern Web Architecture. Retrieved from http://www.ics.uci.edu/~fielding/pubs/webarch_icse2000.pdf

Fischer-Hübner, S., Pettersson, J. S., Bergmann, M., Hansen, M., Pearson, S., & Casassa-Mont, M. (2008). *Digital Privacy – Theory, Technologies, and Practices* (Aquisti, , Eds.). Auerbach Publications.

Fischer-Hübner, S., & Pettersson, J. S. (Eds.). (2004). Evaluation of early prototypes. PRIME deliverable D6.1.b.

Fischer-Hübner, S., Köffel, Ch., Wästlund, E., & Wolkerstorfer, P., (2009). PrimeLife HCI Research Report, Version V1. PrimeLife EU FP7 Project Deliverable D4.1.1.

Fisher, W. R. (1987). Technical logic, rhetorical logic, and narrative rationality. Argumentation: *An International.* [Dordrecht]. *Journal. on Reasoning, 1*(1), 3–21.

Fitts, P. M. (1954). The information capacity of the human motor system in controlling the amplitude of movement. *Journal of Experimental Psychology, 47*(6), 381–391. doi:10.1037/h0055392

Fitts, P. M. (1954). The information capacity of the human motor system in controlling the amplitude of movement. *Journal of Experimental Psychology, 47*(6), 381–391. doi:10.1037/h0055392

Fleishacker, S. (1999). From Cultural Diversity to Universal Ethics: Three Models. *Cultural Dynamics, 11*(1), 105–128. doi:10.1177/092137409901100107

Flood, R. L., & Ulrich, W. (1990). Testament to conversations on critical systems: Thinking between two systems practitioners. *Systems Practice, 3*(1), 7–29. doi:10.1007/BF01062819

Flood, R. L. (1989). Liberating systems theory: A summary and literature review. Proceedings of the ISSS Int. Society for the Systems Sciences, *33rd Annual Conference: Vol. 2*, Edinburgh, Scotland (With a bibliography of 34 entries.)

Floridi, L. (2007). A Look into the Future Impact of ICT on Our Lives. *Journal of the Information Society, 23*(1), 59–64. doi:10.1080/01972240601059094

Følstad, A. (2008). Living Labs for Innovation and Development of Information and Communication Technology: A Literature Review. *The Electronic Journal for Virtual Organisations and Networks, 10*, 100–131.

Forlines, C., Wigdor, D., Shen, C., & Balakrishnan, R. (2007). Direct-touch vs. mouse input for tabletop displays. In *Proceedings of the 2007 SIGCHI conference on human factors in computing systems*, (pp. 647-656) USA

Forsgren, O. (1988). *Samskapande datortillämpningar [Constructive computer applications]* (Doctoral diss., Report UMADP-RRIPCS-3.88.). University of Umeå, Inst. of Information Processing.

Forsgren, O. (1989). The first "co": A prototype of a learning co-constructor." Proceedings of the ISSS Int. Society for the Systems Sciences, *33rd Annual Conference, Vol. 1*, Edinburgh, Scotland.

Forsgren, O., & Ivanov, K. (1989, April). *From hypertext to hypersystem*. Prepared for the EMCSR 90, Tenth European Meeting on Cybernetics and Systems Research, Vienna, Austria. 1990. Umeå University, Inst. of Information Processing.

Forsythe, D. (1993). The construction of work in artificial intelligence. *Science, Technology & Human Values, 18*(4), 460–479. doi:10.1177/016224399301800404

Fort, T. (2001). *Ethics and Governance: Business as Mediating Institutions*. New York: Oxford University Press.

Franklin, U. M. (1999). *Real World Technology* (Rev. edition). Concord, ON: House of Anansi Press.

Frauenfelder, M. (2005). *The computer*. London: Carlton Books.

Freire, P. (1972). *Pedagogy of the Oppressed*. Middlesex, UK: Penguin Books.

Frese, M., & Zapf, D. (1988). Methodological Issues in the Study of Work Stress: Objective vs Subjective Measurement of Work Stress and the Question of Longitudinal Studies . In Cooper, C. L., & Payne, R. (Eds.), *Causes, Coping and Consequences of Stress at Work* (pp. 375–411). New York: John Wiley & Sons Ltd.

Frey, L. A., White, K. P., & Huchinson, T. E. (1990). Eye-Gaze word processing. *IEEE Transactions on Systems, Man, and Cybernetics, 20*, 944–950. doi:10.1109/21.105094

Friedman, T. L. (2006). *The world is flat* (2nd ed.). London: Penguin Books Limited.

Friedman, A. L., & Dominic, S. C. (1991). *Computer Systems Development: History, Organisation and Implementation*. New York, NY: John Wiley.

Frost, R. (1920). *Collected Poems, prose and plays, 7*. New York: Library of America.

Frost, S. H., & Paul, M. J. (2003). Bridging the disciplines: Interdisciplinary discourse and faculty scholarship. *The Journal of Higher Education, 74*, 119–143. doi:10.1353/jhe.2003.0013

FSO - Federal Statistical Office. (2008). *Environmental Accounting. Swiss Confederation*. Neuchatel.

Fuénmayor, R. (1989). Interpretive systemology: A critical approach to interpretive systems thinking. Proceedings of the ISSS Int. Society for the Systems Sciences, *33rd Annual Conference: Vol. 2,* Edinburgh, Scotland.

Fuenzalida, V. (2000). *La television pública en América Latina: reforma o privatización*. México: FCE.

Fussell, S. R., Kiesler, S., Sctlock, L. D., Scupelli, P., & Weisband, S. (2004). Effects of Instant Messaging on the Management of Multiple Project Trajectories. In *Proceedings of CHI 2004* (pp. 191-198), New York: ACM Publications.

Gagne, R. M. (1985). *The conditions of learning: And the theory of instruction* (4th ed.). New York: Holt/Rinehart/Winston.

Galbi, D. A. (2003). *Communications policy, media development, and convergence*. Retrieved from http://www.galbithink.org/media.htm

Gant, D., & Kiesler, S. (2001). Blurring the Boundaries: Cell Phones, Mobility, and the Line between Work and Personal Live . In Brown, B., Green, N., & Harper, R. (Eds.), *Wireless World: Social and Interactional Aspects of the Mobile Age* (pp. 121–131). London: Springer-Verlag.

Garbarino, E. C., & Edell, J. A. (1997). Cognitive effort, affect, and choice. *The Journal of Consumer Research, 24*(2), 147–158. doi:10.1086/209500

Garfinkel, S. L. (2005). *Design Principles and Patterns for Computer Systems That Are Simultaneously Secure and Usable*. PhD Dissertation, Massachusetts Institute of Technology, May 2005.

Garson, B. (1988). *The Electronic Sweatshop: How Computers are Transforming the Office of the Future into the Factory of the Past*. New York: Simon and Schuster.

Garvin, D. A. (1980). *The economics of university behavior*. New York, NY: Academic Press.

Gaver, B., Beaver, J., & Benford, S. (2003). Ambiguity as a resource for design. In G. Cockton & P. Korhonen (Eds.), *Proceedings of the SIGCHI conference on Human Factors in Computing Systems* (pp. 233–240). ACM Conference Proceedings Series. New York: ACM Press.

Geertz, C. (1983). *Local Knowledge: Further Essays in Interpretive Anthropology*. Basic Books.

Geertz, C. (1983). The way we think now: Toward an ethnography of modern thought . In *Local knowledge: Further essays in interpretive anthropology*. New York, NY: Basic Books.

Gibbons, M., Limoges, C., Nowotny, H., Schwartzman, S., Scott, P., & Trow, M. (1994). *The new production of knowledge: The dynamics of science and research in contemporary societies*. London: Sage Publications.

Gibson, M., Jenkings, K. N., Wilson, R., & Purves, I. (2005). Multi-tasking in Practice" Coordinated Activities in the Computer Supported Doctor-Patient Consultation. *International Journal of Medical Informatics*, 74(6), 425–436. doi:10.1016/j.ijmedinf.2005.04.002

Gibson, C. B., & Cohen, S. G. (Eds.). (2003). *The last work - conclusions and implications. Virtual Teams That Work - Creating Conditions for Virtual Team Effectiveness*. San Francisco, CA: Jossey Bass.

Gibson, C. B., & Gibbs, J. L. (2006). Unpacking the concept of virtuality: The effects of geographic dispersion, electronic dependence, dynamice structure and national diversity on team diversity. *Administrative Science Quarterly*, 51(3), 451–495.

Gibson, B. (2007). Enabling an Accessible Web 2.0. *In: W4A2007 - Keynote, Banff, Canada. Co-Located with the 16th International World Wide Web Conference*.

Gibson, D. V., & Ludl, E. J. (1988). Group decision support systems and organizational context. In R.M. Lee, A.M. Cosh & P. Migliarese (Eds.), *Organizational decision support systems*. Amsterdam, NL: North-Holland.

Giddens, A. (1990). *The consequences of modernity*. Cambridge, UK: Polity.

Giddens, A. (2000). *Runaway world*. London, UK: Routledge.

Giddens, A. (1976). *New Rules of Sociological Method: A Positive Critique of Interpretative Sociologies*. London: Hutchinson.

Giddens, A. (1979). *Central Problems in Social Theory: Action, Structure and Contradiction in Social Analysis*. Berkeley, CA: University of California Press.

Giddens, A. (1984). *The Constitution of Society: Outline of the Theory of Structuration*. Berkeley, CA: University of California Press.

Giddens, A. (2000). *Runaway World: How Globalization Is Reshaping Our Lives*. New York: Routledge.

Giddens, A. (1984). *The Constitution of Society*. Los Angeles: Univ California Press.

Giddens, A. (1979). *Central problems in social theory: action, structure and contradiction in social analysis*. Berkeley: University of California Press.

Giddens, A. (1984). *The constitution of society: Outline of the theory of structuration*. Cambridge, UK: Polity Press.

Glenn, F. A., III, Iavecchia, H. P., Ross, L. V., Stokes, J. M., Weiland, W. J., Weiss, D. Z., & Allen, L. (1986). Eyevoicecontrolled interface. In *Proceedings of the Human Factors Society*, (pp. 322-326).

Global Humanitarian Forum. (2009). *The Anatomy of a Silent Crisis*. Geneva. Retrieved June 2, 2009 from http://www.ghf-geneva.org/

Godejord, P. A. (2009). GÅ INN I DIN TID – Fra ide til handling. for Informatikk, HiNe. (English: Getting Involved - From Idea to Action (In Norwegian)). Retrieved from http://www.scribd.com/doc/12777702/Getting-Involved-From-Idea-to-Action-In-Norwegian Government of Canada. Industry Canada. (2000). *Smart Communities*. Report of the National Selection Committee. Retrieved from http://smartcommunities.ic.gc.ca

Godman, D. (1991). *Be as You Are: The Teachings of Sri Ramana Maharshi*. New York: Penguin Book.

Goertzel, B. (2004). Universal Ethics: The Foundations of Compassion in Pattern Dynamics. Retrieved from www.goertzel.org.

Goffman, E. (1974). *Jaget och maskerna* [Eng. The Presentation of Self in Everyday Life]. Stockholm: Rabén & Sjögren.

Gogging, N. L., & Stelmach, G. E. (1990). Age-related Differences in a Kinematic Analysis of Precued Movements. *Canadian Journal on Aging*, 9, 371–385.

Goleman, D. (1995). *Emotional Intelligence*. New York: Bantam Books.

Goleman, D. (2006). *Social Intelligence*. New York: Bantam Books.

Goniak, K. (1996). The Computer Revolution and Problem of Global Ethics. *Science and Engineering Ethics*, 2(2), 177–190. doi:10.1007/BF02583552

Gonzálas, V. M., & Mark, G. (2004). Constant, Constant, Multi-tasking Craziness: Managing Multiple Working Sphere . *CHI*, 6(1), 113–120.

Gonzálas, V. M., & Mark, G. (2005). Managing Currents of Work: Multi-tasking among Multiple Collaborations. In *Proceedings of the 9th European Conference of Computer-supported Cooperative Work (ECSCW '05)* (pp. 143-162), The Netherlands: Springer.

Goodfellow, A., Varnam, R., Rees, D., & Shelly, M. P. (1997). Staff stress on the intensive care unit: a comparison of doctors and nurses. *Anaesthesia*, 52, 1037–1041. doi:10.1111/j.1365-2044.1997.213-az0348.x

Google Wave. (2009). Retrieved December 2009 from http://wave.google.com/

Göranzon, B., Florin, M., & Sällström, P. (1988). Dialogue. *AI & Society*, 2(4), 279–286. doi:10.1007/BF01891362

Gorbov, F. D., & Lebedev, V. I. (1975). *Psychoneurological Aspects of the Work of Operators*. Moscow: Medicine Publishers. (in Russian)

Gordon, T. (1970). *P. E. T. - Parent Effectiveness Training*.

Gould, S. J. (2003). *The hedgehog, the fox, and the magister's pox*. New York, NY: Harmony Books.

Graham, S. (Ed.). (2004a). *The Cybercities Reader*. London: Routledge.

Graham, S. (2004b). From dreams of transcendence to the remediation of urban life . In Graham, S. (Ed.), *The Cybercities Reader* (pp. 1–29). London: Routledge.

Graham, S. (2004c). The Software-Sorted City: Rethinking the "Digital Divide." . In Graham, S. (Ed.), *The Cybercities Reader* (pp. 324–331). London: Routledge.

Graham, S., & Marvin, S. (2004). Planning Cyber-Cities? Integrating Telecommunications into Urban Planning . In Graham, S. (Ed.), *The Cybercities Reader* (pp. 341–347). London: Routledge.

Grandt, M., Pfendler, C., & Mooshage, O. (2003). Empirical comparison of five input devices for anti-air warfare operators. In *Proceedings of the 8th International Command and Control Research and Technology Symposium (ICCRTS) on "Information Age Transformation"*, Washington DC.

Green, H. (1971). Human Values in Technological Society. *Dimensions of American Judaism*, 5, 19–23.

Greenbaum, J. (1993). A design of one's own: towards participatory design in the United States . In Schuler, D., & Namioka, A. (Eds.), *Participatory Design, Principles and Practices* (pp. 27–37). Hillsdale, NJ: Lawrence Erlbaum Associates.

Greenstein, J. S. (1997). Pointing devices. In M. G. Helander, T. K. Landauer, & P. V. Prabhu (Eds.), *Handbook of human-computer interaction* (pp. 1317-1348). Amsterdam: Elsevier Science.

Gregorian, V. (2004). Colleges must reconstruct the unity of knowledge. *The Chronicle of Higher Education*, 4(June), B12.

Gregory, D. (1986). Time-Geography. In R. J. Johnston, D. Gregory & D. M. Smith. *The Dictionary of Human Geography* (pp. 485-487). Oxford: Blackwell Reference.

Gregory, D. (1986). Time-Space Distanciation. In R. J. Johnston, D. Gregory & D. M. Smith. *The Dictionary of Human Geography* (pp. 487-492). Oxford: Blackwell Reference.

Gregory, W. J. (1989). Critical theory and critical systems heuristics: The history and development of an emancipatory systems approach to social change. Proceedings of the ISSS Int. Society for the Systems Sciences, *33rd Annual Conference: Vol.2,* Edinburgh, Scotland.

Greif, I. (Ed.). (1988). *Computer supported cooperative work: A book of readings*. San Mateo, CA: Morgan Kaufman.

Griffin, D. R. (Ed.). (1989). *Archetypal process: Self and divine in Whitehead, Jung, and Hillman*. Evanston, Ill: Northwestern University Press.

Griffin, D. R. (1989). A metaphysical psychology to un-Locke our ailing world . In David, D. R. (Ed.), *Archetypal process: Self and divine in Whitehead, Jung, and Hillman* (pp. 239–250). Evanston, Ill: Northwestern University Press.

Grint, K., Case, P., & Willcocks, L. (1996). Business Process Reengineering Reappraised: The Politics and Technology of Forgetting. In W.J., Orlikowski, G., Walsham, G., & M. Jones (Eds.), *Proceedings of the IFIP WG8.2 Working Conference on Information Technology and Changes in Organizational Work*, December 1995. London, UK: Chapman & Hall.

Grip, A. (1974). *ADB-system och kommunikation (Data processing and communication)*. Lund, Sweden: Hermods-studentlitteratur.

Groeger, J. S., Strosberg, M. A., Halpern, N. A., Raphaely, R. C., Kaye, W. E., & Guntupalli, K. K. (1992). Descriptive analysis of critical care units in the United States. *Critical Care Medicine*, *20*(6), 846–863. doi:10.1097/00003246-199206000-00024

Gross, E. F. (2004). Adolescent Internet use: What we expect, what teens report. *Journal of Applied Developmental Psychology*, *25*(1), 633–649. doi:10.1016/j.appdev.2004.09.005

Groth, D. P. (2004). Information Provenance and the Knowledge Rediscovery Problem. In *Proceedings of the Eighth International Conference on Information Visualization*, (pp. 345-351). Washington: IEEE Computer Society.

Grynbaum, M. M. (2009). Cabbies Stay on Their Phones Despite Ban. *New York Times*. Retrieved August 4, 2009 from http://www.nytimes.com/2009/08/04/nyregion/04taxi.html

Guilford, J. (1967). *The nature of human intelligence*. New York: McGraw-Hill.

Gulbenkian Commission on the Restructuring of the Social Sciences. (1996). *Open the social sciences*. Stanford, CA: Stanford University Press.

Günther, O., & Spiekermann, S. (2005). RFID and the perception of control: The consumer's view, in *Communications of the ACM, 48*(9), 73-76.

Gurses, A. P., Carayon, P., & Wall, M. (2009). Impact of performance obstacles on intensive care nurses' workload, perceived quality and safety of care, and quality of working life. *Health Services Research*, *44*(2), 422–443. doi:10.1111/j.1475-6773.2008.00934.x

Gurstein, M. (2000). *Community Informatics: Enabling Communities with Information and Communication Technologies*. Hershey, PA: Idea Group Publishing.

Gurstein, M. (2003). Effective use: A community informatics strategy beyond the digital divide. *First Monday*, *8*(12). Retrieved from http://firstmonday.org/htbin/cgiwrap/bin/ojs/index.php/fm/article/view/1107/1027.

Gurstein, M. (2007). *What Is Community Informatics (and Why Does It Matter)*? Milan, IT: Polimetrica.

Gurstein, M. (2007). What is Community informatics? (And Why Does It Matter). Polimetrica, Milan. Retrieved from http://eprints.rclis.org/12372/1/WHAT_IS_COMMUNITY_INFORMATICS_reading.pdf

Habermas, J. (1989). *The structural transformation of the public sphere*. Cambridge, UK: Polity.

Habermas, J. (1990). *Die Idee der Universität-Lernprozesse. Eine Art Schadensabwicklung. 1987 Suhrkamp. Frankfurt a.M. Swedish trans*. Umeå, Sweden: K. Nilsson, Umeå University, Inst. of Information Processing.

Hagerstrand, T. (1975). Space, Time and Human Conditions. Dynamic Allocation of Urban Space . In Karlqvist, A., Lundqvist, L., & Snickars, F. (Eds.), *Westmead, Hans* (pp. 3–14). Lexington, MA: Lexington Books.

Hagerstrand, T. (1970). What about People in Regional Science? *Papers and Proceedings of the Regional Science Association, 24,* 7-21.

Hahn, U., & Jarke, M. (1988). A multi-agent reasoning model for negotiation support. Organizational decision support systems. In R.M. Lee, A.M. Cosh & P. Migliarese (Eds.), *Organizational decision support systems.* Amsterdam, NL: North-Holland.

Haigh, T. (2006). Remembering the Office of the Future: The Origins of Word Processing and Office Automation. *IEEE Annals of the History of Computing, 4*(5), 6–31. doi:10.1109/MAHC.2006.70

Hakanen, J., Bakker, A. B., & Schaullefi, W. B. (2006). Burnout and work engagement among teachers. *Journal of School Psychology, 43*(3), 495–513. doi:10.1016/j.jsp.2005.11.001

Halpern, N. A., Pastores, S. M., & Greenstein, R. J. (2004). Critical care medicine in the United States 1985-2000: An analysis of bed numbers, use, and costs. *Critical Care Medicine, 32*(6), 1254–1259. doi:10.1097/01.CCM.0000128577.31689.4C

Halverson, C. (2002). Activity Theory and Distributed Cognition: Or What Does CSCW Need to Do with Theories? *Computer Supported Cooperative Work, 11*(1/2), 243–267. doi:10.1023/A:1015298005381

Han, J. (2006). Multi-Touch Interaction Research. Retrieved December 2009 form http://cs.nyu.edu/~jhan/ftirtouch/

Han, J. Y. (2005). Low-cost multi-touch sensing through frustrated total internal reflection. In *Proceedings of the 18th Annual ACM Symposium on User Interface Software and Technology* (pp. 115-118). New York: ACM Press.

Hancock, P. A., Hancock, G. M., & Warm, J. S. (2009). Individuation: the N = 1 revolution. *Theoretical Issues in Ergonomics Science, 10*(5), 481–488. doi:10.1080/14639220903106387

Handy, C. (1995). Trust and the Virtual Organization. *Harvard Business Review, 73*(3), 40–50.

Hansen, K. K., Larsen, C. F., & Olsen, J. B. (2006). P2P: Information Exchange & Knowledge Production. Retrieved from http://rudar.ruc.dk/bitstream/1800/2941/1/P2P%20Production.pdf

Hanson, C. W., Deutschman, C. S., Anderson, H. L., Reilly, P. M., Behringer, E. C., Schwab, C. W., & Price, J. (1999). Effects of an organized critical care service on outcomes and resource utilization: A cohort study. *Critical Care Medicine, 27*(2), 270–274. doi:10.1097/00003246-199902000-00030

Hanson, M. (2004). *Det flexibla arbetets villkor [The conditions for flexible work].* Doctoral Thesis. National Institute for Working Life. Stockholms University.

Haraway, D. J. (1991). *Simians, Cyborgs, and Women: The Reinvention of Nature.* New York: Routledge.

Hardin, G. (1968). The Tragedy of the Commons. *Science, 62,* 1243–1248.

Harper, R., Rodden, T., Rogers, Y., & Sellen, A. (Eds.). (2008). *Being Human: Human-Computer Interaction in the year 2020.* Cambridge, UK: Microsoft Research Ltd.

Harper, R. (2001). The mobile interface: old technologies and new arguments. In Brown, B., Green, N., & Harper, R. (Eds.), *Wireless World: Social and Interactional Aspects of the Mobile Age* (pp. 207–223). London: Springer-Verlag.

Harr, R. (2009). *Striking a balance: managing collaborative multitasking in computer-supported cooperation.* Doctoral dissertation, Department of Informatics, Umeå University, Sweden.

Harris, T. A. (1969). *I'm OK - You're OK.* Quill.

Harris, J. (2006). No distaste for paste (Why the UI, Part 7). Retrieved December 2009 from http://blogs.msdn.com/jensenh/archiove/2006/04/07/570798.aspx

Harvey, O. J., Hunt, D. E., & Shroder, H. M. (1961). *Conceptual Systems and Personality Organization.* New York: Wiley.

Harvey, O. J. (1966). Experience, Structure, Flexibility, and Creativity . In Harvey, O. J. (Ed.), *Experience, Structure, and Adaptability.* New York: Springer.

Hawkes, J. (2001). *The fourth pillar of sustainability: culture's essential role in public planning, The Cultural Development Network*, Australia, [Online]. Retrieved April 17, 2008 from http://www.cultureandcommunities. ca/downloads/Salons/Salon3-handout.pdf

Hawthorn, D. (1998). Psychophysical Aging and Human Computer Interface Design. In *Proceedings of the Australasian Computer Human Interaction Conference.*

Hay, D., & Oken, D. (1977). The pscyhological stresses of intensive care unit nursing . In Moos, R. H. (Ed.), *Coping with physical illness* (pp. 381–396). New York: McGraw Hill.

Haythornthwaite, C., Bowker, G., Bruce, B., Lunsford, K., Kazmer, M., Brown, J., et al. (2003). Technical Report: *Challenges in the Practice and Study of Distributed, Interdisciplinary, Collaboration.* Retrieved from http://www. igi-global.com/Bookstore/Chapter.aspx?TitleId=27290

Hearn, G., Foth, M., & Gray, H. (2008). Applications and implementations of new media in corporate communications. An action research approach. *Corporate Communications: An International Journal, 14*(1), 49–61. doi:10.1108/13563280910931072

Heeks, R. (2002). Information Systems and Developing Countries: Failure, Success, and Local Improvisations. *The Information Society, 18*(2), 101–112. doi:10.1080/01972240290075039

Heidegger, M. (1962). *Being and Time.* (translated by J. Macquarrie). New York, NY: Harper & Row: New York.

Heiskanen, E., Halme, M., Jalas, M., Kärnä, A., & Lovio, R. (2001). *Dematerialisation: The Potential of ICT and Services.* Helsinki, Finland: Ministry of the Environment.

Hempel, P. S. (2004). Preparing the HR profession for technology and information work. *Human Resource Management, 43*(2-3), 163–177. doi:10.1002/hrm.20013

Hempel, J. (2007). Tapping the Wisdom of the Crowd. *Business Week Online,* 27.

Hendrick, H. W. (1979). Differences in Group Problem-Solving Behavior and Effectiveness as a Function of Abstractness. *The Journal of Applied Psychology, 64*(5), 518–525. doi:10.1037/0021-9010.64.5.518

Hendrick, H. W. (1990). Perceptual Accuracy of Self and Others and Leadership Status as Functions of Cognitive Complexity . In Clark, K. E., & Clark, M. B. (Eds.), *Measures of leadership* (pp. 511–520). West Orange, NJ: Leadership Library of America.

Hendrick, H. W. (1981). Abstractness, Conceptual Systems, and the Functioning of Complex Organizations . In England, G., Negandhi, A., & Wilpert, B. (Eds.), *The Functioning of Complex Organizations* (pp. 25–50). Cambridge, MA: Oelgeschalger, Gunn & Hain.

Hendrick, H. W. (1986). Matching Individual and Job Complexity: Validation of Stratified Systems Theory. In *Proceedings of the Human Factors Society 30th Annual Meeting* (pp. 999-1001). Santa Monica, CA: Human Factors Society.

Henning, R. A., Jacques, P., & Kissel, G. V. (1997). Frequent short rest breaks from computer work: Effects on productivity and well-being at two field sites. *Ergonomics, 40*(1), 78–91. doi:10.1080/001401397188396

Herman, R., Ardeni, S. A., & Ausubel, J. H. (1990). Dematerialization. *Technological Forecasting and Social Change, 38,* 333–347. doi:10.1016/0040-1625(90)90003-E

Hertel, G., Geister, S., & Konradt, U. (2005). Managing virtual teams: A review of current empirical research. *Human Resource Management Review, 15,* 69–95. doi:10.1016/j.hrmr.2005.01.002

Herzog, A. (2007). *Usable Security Policies in Runtime Environments.* Linköping Studies in Science and Technology, Dissertation No. 1075. Linköping University.

Heylighen, F., & Joslyn, C. (2001). Cybernetics and second order cybernetics. In *Encyclopaedia of Physical Science & Technology* (3rd ed., pp. 155-170), 4.

Hilty, L. M. (2008a). *Information Technology and Sustainability: Essays on the Relationship between ICT and Sustainable Development*. Norderstedt, DE: Books on Demand.

Hilty, L. M., Arnfalk, P., Erdmann, L., Goodman, J., Lehmann, M., & Wäger, A. P. (2006a). The Relevance of Information and Communication Technologies for Environmental Sustainability - A Prospective Simulation Study. *Environmental Modelling & Software, 21*(11), 1618–1629. doi:10.1016/j.envsoft.2006.05.007

Hilty, L. M., & Köhler, A., Von Schéele, F., Zah, F., & Ruddy, T. (2006b). Rebound Effects of Progress in Information Technology. *Poiesis & Praxis . International Journal of Technology Assessment and Ethics of Science, 4*(1), 19–38.

Hilty, L. M. (2008b). Emerging Risks in Information Infrastructures – A Technology Assessment Perspective. In *Proceedings of IDRC 2008, International Disaster Reduction Conference*, Davos, Switzerland.

Himanen, P. (2001). *The Hacker Ethic and the Spirit of the Information Age*. New York: Random House.

Hinckley, K. (2008). Input technologies and techniques . In Sears, A., & Jacko, J. A. (Eds.), *The human-computer interaction handbook: fundamentals, evolving technologies, and emerging applications* (p. 161). Taylor & Francis CRC Press.

Hinds, P. J., & Kiesler, S. (1995). Communication across boundaries: Work, structure, and the use of communication technologies in a large organization. *Organization Science, 6*, 373–393. doi:10.1287/orsc.6.4.373

Hinds, P. J., & Weisband, S. P. (2003). Knowledge sharing and shared understanding in virtual teams . In Gibson, C. B., & Cohen, S. G. (Eds.), *Virtual Teams That Work* (pp. 21–36). San Francisco, CA: Jossey-Bass.

Hirschheim, R., Klein, H. K., & Lyytinen, K. (1996). Exploring the Intellectual Structures of Information Systems Development: A Social Action Theoretic Analysis. *Accounting . Management and Information Technologies, 6*(1-2), 1–64. doi:10.1016/0959-8022(96)00004-5

Hirschheim, R., & Klein, H. K. (1989). Four paradigms of information systems development. *CACM, 32*(10), 1199–1216.

Hischier, R., & Hilty, L. M. (2002). Environmental Impacts of an International Conference. *Environmental Impact Assessment Review, 22*(5), 543–557. doi:10.1016/S0195-9255(02)00027-6

Hislop, D. (2008). Conceptualizing knowledge work utilizing skill and knowledge-based concepts. *Management Learning, 39*(5), 579–596. doi:10.1177/1350507608098116

Hjortskov, N., Rissen, D., Blangsted, A. K., Fallentin, N., Lundberg, U., & Sogaard, K. (2004). The effect of mental stress on heart rate and blood pressure during computer work. *European Journal of Applied Physiology, 92*(1-2), 84–89. doi:10.1007/s00421-004-1055-z

Hoare, C. A. R. (1975). Software Design: a Parable. *Software World, 5*(9 &10), 53–56.

Hodges, S., Izadi, S., Butler, A., Rrustemi, A., & Buxton, B. (2007). ThinSight: versatile multi-touch sensing for thin form-factor displays. In *Proceedings of the 20th annual ACM symposium on User interface Software and Technology*. USA, Newport, Rhode Island.

Hofkirchner, W., & Maier-Rabler, U. (2004). The Ethos of the Great Bifurcation. *International Journal of Information Ethics, 2*(11), 1–11.

Hofkirchner, W. (Ed.). (1997). Vladimir I. Vernadskij, Der Mensch in der Biosphäre, Zur Naturgeschichte der Vernunft. Wien, AU: Peter Lang.

Hofkirchner, W., & Fuchs, C. (2003). The Architecture of the Information Society. In J. Wilby. & J. K. Allen (Eds.), *Proceedings of the 47th Annual Conference*, ISSS (pp. 1-10). The International Society of the Systems Sciences.

Hofkirchner, W., Fuchs, C., Raffl, C., Schafranek, M., Sandoval, M., & Bichler, R. (2007). ICTs and Society – The Salzburg Approach. Towards a Theory for, about, and by means of the Information Society. In ICT&S Center Research Paper Series, 3. Retrieved from http://icts.sbg.ac.at/media/pdf/pdf1490.pdf

Högg, R., Meckel, M., Stanoevska-Slabeva, K., & Martignoni, R. (2006). 2.0 Communities . In *Proceedings of GeNeMe Conference* (pp. 23–37). Dresden, Germany: Overview of Business Models for Web.

Hollan, J., Hutchins, E., & Kirsh, D. (2000). Distributed Cognition: Toward a New Foundation for Human-Computer Interaction Research. *ACM Transactions on Computer-Human Interaction*, 7(2), 174–196. doi:10.1145/353485.353487

Hollan, J., & Stornetta, S. (1992). Beyond being there. In *Proceedings of the ACM CHI Conference.* May 3 -7, (pp. 119-125).

Hollnagel, E. (Ed.). (2003). *Handbook of cognitive task design*. London: Lawrence Erlbaum Ass.

Hollnagel, E. (2003a). Prolegomenon to cognitive task design . In Hollnagel, E. (Ed.), *Handbook of cognitive task design* (pp. 3–15). London: Lawrence Erlbaum Ass.

Holst, M., & Ståhlbröst, A. (2006). Enriching the Process of Appreciating Needs with Storytelling. *International Journal of Technology . Knowledge and Society*, 2(4), 61–68.

Holst, M., & Mirijamdotter, A. (2006). Framing Multi-Disciplinary Teams: Sense Making Through the POM-model. In A. Basden, A. Mirijamdotter, & S. Strijbos (Eds.), *12th Annual CPTS Working Conference - Integrating Visions of Technology* (pp. 111-131). Maarssen, The Netherlands.

Holton, J. (2001). Building trust and collaboration in a virtual team. *Team Performance Management: An International Journal*, 7(3/4), 36–47. doi:10.1108/13527590110395621

Holzman, P., & Klein, G. (1954). Cognitive-system principles of levelling and sharpening: Individual differences in visual time-error assimilation effects. *The Journal of Psychology*, 37, 105–122.

Homes, D. (2004). Cybercommuniting on an Information Superhighway: The Case of Melbourne's CityLink . In Graham, S. (Ed.), *The Cybercities Reader* (pp. 341–347). London: Routledge.

Hongladarom, S., & Ess, C. (Eds.). (2007). *Information Technology Ethics: Cultural Perspectives*. Hershey, PA: Idea Group Inc.

Hongladarom, S. (2001). Cultures and Global Justice. *Polylog: Forum for Intercultural Philosophizing*, 2, 1–34.

Hongladarom, S. (2007). Information Divie, Information Flow and Global Justice. *International Review of Information Ethics*, 7, 1–5.

Hoonakker, P. L. T., Carayon, P., Douglas, S., Schultz, K., Walker, J., & Wetterneck, B. T. (2008). Communication in Intensive Care Units and the Relation with Quality of Care and Patient Safety . In Snelwar, L. I., Mascia, F. L., & Montedo, U. B. (Eds.), *Human Factors in Organizational Design and Management, IX* (pp. 715–721). Santa Monica, CA: IEA Press.

House, J. S., Landis, K. R., & Umberson, D. (1988). Social Networks and Mortality . *Science*, 241, 540–545. doi:10.1126/science.3399889

Huang, J., & Fox, M. S. (2004, May). Uncertainty in Knowledge Provenance. In *Proceedings of the 1st European Semantic Web Symposium*, Heraklion, Greece (LNCS).

Huckauf, A., & Urbina, M. (2007). Gazing with pEYE: new concepts in eye typing. In *Proceedings of the 4th symposium on Applied perception in graphics and visualization* (pp.141-141).

Hunt, D. E. (1966). A Conceptual Systems Change Model and its Application to Education . In Harvey, O. J. (Ed.), *Experience, Structure and Adaptability*. New York: Springer.

Hutcheson, F. (1729). *An Inquiry Concerning Moral Good and Evil.* Retrieved from www.encylopedia.com/doc/1E1-Hutcheso.html

Hutchins, E. (1996). *Cognition in the Wild*. Boston, MA: MIT Press.

Hutchinson, T. E., White, K. P., Martin, W. N., Reichert, K. C. & Frey, L. A. (1989). Human-Computer Interaction Using Eye-Gaze Input. *IEEE Transactions on systems, man, and cybernetics*.

Huws, U. (2003). *The Making of a Cybertariat: Virtual Work in a Real World*. New York: Monthly Review Press.

Hyman, I.E., Boss, S.M., Wise, B.M., McKenzie, K.E., & Caggiano, J.M. (2009). Did You See the Unicycling Clown? Inattentional Blindness while Walking and Talking on a Cell Phone, *Applied Cognitive Psychology*. Published online in Wiley InterScience.doi: 10.1002/acp.1638

Iacono, C. S., & Weisband, S. (1997). Developing trust in virtual teams. *Thirtieth Hawaii International Conference on System Sciences*. Wailea, HI.

IBM. (2008). *Putting the Power of Web 2.0 into Practice – How Rich Internet Applications can deliver Tangible Business Benefits*. IBM Corporation, Cambridge, USA. Available at: ftp://ftp.software.ibm.com/software/lotus/lotusweb/product/expeditor/LOW14003-USEN-00.pdf [last accessed 04.08.09]

Intelligent Community Forum (ICF). (2008). *Intelligent Community Indicators*. Retrieved from http://www.intelligentcommunity.org/index.php?submenu=Research&src=gendocs&ref=Research_Intelligent_Community_Indicators&category=Research

Iqbal, S. T., Adamczyk, P. D., Zheng, X. S., & Bailey, B. P. (2005). *Towards an Index of Opportunity: Understanding Changes in Mental Workload during Task Execution*. *CHI 2005* (pp. 311–320). New York: ACM Publications.

Iqbal, S. T., & Horvitz, E. (2007). Disruption and Recovery of Computing Tasks: Field Study, Analysis, and Directions. [New York: ACM Publications.]. *CHI, 2007,* 677–686.

Iqbal, S. T., & Bailey, B. P. (2005). Investigating the Effectiveness of Mental Workload as a Predictor of Opportune Moments for Interruption. In *Proceedings of the CHI 2005* (pp. 311-320). New York: ACM Publications.

Iqbal, S. T., & Bailey, B. P. (2006). Leveraging Characteristics of Task Structure to Predict the Cost of Interruption. In *Proceedings of the CHI 2006* (pp. 741-750). New York: ACM Publications.

Irons, L. R., Robert, K., & Bielema, Ch. L. (2002). Blended Learning and Learner Satisfaction. Keys to user acceptance. *USDLA Journal, 16*(12). O`Toole, J.M., & Douglas J. A. (2003) The impact of Blended Learning on Student Outcomes: Is there Room on the Horse for Two? *Journal of Educational Media, 28*(2/3), 179–191.

IRRIIS Consortium. (2006). *Integrated Risk Reduction of Information-based Infrastructure Systems*. Retrieved May 18, 2008 from http://www.irriis.eu

Isenmann, R. (2008). Sustainable Information Society. In Quingley, M. (Ed.), *Encyclopedia of Information Ethics* (pp. 622–630). Hershey, PA: IGI Global.

Ito, M. (2005). Mobile Phones, Japanese Youth, and the Re-Placement of Social Contact. In Ling, R., & Pedersen, P. (Eds.), *Mobile Communications: re-negotiation of the Social Sphere*. London: Springer -Verlag.

Ivanov, K. (1988). Expert-support systems: The new technology and the old knowledge. *Systems Research, 5*(2), 293–100.

Ivanov, K. (1989). Computer applications and organizational disease. The well-being of organizations. In Churchman, C. W. (Ed.), *The well-being of organizations* (pp. 283–312). Salinas, CA: Intersystems.

Ivanov, K. (1987). Public records and trade-offs. Legal Informatics. In Tuominen, P. (Ed.), *The Inst. for Nordic Law at the University of Lapland. Lapland, FI: Rovaniemi*.

Ivanov, K. (1972). *Quality-control of information: On the concept of accuracy of information in data banks and in management information systems* (Doctoral thesis.) The University of Stockholm and The Royal Institute of Technology, Stockholm, Sweden.

Ivanov, K. (1986). *Systemutveckling och rättssäkerhet: Om statsförvaltningens datorisering och de långsiktiga konsekvenserna för enskilda och företag [Systems development and rule of law]*. Stockholm, SE: SAF:s Förlag.

Ivanov, K. (1987). Rule of law in information systems research: The role of ethics in knowledge-building procedures, especially in the updating of inference networks. In P. Järvinen (Ed.), *Proceedings of the Tenth Information Systems Research Seminar in Scandinavia*, Tampere-Vaskivesi, FI: University of Tampere.

Ivanov, K. (1989). Is the AI society a symptom of a cultural crisis? Proceedings of the ISSS Int. Society for the Systems Sciences, *33rd Annual Conference, Vol. 3.* Edinburgh, Scotland.

Iwase, H., & Murata, A. (2003). Design proposals to assist older adults in using a computer mouse. *IEICE Transactions on Information and Systems . E (Norwalk, Conn.), 86-D,* 141–145.

Iwase, H., & Murata, A. (2002). Empirical study on improvement of usability - for touch-panel for elderly - comparison of usability between touch-panel and mouse. *Systems, Man and Cybernetics, IEEE International Conference* (pp. 252-257).

Izard, J. (1995). *Trial testing and item analysis*. Victoria, Australia: International Institute of Educational Planning.

Izard, J. (1999). *Some potential difficulties in educational research studies (and how to avoid them)*. Philippines: The Third Elementary Education Project.

Izard, J., & McKay, E. (2004). Automated educational/academic skills screening: Using technology to avoid or minimise effects of more formal assessment. In P.L. Jeffrey (Ed.), *Proceedings of the Australian Association for Research Education (AARE 2004): Positioning education research.* Melbourne. Retrieved from http://www.aare.edu.au/04pap/iza04951.pdf

Jackson, S. E., & Schuler, R. S. (1985). A meta-analysis and conceptual critique of research on role ambiguity and role conflict in work settings. *Organizational Behavior and Human Decision Processes, 36,* 16–78. doi:10.1016/0749-5978(85)90020-2

Jackson, M. C. (1989). The critical kernel in modern systems thinking. Proceedings of the ISSS Int. Society for the Systems Sciences, *33rd Annual Conference, Vol. 2.* Edinburgh, Scotland.

Jacob, R. J. K. (1991). The use of eye movements in human computer interaction techniques: What you look at is what you get. *ACM Transactions on Information Systems, 9,* 152–169. doi:10.1145/123078.128728

Jacob, R. J. K. (1993). Eye movement-based human-computer interaction techniques: Toward non-command interfaces. *Advances in Human-Computer Interaction, 4,* 151–180.

Jacucci, C., Jacucci, G., Wagner, I., & Psik, T. (2005). A manifesto for the performative development of ubiquitous media. In *Proceedings of The Fourth Decennial Aarhus Conference* (pp. 19–28). Denmark: ACM Press.

Janelle, D. G. (1969). Spatial Reorganization: A Model and Concept. *Annals of the Association of American Geographers. Association of American Geographers, 59*(2), 348–364. doi:10.1111/j.1467-8306.1969.tb00675.x

Jansson, M., Mörtberg, C., & Berg, E. (2007). Old dreams, new means: an exploration of visions and situated knowledge in information technology. *Gender, Work and Organization, 14*(4), 371–387. doi:.doi:10.1111/j.1468-0432.2007.00349.x

Jansson, E. (2005). *Working Together when Being Apart. An analysis of distributed Collaborative Work through ICT from Psychosocial and Organisational Perspective.* Doctoral dissertation at Department of Computer and System Sciences, IT University, Royal Institute of Technology, Stockholm.

Jansson, E., & Bradley, G. (2004). Sustainability in Collaborative Network Structures – with focus on the Psychosocial Work Environment in Distributed Teams. In *Proceedings of the CIRN conference on Sustainability and Technology: What does this Mean for Community Informatics, 1* (pp. 271-283). Prato, Italy, 29 September–1 October Community, 2004.

Jansson, M., Mörtberg, C., & Mirijamdotter, A. (2008). Participation in e-home healthcare @ North Calotte. In K. Tollmar & B. Jönsson (Eds.), *Proceedings of the 5th Nordic Conference on Human–Computer Interaction: Building Bridges* (pp. 192–200). ACM Conference Proceedings Series. New York: ACM Press.

Jarrett, C. (2007). Problems and Joys of Reading Research Papers for Practitioner Purposes. *Journal of Usability Studies, 3*(1), 1–6.

Jarrick, A. (2005). *Behovet att behövas* [The need to be needed]. Stockholm, Sweden: SNS Förlag.

Jarvenpaa, S. L., Knoll, K., & Leidner, D. E. (1998). Is anybody out there? Antecedents of trust in global virtual teams. *Journal of Management Information Systems, 14*(4), 29–64.

Jarvenpaa, S. L., & Leidner, D. E. (1998). Communication and Trust in Global Virtual Teams. *Journal of Computer-Mediated Communication, 3*(4).

Jarvenpaa, S. L., & Leidner, D. E. (1999). Communication and trust in global virtual teams. *Organization Science, 10*(6), 791–815. doi:10.1287/orsc.10.6.791

Järvenpää, E., & Immonen, S. (2002). Tietointensiivisten organisaatioiden dynamiikka: Tietotyö, johtaminen ja organisaatioiden verkostot. Working paper no. 28/Work and organisational psychology. Helsinki University of Technology.

Jedeskog, G. (1994). *Datorn i undervisningen [Computers in education]*. Liber Distribution, Stockholm, Skolverket rapport, nr 94:84.

Jensen, R. (1999). *The dream society*. New York/London, NY/UK: McGraw-Hill.

Jeong, S. H., & Fishbein, M. (2007). Predictors of Multitasking with Media: Media Factors and Audience Factors. *Media Psychology, 10*(3), 364–384.

Jha, A. K., Orav, E. J., Ridgway, A. B., Zheng, J., & Epstein, A. M. (2008). Does the Leapfrog program help identify high-quality hospitals? *Joint Commission Journal on Quality and Patient Safety, 34*(6), 318–325.

Johnson, P., May, J., & Johnson, H. (2003). Introduction to Multiple and Collaborative Tasks. *ACM Transactions on Computer-Human Interaction, 10*(4), 277–280. doi:10.1145/966930.966931

Johnson, D. G. (2004). *Computer Ethics* (3rd ed.). New Jersey, NJ: Prentice Hall.

Johnson, S. (2006, December 16). It's All About Us. *Time.* Retrieved from http://www.time.com/time/magazine/article/0,9171,1570717,00.html

John-Steiner, V., Weber, R., & Minnis, M. (1998). The challenge of studying collaboration. *American Educational Research Journal, 35*(4), 773–783.

Johnston, J., Eloff, J. H. P., & Labuschagne, L. (2003). Security and human computer interfaces. *Computers & Security, 22*(8), 675–684. doi:10.1016/S0167-4048(03)00006-3

Joint Commission on Accreditation of Healthcare Organizations (JCAHO). (2007). Sentinel events statistics, March 31, 2007. Retrieved August 7, 2007, from http://www.jointcommission.org/SentinelEvents/Statistics/

Jones, M. R., & Karsten, H. (2008). Giddens's Structuration Theory and Information Systems Research. *Management Information Systems Quarterly, 32*(1), 125–137.

Jones, M. R., & Karsten, H. (2003). *Review: Structuration Theory and Information Systems Research*. Judge Institute of Management Working Paper. Cambridge: Cambridge University Press.

Jonscher, C. (1983). Information resources and economic productivity. *Information Economics and Policy, 1*(1), 13–35. doi:10.1016/0167-6245(83)90016-1

Jönsson, S. (1991). Action Research. In H.-E. Nissen, H. K. Klein, & R. Hirschheim (Eds.) *Information Systems Research: Contemporary Approaches and Emergent Traditions* (pp. 371-396). Amsterdam, NL: North-Holland.

Jordan, P. W. (2002). *An Introduction to Usability*. London: Taylor & Francis.

Kagan, J. (1965). Individual differences in the resolution of response uncertainty. *Journal of Personality and Social Psychology, 2*(2), 154–160. doi:10.1037/h0022199

Kalin, J. (1970). In Defense of Egoism. In D. Gauthin (Ed.) *Morality and Rational Self-Interest*, New York: Prentice Hall.

Kammerer, Y., Scheiter, K., & Beinhauer, W. (2008). Looking my way through the menu: The impact of menu design and multimodal input on gaze-based menu selection. In *Proceedings of the 2008 Symposium on Eye Tracking Research & Applications – ETRA* (pp. 213-220).

Kankainen, A., & Oulasvirta, A. (2003). Design Ideas for Everyday Mobile and Ubiquitous Computing Based on Qualitative User Data. In N. Carbonell, & Stephanidis (Eds.), *User Interface for All* (LNCS 2615, pp. 458-464).

Kanstrup, A. M., & Christiansen, E. (2006). Selecting and evoking innovators: combining democracy and creativity. In A. Mørch, K. Morgan, T. Bratteteig, G. Ghosh & D. Svanæes (Eds.), *Proceedings of the 4th Nordic Conference on Human–Computer Interaction: Changing Roles* (pp. 321-330). ACM Conference Proceedings Series. New York: ACM Press.

Kant, I. (1981). *Grounding for the Metaphysics of Morals* (Ellington, J. W., Trans.). Indianapolis: Hackett Publishing Company.

Kant, I. (1989). *Scritti di filosofia della religione* (Trans. essays from the German, by G. Riconda). Milan, IT: Mursia.

Karasek, R. (1979). Job demands, job decision latitude and mental strain: implications for job redesign. *Administrative Science Quarterly, 24*(2), 285–308. doi:10.2307/2392498

Karasek, R., & Theorell, T. (1990). *Healthy work: Stress, Productivity and the Reconstruction of working life*. New York: Basic Books.

Karasti, H. (2001). *Increasing sensitivity towards everyday work practice in system design*. Dissertation, University of Oulu, Oulu.

Kassebaum, E. A., Eslambolchi, S., Korukonda, S. K., Garber, N. J., & Miller, J. S. (2007). The impact of red light cameras (photo-red enforcement) on crashes in Virginia. *The Virginia Transportation Research Council.* Retrieved from http://www.virginiadot.org/vtrc/main/online_reports/pdf/07-r2.pdf

Kato, H. (2006). Japanese Youth and the Imagining of Keitai. In Ito, M., Okabe, D., & Matsuda, M. (Eds.), *Personal, Portable, Pedestrian: Mobile Phones in Japanese Life* (pp. 103–119). Cambridge, MA: MIT Press.

Kawakami, N., Roberts, C.R., & Haratani, T. (1995). Job stress characteristics of computer work in Japan. *Advances in Human Factors/Ergonomics, 20*(2), 705-710.

Keen, P., & Tan, M. (2007). Knowledge Fusion: A framework for extending the rigor of knowledge management. *International Journal of Knowledge Management, 3*(4), 1–17.

Kelloway, E. K., & Barling, J. (2000). Knowledge work as organizational behaviour. *International Journal of Management Reviews, 2*(3), 287–304. doi:10.1111/1468-2370.00042

Khakhar, D. (Ed.). (2004). *WITFOR 2003 (WORLD IT FORUM) White Book*. Key note contributions and panel discussions from the 8 commissions. Luxemburg: IFIP Press.

Kim, S.-G., Kim, J.-W., & Lee, C.-W. (2007). Implementation of multi-touch tabletop display for HCI. In Jacko, J. (Ed.), *Human-Computer Interaction, Part II* (pp. 854–863). Heidelberg, Deutschland: Springer-Verlag Berlin.

King, L. A., & Hicks, J. A. (2007). What Ever Happened to "What Might Have Been" (section on "Happiness and Complexity: Two Sides of Maturity")? *The American Psychologist, 62*(7), 625–636. doi:10.1037/0003-066X.62.7.625

King, M., & Majchrzak, A. (2003). Technology Alignment and Adaptation for Virtual Teams Involved in Unstructured Work. In Gibson, C. B., & Cohen, S. G. (Eds.), *Virual Teams That Work* (pp. 265–291). San Francisco, CA: Jossey-Bass.

Kittinger, R. (n.d.). *Web 2.0 - Social Behavior of Internet Users*. Retrieved May 8, 2009 from http://www.auburn-media.com/pdf/kittinger_web_2.0.pdf

Klein, J. Th. (1980). *Interdisciplinarity: History, theory and practice*. Detroit, MI: Wayne State University Press.

Kline, D., & Burstein, D. (2005). *Blog! How the newest media revolution is changing politics, business, and culture*. New York: CDS Books.

Kling, R. (1999/2007). What Is Social Informatics and Why Does It Matter? *The Information Society, 23*(4), 205–220. doi:10.1080/01972240701441556

Kling, R., & Scaachi, W. (1982). The Social Web of Computing: Computer Technology as Social Organization. *Advances in Computer, 21*, 2–90.

Kluge, E.-H. (2003). *A Handbook of Ethics for Health Informatics Professionals*. London: Health Informatics Committee, British Computer Society.

Knaus, W. A., Draper, E. A., Wagner, D. P., & Zimmerman, J. E. (1986). An evaluation of outcome from intensive care in major medical centers. *Annals of Internal Medicine, 104*, 410–418.

Knights, D., & McCabe, D. (1998). When "Life is but a Dream": Obliterating Politics through Business Process Reengineering? *Human Relations, 51*(6), 761–798. doi:10.1177/001872679805100604

Knights, D., & Vurdubakis, T. (2005). Information Technology as Organization/Disorganization [Editorial]. *Information and Organization, 15*, 181–184. doi:10.1016/j.infoandorg.2005.06.002

Köffel, Ch., Wästlund, E., & Wolkerstorfer, P. (2008). PRIME IPv3 Usability Test Report V1.2.

Kohiyama, K. (2006). A Decade in the Development if Mobile Communications in Japan (1993-2002) . In Ito, M., Okabe, D., & Matsuda, M. (Eds.), *Personal, Portable, Pedestrian: Mobile Phones in Japanese Life* (pp. 61–74). Cambridge, MA: MIT Press.

Kolata, G. (1993, June 29). Scientist at Work: Andrew Wiles; Math Whiz Who Battled 350-Year-Old Problem. *New York Times*. Retrieved from http://www.nytimes.com/1993/06/29/science/scientist-at-work-andrew-wiles-math-whiz-who-battled-350-year-old-problem.html?scp=8&sq=&pagewanted=all

Korunka, C., & Vitouch, O. (1999). Effects of the implementation of information technology on employees' strain and job satisfaction: a context-depemdent approach. *Work and Stress, 34*(4), 341–363.

Kramer, R. M. (1999). Trust and distrust in organizations: Emerging perspectives, enduring questions. *Annual Review of Psychology, 50*, 569–598. doi:10.1146/annurev.psych.50.1.569

Kraut, R. E., Galegher, J., Fish, R. S., & Chalfonte, B. (1992). Task requirements and media choice in collaborative writing. *Human-Computer Interaction, 7*(4), 375–407. doi:10.1207/s15327051hci0704_2

Kretzman, J. P., & McKnight, J. L. (1993). *Building Communities From The Inside Out: A Path Toward Finding and Mobilizing A Community's Assets*. Chicago, IL: ACTA Publication.

Kubisch, A. C. (1997). *Voices from the Field: Learning from the Early Work of Comprehensive Community Initiatives*. Washington, DC: Aspen Institute.

Kuehn, B. M. (2007). No end insight to nursing shortage: Bottleneck at nursing schools a key factor. *Journal of the American Medical Association, 298*(14), 1623–1625. doi:10.1001/jama.298.14.1623

Kuhn, T. (1996). *The Structure of Scientific Revolutions*. Chicago, IL: University of Chicago Press.

Kuo, Y.-F., & Chen, L.-S. (2004). Individual demographic differences and job satisfaction among information technology personnel: an empirical study in Taiwan. *International Journal of Management, 21*(2), 221–231.

Kuorinka, I., Forcier, L., Hagberg, M., Silverstein, B., & Wells, R. Smith. M., Hendrick, H., Carayon, P., & Perusse, M. (1995). *Work Related Musculoskeletal Disorders (WMDSs): A Reference Book for Prevention*. London: Taylor & Francis.

Ladd, J. (1991). Collective and Individual Moral Responsibility in Engineering: Some Questions . In Johnson, D. (Ed.), *Ethical Issues in Engineering*. New Jersey, NJ: Prentice Hall.

Ladmiral, J. R. (1984). J. Habermas. In D. Huisman (Ed.), *Dictionnaire des philosophes*. Paris, FR: Presses Universitaires de France.

Lafferty, W. M., Aall, C., Lindseth, G., & Nordland, I. T. (Eds.). (2006). *Lokal Agenda 21 i Norge: Så mye hadde vi - så mye ga vi bort – så mye har vi igjen* [Local Agenda 21 in Norway], Unipub forlag, Oslo.

Lakoff, G. (1987). *Women, Fire, and Dangerous Things: What categories reveal about the mind*. Chicago, IL: The University of Chicago Press.

Lamb, R., & Kling, R. (2003). Reconceptualising Users as Social Actors in Information Systems Research. *Management Information Systems Quarterly, 27*(2), 197–235.

Lamothe, L. (1999). Hospital reconfiguration: A professinal challenge. *Ruptures, 6*, 132–149.

Landay, J. (2009). I Give Up on CHI/UIST. Blog entry, November 7, 2009. Available at: http://dubfuture.blogspot.com/2009/11/i-give-up-on-chiuist.html (checked November 10, 2009)

Landes, M. (2005). *A case in interdisciplinarity: The product design program at Stanford. Unpublished seminar paper prepared for Education 357X*. Interdisciplinarity in Higher Education.

Langefors, B., & Sundgren, B. (1975). *Information systems architecture*. New York, NY: Petrocelli/Charter.

Larsman, P., Thorn, S., Sogaard, K., Sandsjo, L., Sjogaard, G., & Kadefors, R. (2009). Work related perceived stress and muscle activity during standardized computer work among female computer users. *Work – A Journal of Prevention Assessment and Rehabilitation, 32*(2), 189-199.

Lasch, C. (1977). *Haven in a heartless world: The family besieged*. New York, NY: Basic Books.

Lastra, S. (2001). Harvesting community knowledge. In *Proceedings of the 34th Hawaii International Conference on System Sciences*, Los Alamitos CA, IEEE Computer Society.

Lastra, S. (2004). The Power of Community Events for Designing Participatory Community ICTs. *PDC04: The Eighth Participatory Design Conference*, July 27 – 31 Toronto, Canada.

Lastra, S. (2006). *Making sense of community informatics: The development and application of the Community Event Research Method*. Ph.D. dissertation, University of Illinois at Urbana-Champaign, United States -- Illinois. Retrieved October 4, 2009, from Dissertations & Theses: Full Text. (Publication No. AAT 3242911).

Latour, B. (1993). *We have never been modern*. Cambridge, MA: Harvard University Press.

Laurell, K. (2005). *Headache in school children: Epidemiology, Pain Comorbidity and Psychosocial Factors*. Ph D Thesis. Department of Neuroscience, Uppsala University.

Lawless, E. (1993). *Holy Women, Wholly Women: Sharing Ministries of Wholeness through Life Stories and Reciprocal Ethnography*. Philadelphia, PA: University of Pennsylvania Press.

Lawless, E. (2000). Reciprocal ethnography: No one said it was easy. *Journal of Folklore Research, 37*(2/3), 197–205.

Le Blanc, P. M., de Jonge, J., de Rijk, A. E., & Schaufeli, W. B. (2001). Well-being of intensive care nurses (WEBIC): a job analytic approach. *Journal of Advanced Nursing, 36*(3), 460–470. doi:10.1046/j.1365-2648.2001.01994.x

LeBourgeois, MK., Gainnotti, F., Cortesi, F., Wolfson, AR., & Harsch, J. (2005). *The relationship between reported sleep quality and sleep hygiene in Italian and American adolescents* (pp. 257-265). Pediatrics: 115 (1rst).

Lee, S., Hwang, T., & Lee, H. H. (2006). Corporate blogging strategies of the Fortune 500 companies. *Management Decision, 44*(3), 316–334. doi:10.1108/00251740610656232

Leeson, P. T. (2007). Balkanization and assimilation: Examining the effects of state-created Homogeneity. *Review of Social Economy, 65*(2), 141–164. doi:10.1080/00346760600709960

Leitner, P., & Grechenig, T. (2008). Social Networking Sphere: a Snapshot of trends, functionalities and revenue models. In *Proceedings of the IADIS International Conference on Web Based Communities* (pp. 187-191), Amsterdam, The Netherlands.

Lenhart, A. (2005). *Protecting teens online. Pew Internet and American Life Project.* Retrieved March 2010 from www.pewinternet.org

Lennerlöf, L., & Aronsson, G. (1991). *Människan i arbetslivet* [The individual in working life]. Stockholm, Sweden: Nordstedts Juridik AB.

Leontiev, A. N. (1971). *Needs, Motivations, Emotions.* Moscow: Moscow University Press. (in Russian)

Levén, P., & Nordström, T. (1989, March). Socially responsive systems. Presented at the conference Support, society and culture: Mutual uses of cybernetics and science, *The Int. Federation for Cybernetics*, Amsterdam. Report UMADP-WPIPCS 22.89, Umeå university, Inst. of Information Processing, Umeå, Sweden.

Levi, L. (1972). *Stress and Distress in Response to Psychosocial Stimuli.* New York: Pergamon Press.

Levi, L. (2001). *Stress och Hälsa [Stress and Health].* Stockholm, SE: Skandia.

Lévy, P. (1997). *Collective Intelligence, Mankind's Emerging World in Cyberspace.* New York: Plenum Trade.

Lew, G. S. (2009). What Do Users Really Do? Experience Sampling in the 21st Century. *HCI International 2009.* San Diego, USA.

Lewandowski, J. D. (2003). Thematizing Embeddedness: Reflexive Sociology as Interpretation. *Philosophy of the Social Sciences, 30*(1), 49–66. doi:10.1177/004839310003000103

Lewicki, R. J., & Bunker, B. B. (Eds.). (1996). *Developing an maintaing trust in work relationships. Trust in organizations: Frontiers of theory and research.* Thousand Oaks, CA: Sage.

Lewis, R. (2001). Redesigning the Workplace. The North American Factory in the Interwar Period. *Technology and Culture, 42*(3), 665–684. doi:10.1353/tech.2001.0172

Lewis, D. (2006). *What is Web 2.0.* Crossroads ACM Student Magazine.

Lewis, C. S. (1988). *Christian reflections* (Walter Hooper, Ed. First published in 1967). Glasgow, UK: Collins.

Lichbach, M. I. (1996). *The cooperator's dilemma.* Ann Arbor: University of Michigan Press.

Licoppe, C., & Heurtin, J. P. (2001). Managing One's Availability to Telephone communication through Mobile Phones. *Personal and Ubiquitous Computing, 5*(2), 98–108. doi:10.1007/s007790170013

Liepmann, D., Beauducel, A., Brocke, B., & Amthauer, R. (1999, 2001). *Intelligenz-Struktur-Test 2000 R*, Göttingen, Deutschlang: Hogrefe Verlag.

Lim, S. (2008). Job ssatisfaction of information technology workers in academic libraries. *Library & Information Science Research, 30*, 115–121. doi:10.1016/j.lisr.2007.10.002

Lin, H.-H., & Chang, T.-W. (2007). *A camera-based multi-touch interface builder for designers. Human-Computer Interaction.* HCI Applications and Services.

Linebaugh, P. (2001). 'The Red-Crested Bird and Black Duck'—a Story of 1802: Historical Materialism, Indigenous People, and the Failed Republic. *The Republic Journal, 2*(Spring/Summer), 104–125.

Linger, H. (2006). Supporting collaborative knowledge work: A methodology for developing ICT tools for biomedical research. *Neural Networks, 3931*, 261–271.

Liskov, B. (1981). Biography of Kristen Nygaard. In R. L. Wexelblat, (Ed.) *History of Programming Languages I*. New York: ACM. Retrieved from http://doi.acm.org/10.1145/800025.1198397

Lloyd, K. M., & Auld, C. J. (2001). The role of leisure in determining quality of life: issues of content and measurement. *Social Indicators Research, 57*(3), 42–71.

Lloyd, W. F. (1833). *Two lectures on the checks to population*. Oxford, UK: Michaelmas.

Loh, L., Sankar, C. S., & Yeong, W. Y. (1995). Job orientation, perceptions, and satisfaction: a study of information technology professionals in Singapore. *Information & Management, 29*, 239–250. doi:10.1016/0378-7206(95)00022-X

Lohmann, S. (2003). *How universities think. Unpublished manuscript*. Department of Political Science, University of California.

London Knowledge Lab. (2008). Education 2.0? Designing the web for teaching and learning. A Commentary by the Technology Enhanced Learning phase of the Teaching and Learning Research Programme. Retrieved July 8, 2009 from http://www.tlrp.org/pub/documents/TELcomm.pdf

Lounsbury, J. W., Moffitt, L., Gibson, L. W., Drost, A. W., & Stevens, M. (2007). An investigation of personality traits in relation to job and career satisfaction of information technology professionals. *Journal of Information Technology, 22*, 174–183. doi:10.1057/palgrave.jit.2000094

Lovelock, J. (1987). *Gaia*. Oxford, UK: Oxford University Press.

Luczak, H., & Frenz, M. (2008). Kompetenz - Erwerb, Erhalt, Ausbau, In Heinz Kowalski, CW Haarfeld (Hrsg), *Stärkung der persönlichen Gesundheitskompetenz im Betrieb - Bis 67 fit im Job* (pp. 19-59): Köln, Deutschland.

Luczak, H., & Stemann, M. (2008). Ergonomic Design and Intervention Strategies in Health Promotion for Ageing Workforces, In Conrad, H.; Heindorf, V.; Waldenberger, F., Palgrave Macmillan (Hrsg) (2008). *Human Resource Management in Ageing Societies* (pp. 144-156): Hampshire, UK: Palgrave.

Lukes, S. (2004). Durkheim, Emile (1858–1917). In N. J. Smelser & P. Baltes, *International Encyclopedia of the Social & Behavioral Sciences* (pp. 3897-3903). Oxford, UK: Elsevier Science Ltd.

Lundquist, T., & Huston, M. M. (1990). Information rich environments for continuous organic development—CODE. *Manuscript. Submitted to the J. of Applied Systems Analysis*. Luleå Institute of Technology and Texas Women's University.

Luria, A. R. (1968). *The mind of a mnemonist; a little book about a vast memory*. New York: Basic Books.

Luria, A. R. (1972). *The man with a shattered world; the history of a brain wound*. New York: Basic Books.

Luria, A. R. (1979). *The Making of Mind*. Cambridge, MA: Harvard University Press.

Macgregor, G. (2005). The nature of information in the twenty-first century: Conundrums for the informatics community? *Library Review, 54*(1), 10–23. doi:10.1108/00242530510574129

Macklin, R. (1999). *Against Relativism*. New York: Oxford University Press.

Maines, D. R. (1977). Social Organization and Social Structure in Symbolic Interactionist Thought. *Annual Review of Sociology, 3*, 235–259. doi:10.1146/annurev.so.03.080177.001315

Mäki, E., Järvenpää, E., & Hämäläinen, L. (2001). Managing knowledge processes in knowledge intensive work. In *Proceedings of the 2nd ECKM 2001 - CA The 2nd European Conference on Knowledge Management*. Bled School of Management, Slovenia, November 8-9, 2001.

Malena, C., & Finn Heinrich, V. (2007). Can we measure civil society? A proposed methodology for international comparative research. *Development in Practice, 17*(3), 338–352. doi:10.1080/09614520701336766

Malone, T. W. (2004). *The Future of Work: How the New Order of Business Will Shape Your Organization, Your Management Style, and Your Life.* Cambridge, MA: Harvard Business School Press.

Mandke, V. V., & Nayar, M. K. (2004). Beyond Quality: the Information Integrity Imperative. *Total Quality Management and Business Excellence, 15*(5-6), 645–654. doi:10.1080/14783360410001680134

Manning, P. K. (1996). Information Technology in the Police Context: The "Sailor" Phone. *Information Systems Research, 7*(1), 52–62. doi:10.1287/isre.7.1.52

Mansilla, V. B., & Gardner, H. Assessing interdisciplinary work at the frontier. An empirical exploration of "symptoms of quality". Available from http://www.inter-disciplines.org/ interdisciplinarity/papers/6; INTERNET.

March, J. G. (1991). *Exploration and exploitation in organizational learning.* Organization Science [Special Issue: Organizational Learning Papers in Honor of (and by) James G. March] 2, 71–87.

Mark, G. (2009). The Effects of Perpetual Distraction. *New York Times.* Retrieved 22 October 2009 from, http://roomfordebate.blogs.nytimes.com/2009/10/14/does-the-brain-like-e-books/

Mark, G., Gudith, D., & Klocke, U. (2008). The Cost of Interrupted Work: More Speed and Stress. In *Proceedings of the 26th SIGCHI Conference on Human Factors in Computing Systems* (pp. 107-110). New York: ACM Publications.

Markopoulos, P., & Rauterberg, G. W. M. (2000). Living Lab: A White Paper. IPO Annual Progress Report (pp. 53-65).

Marschall, D. (2002). Internet Technologists as an Occupational Community: Ethnographic Evidence. *Information Communication and Society, 5*(1), 51–60. doi:10.1080/13691180110117659

Martin, S. B. (1999). Employment in the information age. Information technology and information work. *The Journal of Policy . Regulation and Strategy for Telecommunications and Media, 2*(3), 271–283.

Martin, D. C. (1997). Empowering Educators and Parents: Content Advisories for the Internet. In *Proceedings of the ITiCSE.* ACM.

Martinez, M. (2000). Foundations for personalized web learning environments. *ALN Magazine - A publication of the Sloan Consortium, 4*(2).

Martins, L. L., Gilson, L. L., & Maynard, T. (2004). Virtual teams: What do we know and where do we go from here? *Journal of Management, 30*(6), 805–835. doi:10.1016/j.jm.2004.05.002

Maslach, C. (1993). *Burnout: A multidimensional perspective. In professional burnout: Recent development in theory and research* (pp 19-32). Series in applied psychology: Social issues and questions. Philadelphia, PA: Taylor & Francis.

Massy, W. F., & Robert, Z. (1994). Faculty discretionary time: Departments and the academic ratchet. *The Journal of Higher Education, 65*, 1–22. doi:10.2307/2943874

Mayer, R. C., Davis, J. H., & Schoorman, E. F. (1995). An integrative model of organizational trust. *Academy of Management Review, 20*(3), 709–734. doi:10.2307/258792

Mayer, R. E. (Ed.). (2005). *The Cambridge handbook of multimedia learning.* Cambridge, UK: Cambridge University Press.

McCarthy, J., & Wright, P. (2004). *Technology as Experience.* Cambridge, MA: MIT Press.

McChesney, R. (2004). *The problem of the media: U.S. Communication politics in the 21st century.* Chicago, IL: Monthly review.

McFarlane, D. C., & Latorella, K. A. (2002). The Scope and Importance of Human Interruption in Human-Computer Interaction Design. *Human-Computer Interaction, 17*(1), 1–61. doi:10.1207/S15327051HCI1701_1

McFarlane, A., Sparrowhawk, A., & Heald, Y. (2005). *Report on the educational use of games*. TEEM: Teachers Evaluating Educational Media. Retrieved August 31, 2006 from http://www.teem.org.uk/publications

McIver, W., Jr. (2003). A Community Informatics for the Information Society. In S. O'Siochrú and B. Girard (Eds.) *Communicating in the Information Society*. Geneva, Switzerland: United Nations Research Institute for Social Development (UNRISD), 2003. Retrieved May 12, 2008 from http://www.unrisd.org/80256B3C005BCCF9/(http Publications)/5DCA28E932BB8CFDC1256E240029A0 75?OpenDocument&panel=additional

McIver, W., Jr. (2006, November). Community Informatics and Human Development. In *Proceedings International Workshop on Community Informatics*, (COMINF'06). Montpellier, France. NRC 48767.

McKay, E. (1999). An investigation of text-based instructional materials enhanced with graphics. *Educational Psychology, 19*(3), 323–335. doi:10.1080/0144341990190306

McKay, E. (2000b). Measurement of cognitive performance in computer programming concept acquisition: Interactive effects of visual metaphors and the cognitive style construct. *Journal of Applied Measurement, 1*(3), 257–286.

McKay, E. (Ed.). (2007a). *Enhancing learning through human-computer interaction*. Hershey, PA: Idea Group Reference.

McKay, E. (2007b). Planning effective HCI to enhance accessibility. *Universal Access in the Information Society, 6*, 77–85. doi:10.1007/s10209-007-0070-3

McKay, E. (2000a). *Instructional strategies integrating the cognitive style construct: A meta-knowledge processing model (contextual components that facilitate spatial/logical task performance)*. Unpublished PhD Thesis, Deakin Univ., Australia. Retrieved from http://tux.lib.deakin.edu. au/adt-VDU/public/adt-VDU20061011.122556/.

McKay, E., & Izard, J. (2004). Automated educational skills evaluation: A systems design case study. In E. McKay (Ed.), *Proceedings of the International Conference on Computers in Education - Acquiring and Constructing Knowledge through Human-Computer Interaction: Creating new visions for the future of learning*. Melbourne Exhibition Centre, Australia: Common Ground Publishing, *1*(3), 1051-1061.

McKay, E., & Merrill, M. D. (2003). Cognitive skill and web-based educational systems. In E. McKay (Ed.), *Proceedings of the eLearning Conference on Design and Development: Instructional Design - Applying first principles of instruction*, (pp.96-108). Melbourne: Informit Library: Australasian Publications. Retrieved from http://www.informit.com.au/

McKay, E., Thomas, T., & Martin, J. (2004). Work search prototype design: Human-computer interaction for vocational rehabilitation. In V. Uskov (Ed.), Paper presented at the *International Association of Science and Technology for Development - Computers and Advanced Technology in Education (CATE 2004)* (pp.167-172). Anaheim: ACTA Press.

McMurtrey, M. E., Grover, V., Teng, J., & Lightner, N. (2002). Job satisfaction on information technology workers: the impact of career orientation and task automation in a case environment. *Journal of Management Information Systems, 9*(2), 273–302.

McRobb, S., & Rogerson, S. (2004). Are They Really Listening? An investigation into published online privacy policies. *Information Technology & People, 17*(4), 442–461. doi:10.1108/09593840410570285

Mehta, N. (1982). *A flexible machine interface*. M.A.Sc. Thesis, Department of Electrical Engineering, University of Toronto, Canada.

Melguizo, T., & Myra, H. S. (2005). *A prestige model of the determinants of full-time faculty salaries at four-year institutions in the U.S.* Unpublished manuscript.

Melville, N., Kraemer, K., & Gurbaxani, V. (2004). Information technology and organisational performance: An integrative model of IT business value. *Management Information Systems Quarterly, 45*(2), 283–322.

Melvin, W. S., Needleman, B. J., Krause, K. R., Schneider, C., Wolf, R. K., Michler, R. E., & Ellison, E. C. (2002). Computer-enhanced robotic telesurgery. *Surgical Endoscopy, 16*(12), 1790–1792. doi:10.1007/s00464-001-8192-9

Merrill, M. D. (2003). Keynote address: Does your instruction rate 5 stars? In E. McKay, (Ed.), *Proceedings of the eLearning Conference on Design and Development: Instructional Design - Applying first principles of instruction*, (pp.13-14). Melbourne: Informit Library: Australasian Publications. Retrieved from http://www.informit.com.au/

Messer-Davidow, E. (2002). *Disciplining feminism: From social activism to academic discourse*. Durham, NC: Duke University Press.

Messeter, J., Brandt, E., Hasle, J., & Johansson, M. (2004). *Contextualizing mobile IT. Designing Interactive Systems* (pp. 27–36). Cambridge, MA: MIT Press.

Meyer, H. (2005, January). The nature of information and its effective use in rural development. *Information Research, 10*(2). Retrieved October 20, 2006 from http://informationr.net/ir/10-2/paper214.html

Micire, M., Drury, J. J., Keyes, B., & Yanco, H. A. (2009). Multi-touch interaction for robot control. *Submitted for Conference publication. IUI 2009 Workshop*, Florida.

Midgley, G. (1989). Critical systems: The theory and practice of partitioning methodologies. Proceedings of the ISSS Int. Society for the Systems Sciences, *33rd Annual Conference, Vol.2*, Edinburgh, Scotland.

Miezio, K., Smith, M. J., & Carayon, P. (1987). Electronic Performance Monitoring: Behavioral and Motivational Issues. In S.S. Asfour (Ed.), *Trends in Ergonomics/Human Factors IV*, (pp. 253-257) Amsterdam, NL: North Holland.

Miliband (1973). Poulantzas and the Capitalist State. *New Left Review*, I, 82-92.

Miller, G. (1956). The magical number seven, plus or minus two: Some limits on our capacity for processing information. *Psychological Review, 63*(1), 81–97. doi:10.1037/h0043158

Minton, L., Boyle, R., & Dimitrova, V. (2004). If diversity is a problem could e-learning be part of the solution? A case study. In *Proceedings of the ITiCSE'04 Conference* (pp. 42-46). ACM.

Miranda, D. R. (1992). Critically examining intensive care. *International Journal of Technology Assessment in Health Care, 8*(3), 444–456. doi:10.1017/S0266462300013738

Miranda, P., Chen, N.-S., & Isaías, P. (2005). Design, Implementation and Evaluation of a Virtual Conference. In *Proceedings of the IADIS International Conference e-Society 2005* (pp. 59-68), Qawra, Malta.

Mirijamdotter, A., Somerville, M. M., & Holst, M. (2006). An Interactive and Iterative Evaluation Approach for Creating Collaborative Learning Environments. [EJISE]. *The Electronic Journal of Information Systems Evaluation, 9*(2), 83–92.

Mitroff, I. I. (1988, Winter). Crisis management: Cutting through the confusion. *Sloan Management Review*, 15–20.

Mitroff, I. I. (1990). *Can appropriate technology help in the battle against crises? Computer software for crisis management. Submitted for publication to Security Management Review*. University of Southern California, Graduate School of Business, Center for Crisis Management.

Mondin, B. (1988). *Scienze umane e teologia*. Roma, IT: Urbaniana University Press.

Moon, S., & Sauter, S. (Eds.). (1996). *Beyond Biomechanics: Psychosocial Aspects of Cumulative Trauma Disorders*. London: Taylor & Francis.

Moor, J. H. (1985). What is Computer Ethics? *Metaphilosophy, 4*(16), 266–275. doi:10.1111/j.1467-9973.1985.tb00173.x

More, T. (1961). *Utopia*. (P. Turner, Translation - Original work published 1516). London: Penguin Books.

Moreau, L., Groth, P., Miles, S., Vazquez-Salceda, J., Ibbotson, J., & Jiang, S. (2008). The provenance of electronic data. *Communications of the ACM, 51*(4), 52–58. doi:10.1145/1330311.1330323

Morgenstern, O. (1963). *On the accuracy of economic observations.* Princeton, NJ: Princeton University Press.

Mork, P. J., & Westgaard, R. H. (2007). The influence of body posture, arm movement, and work stress on trapezius activity during computer work. *European Journal of Applied Physiology, 101*(4), 445–456. doi:10.1007/s00421-007-0518-4

Morozov, E. (2009). Censoring cyberspace. *RSA Journal,* 20-23.

Morris, C. (1946). *Signs, language und behaviour.* New York: Prentice-Hall.

Morris, M., Huang, A., Paepcke, A., & Winograd, T. (2006). Cooperative gestures: Multi-user gestural interactions for co-located groupware. *CHI 2006,* Montréal, Québec, Canada.

Mörtberg, C., & Elovaara, P. (in press). Attaching people and technology: between e and government . In Booth, S., Goodman, S., & Kirkup, G. (Eds.), *Gender Issues in Learning and Working with Information Technology: Social Constructs and Cultural Context.* Hershey, PA: IG Global.

Mörtberg, C., Stuedahl, D., & Elovaara, P. (forthcoming). Designing for sustainable ways of living with technologies . In Wagner, I., Bratteteig, T., & Stuedahl, D. (Eds.), *Exploring Digital Design Multi-disciplinary Design Practices.* Berlin-Heidelberg, DE: Springer Verlag.

Moss, J., Xiao, Y., & Zubaidah, S. (2002). The operating room charge nurse: Coordinator and communicator. *J Am Med Inform Assoc, 9*(Nov - Dec Suppl), S70-74.

Müller-Stich, B., Reiter, M., Mehrabi, A., Wente, M. N., Fischer, L., Köninger, J., & Gutt, C. N. (2009). No relevant difference in quality of life and functional outcome at 12 months' follow-up—a randomised controlled trial comparing robot-assisted versus conventional laparoscopic Nissen fundoplication. *Langenbeck's Archives of Surgery, 394*(3), 441–446. doi:10.1007/s00423-008-0446-8

Mumford, L. (1964). *The Myth of the Machine, The Pentagon of Power.* New York: Harcourt Brace Jovanovich.

Munipov, V. M. (1978). Applied Ergonomics in the USSR. *Applied Ergonomics, 9*(4), 215–222. doi:10.1016/0003-6870(78)90082-0

Munipov, V. M. (1979). Ergonomics as a Factor in Social and Economic Development. *Ergonomics, 22*(6), 607–611. doi:10.1080/00140137908924645

Munipov, V. M. (1992). Chernobyl Operators: Criminals or Victims? *Applied Ergonomics, 23*(5), 337–342. doi:10.1016/0003-6870(92)90295-7

Munipov, V. M., & Zinchenko, V. P. (2001). *Human-Centered Ergonomic Design of Tool, Technology, Hardware, Software and Environment.* Moscow: Logos. (in Russian)

Munipov, V. M. (1991). Human engineering analysis of Chernobyl Accident . In Kumashiro, M., & Megan, E. D. (Eds.), *Towards human work: Solution to problems in Occupational Health and Safety.* London: Taylor and Francis.

Munipov, V. M. (Ed.). (1983). *Ergonomics: Principles and Recommendations. A Manual* (in Russian). Moscow, RU: VNIITE.

Munipov, V. M. (1976). Ergonomics and psychological science, (in Russian). *Questions of psychology,* 5, 3-17.

Murata, A. (2006). Eye-Gaze Input Versus Mouse: Cursor Control as a Function of Age. *International Journal of Human-Computer Interaction, 21,* 1–14.

Naegele, G. (2004). *Zwischen Arbeit und Rente: Gesellschaftliche Chancen und Risiken älterer Arbeitnehmer.* Augsburg, Deutschland: Maro-Verlag.

Nagata, S. F. (2003). Multitasking and Interruptions during Mobile Web Tasks. In *Proceedings of the 47th annual meeting of the Human Factors and Ergonomics Society* (pp. 1341-1345). Retrieved 21 September 2009 from, http://interruptions.net/literature/Nagata-HFES03.pdf

Nair, S. N., Lee, C. C., & Czaja, S. J. (2005). Older adults attitudes toward computers: Have they changed with recent advances in technology? In *Proceedings of the 49th Annual Meeting of Human Factors and Ergonomics Society* (pp. 154–157).

Nakatani, L. H., & Rohrlich, J. A. (1983). Soft machines: A philosophy of user-computer interface design. In *Proceedings of the ACM Conference on Human Factors in Computing Systems* (pp. 12-15). New York: ACM Press.

Nanavati, A. A., & Bias, R. G. (2005). Optimal Line Length in Reading--A Literature Review . *Visible Language*, *39*(2), 121–145.

Nance, K. L., & Strohmaier, M. (1994). *Ethical accountability in the cyberspace. Ethics in the computer age* (pp. 115–118). New York: ACM.

Nardi, B., Whittaker, S., & Schwarz, H. (2002). NetWORKers and their Activity in Intensional Networks. *Computer Supported Cooperative Work*, *11*(1-2), 205–242. doi:10.1023/A:1015241914483

Nardi, B., Whittaker, S., & Bradner, E. (2000). Interaction and Outeraction: Instant Messaging in Action. In *Proceedings of the 2000 ACM Conference on Computer Supported Cooperative Work* (pp. 79-88). Philadelphia, PA: ACM Press.

National Academy of Sciences, National Academy of Engineering, and Institute of Medicine. (2005). *Facilitating interdisciplinary research*. Washington, DC: The National Academies Press.

National Institute of Medicine. (2003). *Enhancing the vitality of the National Institutes of Health: Organizational change to meet new challenges*. Washington, DC: National Academies Press.

National Institute on Aging & National Institutes of Health. Washington. (2007). Why Population Aging Matters: A Global Perspective. Retrieved February 12, 2008 from http://www.nia.nih.gov/NR/rdonlyres/9E91407E-CFE8-4903-9875-D5AA75BD1D50/0/WPAM.pdf

Neerincx, M. A. (2003). Cognitive Task Load analysis: allocating tasks and designing support . In Hollnagel, E. (Ed.), *Handbook of cognitive task design* (pp. 283–305). London: Lawrence Erlbaum Ass.

Neumann, P. G. (1995). *Computer Related Risks*. New York: ACM Press.

Newell, A., & Simon, H. A. (1972). *Human problem solving*. Englewood Cliffs, NJ: Prentice-Hall, Inc.

Niebuhr, R. (1986). *The essential Reinhold Niebuhr: Selected essays and addresses* (Ed. and intr. by R. McAfee Brown). New Haven/London, CI/UK: Yale University Press.

Nielsen, J. (1994). Heuristic evaluation. In Nielsen & Mack (Eds.), *Usability Inspection Methods*. New York: John Wiley & Sons. Retrieved from http://www.useit.com/papers/heuristic/heuristic_list.html

Nielsen, J. (2003, October 13). Web guru fights info pollution. *BBC News Online*. Retrieved October 24, 2006 from http://news.bbc.co.uk/2/hi/technology/3171376.stm

Nielsen, J. (2004). Jacob Nielsen's Alertbox, User Education Is Not the Answer to Security Problems. Retrieved from http://www.useit.com

Niles, D. P. (2003). Justice, Peace and the Integrity of Creation. In Ecumenical Dictionary. Retrieved from http://www.wcc-coe.org/wcc/who/dictionary-article11.html

Nilsson, K. (1989). Designing for creativity: Toward a theoretical basis for the design of interactive information systems. *Proceedings of the 12th IRIS Conference - Information Systems Research in Scandinavia*, Skagen, Denmark. Aalborg University, Inst. of Electronic Systems. Aalborg. Report UMADP—WPIPCS 20:89, Umeå university, Inst. of Information Processing. Also as report UMADP-RRIPCS-8.89, University of Umeå, Inst. of Information Processing.

Norman, D. (2004). *Emotional design: Why we love (or hate) everyday things*. New York: Basic Books.

Norris, A. C. (2002). *Essentials of Telemedicine and Telecare*. New York: John Wiley & Sons.

Norum, K. E. (2001). Appreciative Design. *Systems Research and Behavioral Science*, *18*(4), 323–333. doi:10.1002/sres.427

Nyberg, A. (2008). *Att studera digitala artefakter i människors vardagsliv*. (English title: On the exploration of people's attitudes to digital artefacts) PhD Thesis. Umeå University. Sweden: Department of Informatics. Umeå.

O'Conaill, B., & Frohlich, D. (1995). Timespace in the Workplace: Dealing with Interruptions. In *Proceedings of CHI 1995*. Retrieved from http://old.sigchi.org/chi95/Electronic/documnts/shortppr/boc_bdy.htm

O'Neil, D. (2001). Merging theory with practice: Toward an evaluation framework for community informatics. *Internet Research 2.0*: INTERconnections. The Second International Conference of the Association of Internet Researchers, University of Minnesota. Available at http://www.ehealthstrategies.com/files/eval_comm_inf.pdf.

Oborne, D. (1985). *Computers at work*. London: John Wiley & Sons Ltd.

Odajnyk, V. W. (1976). *Jung and politics: The political and social ideas of C.G. Jung*. New York, NY: Harper & Row.

OECD. (2008). *Measuring material flows and resource productivity. Synthesis report*. Paris, France: Organisation for Economic Cooperation and Development.

OECD. (2009). Investment in ICT. Science and technology. OECD Factbook. Retrieved March 5, 2010 from http://puck.sourceoecd.org/pdf/factbook2009/3020090 11e-07-02-02.pdf

Oh, H., Rizo, C., Enkin, M., & Jadad, A. (2005). What is eHealth? (3): A Systematic Review of Published Definitions. *Journal of Medical Internet Research*, *7*(1), e1. doi:10.2196/jmir.7.1.e1

Oldenburg, R. (1997). *The Great Good Place*. New York: Paragon House. (Original work published 1989)

O'Leary, M. B., & Cummings, J. N. (2007). The spatial, temporal, and configurational characteristics of geographic dispersion in teams. *Management Information Systems Quarterly*, *31*(3), 433–452.

Oliga, J. C. (1990). Power-ideology matrix in social systems control. *Systems Practice*, *3*(1), 31–49. doi:10.1007/BF01062820

Oliga, J. C. (1989). Ideology and systems emancipation. School of Accountancy and Commerce, Nanyang Technological Institute, Singapore. ISSS Int. Society for the Systems Sciences, *33rd Annual Conference*, Edinburgh, Scotland, 2-7 July 1989.

Olson, E. (2006). Families-Agents of Social Development . In *Proceedings of International Seminar*. Vienna, Austria: Families Agents of Social Development.

Olson, M. (1965). *The logic of collective action*. Cambridge, MA: Harvard University Press.

Olwal, A., Feiner, S., & Heyman, S. (2008). Rubbing and tapping for precise and rapid selection on touch-screen displays. In *Proceedings of the 2008 SIGCHI conference on Human Factors in computing systems* (pp. 295-304), Italy.

Ophir, R., Nass, C., & Wagner, A. D. (2009). Cognitive Control in Media Multitaskers. *Proceedings of the National Academy of Sciences of the United States of America*, *106*(37), 15583–15587. doi:10.1073/pnas.0903620106

O'Reilly, T. (2005). *What is Web 2.0? Design Patterns and Business Models for the Next Generation of Software*. Retrieved April 8, 2009 from http://oreilly.com/web2/archive/what-is-web-20.html

Orlikowski, W. J. (2000). Using Technology and Constituting Structures: A Practice Lens for Studying Technology in Organizations. *Organization Science*, *11*(4), 404–428. doi:10.1287/orsc.11.4.404.14600

Orlikowski, W. J. (2005). Material Works: Exploring the Situated Entanglement of Technological Performativity and Human Agency. *Scandinavian Journal of Information Systems*, *17*(1), 183–186.

Orlikowski, W. (1995). *Action and Artifact: The Structuring of Technologies-in-Use*. Retrieved 20 October, 2003, from http://hdl.handle.net/1721.1/2600

Orlikowski, W. J. (1993). Learning from Notes: Organizational Issues in Groupware Implementation. In *Proceedings of the 1992 ACM Conference on Computer-Supported Cooperative Work*, Toronto, Canada.

Orth-Gomér, K. (Ed.). (2007). *Job strain and risk of recurrent coronary events*. Journal of the American Medical Association.

Orth-Gomér, K., Wamala, S. P., Horsten, M., Schenck-Gustafsson, K., Schneiderman, N., & Mittleman, M. A. (2000). Marital stress worsens prognosis in women with coronary heart disease . *Journal of the American Medical Association, 284*, 3008–3014. doi:10.1001/jama.284.23.3008

Orth-Gomér, K., & Perski, A. (Eds.). (2008). *Preventiv medicin – Teori och praktik (Preventive Medicine – Theory and Practice)* (First published in 1999). Stockholm, SE: Studentlitteratur.

Ostberg, O., & Nilsson, C. (1985). Emerging technology and stress . In Cooper, C. L., & Smith, M. I. (Eds.), *Job Stress and Blue-Collar Work* (pp. 149–169). New York: John Wiley & Sons.

Ostrom, E. (2000). Collective action and the evolution of social norms. *The Journal of Economic Perspectives, 14*, 137–158. doi:10.1257/jep.14.3.137

Ostrom, E., Gardner, R., & Walker, J. (1995). *Analysing long-enduring, self-organised, and self-governing CPRs*. Ann Arbor, MI: University of Michigan Press.

Ottmann, H. (1982). Cognitive interests and self-reflection . In Thompson, J. B., & Held, D. (Eds.), *Habermas: Critical debates* (pp. 79–97). London, UK: Macmillan.

Paas, F., Renkl, A., & Sweller, J. (2003). Cognitive Load Theory and Instructional Design: Recent Developments. *Educational Psychologist, 38*(1), 1–4. doi:10.1207/S15326985EP3801_1

Pagliari, C., Sloan, D., Gregor, P., Sullivan, F., Detmer, D., & Kahan, JP. (2005). What is eHealth? (4): A Scoping Exercise to Map the Field. *Journal of Medical Internet Research, 7*(1), e.

Pak, R., McLaughlin, A. C., Lin, C. C., Rogers, W. A., & Fisk, A. D. (2002). An age-related comparison of a touch screen and a novel input device. In *Proceedings of the Human Factors and Ergonomics Society 45th Annual Meeting*.

Palme, J. (1997). *User influence on software design may give less good software*. Computer Mediated Communication.

Palme, J. (1975). *Interactive Software for Humans* (An abbreviated version was published in *Management Informatics, 7*(1976), pp. 4-16).

Palme, J. (2000). *A personal history of CMC* (Honorary publication dedicated to Yvonne Wærn on Her Retirement).

Pang, N., Denison, T., Williamson, K., Johanson, G., & Schauder, D. (2008). Augmenting Communities with Knowledge Resources: The Case of the Knowledge Commons in Public Libraries . In Aurigi, A., & De Cindio, F. (Eds.), *Augmented Public Spaces: Articulating the Physical and Electronic City* (pp. 185–199). Ashgate Publishing.

Pang, N., & Schauder, D. (2007). The Culture of Information Systems in Knowledge-Creating Contexts: The Role of User-Centred Design. *Informing Science: The International Journal of an Emerging Discipline, 10*(Monograph), 203-235.

Pang, N., Schauder, D., Quartly, M., & Dale-Hallett, L. (2006). User-centred design, e-research, and adaptive capacity in cultural institutions: The case of the women on farms gathering collection. In C. Khoo, D. Singh & A. Chaudhry (Eds.), *Proceedings of the Asia-Pacific Conference on Library & Information Education & Practice* (A-LIEP 2006) (pp. 526-535). Singapore.

Paoletti, I. (2009). Communication and Diagnostic Work in Medical Emergency Calls in Italy. *Computer Supported Cooperative Work*, *18*(2-3), 229–250. doi:10.1007/s10606-009-9091-1

Parillo, J. (1995). A silver anniversary for the Society of Critical Care Medicine - Visions of the past and future: The presidential address from the 24th Educational and Scientific Symposium of the Society of Critical Care Medicine. *Critical Care Medicine*, *23*(4), 607–612.

Park, D. C., & Schwarz, N. (2000). *Cognitive Aging: A Primer*. London: Psychology Press.

Parker-Pope, T. (2009a, January 13). A Problem of the Brain, Not the Hands: Group Urges Phone Ban for Drivers. *New York Times*. Retrieved 17 August 2009 from, http://www.nytimes.com/2009/01/13/health/13well.html

Parker-Pope, T. (2009b). What Clown on a Unicycle? Studying Cellphone Distraction. *New York Times*. Retrieved 23 October 2009 from http://well.blogs.ytimes.com/2009/10/22/what-clown-on-a-unicycle-studying-cell-phone-distraction/

Parush, A. (2006). Practice and Research in Human Computer Interaction: Towards a common ground. *Interaction*, *13*(6), 61–62. doi:10.1145/1167948.1167994

Pask, G., & Scott, B. C. E. (1972). Learning strategies and individual competence. *International Journal of Man-Machine Studies*, *4*, 217–253. doi:10.1016/S0020-7373(72)80004-X

Patnaik, D., & Becker, R. (1999). Needfinding: The Why and How of Uncovering People's Needs. *Design Management Journal*, *10*(2), 37–43.

Patrick, A. S., & Kenny, S. (2003). *From Privacy Legislation to Interface Design: Implementing Information Privacy in Human-Computer Interaction*. Privacy Enhancing Technologies Workshop (PET2003), Dresden/Germany.

Patrick, A. S., Kenny, S., Holmes, C., & van Breukelen, M. (2003). Human Computer Interaction. In van Blarkom, G.W., Borking, J.J., & Olk, J.G.E. (Eds.), *Handbook for Privacy and Privacy-Enhancing Technologies* (pp. 249-290). PISA project.

Paul, D. L., & McDaniel, R. R. (2004). A field study of the effect of interpersonal trust on virtual collaborative relationship performance. *Management Information Systems Quarterly*, *28*(2), 183–227.

Pearce, C., Duan, K., Arnold, M., Phillips, C., & Trumble, S. (2009). Doctor, Patient and Computer—A Framework for the New Consultation. *International Journal of Medical Informatics*, *78*(1), 32–38. doi:10.1016/j.ijmedinf.2008.07.002

Pearson, S. (2006). Towards Automated Evaluation of Trust Constraints. In *Trust Management* (LNCS 3986, pp. 252-266).

Pedersen, J. (1998) *Informationstekniken i skolan* [Information technology in school]. Stockholm, SE: Skolverket.

Peirce, C. S. (1891). The architecture of Theories. *The Monist*, *1*(2), 161–176.

Pennathur, P. R., Bisantz, A. M., Fairbanks, R. J., Perry, S. J., & Wears, R. L. (2007). *Assessing the Impact of Computerization on Work Practice: Information Technology in Emergency Departments*. Presented at the Human Factors and Ergonomics Society 51st Annual Meeting, Baltimore, Maryland, October, 2007.

Pennock, R. (2009). Going Movile. *Nature*, *461*(22). Retrieved October 21, 2009 from http://www.nature.com/naturejobs/2009/091022/pdf/nj7267-1157a.pdf

Perrow, C. (1999). *Normal Accidents: Living with High Risk Technologies* (Updated ed.). Princeton, NJ: Princeton University Press.

Perry, M., O'Hara, K., Sellen, A., Brown, B., & Harper, R. (2001). Dealing with Mobility: Understanding Access Anytime, Anywhere. *AMC Transaction on Computer-Human Interaction*, *8*(4), 323–347. doi:10.1145/504704.504707

Pettersson, J. S. (Ed.). (2008). HCI Guidelines. PRIME deliverable D6.1.f.

Pettersson, J. S., Fischer-Hübner, S., & Bergmann, M. (2006). Outlining Data Track: Privacy-friendly Data Maintenance for End-users. In *Proceedings of the 15th International Conference on Information Systems Development (ISD 2006)*, Budapest, 31st August - 2nd September 2006. Springer Scientific Publishers.

Pettersson, J. S., Fischer-Hübner, S., Danielsson, N., Nilsson, J., Bergmann, M., Clauß, S., et al. (2005). Making PRIME usable. *SOUPS 2005 Symposium on Usable Privacy and Security*, Carnegie Mellon University, July 6-8 July, 2005, Pittsburgh. Available in ACM Digital Library.

Pfeiffer, J. W., & Jones, J. E. (1969). *A Handbook of Structured Experiments for Human Relations Training (Vol. 1)*. Iowa City, IA: University Associates Press.

Pfitzmann, A., & Hansen, M. (2008, February 15). Anonymity. Unlinkability, Undetectability, Unobservability, Pseudonymity, and Identity Management – A Consolidated Proposal for Terminology, Version v0.31. Retrieved from http://dud.inf.tu-dresden.de/literatur/Anon_Terminology_v0.31.doc#_Toc64643839

Piaget, J. (1948). *The Moral Judgment of the Child*. Glencoe, IL: Free Press.

Pickering, J. A. (1985). Touch-sensitive screens: the technologies and their application. *International Journal of Man-Machine Studies*, *25*, 249–269. doi:10.1016/S0020-7373(86)80060-8

Pinheiro da Silva, P., Deborah, S., McGuinness, D. L., & McCool, R. (2003). Knowledge Provenance Infrastructure. *A Quarterly Bulletin of the Computer Society of the IEEE Technical Committee on Data Engineering*, *26*(4), 26–32.

Pinsonneault, A., & Caya, O. (2005). Virtual teams: What we know, what we don't know. *International Journal of e-Collaboration*, *1*(3), 1–16.

Pirsig, R. (1974). *Zen and the art of motorcycle maintenance*. New York, NY: Bantam Books.

Pitkin, B. (2001). Community Informatics: hope or hype. In *Proceedings of the 34th Hawaii International Conference on System Sciences*. Retrieved from http://csdl.computer.org/comp/proceedings/hicss/2001/0981/08/09818005.pdf

Pitrella, F. D., & Käppler, W.-D. (1988). *Identification and Evaluation of Scale Design Principles in the Development of the Sequential Judgment, Extended Range Scale. Forschungsinstitut für Anthropotechnik. FAT-Bericht Nr. 80*. Wachtberg.

Poole, J. (2006). E- learning and e-learning styles: students' reactions to web-based Language and Style at Blackpool and the Fylde College. *Language and Literature*, *15*, 307. doi:10.1177/0963947006066129

Poulantzas, N. (1969). The Problem of the Capitalist State. *New Left Review*, *I*(58), 68–78.

Powell, A., Piccoli, G., & Ives, B. (2004). Virtual teams: A review of current literature and directions for future research. *The Data Base for Advances in Information Systems*, *35*(1), 6–36.

Preece, J., Rogers, Y., & Sharp, H. (2007). *Interaction design: beyond human – computer interaction*. New York: Wiley.

Preece, J., Rogers, Y., Sharp, H., Benyon, D., Holland, S., & Carey, T. (1994). *Human-computer interaction*. Harlow, UK: Addison-Wesley.

Priest, H. A., Stagl, K. C., Klein, C., & Salas, E. (2006). Virtual teams: Creating context for distribuited teamwork . In Bowers, C., Salas, E., & Jentsch, F. (Eds.), *Creating high-tech teams - Practical guidance on work performance and technology* (pp. 185–212). Washington, DC: American Psychological Association. doi:10.1037/11263-009

Progoff, I. (1973). *Jung's psychology and its social meaning* (Original ed., 1953), Garden City, NY: Anchor Press/Doubleday.

Pronovost, P. J., Angus, D. C., Dorman, T., Robinson, K. A., Dremsizov, T. T., & Young, T. L. (2002). Physician staffing patterns and clinical outcomes in critically ill patients - A systematic review. *Journal of the American Medical Association*, *288*(17), 2151–2162. doi:10.1001/jama.288.17.2151

Pronovost, P. J., Jenekes, M. W., Dormant, T., Garrett, E., Breslow, M., & Rosenfeld, B. A. (1999). Organizational characterisitcs of intensive care units related to outcomes of abdominal aortic surgery. *Journal of the American Medical Association, 281*(14), 1310–1317. doi:10.1001/jama.281.14.1310

Putz-Anderson, V. (Ed.). (1988). *Cumulative Trauma Disorders-A Manual for Musculoskeletal Diseases of the Upper Limbs*. London: Taylor & Francis.

Pye, G., & Warren, M. J. (2006). Striking a Balance Between Ethics and ICT Governance. *Australian Journal of Information System, 13*(2), 201–207.

Pyöriä, P. (2005). Information technology, human relations and knowledge work teams. *Team Performance Management, 11*(3/4), 104–112. doi:10.1108/13527590510606307

Quan-Haase, A., & Cothrel, J. (2003). Uses of Information Sources in an Internet-era Firm: Online and Offline. In M.H. Huysman, E. Wenger & V. Wulf (Eds.), *Proceedings of the First International Conference on Communities and Technologies*, Amsterdam, Holland, 19-21 September, Kluwer Academic Publishers, Dordrecht. Retrieved October 3, 2009 from http://www.iisi.de/fileadmin/IISI/upload/C_T/2003/quanhaase-cothrel.pdf

Quan-Haase, A., Cothrel, J., & Wellman, B. (2005). Instant Messaging for Collaboration: A Case Study of a Hightech Firm. *Journal of Computer-Mediated Communication, 10*(4). Retrieved October 3, 2009 from http://jcmc.indiana.edu/vol10/issue4/quan-haase.html

Quinn, R. (2005). Flow in knowledge work: high performance experience in the design of national security technology. *Administrative Science Quarterly, 50*(4), 610–641.

Qureshi, S., & Keen, P. (2005). Activating Knowledge through Electronic Collaboration: vanquishing the knowledge paradox. *IEEE Transactions on Professional Communication, 48*(1), 40–54. doi:10.1109/TPC.2004.843296

Rabin, R. C. (2009, January 30). When Talking on the Phone May Endanger a Child. *New York Times*. Retrieved September 17, 2009 from http://www.nytimes.com/2009/01/30/health/30phone.html

Radhakrishnan, S., & Moore, Ch. A. (1957). *A Sourcebook in Indian Philosophy*. Princeton, NJ: Princeton University Press.

Raghavan, V. V., Sakaguchi, T., & Mahaney, R. (2008). An empirical investigation of stress factors in information technology professionals. *Information Resources Management Journal, 21*(2), 38–62.

Rainey, T. G., & Shapiro, M. J. (2001). Critical care medicine for the 21st century. *Critical Care Medicine, 29*(2), 436–437. doi:10.1097/00003246-200102000-00040

Rapoport, J., Teres, D., Steingrub, J., Higgings, T., McGee, W., & Lemeshow, S. (2000). Patient characteristics and ICU organizational factors that influence frequency of pulmonary artery catheterization. *Journal of the American Medical Association, 283*(3), 259–2567.

Raskin, J. (2000). *The Humane Interface – New Directions for Designing Interactive Systems*. New York: ACM Press.

Rau, P.-L. P., & Hsu, J.-W. (2005). Interaction devices and web design for novice older users. *Educational Gerontology, 31*, 19–40. doi:10.1080/03601270590522170

Rawlings, A., Woodland, J. H., Vegunta, R. K., & Crawford, D. L. (2007). Robotic versus laparoscopic colectomy. *Surgical Endoscopy, 21*(10), 1701–1708. doi:10.1007/s00464-007-9231-y

Rayner, K. (1998). Eye Movements in Reading and Information Processing: 20 Years of Research. *Psychological Bulletin, 124*(3), 372–422. doi:10.1037/0033-2909.124.3.372

Reason, P., & Bradbury, H. (2002). Introduction: Inquiry and participation in search of a world worthy of human aspiration. In Reason, P., & Bradbury, H. (Eds.), *Handbook of Action Research: Participative Inquiry and Practice* (pp. 1–14). Thousand Oaks, CA: SAGE Publications.

Reid, M. F., Riemenschneider, C. K., Allen, M. W., & Armstrong, D. (2008). Information technology employees in state government – A study of affective organizational commitment, job involvement and job satisfaction. *American Review of Public Administration, 38*(1), 41–61. doi:10.1177/0275074007303136

Rekimoto, J. (2002). Smartskin: An infrastructure for freehand manipulation on interactive surfaces. In *Proceedings of the 2002 SIGCHI Conference on Human Factors in Computing Systems*, USA.

Renfrew, C., & Bahn, P. (2004). *Archaeology: theories, methods and practice*. London: Thames and Hudson.

Rennecker, J., & Godwin, L. (2005). Delays and Interruptions: A Self-Perpetuating Paradox of Communication of Technology Use. *Information and Organization, 15*(3), 247–266. doi:10.1016/j.infoandorg.2005.02.004

Reynolds, H. N., Haupt, M. T., Thill-Baharozian, M. C., & Carlson, R. W. (1988). Impact of critical care pysician staffing on patients with septic shock in a university hospital medical intensive care unit. *Journal of the American Medical Association, 260*(23), 3446–3450. doi:10.1001/jama.260.23.3446

Rice, R. E. (1992). Task analyzability, use of new media, and effectiveness: A multi-site exploration of media richness. *Organization Science, 3*(4), 475–500. doi:10.1287/orsc.3.4.475

Rice, R. E., & Shook, D. E. (1990). Voice messaging, coordination, and communication. In Galegher, J., Kraut, R. E., & Egido, C. (Eds.), *Intellectual Teamwork: Social and Technological Foundations of Cooperative Work* (pp. 327–350). Hillsdale, NJ: Lawrence Erlbaum Associates.

Richmond, A., & Skitmore, M. (2006). Stress and coping; a study of project managers in a large ICT organization. *Project Management Journal, 37*(5), 5–16.

Richtel, M. (2009a, September 8). Text Driving Now an Issue in the Back Seat. *New York Times*. Retrieved August 17, 2009 from http://www.nytimes.com/2009/09/09/technology/09distracted.html

Richtel, M. (2009b, August 29). Utah Gets Tough with Texting Drivers. *New York Times*. Retrieved August 17, 2009 from http://www.nytimes.com/2009/08/29/technology/29distracted.html

Richtel, M. (2009c, August 17). Drivers and Legislators Dismiss Cellphone Risks. *New York Times*. Retrieved August 17, 2009 from http://www.nytimes.com/2009/07/19/technology/19distracted.html

Richtel, M. (2009d, August 17). In Study, Texting Lifts Crash Risk by Large Margin. *New York Times*. Retrieved 17 August 2009, http://www.nytimes.com/2009/07/28/technology/28texting.html

Richtel, M. (2009e, July 21). U.S. Withheld Data on Risks of Distracted Driving. *New York Times*. Retrieved September 17, 2009 from http://www.nytimes.com/2009/07/21/technology/21distracted.html

Richtel, M. (2009f, July 29). Senators Seek a Ban on Texting and Driving. *New York Times*. Retrieved September 17, 2009 from http://www.nytimes.com/2009/07/30/technology/30distracted.html

Richtel, M. (2009g, October 1). At 60 M.P.H., Office Work is High Risk. *New York Times*. Retrieved October 1, 2009 from http://www.nytimes.com/2009/10/01/technology/01distracted.html

Riding, R. (1993). *A trainer's guide to learning design: Learning methods project report, Assessment Research Unit*. Birmingham, UK: University of Birmingham.

Riding, R., & Cheema, I. (1991). Cognitive styles - an overview and integration. *Educational Psychology, 11*(3&4), 193–215. doi:10.1080/0144341910110301

Riding, R. J., & Caine, R. (1993). Cognitive style and GCSE performance in mathematics, English language and French. *Educational Psychology, 13*(1), 59–67. doi:10.1080/0144341930130107

Riding, R. J., & Mathais, D. (1991). Cognitive styles and preferred learning mode, reading attainment and cognitive ability in 11-year-old children. *Educational Psychology, 11*(3 & 4), 383–393. doi:10.1080/0144341910110312

Riding, R. J., & Rayner, S. (1998). *Cognitive styles and learning strategies*. UK: Fulton.

Ries, M. (2009). Tele-ICU: A new paradigm in critical care. *International Anesthesiology Clinics, 47*(1), 153–170. doi:10.1097/AIA.0b013e3181950078

Riis, U. Jedeskog, (1997) *Pedagogik, teknik eller ekonomi? [Teaching, technology or economy?]*. Repro-centralen HSC, Uppsala Universitet, Sweden.

Riley, P. (1986). *The general will before Rousseau: The transformation of the divine into the civic*. Princeton, NJ: Princeton University Press.

Riley, P. (1983). Marx and morality: A reply to Richard Miller . In Pennock, J. R., & Chapman, J. W. (Eds.), *Marxism* (pp. 33–53). New York/London, NY/UK: New York University Press.

Riviere, C. N., & Thakor, N. V. (1996). Effects of age and disability on tracking tasks with a computer mouse: Accuracy and linearity. *Journal of Rehabilitation Research and Development, 33*(1), 6–15.

Robbin, A. (2007). Rob Kling In Search of One Good Theory. *The Information Society, 23*(4), 235–250. doi:10.1080/01972240701444154

Robbin, A. (2010). Theorizing ICT and society: A Preliminary Inquiry into the Methodologies Employed in Research on ICTs and Society: Prologue (An Alternate View of Knowledge Negotiation). *Triple C: Cognition, Communication, Co-operation, 8*(2). Retrieved July 19, 2010, from http://triple-c.at/index.php/tripleC/article/view/171/182

Robbins, S. R. (1983). *Organization Theory: The Structure and Design of Organizations*. Englewood Cliffs, NJ: Prentice Hall.

Robertson, M., & Rahimi, M. (1990). A systems analysis for implementing video display terminals. *IEEE Transactions on Engineering Management, 37*, 55–62. doi:10.1109/17.45270

Robertson, M. M., & Courtney, T. K. (2004). Solving office work systems performance problems- a systems analysis approach. *Theoretical Issues in Ergonomic, 5*(3), 181–197. doi:10.1080/1463922021000032320

Robertson, M. M., & Kleiner, B. (2002). Macroergonomic methods: Assessing work system processes . In Hendrick, H., & Kleiner, B. (Eds.), *Macroergonomics Theory, Methods, and Applications*. New Jersey: Lawrence Erlbaum Associates.

Robertson, M. M. (2005). Systems analysis tool (SAT). In Stanton, N. Hedge, A., Brookhuis, K., Salas, Ed., Hendrick, H. (Eds.), *Handbook of Human Factors and Ergonomics methods*. CRC Press.

Robertson, M., & Bradley, G. (1997). Competence development in ten high tech companies in Silicon Valley. In Salvendy, G. & Smith, M. J. & Koubek, R.J. (Eds.). *Design of Computing Systems. Proceedings of the Seventh International Conference on Human-Computer Interaction*, San Francisco, California, USA, August 24-29, 1997. Amsterdam/Lausanne/New York/Oxford/Shannan/Tokyo: Elsevier

Robinson, M. (1989, March). Double level languages and cooperative working. Support, society and culture: Mutual uses of cybernetics and science. *The International Federation for Cybernetics*. Amsterdam, The Netherlands.

Rogers, W. A., Cabera, E. F., Jamieson, B. A., & Rousseau, G. K. (1995). Automatic teller machines and older adults: Usage patterns and training needs. In *Proceedings of the 103 Annual Convention of the American Psychological Association*.

Rogerson, S., & Bynum, T. W. (1995). Cyberspace: The Ethical Frontier . *Times Higher Education Supplement, 1179*(9), 4.

Rogerson, S. (2007). E- Inclusion Ethics. *ETHICOL in the IMIS Journal, 17*(7).

Rosenfeld, B. A., Dorman, T., Breslow, M. J., Pronovost, P., Jenckes, M., & Zhang, N. (2000). Intensive care unit telemedicine: Alternate paradigm for providing continuous intensivist care. *Critical Care Medicine, 28*(12), 3925–3931. doi:10.1097/00003246-200012000-00034

Rothberg, H. N., & Erickson, G. S. (2004). *From Knowledge to Intelligence: Creating Competitive Advantage in the Next Economy*. Oxford, UK: Elsevier Butterworth-Heinemann.

Rothman, J., & Tropman, J. E. (1970). Models of Community Organization and Macro Practice Perspectives: Their Mixing and Phasing . In Cox, F. M. (Ed.), *Strategies of Community Organization* (pp. 3–26). Itasca, Ill: FE Peacock.

Rousseau, D. M., Sitkin, S. B., Burt, R. S., & Camerer, C. (1998). Not so different after all: A cross-discipline view of trust. *Academy of Management Review, 23*(3), 393–404.

Rowe, D., & Gray, J. J. (2000). *The Hilbert Challenge*. Oxford: Oxford University Press.

Ruble, D. A. (1997). *The Event Model, Practical Analysis and Design for Client Server & GUI Systems* (pp. 79–115). Upper Saddle River, NJ: Prentice Hall.

Rullo, A. (2008). The soft qualities of interaction. *ACM Transactions on Computer-Human Interaction, 15*(4), 17. doi:10.1145/1460355.1460359

Sachs, L. (1999). *Angewandte Satistik, Anwendung statistischer Methoden*. Heidelberg, Deutschland: Springer Verlag.

Sacks, O. (1970). *The Man Who Mistook His Wife For A Hat: And Other Clinical Tales*. New York: Touchstone.

Sadler, K., Robertson, T., Kan, M., & Hagen, P. (2006). Balancing Work, Life and Other Concerns: A Study of Mobile Technology Use by Australian Freelancers. In *Proceedings of the 2006 NordiCHI conference: Changing Roles* (pp. 413-416). Oslo, Norway.

Salanova, M., Cifre, E., & Martin, P. (2004). Information technology implementation styles and their relation with workers' subjective well-being. *International Journal of Occupations and Production Management, 24*(1), 42–54. doi:10.1108/01443570410510988

Saleem, J., Russa, A., Justice, C. F., Hagga, H., Ebrighte, P. R., Woodbridge, P. A., & Doebbeling, B. N. (2009). Exploring the Persistence of Paper with the Electronic Health Record. *International Journal of Medical Informatics, 78*(9), 618–628. doi:10.1016/j.ijmedinf.2009.04.001

Salvendy, G., & Smith, M. I. (Eds.) (1981). *Machine-Pacing and Occupational Stress*. London: Taylor & Francis.

Sandberg, Å., & Augustsson, F. (2002). *Interactive Media in Sweden – The Second Interactive Media, Internet and Multimedia Industry Survey*. Stockholm: National Institute for Working Life.

Santos, A. (2004). Do community technology centers decrease social inequities? Results of a nationwide qualitative study to evaluate the plazas communitarieas project in Mexico. In E. McKay, (Ed.), *Proceedings of the International Conference on Computers in Education - Acquiring and Constructing Knowledge Through Human-Computer Interaction: Creating new visions for the future of learning* (pp.1133-1144.), Melbourne Exhibition Centre, Australia: Common Ground Publishing.

Sassen, S. (1991). *The Global City: London, Tokyo, New York*. New Jersey: Princeton University Press.

Scarbrough, H. (1999). Knowledge as Work: Conflicts in the Management of Knowledge Workers. *Technology Analysis and Strategic Management, 11*(1), 5–16. doi:10.1080/095373299107546

Schaffers, H., Cordoba, M., Hongistro, P., Kallai, T., Merz, C., & Rensburg, J. (2007). Exploring Business Models for Open Innovation in Rural Living Labs. In *Proceedings of the 13th International Conference on Concurrent Enterprising* (pp. 49-56). Sophia-Antipolis, France.

Schank, R. C. (1982). *Dynamic memory*. Cambridge, UK: Cambridge University Press.

Schank, R. C., & Abelson, R. P. (1977). *Scripts, plans, goals, and understanding: An inquiry into human knowledge structures*. Hillsdale, NJ: Lawrence Erlbaum Associates.

Schauer, T. (2003). *The Sustainable Information Society: Vision and Risks*. Ulm, DE: Universitätsverlag.

Schechter, D. (1989). For whom and to do what? Questions for a liberating systems theory. Proceedings of the ISSS Int. Society for the Systems Sciences, *33rd Annual Conference, Vol.2*, Edinburgh, Scotland.

Schechter, S. E., Dhamija, R., Ozment, A., & Fischer, I. (2007). The Emperor's New Security Indicators: An evaluation of web site authentication and the effect of role playing on usability studies. *IEEE Symposium on Security and Privacy*, May 20-27, 2007, Oakland, California.

Scheler, M. (1957). *Der Bourgeois und die religiöse Mächte (Vol. 3)*. Bern-München, DE: Gesammelte Werke.

Scheler, M. (1988). *Lo spirito del capitalismo; e altri saggi* (Trans. collection of essays from German orig.). Guida, IT: Napoli.

Schiller, H. (1993). Public way of private road? *Nation (New York, N.Y.), 12*, 64–66.

Schlager, E. (2002). Rationality, cooperation, and common pool resources. *The American Behavioral Scientist, 45*(5), 801–819. doi:10.1177/0002764202045005005

Schleifer, L. M., Spalding, T. W., Kerick, S. E., Cram, J. R., Ley, R., & Hatfield, B. D. (2008). Mental stress and trapezius muscle activation under psychomotor challenge: A focus on EMG gaps during computer work. *Psychophysiology, 45*(3), 356–365. doi:10.1111/j.1469-8986.2008.00645.x

Schmidt-Bleek, F. (2009). *The Earth: Natural Resources and Human Intervention*. London: Haus Publishing Limited.

Schneider, F. (2006, November 6). *Collaboration - some thoughts concerning new ways of learning and working together*. Centre for Research Architecture. Retrieved March 7, 2007, from http://roundtable.kein.org/node/525

Schneider, N., Vetter, S., Kausch, B., & Schlick, C. (2009). Age-differentiated Visualization of Network Plans for Project Management Software. *17th World Congress on Ergonomics,* Beijing.

Schrier, K., & Kinzer, Ch. (2008). Using Digital Games to Develop Ethical Teachers . In Glibson, D., & Baek, Y. (Eds.), *Digital Simulations for Improving Education: Learning Through Artifial Teaching Environment* (pp. 308–333). Hershey, PA: IGI Global.

Schuler, D., & Day, P. (2004). *Community Practice in the Network Society: Local Action/ Global Interaction*. London: Routledge.

Schultze, U., & Boland, R. J. Jr. (2000). Knowledge management technology and the reproduction of knowledge work practices. *The Journal of Strategic Information Systems, 9*, 193–212. doi:10.1016/S0963-8687(00)00043-3

Scott, K. M. (2009). Is Usability Obsolete? *Interaction, 16*(3), 6–11. doi:10.1145/1516016.1516018

Scott, S. D., & Carpendale, S. (2006). Investigating tabletop territoriality in digital tabletop work. *Technical Report 2006* (pp. 836-826). Department of Computer Science, University of Calgary, Canada.

Searle, J. R. (1969). *Speech Acts – An essay in the philosophy of language*. London: Cambridge University Press.

Seligman, M. E. P. (1975). *Helplessness: On depression, development and death*. San Francisco, SF: W.H. Freeman & Company.

Selye, J. (1956). *The Stress of Life*. New York: McGraw Hill.

Sen, A. (1999). *Development as Freedom*. Oxford: Oxford University Press.

Sen, A. (2002). *Rationality and Freedom*. Cambridge, MA: Harvard University Press.

Sen, A. (2003). Development and Capability Expansion . In Fukuda-Parr, S., & Shiva Kumar, A. K. (Eds.), *Readings in Human Development*. Oxford: Oxford University Press.

Sen, A. (2000). *Why Human Security. International Symposium Human Security*, Tokyo, 28 July, 2000. Retrieved June 17, 2009 http://indh.pnud.org.co/files/rec/SenWhyHS.pdf

Senge, P. (1990). *The fifth discipline: The art and practices of the learning organization*. New York: Random House.

Sengpiel, M., Struve, D., Dittberner, D. & Wandke, H. (2008). Entwicklung von Trainingsprogrammen für ältere Benutzer von IT- Systemen. *Wirtschaftspsychologie aktuell*, 10, 94-105.

Seppälä, P. (2001). Experience of stress, musculoskeletal discomfort, and eyestrain in computer-based office work: A study in municipal workplaces. *International Journal of Human-Computer Interaction*, 13(3), 279–304. doi:10.1207/S15327590IJHC1303_1

Sewell, W. H. (1992). A Theory of Structure: Duality, Agency, and Transformation. *American Journal of Sociology*, 98(1), 1–29. doi:10.1086/229967

Shami, T. A. (2008). Living Labs: Good Practices in Europe . In Schumacher, J., & Niitamo, V. P. (Eds.), *European Living Labs - A New Approach for Human Centric Regional Innovation* (pp. 15–30). Berlin, DE: Wissenschaftlicher Verlag.

Shani, A. B., Sena, J., & Stebbing, M. W. (2000). Knowledge work teams and groupware technology: learning from Seagate's experience. *Journal of Knowledge Management*, 4(2), 111–124. doi:10.1108/13673270010336602

Shannon, C. E., & Weaver, W. (1949). *A Mathematical Theory of Communication*. Eleventh edition, 1967. Urbana, IL: University of Illinois Press.

Shapiro, D. (2005). Participatory design: the will to succeed. In O. W. Bertelsen, N. O. Bouvin, P. G. Krogh & M. Kyng (Eds.), *Proceedings of the 4th Decennial Conference on Critical Computing: Between Sense and Sensibility* (pp. 29–38). New York: ACM Press.

Sharit, J., Czaja, S. J., & Nair, S. N. (1998). Subjective experiences of stress, workload, and bodily discomfort as a function of age and type of computer work. *Work and Stress*, 12(2), 125–144. doi:10.1080/02678379808256855

Sheikh, A., & Gatrad, A. R. (Eds.). (2000). *Caring for Muslim Patients*. Oxford, UK: Radcliffe Medical Press.

Sherman, F. T. (2001). Functional assessment – Easy-to-use screening tools speed initial office work-up. *Geriatrics*, 56(8), 36–40.

Shneiderman, B. (1998). *Designing the User Interface* (Wesley, A., Ed.).

Shortell, S. M., & Rousseau, D. M. (1989). *The Organization and Management of Intensive Care Units*. University of California-Berkeley.

Shortell, S. M., Rousseau, D. M., Gillies, R. R., Devers, K. J., & Simons, T. L. (1991). Organizational assessment in intensive care units (ICUs): construct development, reliability, and validity of the ICU nurse-physician questionnaire. *Medical Care*, 29(8), 709–726. doi:10.1097/00005650-199108000-00004

Shortell, S. M., Zimmerman, J. E., Rousseau, D. M., Gillies, R. R., Wagner, D. P., & Draper, E. A. (1994). The performance of intensive care units - does good management make a difference. *Medical Care*, 32(5), 508–525. doi:10.1097/00005650-199405000-00009

Sibert, L. E., & Jacob, R. J. K. (2000). Evaluation of eye gaze interaction. In . *Proceedings, CHI2000*, 282–288.

Sider, R. (2001). Book review: *Development as Freedom Amarta Sen*. Retrieved June 12, 2009 from http://www.leaderu.org/ftissues/ft0101/reviews/sider.html

Siegrist, J. (1996). Adverse health effects of high-effort/low-reward conditions. *Journal of Occupational Health Psychology*, 1(2), 27–41. doi:10.1037/1076-8998.1.1.27

Siirak, V. (2002). Multi-media and the internet as educational tools for solving the problems of ergonomics and safety . In *Human Factors in Transportation, Communication, Health and the Workplace* (pp. 471–472). The Netherlands: Shaker Publishing.

Siirak, V. (2000). Influencing behaviour through learning of ergonomics knowledge in Cyberspace: a new millennium strategy to the reduction of health risks and accidents at working environment in Estonia. In K.E. Fostervold & T. Endestad (Eds.), *At the gateway to Cyberspace-ergonomic thinking in a new millennium* (pp. 225-228). Oslo, NO: Nordiska Ergonomisällskapet.

Siirak, V. (2001). New challenge for ergonomics and human factors education in technical universities. In *Proceedings of NES 2001 Nordic Ergonomics Society 33rd Annual Congress* (pp. 210-212). University of Tampere, Finland.

Siirak, V. (2002). Experience of new teaching strategies of occupational health and ergonomics at Tallinn Technical University. In *Proceedings of 6th International Conference Scientific Committee on Education and Training in Occupational Health Ideas that Sizzle* (pp. 224-226). Baltimore, Maryland, USA.

Siirak, V. (2003), Computer Based Learning as an Effective Tool for Prevention of Chemical Risks - CD ROM. In *Proceedings of 8th International Symposium of ISSA Research Section*, Athens, Greece E.L.I.N.Y.A.E. (Hellenic Institute for Occupational Health and Safety)

Siirak, V. (2004). New Challenges for Human Factors and Ergonomics Education in Technical Universities- CD ROM. In *Proceedings of WorkCongress6: 6th International Congress on Work Injuries, Prevention, Rehabilitation and Compensation*, Rome. Italy. INAIL. Italian Workers Compensation Authority. Italian Workcover. Directorate of Communication. External Communication and International Relations Unit. Piazzale Giulio Pastore 6. I-0014 Rome RM, EUROPEAN UNION.

Siirak, V. (2005). Some experience of computer based learning in occupational health and safety education for future engineers. In *Proceedings of the 1st International Conference on Interdisciplinarity in Education ICIE 2005* (pp. 91-96). National Technical University of Athens, Athens, Greece.

Siirak, V. (2006). Some experience of ECTAS education for crossing international, cultural and social borders. Ioannides. In *Proceedings of the 2nd International Conference on Interdisciplinarity in Education ICIE 2006* (pp. 113-117). National Technical University of Athens, Athens, Greece.

Siirak, V. (2007). Experiencing Education in Engineering, Computer Technology and Applied Science for Crossing International, Cultural and Social Borders. In *Proceedings of 3rd International Conference on Interdisciplinarity in Education ICIE`07 as International Forum for Multi-Culturality, Multi-Ethnicity and Multi-Disciplinarity in European Higher Education and Research MULTIFORUM`07* (pp. 114-119). Athens, Greece.

Siirak, V. (2007). Experiencing the Computer Based Learning in Occupational Health and Safety Education for Future Engineers. In *Proceedings of 3rd International Conference on Interdisciplinarity in Education ICIE`07 as International Forum for Multi-Culturality, Multi-Ethnicity and Multi-Disciplinarity in European Higher Education and Research MULTIFORUM`07* (pp.276-279). National Technical University of Athens, Athens, Greece.

Siirak, V. (2008). Moodle e-learning environment – an effective tool for a development of a learning culture. In *Proceedings of International Symposium Hazards XX: Process Safety and Environmental Protection- Harnessing Knowledge _ Challenging Complacency* (pp.290-296). Manchester, UK.

Siirak, V., & Kristjuhan, U. (2000). Changing Paradigms for Ergonomics and Safety Educational Technology in Estonia. In *Proceedings of the Second International Conference ERGON-AXIA 2000 - Ergonomics and Safety for Global Business Quality and Productivity* (pp. 293-296). Warsaw, Poland.

Silverman, D. (2001). *Interpreting Qualitative Data: Methods for Analysing Talk, Text and Interaction*. Thousand Oaks, CA: SAGE Publications.

Silverstein, B., Fine, L., & Armstrong, T. (1987). Occupational factors and the carpal tunnel syndrome. *American Journal of Industrial Medicine, 11*, 343–358. doi:10.1002/ajim.4700110310

Simon, H. A. (1957). *Models of Man: social and rational.* New York: John Wiley & Sons.

Simon, H. A. (1960). *The New Science of Management Decision.* New York, NY: Harper & Row Pub.

Simpson, G. (1951). Science as morality. *Philosophy of Science, 18*(2), 132–143. doi:10.1086/287139

Smedje, G. (2000). *The indoor environment of schools: Respiratory effects and air quality.* Ph D Thesis, Institutionen för medicinska vetenskap, Uppsala University, Uppsala, Sweden.

Smith, M. J., & Carayon, P. C. (1995). New technology, automation and work organization: Stress problems and improved technology implementation strategies. *The International Journal of Human Factors in Manufacturing, 5*, 99–116. doi:10.1002/hfm.4530050107

Smith, M. J., & Sainfort, P. C. (1989). A balance theory of job design for stress reduction. *International Journal of Industrial Ergonomics, 4*, 67–79. doi:10.1016/0169-8141(89)90051-6

Smith, M. W., Sharit, J., & Czaja, S. J. (1999). Aging, motor control, and the performance of computer mouse tasks. *Human Factors, 41*(3), 389–396. doi:10.1518/001872099779611102

Smith, M. J. (1985). Machine-paced work and stress . In Cooper, C. L., & Smith, M. J. (Eds.), *Job Stress and Blue-Collar Work* (pp. 51–64). New York: John Wiley & Sons.

Smith, M. J., & Carayon, P. C. (1996). Work Organization, Stress and Cumulative Trauma Disorders . In Moon, S., & Sauter, S. (Eds.), *Beyond Biomechanics: Psychosocial Aspects of Cumulative Trauma Disorders* (pp. 23–42). London: Taylor & Francis.

Smith, M. J. (1987). Occupational stress . In Salvendy, G. (Ed.), *Handbook of Human Factors* (pp. 844–860). New York: John Wiley & Sons.

Smith, M. J., Carayon, P., Eberts, R., & Salvendy, G. (1992). Human-Computer interaction . In Salvendy, G. (Ed.), *Handbook of Industrial Engineering* (pp. 1107–1144). New York: John Wiley & Sons.

Smith, M. J., & Amick, B. C. III. (1989). Electronic Monitoring at the Workplace: Implications for Employee Control and Job Stress . In Sauter, S., & Hurrell, J. (Eds.), *Job Control and Worker Health* (pp. 275–288). Chichester, UK: John Wiley and Sons, Ltd.

Smith, A. (1759). The Theory of Moral Sentiments. In A. Smith (Ed.), *Moral and Political Philosophy* (hH. Schneider, New York, NY: Harper & Row. (1948 & 1978).

Smith, M. J., Carayon, P., & Miezio, K. (1986). Motivational, Behavioral and Psychological Implications of Electronic Monitoring of Worker Performance. *Prepared for the Office of Technology Assessment.* United States Congress. Washington, DC: Office of Technology Assessment, U.S. Congress

Snow, C. P. (1998). *The two cultures.* Cambridge, UK: Cambridge University Press. (Original work published 1959)

Söderström, M., Jeding, K., Ekstedt, M., Kecklund, G., & Åkerstedt, T. (2003). *Arbetsmiljö, stress och utbrändhet inom ett företag i IT-branschen.*[The working environment, stress and burnout in a company in the IT sector] 312(pp. 1-54).

Solow, R. M. (1987). We'd better watch out. *New York Times Book Review, 12*(2), 36-50.

Som, C., Hilty, L. M., & Ruddy, T. F. (2004). The Precautionary Principle in the Information Society. *Human and Ecological Risk Assessment, 10*(8), 787–799. doi:10.1080/10807030490513801

Sonnetag, S., & Bayer, U. (2005). Switching off mentally: Predictors and Consequences of Psychological Detachment from Work During off-job time. *Journal of Occupational Health Psychology, 10*(4), 393–414. doi:10.1037/1076-8998.10.4.393

Sonnier, I. L. (1989). *Affective education: Methods and techniques*. New Jersey: Educational Technology Publications.

SOU 2006:77. Statens Offentliga Utredningar. Ungdomar, stress och psykisk ohälsa.www.regeringen.se

Soukoreff, R. W., & MacKenzie, I. S. (2004). Towards a standard for pointing device evaluation, perspectives on 27 years of Fitts' law research in HCI. *International Journal of Human-Computer Studies, 61*, 751–789. doi:10.1016/j.ijhcs.2004.09.001

Soundcloud (2009). *Who We Are*. Retrieved July 11, 2009, from http://soundcloud.com/pages/who-we-are

Srivastava, L. (2005). Mobile phones and the evolution of social behavior. *Behaviour & Information Technology, 24*(2), 111–129. doi:10.1080/01449290512331321910

Ståhlbröst, A., & Holst, M. (2006). Appreciating Needs for Innovative IT Design. *International Journal of Knowledge . Culture and Change Management, 6*(4), 37–46.

Ståhlbröst, A., & Bergvall-Kåreborn, B. (2008). FormIT - An Approach to User Involvement . In Schumacher, J., & Niitamo, V. P. (Eds.), *European Living Labs- A New Approach for Human Centric Regional Innovation* (pp. 63–76). Berlin, DE: Wissenschaftlicher Verlag.

Ståhlbröst, A. (2004). Exploring the Testbed Field. In *27th Information Systems Research Seminars in Scandinavia, IRIS 27*, Falkenberg, Sweden.

Ståhlbröst, A. (2008). *Forming Future IT - The Living Lab Way of User Involvement*. Department of Business Administration and Social Sciences. PhD Thesis. Luleå, Luleå University of Technology, Sweden.

Staley, A. (2005). Students`Perspectives of Moodle, Digital Future. *The Newsletter of the Learning Technology Development Unit, 2*, 2–3.

Stamp, G. (1981). Levels and Types of Managerial Capability. *Journal of Management Studies, 18*(4), 277–297. doi:10.1111/j.1467-6486.1981.tb00103.x

Benton Foundation. (2004). Defining the Technology Gap: from Losing Ground Bit by Bit: Low-Income Communities in the Information Age . In Stephen, G. (Ed.), *The Cybercities Reader* (pp. 306–308). London, UK: Routledge.

Stevenson, W. B. (1993). Organizational Design . In Golembiewski, R. T. (Ed.), *Handbook of Organizational Behavior*. New York: Marcel Dekker.

Stillman, L. (2008). Gunilla Bradley: Social and Community Informatics: Humans on the Net [Review]. *Information Communication and Society, 11*(3), 433–438.

Stillman, L., Kethers, S., French, R., & Lombard, D. (2009). Adapting Corporate Modelling for Community Informatics. *VINE: The Journal of Information and Knowledge Management Systems, 39*(3), 259–274.

Stillman, L., & Stoecker, R. (2008). Community Informatics . In Garson, G. D., & Khosrow-Pour, M. (Eds.), *Handbook of Research on Public Information Technology* (pp. 50–60). Hershey, PA: Idea Group.

Stinchcombe, A. L. (1990). *Information and organizations*. Berkeley, CA: University of California Press.

Stolterman, E. (1989, August). System design methods as creativity "killers". *Proceedings of the 12th IRIS Conference - Information Systems Research in Scandinavia*, Skagen, Denmark. Aalborg University, Inst. of Electronic Systems. Aalborg. Report UMADP—WPIPCS 20:89, Umeå university, Inst. of Information Processing.

Strasnick, T. (1981). Neo-Utilitarian Ethics and Ordinal Representation Assumption. In by J.Pitt. (Ed.) *Philosophy in Economics*, Reidel Publishing.

Strauss, A. L. (1993). *Continual Permutations of Action*. New York: Aldine de Gruyter.

Strauss, A., & Corbin, J. (Eds.). (1997). *Grounded Theory in Practice*. London: SAGE Publications.

Strijbos, S., & Basden, A. (2006). *In Search of an Integrative Vision for Technology*. New York, NY: Springer. doi:10.1007/0-387-32162-4

Stubbs, M., & Martin, I. (2003). Blended Learning One Small Step. *Learning and Teaching in Action, 2*(3).

Stuedahl, D. (2004). Forhandlinger og overtalelser: kunnskapsbygging på tvers av kunnskapstradisjoner i brukermedvirkende design av ny IKT [Negotiations and persuasion. Knowledge building crosses knowledge traditions in participa- tory design IT design], Series of Dissertations No. 34', The Faculty of Education, University of Oslo.

Su, N. M., & Mark, G. (2008). Communication Chains and Multitasking. In *Proceeding of the 26th annual SIGCHI Conference on Human Factors in Computing Systems* (pp. 83-92), New York: ACM Press.

Suchman, L. (1995). Making Work Visible. *Communications of the ACM, 38*(9), 56–61. doi:10.1145/223248.223263

Suchman, L. A. (2007). *Human-Machine Reconfigurations: Plans and Situated Actions* (2nd ed.). Cambridge, UK: Cambridge University Press.

Suchman, L. (2002). Located accountabilities in technology production. *Scandinavian Journal of Information Systems, 14*(2), 91–105.

Sugden, R. (1986). *An Introduction to Game Theory and the Spontaneous Emergence of Cooperation in the Economics of Rights, Cooperation and Welfare.* Oxford, UK: Basil Blackwell.

Sundin, L. (2009). *Work-related social support, job demands and burnout. Studies of Swedish workers, predominantly employed in health care.* Diss. Karolinska Institutet, Stockholm: Universitetsservice.

Svara, J. H. (1997). The Ethical Triangle . In Bowman, J. S. (Ed.), *Public Integrity Annual* (pp. 33–42). Lexington, Ky.: CSG/ASPA.

Sweller, J. (1988). Cognitive Load During Problem Solving: Effects on Learning. *Cognitive Science, 12*(6), 257–285. doi:10.1207/s15516709cog1202_4

Sweller, J. (1994). Cognitive load theory, learning difficulty, and instructional design. *Learning and Instruction, 4*, 293–312. doi:10.1016/0959-4752(94)90003-5

Sweller, J., & Levine, M. (1982). Effects of goal specificity on means-ends analysis and learning. *Journal of Experimental Psychology. Learning, Memory, and Cognition, 8*(5), 463–474. doi:10.1037/0278-7393.8.5.463

Sweller, J. (2005). Implications of cognitive load theory for multimedia learning . In Mayer, R. E. (Ed.), *The Cambridge handbook of multimedia learning.* Cambridge, UK: Cambridge University Press.

Swierstra, T., & Jelsma, J. (2006). Responsibility without Moralism in Technoscientific Design Practice. *Science, Technology & Human Values, 31*(2), 309–332. doi:10.1177/0162243905285844

Szalma, J. L. (2009). Individual differences in human-technology interaction: incorporating variation in human characteristics into human factors and ergonomics research and design. *Theoretical Issues in Ergonomics Science, 10*(5), 381–397. doi:10.1080/14639220902893613

Taha, L. H., & Caldwell, B. S. (1993). Social Isolation and Integration in Electronic Environments. *Behaviour & Information Technology, 12*(5), 276–283. doi:10.1080/01449299308924391

Tang, Z., Weavind, L., Mazabob, J., Thomas, E. J., Chu-Weininger, M. Y. L., & Johnson, T. R. (2007). Workflow in intensive care unit remote monitoring: A time-and-motion study. *Critical Care Medicine, 35*(9), 2057–2063. doi:10.1097/01.CCM.0000281516.84767.96

Taylor, A., & Harper, R. (2003). The Gift of the Gab?: A Design oriented Sociology of young people's use of mobiles. *Computer Supported Cooperative Work*, 267–296. doi:10.1023/A:1025091532662

Teilhard de Chardin, P. (1975). *The Phenomenon of Man.* New York: Harper & Row.

Thargard, P. (1992). *Conceptual revolutions.* New Jersey: Princeton University Press.

The European Union. (2006). *7th Research Framework Programme, 'Science in Society'.* Brussels. Retrieved February 19, 2008 from http://cordis.europa.eu/fp7/home_en.html

Thomas, E. J., & Brennan, T. A. (2000). Incidence and types of preventable adverse events in elderly patients: population based review of medical records. *BMJ (Clinical Research Ed.), 320*(7237), 741–744. doi:10.1136/bmj.320.7237.741

Thomas, E. J., Chu-Weininger, M. Y. L., Wueste, L., Lucke, J. F., Weavind, L., & Mazabob, J. (2007). The impact of a tele-ICU provider attitudes about teamwork and safety climate. *Critical Care Medicine, 35*, A145.

Thomée, S., Eklöf, M., Gustafsson, E., Nilsson, R., & Hagberg, M. (2007). Prevalence of perceived stress, symptoms of depression and sleep disturbances in relation to information and communication technology (ICT) use among young adults – an explorative prospective study. *Computers in Human Behavior, 23*, 1300–1321. doi:10.1016/j.chb.2004.12.007

Thompson, J. B., & Held, D. (Eds.). (1982). *Habermas: Critical debates*. London, UK: Macmillan.

Thompson, J. (2008, December). Don't Be Afraid to Explore Web 2.0. *The Education Digest.*

Tiitta, S. (2003). Identifying elderly people's needs for communication and mobility. *Include 2003.*

Tilghman, Ch. (2005). *Considering interdisciplinarity. Unpublished seminar paper prepared for Education 357X.* Interdisciplinarity in Higher Education.

Timmermans, S. (1999). Closed-Chest Cardiac Massage: The Emergence of a Discovery Trajectory. *Science, Technology & Human Values, 24*(2), 213–240. doi:10.1177/016224399902400202

Tobias, C. L. (1987). Computers and the elderly: A review of the literature and directions for future research. In *Proceedings of the Human Factors Society 31st Annual Meeting* (pp. 866–870), USA.

Toelken, B. (1996). *The Dynamics of Folklore.* Utah: Utah State University Press.

Toffler, A. (1970). *Future Shock.* New York: Bantam Books.

Toffler, A. (1980). *The Third Wave.* London: Collins.

Tognazzini, B. (1992). *Tog on design.* Reading, MA: Addison-Wesley.

Toivonen, M., Smedlund, A., & Järvenpää, E. (2007). *The impacts of information technology on the stock of and flow of a firm's intellectual capital.* In L.A. Joia (Ed.), *Strategies for Information Technology and Intellectual Capital: Challenges and Opportunities* (pp. 111-126). Hershey: Information science reference.

Toll, E. (2000). *A Power of Now: A Guide to Spiritual Enlightenment.* UK: Hodder and Stoughton.

Toll, E. (2005). *A New Earth: Awakening to Your Life's Purpose.* UK: Dotton.

Torres, D. A. (2006). Evaluating a pen-based computer interface for novice older users. *Conference on Computers & Accessibility ASSETS '06*, Portland, Oregon, USA. Association for Computing Machinery.

Toulmin, S. E. (1958). *The Uses of Argument.* London: Cambridge University Press.

Toulmin, S., Rieke, R., & Janik, A. (1978). *An introduction to reasoning.* (A second edition appeared in 1984, page references to the second edition). New York: Macmillan.

Treaster, D., Marras, W. S., Burr, D., Sheedy, J. E., & Hart, D. (2006). Myofascial trigger point development from visual and postural stressors during computer work. *Journal of Electromyography and Kinesiology, 16*(2), 115–124. doi:10.1016/j.jelekin.2005.06.016

Tucker, P., Dahlgren, A., Åkerstedt, T., & Waterhouse, J. (2007). *The impact of free-time activities on sleep, recovery and well-being.* Elsevier.

Turkle, S. (1980). Computers as Rorschah. *Society, 17*(2), 15–24. doi:10.1007/BF02700055

Turner, P. (2006). Critical Reappraisal of Activity Theory. In Karwowski, W. (Ed.), *International Encyclopedia of Ergonomics and Human Factors* (2nd ed., *Vol. 1*). London: Taylor and Francis.

Turner, S. (2000). What are disciplines? And how is interdisciplinarity different? In Weingart, P., & Stehr, N. (Eds.), *Practicing Interdisciplinarity*. Toronto, CA: University of Toronto Press Inc.

Turner, C. W., Zavod, M., & Yurcik, W. (2001). Factors that Affect the Perception of Security and Privacy of E-commerce Web Sites. In *Proceedings of the Fourth International Conference on Electronic Commerce Research*, Dallas, TX.

U.S. Congress, Office of Technology Assessment. (1987). *The Electronic Supervisor: New Technology, New Tensions. OTA-CIT-333*. Washington, DC: U.S. Government Printing Office.

U.S. Department of Transportation. National Safety Board 2008, Driver Electronic Device Use in (2007), Research Note DOT HS 810 963, U.S. Department of Transportation, Washington, DC, June. Retrieved September 17, 2009, http://www-nrd.nhtsa.dot.gov/Pubs/810963.PDF

Ulrich, W. (1994). *Critical Heuristic of Social Planning: A New Approach to Practical Philosophy, (First published 1983)*. Chichester, UK: Wiley.

Ulrich, W. (1987). Critical heuristics of social systems design. *European Journal of Operational Research, 31*(3), 276–283. doi:10.1016/0377-2217(87)90036-1

Ulrich, W. (1983). *Critical heuristic of social planning*. Bern, CH: Paul Haupt.

Ulrich, W. (1989). Liberating systems theory: Four key strategies. Proceedings of the ISSS Int. Society for the Systems Sciences, *33rd Annual Conference, Vol. 2*, Edinburgh, Scotland.

Umemuro, H. (2004). Lowering elderly Japanese users' resistence towards computers by using touchscreen technology. *Universal access in the information society, 3*, 276-288.

Undén, A.-L., & Orth-Gomér, K. (1991). The measurement of social supports. *Social Science & Medicine, 24*(1), 83–94.

UNESCO. (2005). *Towards Knowledge Societies*. Paris, France. Retrieved October 11, 2007 from http://unesdoc.unesco.org/images/0014/001418/141843e.pdf

UN-HABITAT. (2006). *2006 Annual Report of the Cities Alliance*. Retrieved January 5, 2008 from http://www.citiesalliance.org/publications/annual-report/2006-annual-report.html

United Nations Environment Programme. (2009). *UNEP Year Book* 2009. Nairobi. Retrieved June 3, 2009 from http://www.unep.org/geo/yearbook

United Nations Food and Agricultural Organisation. (2001). *Feeding the Cities*. Rome. Retrieved June 3, 2009 from http://www.fao.org/fcit/docs/introduction_en.pdf

United Nations Food and Agricultural Organisation. (2006). *Food Security*. Retrieved June 5, 2009 from ftp://ftp.fao.org/es/ESA/policybriefs/pb_02.pdf

United Nations Food and Agricultural Organisation. (2009). *Climate Change and Food Safety*, Rome. Retrieved June 7, 2009 from http://www.fao.org/ag/agn/agns/files/HLC1_Climate_Change_and_Food_Safety.pdf

United Nations Habitat. (2006). *Report World Urban Forum*. Retrieved February 4, 2008 http://www.un-habitat.org/downloads/docs/4077_70142_WUF3-Report-final%20%20dm1%2023%20june.REV.1.pdf

United Nations. (2005). *World Urbanization Prospects*. Retrieved February 7, 2008 from http://www.un.org/esa/population/publications/WUP2005/2005wup.htm

United Nations. (2007). *Human Development Report 2006*. New York. Retrieved November 28, 2007 from http://hdr.undp.org/en/media/hdr06-complete.pdf

United Nations. (2007). *Inter Government Panel on Climate Change*. Fourth Assessment Report. Valencia. Summary for Policy Makers. Retrieved June 3, 2009 from http://www.ipcc.ch/pdf/assessment-report/ar4/syr/ar4_syr_spm.pdf

United Nations. (2007). *Resolution 62 / 111A General Assembly*. New York. Retrieved May 12, 2008 from http://daccessdds.un.org/doc/UNDOC/GEN/N07/470/43/PDF/N0747043.pdf?OpenElement

United Nations. (2007). *State of the World's Cities*. New York. Retrieved May 12, 2008 from http://www.un.org/Pubs/chronicle/2006/issue2/0206p24.htm

United Nations. (2008). *Information Economy Report 2007-2008 Science & technology for development: the new paradigm of ICT*. New York. Retrieved February 13, 2008 from http://www.unctad.org/Templates/webflyer.asp?docid=9479&intItemID=1397&lang=1&mode=toc

US DHHS HRSA. (2006). *Report to congress the critical care workforce: a study of the supply and demand for critical care physicians*. Washington, D. C.: US Department of HHS HRSA.

Valovic, Th. (2000). *Digital Mythologies: the hidden complexities of the Internet*. New Jersey: Rutgers.

Van den Berg, P. T., & Schalk, R. (1997). Type A behavior, well-being, work overload and role-related stress in information work. *Journal of Social Behavior and Personality, 12*(1), 175–187.

Van den Hoven, J. (2007). *The Information Society: Innovations, Legitimacy, Ethics and Democracy. IFIP International Federation for Information Processing, 233* (Goujon, P., Lavelle, S., Duquenoy, P., Kimppa, K., & Laurent, V., Eds.). Boston, MA: Springer.

Van den Hoven, J. (1996). Computer Ethics and Moral Methodology. In P. Barroso, S. Rogerson & T. Bynum (Eds.) *Values and Social Responsibilities of Computer Science,* Proceedings of ETHICOMP 96. Computence Univesity Press: pp.444-453.

van Dongen, C. (1996). Quality of life and self-esteem in working and non-working persons with mental illness. Community . *Mental Health, 32*(6), 535–549.

Varela, F. J. (1979). *Principles of Biological Autonomy*. New York: North Holland.

Vasilyuk, F. (1988). *The psychology of experiencing*. Moscow: Progress Publishers.

Vattimo, G. (1990). *La sociedad transparente*. Barcelona, ES: E: Paidos.

Vaughan, D. (1996). *The Challenger Launch Decision: Risky Technology, Culture, and Deviance at NASA*. Chicago: University of Chicago Press.

Vercruyssen, M. (1996). Movement control and speed of behavior . In Fisk, A. D., & Rogers, W. A. (Eds.), *Handbook of Human Factors and the Older Adult* (pp. 55–86). San Diego, CA: Academic Press.

Verhulst, S. G. (2004). About scarcities and intermediaries: the regulatory paradigm shift of digital content reviewed . In Lievwrouv, L., & Livingstone, S. (Eds.), *Handbook of new media* (pp. 432–437). New York: Sage Publications.

Vetandets Värld. (2006). *(In Swedish broadcasting, audio). Den mänskliga faktorn som förklaring till olyckshändelser. Vetandets värld*. Sveriges Radio.

Vignau, J., Bailly, D., Duhamel, A., & Vervaecke, P., Beuscart, & R., Collinet, C. (1997). Epidemiologic study of sleep quality and troubles in French secoundary school adolescents. *The Journal of Adolescent Health, 21*(5), 343–350. doi:10.1016/S1054-139X(97)00109-2

Vincent, J. L., Suter, P., Bihari, D., & Bruining, H. (1997). Organization of intensive care units in Europe: lessons from the EPIC study. *Intensive Care Medicine, 23*, 1181–1184. doi:10.1007/s001340050479

Vink, P., & Kompier, M. A. J. (1997). Improving office work: a participatory ergonomic experiment in a naturalistic setting. *Ergonomics, 40*(4), 435–449. doi:10.1080/001401397188071

Visvanathan, S. (1991). Mrs Brundtland lovely non-magical cosmos, *Lokayan Bulletin, 9*(1). *Alternatives*, 3.

Von Buskirk, E. (2009). SoundCloud Threatens MySpace as Music Destination for Twitter Era. *Wired*. Retrieved from http://www.wired.com/epicenter/2009/07/soundcloud-threatens-myspace-as-music-destination-for-twitter-era/

Von Hippel, E. (1986). Lead User: A Source of Novel Product Concepts. *Management Science, 32*(7), 791–805. doi:10.1287/mnsc.32.7.791

Von Hippel, E., & Katz, R. (2002). Shifting Innovation to Users via Toolkits. *Management Science, 48*(7), 821–833. doi:10.1287/mnsc.48.7.821.2817

Von Weizsäcker, E. U., & Lovins, A. B. L., & Lovins, L. H. (1997). *Factor Four: Doubling Wealth, Halving Resource Use – A Report to the Club of Rome*. London: Earthscan.

Wackernagel, M., & Rees, W. E. (1996). *Our Ecological Footprint: Reducing Human Impact on the Earth*. Philadelphia, PA: New Society Publishers.

Wajcman, J. (2000). Reflections on gender and technology studies. In what state is the art? *Social Studies of Science, 30*(3), 447–464. doi:.doi:10.1177/030631200030003005

Wajcman, J. (2001). Gender and Technology. In *International Encyclopedia of the Social & Behavioral Sciences* (pp. 5976-5979). Oxford, UK: Elsevier Science Ltd.

Walker, B. N., & Kramer, G. (2006). Sonification . In Karwowski, W. (Ed.), *International Encyclopedia of Ergonomics and Human Factors*. Boca Raton, FL: Taylor & Francis. doi:10.1201/9780849375477.ch195

Walker, N., Philbin, D. A., & Spruell, C. (1996). The use of signal detection theory in research on age-related differences in movement control . In Rogers, W. A., Fisk, A. D., & Walker, N. (Eds.), *Aging and skilled performance. Advances in theory and applications* (pp. 45–64). New Jersey: Lawrence Erlbaum Associates.

Wallgren, L. G., & Johansson Hanse, J. (2007). Job characteristics, motivators and stress among information technology consultants: A structural equation modelling approach. *International Journal of Industrial Ergonomics, 37*, 51–59. doi:10.1016/j.ergon.2006.10.005

Walther, J. B., & Burgoon, J. (1992). Relational communication in computermediated interaction. *Human Communication Research, 19*, 50–88. doi:10.1111/j.1468-2958.1992.tb00295.x

Ware, C., & Mikaelin, H. H. (1987). An evaluation of an eye tracker as a device for computer input. In *Proc. ACM CHI'87* (pp. 183-188).

Wasko, M. M., & Faraj, S. (2005). Why should I share? Examing Social Capital and Knowledge Contribution in Electronic Networks of Practice. *Management Information Systems Quarterly, 29*(1), 35–37.

WCED – World Commission on Environment and Development. (1987). *Our Common Future*. London: Oxford University Press.

Weaver, P., Lambrou, N., & Walkley, M. (2002). *Practical Business Systems Development using SSADM: A complete tutorial guide* (3rd ed.). Pearson Education Ltd., Edinburgh Gate.

Weeks, J. (2004). *Unpopular Culture: The Ritual of Complaint in a British Bank*. Chicago: University of Chicago Press.

Weick, K. E. (1990). The Vulnerable System: An Analysis of the Tenerife Air Disaster. *Journal of Management, 16*(3), 571–593. doi:10.1177/014920639001600304

Weick, K. E., & Sutcliffe, K. M. (2007). *Managing the unexpected: resilient performance in an age of uncertainty* (2nd ed.). San Francisco: Jossey-Bass.

Weingart, P. (2000). Interdisciplinarity: The paradoxical discourse . In Weingart, P., & Stehr, N. (Eds.), *Practicing interdisciplinarity*. Toronto, CA: University of Toronto Press Inc.

Weininger, O. (1903). *Geschlecht und Character: Eine prinzipielle Untersuchung* ((Page refs. to Ital. trans. *Sesso e carattere*. Milano: Feltrinelli/Bocca, 1978). Wien/Leipzig, AU: Braumüller.

Weizenbaum, J. (1976). *Computer Power and Human Reasoning: From Judgement to Calculation*. San Francisco, SF: W.H. Freeman.

Wenger, N., Chesney, M., & Orth-Gomér, K. (Eds.). (1998). *Women, stress and heart disease*. New Jersey: Erlbaum Association.

Wenger, E. (n.d.). Communities of practice a brief introduction. Retrieved April 8, 2009 from http://www.ewenger.com/theory/index.htm [last accessed 04.08.09

Wertsch, J. (Ed.). (1981). *The Concept of Activity in Soviet Psychology*. New York: Sharpe Inc.

Whitaker, R. (1992). *Venues for Contexture: A critical analysis and enactive reformulation of group decision support systems*. (Diss.) Research Reports in Information Processing and Computer Science: Nr. UMADP-RRIPCS 15.92, Umeå University, Sweden.

White, M., & Dorman, S. M. (2001). Receiving social support online: implications for health education. *Health Education Research, 16*(6), 693–707. doi:10.1093/her/16.6.693

Whitehouse, D. (2009) Book review. The Medicalization of Cyberspace. In *Journal of Information, Communication and Ethics*. February 2009. 7 (2/3), 211-213.

Whitehouse, D., & Duquenoy, P. (2009). Applied Ethics and eHealth: Principles, Identity, and RFID. In V. Matyáš et al. (Eds.) *IFIP AICT 298* (pp. 43-55). Laxenburg, AU: IFIP Press.

Wickens, C. D., Lee, J. D., Liu, Y., & Gordon Becker, S. E. (2004). *An Introduction to Human Factors Engineering*. Upper Saddle River, NJ: Pearson Prentice Hall.

Widgor, D., Penn, G., Ryall, K., Esenther, A., & Shen, C. (2007). Living with a tabletop: analysis and observations of long term office use of a multi-touch table. *Second Annual IEEE International Workshop on Horizontal Interactive Human-Computer System.*

Wiener, N. (1948). *Cybernetics: Control and Communication in Animal and the Machine*. London/New York, UK/NY: John Wiley & Sons.

Wiener, N. (1954). *The Human Use of Human being*. Boston, MA: Houghton Miffins.

Wikipedia (2009b). History of the automobile. Retrieved December 2009 from http://en.wikipedia.org/wiki/History_of_the_automobile

Wikipedia. (2009a). Fax. Retrieved December 2009 from http://en.wikipedia.org/wiki/Fax

Wilson, E. O. (1999). *Consilience: The unity of knowledge*. New York, NY: Vintage Books.

Winner, L. (1989). *The whale and the reactor: a search for limits in the age of high technology*. Chicago, IL: Chicago University Press.

Winograd, T. (1988). Where the action is. *BYTE, 13*(13), 256A–258.

Winograd, T., & Flores, F. (1986). *Understanding Computers and Cognition: A new foundation for design*. New Jersey: Ablex Publishing Corporation.

Wissner, A. (1994). Organization anthropotechnological contingencies an analytical approach. In G.E. Bradley & H. W. Hendrick (Eds.), *Human Factors in organizational design and management* (pp.613-617). Amsterdam, NL: North-Holland.

Witkin, H. A., Dyke, R. B., Patterson, H. F., Goodman, D. R., & Kemp, D. R. (1962). *Psychological differentiation*. New York: Wiley.

Witterseh, T., Wyon, D. P., & Clausen, G. (2004). The effects of moderate heat stress and open-plan office noise distraction on SBS symptoms and on the performance of office work. *Indoor Air, 14*(8), 30–40. doi:10.1111/j.1600-0668.2004.00305.x

Wobbrock, J. O., Rubinstein, J., Sawyer, M. W., & Duchowski, A. T. (2008). Longitudinal Evaluation of Discrete Consecutive Gaze Gestures for Text Entry. In *Proceedings of the Eye Tracking Research & Application Symposium* (pp. 11–18), ETRA.

Woerner, S. L., Yates, J., & Orlikowski, W. J. (2007). Conversational Coherence in Instant Messaging and Getting Work Done. *40th Annual Hawaii International Conference on System Sciences (HICSS'07)*, 3-6 January, Big Island Hawaii. http://doi.ieeecomputersociety.org/10.1109/HICSS.2007.152

Wojtyla, K. (1980). *I fondamenti dell'ordine etico*. Città del Vaticano, IT: Libreria Editrice Vaticana. [1] This article is a revised version. The original article was first published in 1991 in the *Journal of Applied Systems Analysis*.

Wolton, D. (1999). *Internet et après? Une théorie critique des nouveaux medias*. Paris, FR: Flammarion.

Woolston, C. (2002). *Why unemployment is bad for your health*. Principle Health News.

World Bank. (2006). *The Global Burden of Disease and Risk Factors*. Oxford: Oxford University Press.

WSIS (World Summit on the Information Society). (2003) *Geneva 2003 and Tunis 2005 Declarations of Principles. Building the Information Society: A Global Challenge in the New Millennium*, [Online] Retrieved July 15, 2008 from http://www.itu.int/dms_pub/ itu-s/md/03/wsis/doc/S03-WSIS-DOC-0004!!PDF-E.pdf

Wu, A. W., Pronovost, P. J., & Morlock, L. (2002). ICU incident reporting systems. *Journal of Critical Care, 17*(2), 86–94. doi:10.1053/jcrc.2002.35100

Wu, M., & Balakrishnan, R. (2003). Multi-finger and whole hand gestural interaction techniques for multi-user tabletop displays. In *Proceedings of the UIST '03 Vancouver* (pp. 193-202). BC, Canada.

Wu, M., Shen, C., Ryall, K., Forlines, C., & Balakrishnan, R. (2006). Gesture registration, relaxation, and reuse for multi-point direct-touch surfaces. In *Proceedings of the First IEEE International Workshop on Horizontal Interactive Human-Computer Systems* (pp. 185-192), Washington, DC.

Xiao, M., Hyppolite, J. R., Pomplun, M., Sunkara, S., & Carbone, E. (2005). Compensating for the Eye-Hand Span Improves Gaze Control in Human-Computer Interfaces. In *Proceedings of the HCI 2005*.

Yarnold, P. R., Stewart, M. J., Stille, F. C., & Martin, G. J. (1996). Assessing functional status of elderly adults via microcomputer. *Perceptual and Motor Skills, 82*, 689–690.

Yee, K.-P. (2002). User interaction design for secure systems. In [Springer-Verlag.]. *Proceedings of the International Conference on Information and Communications Security, ICIC, 02*, 278–290.

Zajicek, M. (2007). Web 2.0: Hype or Happiness? *W4A2007 – Keynote, May 07–08, 2007*, Banff, Canada. Co-Located with the 16th International World Wide Web Conference.

Zawada, E. T. J., Herr, P., Larson, D., Fromm, R., Kapaska, D., & Erickson, D. (2009). Impact of an intensive care unit telemedicine program on a rural health care system. *Postgraduate Medicine, 121*(3), 160–170. doi:10.3810/pgm.2009.05.2016

Zeihe, T. (1986). *Ny ungdom [New youth]*. Stockholm, SE: Nordstedts.

Zhai, S., Morimoto, C., & Ihde, S. (1999). Manual and Gaze Input Cascaded (MAGIC) Pointing. *Proc. ACM CHI'99* (pp. 246-253).

Zijlstra, F. R. H., Roe, R. A., Leonora, A. B., & Krediet, I. (1999). Temporal Factors in Mental Work: Effects of Interrupted Activities. *Journal of Occupational and Organizational Psychology, 72*, 163–185. doi:10.1348/096317999166581

Zijlstra, F. R. H., & Sonnentag, S. (2006). After work is done: Psychological perspectives on recovery from work. *European Journal of Work and Organizational Psychology, 15*(2), 129–138. doi:10.1080/13594320500513855

Zinchenko, V. P., & Munipov, V. M. (1976). Man and Modern Production. [Moscow: USSR Academy of Sciences.]. *Social Sciences, 4*.

Zinchenko, V. P., & Munipov, V. M. (1989). *Fundamentals of Ergonomics*. Moscow: Progress.

Zinchenko, V. P. (Ed.). (1970-1986). *Works of VNIITE* (in Russian). Series 1-32. Moscow: VNIITE.

Zinchenko, V.P., Gordon V.M. & Munipov, V.M. (1973). Study of Visual Thinking (in Russian). *Soviet Psychology*, XII(2).

Zöllner, M., Keil, J., Behr, J., Gillich, J., Gläser, S., & Schöls, E. (2008). Coperion 3D - A virtual factory on the tabletop. 5th Intuition 2008. *Proceedings: Virtual Reality in Industry and Society: From Research to Application*, Italy.

Zuboff, S. (1988). *In the Age of the Smart Machine: The Future of Work and Power*. New York: Basic Books.

Zuboff, S. (1988). *In the Age of the Smart Machine. The Future of Work and Power*. Oxford, UK: Heineman.

About the Contributors

Darek M. Haftor, PhD, (prev. Darek M. Eriksson) is currently an associate professor at the Stockholm University School of Business, Stockholm, Sweden. He has studied the sciences and arts at various universities in Europe and North America, and received his doctorate in Industrial Organization at Chalmers University of Technology, Sweden. He has spent fifteen years in various managerial positions in the private industry sector, and has worked in Europe and the Middle East. Previously, he has held several academic positions in Sweden, including the Mid Sweden University, the Luleå University of Technology, and at the Linnaeus University where he is currently affiliated as a senior researcher. Darek is now mainly occupied with research and teaching, and he is also the Director of Executive Education at the Stockholm University School of business. His research addresses two main frontiers: the structure and dynamics of information-based organizations and their operations, and the normative conditions inherent in the design, development and change of any human affairs.

Anita Mirijamdotter is Professor and Head of the Information Systems Research group at the School of Computer Science, Physics, and Mathematics, Linnaeus University. She also holds the position as Vice-Dean of the Faculty of Science and Engineering which includes leading the committee work for First and Second Cycle Education. Additional honorary tasks are: board member for the international research collaboration in the Centre for Philosophy, Technology and Social Systems (CPTS); board member for the cross-disciplinary area Mathematical Modeling and Systems Collaboration within the Linnaeus University; and member of the Leadership team of the Swedish Research School of Management and IT (MIT). Anita has served as a referee in academic conferences and journals and contributed to more than forty conference- and journal publications. Her research focus is mainly in areas related to: information and communication technology (ICT) impact on (or implications for) organisational processes, and interactive and human centric methods for need-finding, evaluating, valuing and learning.

***

Sara Alander, MSc in Environmental Planning and Design, PhD in Gender and Technology. Her research interests are in the relationship between technology and society with a particular focus on sustainable development, not only in an ecological, resource saving way but also in regard to social, economic and cultural aspects such as health, social care, participation, creativity and understanding. Her research shows how awareness of diversity, the multiplicity of perspectives and visions that continue to influence the use of technology and technology development enhances the opportunities to understand and integrate situated knowledges in making the changes required for sustainable development.

Sebastiano Bagnara, Chair of Cognitive Psychology at the Department of Architecture and Urban Planning University of Sassari at Alghero. He was General Secretary of International Ergonomics Association, Head of the Department of Communication Sciences at the University of Siena, chair of Cognitive Ergonomics and Psychology at Department of Design at the Politecnico of Milan, Director of the Institute of Psychology of the National Research Council, President of the European Association of Cognitive Ergonomics and of the Italian Society of Ergonomics. He is member of a number of scientific and professional societies and of the editorial board of several international scientific journals. He is Associate Editor of Theoretical Issues in Ergonomic Sciences. He is the co-editor (with Gillian Crampton Smith) of the book "Theories and practice in interaction design".

Jacques Berleur is an emeritus professor at the Computer Science Faculty <http://www.info.fundp. ac.be/index_eng.html> of the University of Namur <http://www.fundp.ac.be/fundp_eng.html> (Belgium) where he was a professor from 1972. He continues to be interested in, and specialized in, the fields of "Computers and Rationality", "Computers and Society" and "Ethics of Computing". His research interests have included the epistemology of computing, technology assessment in the field of development and use of information and communication technology, social informatics <http://www.slis.indiana.edu/SI/index.html>, and the ethics of computing. He was previously co-director of the Cellule Interfacultaire de Technology Assessment (CITA)<http://www.info.fundp.ac.be/CITA>, an interdisciplinary research team that focuses on the assessment of information and communication technology. He was President of his University, which is a Catholic University, for 9 years (1984-1993) <http://www.sjweb.info/education/index.htm>, and a European advisor to the Jesuit Advisory Committee for Higher and University Education of the Society of Jesus in Rome (1994-1997). He was involved as a Belgian expert to several initiatives co-financed by the European Commission including the FAST Programme (Forecasting and Assessment for Science and Technology) and the MONITOR Programme (1989-93). He co-authored the first "Science and Technology Assessment Report" to the European Parliament. He is co-founder of the European Association for Society, Science and Technology (ESST <http://www.sv.uio.no/esst>), a consortium of fifteen European Universities which has created common masters curricula in "Society, Science and Technology". He is a corresponding member of the "Académie Européenne des Sciences, des Arts et des Lettres" in Paris since 1993. He is a longstanding member of the International Federation for Information Processing, and helped to found Technical Committee 9 on Computers and Society, working group 9.2 on social accountability and computing, and special interest group 9.2.2 on the IFIP framework on ethics. He is author of around 200 papers <http://www.info.fundp.ac.be/~jbl/papers.html> and has authored and co-edited several well-known books which provided many of the foundations to the two fields known today as computers and society and the ethics of computing <http://www.info. fundp.ac.be/~jbl/books.html>.

Birgitta Bergvall-Kåreborn, PhD, is professor in Social Informatics at Luleå University of Technology, where she also earned her Ph.D. Her current research interests concern participatory design in distributed and open environments; human centric and appreciative methodologies and methods for design, evaluation and learning; and, the relation between IT-use and IT-design. She has contributed to the field of participatory design with more than thirty conference- and journal publications, and served as a referee in a number of academic conferences and journals.

Gunilla Bradley, PhD, is Professor emerita at School of ICT, Royal Institute of Technology (KTH). She is an interdisciplinary scholar that has focused her lifelong research in the interplay between ICT, Human Beings, and Society. Beginning in 1973, Prof. Bradley who has a broad background in the social and behavioral sciences, initiated and led cross-disciplinary research programs on computerization and working life at Stockholm University. This program was conducted for twenty years. Gunilla Bradley was one of the first to do interdisciplinary studies with Computer Science and ICT related disciplines on psychosocial, motivational and emotional changes, and additionally, organizational, institutional and, societal changes emerging of the interrelations between ICT, Society, and Human Beings. Prof. Bradley's positions have been placed in several institutions in Sweden as well as abroad, e.g., professor of Technology and Social Change at Royal Institute of Technology, professor of Informatics at Umeå University and Mid Sweden University, professor of Informatics at KTH, guest professor at the Centre for ICT & Society in Salzburg Austria, visiting professor at Stanford University USA in two periods. Her positions and engagement in academia has led to the establishment of a worldwide network of renowned scholars from a variety of fields that are inspired by professor Bradley's pioneering work. These fields range from: Human Work Science, Social Informatics, Human-Computer Interaction, Media Technology, Computer Science, Communications. Prof. Bradley has authored more than 200 publications during the last 30 years and is the author of 13 books.

Barrett S. Caldwell, PhD, Associate Professor, Schools of Industrial Engineering / Aeronautics & Astronautics, Purdue University. Prof. Caldwell has two undergraduate degrees from MIT (1985) and a PhD (1990) in social psychology from the University of California-Davis. His research lab, known as GROUPER, studies *how people get, share, and use information well*. Prof. Caldwell's research efforts have resulted in over 100 scientific publications; projects since 2000 have been funded by sources including Motorola, NASA, the Regenstrief Center for Healthcare Engineering, and the United Space Alliance. He has been honored to lecture at Mid-Sweden University in Östersund, and Luleå University, and involved in international exchange discussions at KTH and Linköping Institute of Technology.

Pascale Carayon, PhD, is Procter & Gamble Bascom Professor in Total Quality and Associate Chair in the Department of Industrial and Systems Engineering and the Director of the Center for Quality and Productivity Improvement (CQPI) at the University of Wisconsin-Madison. She received her Engineer diploma from the Ecole Centrale de Paris, France, in 1984 and her Ph.D. in Industrial Engineering from the University of Wisconsin-Madison in 1988. Her research examines systems engineering, human factors and ergonomics, sociotechnical engineering and occupational health and safety, and has been funded by numerous US federal agencies, various foundations and private industry. She is the North American editor for *Applied Ergonomics*, and a member of the editorial boards of the *Journal of Patient Safety, Behaviour and Information Technology*, and *Work and Stress*. She is a Fellow of the Human Factors and Ergonomics Society and the International Ergonomics Association. Website: http://www.engr.wisc. edu/ie/faculty/carayon_pascale.html

Peter Crowley, born in 1943 in Dublin. Doctor of Philosophy, University College Dublin. Psychology Graduate, University of Duesseldorf, Germany. Communication Science Graduate, University of

Salzburg. Former lecturer Adlerian Institute for Individual Psychology Duesseldorf. Current NGO affiliate representative to the United Nations. Chairperson Vienna NGO Committee on the Family at the United Nations Office in Vienna, 1998 – 2004 and current Deputy Chairperson. Editor, 'Documenting Contributions of Civil Society Organisations to the Well-Being of Families', financed by the United Nations Trust Fund on Family Activities in 2004. Editor, 'Families International', Quarterly Bulletin of the Vienna NGO Committee.

Ulrika Danielsson, PhD at the Division of Psychology, Department of Social Sciences, Mid Sweden University, Campus Östersund, Sweden. Her main areas of interest in research are the relationships between individuals' psychosocial life environment and their use of ICT, with particular focus on psychosocial health and recovery. The title of her thesis: Relationships Between Information Communication Technology and Psychosocial Life Environment - Students and Young Urban Knowledge Workers in the ICT-Era. Ulrika's personal web site may be reached through: www.miun.se/shv/psy

Tom Denison, PhD is a research associate with the Centre for Community Networking Research, Monash University, Melbourne. Having consulted widely in Australia and Vietnam, his research interests relate to the provision of online services, and the situated use of information and communications technology within the frameworks of social and community informatics. His recent projects include: a cross-cultural study of the drivers for, and barriers to, the adoption of web-based technologies by non-profit organizations in Australia and Italy; and a study of the use of information and communications technology for social cohesion among Chinese and Italian communities in Melbourne, Australia, and the Chinese in Prato, Italy.

Susan Dray, PhD, has worked in the field of Human Factors since 1979. She worked for 14 years industry, on both research and corporate IT systems. Since 1993, as president of Dray & Associates, Inc., she has provided contextual user research, usability evaluation, and interface design consultation for a wide range of products, systems, and applications and has worked in 24 countries. She has given over 100 talks at professional conferences in the U.S., Europe, Africa, and Australia, including invited plenary and keynote speeches. In addition, she has published numerous papers and book chapters. She is Publications Director of the UPA, was the North American editor of *Behaviour and Information Technology*, and co-edited the Business Column of the ACM magazine *<interactions>* for many years. Susan was elected a Fellow of the Human Factors and Ergonomics Society in 1994. She is the 2006 recipient of the ACM-SIGCHI Lifetime Service Award.

Penny Duquenoy has a first degree in Philosophy from the School of Cognitive and Computing Science at Sussex University, UK, and a PhD in Internet Ethics. She is a Principal Lecturer at Middlesex University, London. Penny has been an active researcher in the field of Computer Ethics for a number of years, with more than 40 publications on the ethical implications of ICT. She is also a co-editor of the 2008 book titled *Ethical, Legal and Social Issues in Medical Informatics*. Key areas of research are the ethical implications of intelligent technologies in everyday life (described as 'Ambient Intelligence' in European Union research) and medical informatics. She has acted as an expert ethics evaluator for the European Commission (Information Society and Media Directorate-General) and given invited presentations on ethics and ambient technologies at EU level and internationally. She is a former Chair of IFIP

Working Group 9.2 (Computers and Social Accountability), member of IFIP Special Interest Group 9.2.2 "Taskforce on Ethics" and Manager of the BCS, the Chartered Institute for IT, Ethics Strategic Panel.

Annagreta Dyring was born in Lapland (northern Sweden) and studied Modern Language at Uppsala University, Trinity College in Dublin and the universities of Göttingen and Rome. After working as director of communication at Uppsala University, she was offered to lead the Swedish programme for Public Understanding of Science at the Swedish Council for Planning and Coordination of Research, where her specialization as a journalist in popular science grew. She engaged researchers and artists in the public debate and developed new forms of communicating between researchers and the community in general: debate books, theatre of science, popular science weeks, etc. In the1990s she was the curator for two large popular science exhibitions at the Bundeskunsthalle in Bonn; "ErdSicht" and "Arctic-Antarctica". The combination of Art & Science is her speciality. Annagreta Dyring has participated in a large Multi Media-project in the European Union, and has had a lot of board assignments; for example the Swedish Author's Fund, The National Museum of Science and Technology, The Swedish Species Information Centre and others. She is also a writer. Her latest book "Polardrömmars höga pris" (The High Price of Polar Dreams) was published in 2007. She received The Royal Society of Pro Patria gold medal and the Royal Academy of Engineering Sciences gold medal. The University of Stockholm has appointed her honorary doctor.

Simone Fischer-Hübner has been a Full Professor at the Computer Science Department of Karlstad University, Sweden, since June 2000, where is the head of the PriSec (Privacy & Security) research group. She received Doctoral (1992) and Habilitation (1999) Degrees in Computer Science from Hamburg University. She was a research assistant/assistant professor at Hamburg University (1988-2000) and a Guest Professor at the Copenhagen Business School (1994-1995) and at Stockholm University/ Royal Institute of Technologies (1998-1999). Her research interests include technical, legal and social aspects of IT-security, privacy and privacy-enhancing technologies and identity management and usable security/privacy.

Hal Hendrick is Emeritus Professor of Human Factors and Ergonomics at the University of Southern California (USC). He is a past chair of USC's Human Factors Department and former Executive Director of the University's Institute of Safety and Systems Management. He is a Certified Professional Ergonomist. He holds a Ph.D. in Industrial Psychology and MS in Human Factors from Purdue University, with a minor in Industrial Engineering. He is a Past President of the Human Factors and Ergonomics Society, the International Ergonomics Association, and the Board of Certification in Professional Ergonomics. He is the author or co-author of over 200 professional publications. Hal conceptualized and initiated sub-discipline of macroergonomics.

Wolfgang Hofkirchner, born in 1953 in Vienna, Austria, was educated as Political Scientist and Psychologist. He specialised in the field of Science–Technology–Society. He is interested in information studies, information society research, thinking in complexity, and transdisciplinarity. He is affiliated with the Vienna University of Technology , worked as professor at the University of Salzburg and was visiting professor at different universities in Brazil and Spain. He founded the Unified Theory of Information Research Group and the open-access online journal for a Global Sustainable Information Society, triple-C, is member of numerous scientific societies and published more than 150 contributions.

Lorenz M. Hilty is Prof. Dr. and Head of the Technology and Society Lab (TSL) at Empa, the Swiss Federal Laboratories for Materials Testing and Research, and professor at the University of Zurich. He studied Informatics at the University of Hamburg, where he habilitated in 1997. From 1998 to 2005, he was professor of Information Systems at the University of Applied Sciences Northwestern Switzerland. In parallel with that (since 2000), he was leading Empa's research program "Sustainability in the Information Society", from which the Technology and Society Lab emerged in 2004. In 2009 he was appointed to the newly created chair of "Informatics and Sustainability" at the University of Zurich.

Peter Hoonakker, PhD, is Research Scientist at the Center for Quality and Productivity Improvement at the University of Wisconsin-Madison. Hoonakker's research focuses on the relationship between job and organizational characteristics and quality, safety and health, in different settings such as the construction industry, the public sector, the IT sector, and healthcare. He has published the results of his studies in more than 60 technical reports and nearly 100 conference papers, book chapters, and journal articles.
Website: http://cqpi.engr.wisc.edu/hoonakker

Geraldine Hultkrantz, née Pratchett was born in Hassocks, Sussex, England in 1938 and spent the war years in England. On her father's return from serving as a Naval Mine Disposal Officer in 1946, the family moved to South Africa. Returning to Europe in 1953 they settled in Jersey, Channel Islands. Geraldine joined the WRNS (Women's Royal Naval Service) and served there until her marriage to Professor Åke Hultkrantz in Stockholm in 1960 when she became an English teacher (RSA – teaching English as a second language). She started an English Kindergarten in their house, and taught English for various Adult Education Programmes. Her work entailed translation, checking manuscripts for her husband and other professionals as well as for journals e.g. *Acta Americana*, etc. Geraldine has painted animal portraits as a hobby, designed book covers for some of her husband's books and collaborated with him in *Das Buch der Schamanen: Nord – und Südamerika*, (Luzerne, 2002). Since 2006 Geraldine has been working on many of her late husband's unpublished manuscripts. Two volumes of *The Veils of Religion,* are to be published in Aberdeen. She has also compiled *Shoshone Tales* –a collection of Indian Tales. These should be in book form by Christmas 2010. She has written the *History of the Hultkrantz Family, Lt. R.M. Pratchett, RNVR, M.B.E. World War II Experiences,* (the story of her father's exploits and adventures during WWII). Her first novel – *Time to Tell* – a story of forbidden love during the Occupation of the Channel Islands during WWII has just been released. A sequel is planned. Geraldine's friendship with Gunilla started when Gunilla's children attended English Kindergarten some thirty years ago and has strengthened and grown with the years.

Stina Immonen is D. Sc (Tech). She works as Lecturer at Aalto University School of Science and Technology, Helsinki. Her most recent research initiatives deal with media industry, how technological advancements will affect the media professionals' knowledge work, and how media organisations' flexibility and agility can be improved through organisational development.

Pedro Isaías is an auxiliary professor at the Universidade Aberta (Portuguese Open University) in Lisbon, Portugal, responsible for several courses and director of the master degree program in Electronic Commerce and Internet. He is co-founder and president of IADIS – International Association for Development of the Information Society, a scientific non-profit association. He holds a PhD in Information Management (in the speciality of information and decision systems) from the New University of Lisbon.

Author of several books, papers and research reports, all in the information systems area, he has headed several conferences and workshops within the mentioned area.

Kristo Ivanov is PhD and Professor Emeritus of Informatics at Umeå University, Sweden. He was educated in Brazil, France and Sweden, and worked both as engineer and manager in France, Sweden and the USA. In 1972, he was the first in Sweden to receive a PhD in Informatics (then Electronic Data Processing), from the Royal Institute of Technology, on a thesis that gains relevance for every year: the quality of information. He has held academic positions at Stockholm University, Linkoping University, and Umeå University, all in Sweden; in the latter he founded and managed the Department of Informatics, a nationally and internationally leading institution of its kind. Ivanov's research interests, presented in more than 100 main publications, are focused on the relation between Systems Sciences and its applications to business and government. He is especially interested in the interplay among technical, economic, political, psychological, aesthetical and ethical considerations in the design and use of information technology, including philosophical and theological issues. One main question that dominates the research interest is what directs and should direct the development and application of information technology.

Nicole Jochems studied computer science at the RWTH Aachen University. Since April 2005 she is a research assistant and Ph.D. candidate at the Institute of Industrial Engineering and Ergonomics at RWTH Aachen University. In 2010 she will receive the Dr.-Ing. degree from RWTH Aachen University. Her research interests include human-computer interaction, design of age-based user interfaces and ergonomics.

Eila Järvenpää, D.Sc. (Tech) is a full professor of work psychology and leadership at Aalto University, School of Science and Technology, Dept. of Industrial Engineering and Management in Helsinki. Her research interests include knowledge work, knowledge management, organizational networks, cross-cultural management, and ICT and quality of working life.

Miranda Kajtazi is a PhD candidate in Informatics, at the School of Computer Science, Physics and Mathematics, at Linnaeus University in Sweden. She received a Master Degree in Computer Science from Växjö University and a Bachelor Degree in Computer Science from South East European University. Her research interest concerns one of the most crucial resources of our human and social affairs: Information. Thus, Miranda explores the interplay of social dynamics and technology, by focusing at the causes and consequences of information inadequacy in our global society. She has also worked in industry as a software engineer and a database administrator.

Bernhard Kausch studied mechanical engineering at the Technical University of Munich. His area of specialization was ergonomics and product development. From August 2002 to April 2008, he was research assistant and since May 2008, he is a team lead at the Institute of Industrial Engineering and Ergonomics at RWTH Aachen University.

Sarai Lastra, PhD, is Vice Chancellor of Information Resources and Director of the Virtual Library (http://bibliotecavirtualut.suagm.edu) at Universidad del Turabo (http://ut.pr) in Gurabo, Puerto Rico. She is chair of the Community Informatics Center and a member of the advisory group for the Museum and Center of Humanistic Studies at Universidad del Turabo, and a consultant to various museum and public library projects in Puerto Rico. She teaches information retrieval and school library services at Universidad del Turabo and at the University of Puerto Rico. She holds a Ph.D. from the Graduate School of Library and Information Science at the University of Illinois at Urbana-Champaign, a master's in library science from Dominican University, a master's in quantitative psychology from the University of North Carolina at Chapel Hill, and a bachelors degree in elementary education from Interamerican University of Puerto Rico. Her thesis work titled, 'Making Sense of Community Informatics: The Development and Application of the Community Event Research Method'. Her doctoral research has lead to presentations of the power of community events as research tools at various international conferences. Her research interests are in the areas of the cultural appropriation of information and communication technologies, the development of research methods for community informatics, and the design and use of virtual environments for libraries and museums within the context of Spanish-speaking communities.

Holger Luczak received the Dipl.-Ing, the Dr.-Ing. and the Habilitation degrees from Darmstadt University of Technology, Germany, in 1969, 1974 and 1997, respectively. From 1969 to 1974 he was a research assistant and from 1974 to 1977 an assistant Professor (Oberingenieur) at the Institute of Ergonomics of Darmstadt University. From 1977 to 1983 he was a Full Professor of production engineering at Bremen University of Technology, Germany. He founded the Faculty of Production Engineering and the Bremen Institute of Industrial Engineering and Applied Ergonomics. From 1983 to 1992 he was a Full Professor of Industrial Engineering and Ergonomics at the Faculty of Mechanical Engineering of Berlin University of Technology, Germany. From 1992 to 2005 he was a Full Professor at the Faculty of Mechanical Engineering of RWTH Aachen University of Technology where he was the director of the Institute of Industrial Engineering and Ergonomics as well as the managing director of the Research Institute for Operations Management. He is a member of editorial boards of national and international journals in ergonomics and is an advisory and supervisory council member on several national and international committees.

Eduardo Villanueva - Mansilla (Lima, Peru, 1965) is an associate professor at the Department of Communications, Pontificia Universidad Católica del Perú. He holds a MA in Communications by the same college. His areas of interest are convergent media policies, community informatics and the confluence of digital lifestyles and cultural change in Peru. Currently he is an associate editor of the Journal of Community Informatics, and has been a keynote presenter at several conferences, including CIRN 2008 at Prato, and Felafacs 2009 at Havana. His most recent book, VIda Digital, is set for publication in May 2010 in Peru.

Kerry Mcguire, BS, is a doctoral student of Dr. Pascale Carayon in human factors and patient safety at the University of Wisconsin – Madison. She is also an AHRQ T32 recipient. She received her bachelors in science from Clemson University in 2005 in Industrial Engineering. Since, 2003 she has co-oped at NASA's Johnson Space Center in the Usability and Testing Analysis Facility. Website: http://cqpi.engr.wisc.edu/mcguire

William Mciver, Jr., PhD is a computer scientist. He is a Senior Research Officer in the National Research Council of Canada's Institute for Information Technologies where he is a member of the People-Centred Technologies Group and where he heads the e-Citizen Studio. Bill has research interests in community informatics, communication rights, and development design. He currently heads the Intelligent City project, which is developing location-based services for public transportation and other aspects of communities. Bill is a graduate of Morehouse College and the University of Colorado at Boulder. He is a member of Computer Professionals for Social Responsibility and Engineers Without Borders – Canada, and was a participant in the World Summit on the Information Society.

Elspeth McKay, PhD, FACS, is an active researcher in the School of Business IT and Logistics at the RMITI University, Australia www.rmit.edu.au/staff/elspeth_mckay. Her PhD is in Computer Science and Information Systems, from Deakin University, Geelong, Australia. Elspeth also holds further qualifications in Instructional Design, Computer Education and Business Information Systems. She is passionate about designing effective eLearning resources for the education sector and industry training/reskilling programmes research interests involve investigations of how individuals interpret text and graphics within Web-mediated learning environments. Her work involves developing specialist e-Learning tools implemented through rich internet applications; including: ARPS – an advanced repurposing pilot system, COGNIWARE – a multi-modal e-Learning framework, GEMS – a global eMuseum System, eWRAP – Electronic work readiness awareness programme, EASY – Educational/academic (skills) screening for the young, offering enhanced accessibility through touch screen technologies. Over the last decade Dr McKay has published extensively in the research fields of HCI and educational technology. Her authored books include*: The eLearning Toolkit,* ARK Group, UK, 2009; *The Human-Dimensions of Human-Computer Interaction: Balancing the HCI Equation,* Vol:3 Future of Learning, IOS Press, Netherlands, 2008; *Enhancing Learning Through Human-Computer Interaction: Premier Reference Source.* London: Idea Group Reference, 2007. In recognition of her contribution to the professional practice of information systems research, she was elected as a Fellow of the Australian Computer Society (ACS).

Vladimir Munipov, a leading pioneer of the science of ergonomics in Russia, is an authority on the theory, practice, and history of ergonomics, industrial design, and labor psychology. Munipov was born in 1931 in Asbest city in Ural. He graduated at the science department of the philosophy faculty at the Lomonosov Moscow State University in 1954. In 1962, he was one of the founders of USSR Research Institute of Industrial Design (VNIITE). From 1962 to 1992 he worked in VNIITE. Munipov received PhD in ergonomics in USSR in 1988 and received the professorship in ergonomics in 1990. In 1995, Munipov was elected as academician of the Russian Academy of Education. Today he is professor at the Moscow State University of Radioengineering, Electronics and Automation. Munipov was the author of more than 300 scientific contributions. He is known to professionals throughout the world as the author of the paper "Chernobyl operators: criminals or victims?" published in Applied Ergonomics (1992). He contributed to the chapter on ergonomics published in International Encyclopedia on the Work Safety and Hygiene (Geneva, 1997). He wrote the text book for students of the highest educational institutes "Ergonomics: The Human-centered Ergonomic Design of Tool, Technology, Hardware, Software and Environment" (2001). Munipov was elected to the International Commission on Human Factors in Computerization, and he was member of advisory board of the Handbook on Human Factors (three editions have been issued, USA). He also served as a member of international editorial board of the journals Applied Ergonomics (UK), Ergonomics (UK), Human-Computer Interaction (USA) and others. Munipov was part of prominent professionals on ergonomics in International Encyclopedia of Ergonomics and Human Factors (second edition, 2006).

Christina Mörtberg, PhD, docent/reader, is an associate professor at the Department of Informatics, University of Oslo, Norway and University of Umeå, Sweden. Mörtberg's current research interests can be described in two interrelated areas that link to each other. In the first, systems design, she bases her research on situated perspectives and participatory design approaches and in the second, a theoretical/methodological perspective is in focus where systems design is studied in combination with theory/methodology based on (feminist) science and technology studies. Mörtberg has been involved in numerous national, Nordic, and international research projects throughout the years and has also been one of the founders of several transnational research networks. She has published and continues to publish her research on her own as well as in collaboration with doctoral students and colleagues.

Hans-Erik Nissen is Professor emeritus. Since 1991 he is a senior research fellow at the department of Informatics at Lund University. He graduated in chemistry from the Royal Institute of Technology, Stockholm. For many years he worked in various positions in the Swedish Cellulose Company (SCA). During his seven last years of these he started and headed the first computer center of SCA. He reentered academia at Stockholm University in 1969 to understand what computerized information systems can and cannot offer practitioners. He is since many years a member of IFIP's WG 8.2.

Kristina Orth-Gomér, PhD and MD, is since 1996 professor at Karolinska Institute in Sweden, and emerita since 2008. She was appointed Professor in Behaviour Medicine in 1992, after some years as associate professor at The Institute for Psychosocial Environmental Medicine, Karolinska Institute. She early spent a year as a research associate at the New York Hospital, Cornell Medical School, where she learnt clinical epidemiology, ambulatory stress and EKG monitoring. There she wrote her first scientific paper, an invited review article about psychosocial stress and atherosclerosis (Social science and Medicine). She foresaw and described the complexity and sophistication within the psycho-biological research field. Returning to Stockholm and the Seraphimer Hospital, she completed her medical residency and specialized in internal medicine with focus on cardiology, psychiatry and family medicine. She presented in 1979 her academic thesis, on psychosocial risk factors and cardiac dysrhytmia in men with coronary disease. She found that both stressors at work and a stressed behaviour style increased the coronary risk in men. There were two *distinct* emotional characteristics: depression and distrust. Men with an emotions profile of distrust and depression had an increased risk of malignant cardiac arrhythmia, in turn increasing the risk for sudden cardiac death (Acta Med Scand 1980). She initiated, together with colleagues at Karolinska, the Stockholm Female Coronary Risk study, an extensive investigation of women's stress and heart disease, with a great amount of publications and doctorial dissertations.

Jacob Palme, Professor emeritus at Stockholm university, Department of Computer and Information Science. He has done research on natural-language understanding, programming language design (co-inventor of object oriented languages 1973), computer-mediated communication (early research 1975-1990).

Natalie Pang graduated with a PhD from Monash University's Faculty of Information Technology. Her research is an interdisciplinary study of cultural institution, the commons and participation in the contemporary media environment. Her other research and teaching interests include archival informatics, information management, human-computer interaction, and collaborative records management. A graduate of Melbourne University in Australia and Nanyang Technological University in Singapore,

Natalie has worked in Singapore, Malaysia, and Australia. An active contributor and member of the P2P Foundation, she has also served as an Honorary Research Associate of Museum Victoria, the Victorian Association of Tertiary Libraries and the Centre for Community Networking and Research, Monash University in Australia.

John Sören Pettersson, professor in Information Systems and dean at Karlstad University, holds a PhD in General Linguistics and has his main research interests in Human-Computer Interaction, especially the representation of interactivity in systems development and the usability of privacy-enhancing technology. Member of the board of the Centre for HumanIT at Karlstad University.

Simone Pozzi works as Human Factors and Safety R&D expert in Deep Blue - Consultancy and Research (Rome). He also lectures interaction design at the Department of Architecture and Urban Planning University of Sassari at Alghero. He achieved his master degree (2001) and a PhD (2006), with specialisation in Human-Computer Interaction. He has participated in many international R&D projects in the area of Human Factors and Safety, funded by different organisations, including the EU commission and the European Organisation for Safety in Air Traffic Control (EUROCONTROL). He regularly publishes in peer-reviewed international academic journal (the latest ones are Mind, Culture and Activity; Culture & Psychology; Safety Science; Reliability Engineering and System Safety), and in international conferences (latest ones: EUROCONTROL Annual Safety R&D Seminar, EUROCONTROL INO, SAFECOMP, ISCAR, Symposium on Resilience Engineering).

Alice Robbin is an associate professor of library and information science in the School of Library and Information Science at Indiana University Bloomington. She is co-director of the Rob Kling Center for Social Informatics. Her research interests include information policy, communication and information behavior in complex organizations, and the societal implications of the information age. In addition to her research on the consequences of privacy law and policy for social research, the effects of digital inequality, and information seeking behavior on the Internet, she examines the political controversy over the federal reclassification of standards for racial and ethnic group data.

Michelle M. Robertson, PhD., CPE is a research scientist at the Liberty Mutual Research Institute for Safety and has conducted primarily applied, field intervention research studies in ergonomics and training for more than 17 years. Dr. Robertson also spent 12 years at the University of Southern California where she served on the faculty at the Institute of Safety and Systems Management. She is a Board Certified Professional Ergonomist and holds a Ph.D. in Instructional Technology and a M.S. in Systems Management from the University of Southern California, and a B.A. in Human Factors from the University of California, Santa Barbara. She is a Fellow of the Human Factors and Ergonomics Society and the International Ergonomics Association. She was co-recipient of the National Occupational Research Agenda, Innovative Research Award for Worker Health and Safety.

Simon Rogerson is Director of the Centre for Computing and Social Responsibility at De Montfort University, UK. He is Europe's first Professor in Computer Ethics. He received the 2000 IFIP Namur Award for outstanding contribution to the creation of awareness of the social implications of ICT. In 2005 he was awarded the SIGCAS Making a Difference Award by the ACM. His current research focuses on technological assessment, ethical systems development and qualitative stakeholder analysis.

He is co-editor of the Journal of Information, Communication and Ethics and Society. He conceived and co-directs the ETHICOMP conference series on the ethical impacts of ICT.

Katherine J. Rogers (Sanders) was a graduate student in Industrial Engineering at the University of Wisconsin-Madison working with professors Smith and Carayon at the time this article was written. After graduation Dr. Sanders worked for the university as an expert on improving faculty teaching and career development. She left the university for a successful career as a private consultant. Dr. Sanders recently returned to the university as an assistant Dean for the International Studies Program.

Christopher M. Schlick is Professor of Engineering at RWTH Aachen University and head of the Institute of Industrial Engineering and Ergonomics. He is a member of the management board of the Fraunhofer Institute for Communication, Information Processing and Ergonomics (FKIE). His research interests include modeling and simulation of work and business systems as well as the ergonomic design of human machine interfaces.

Virve Siirak is a Lecturer of Tallinn University of Technology and Chair of Labour Environment and Safety. Virve teaches the course in Working Environment and Ergonomics. She got her education from the University of Tartu, medical faculty, and became a Physician in 1970. She is a university teacher since 1996.

Sangeeta Sharma is Professor of Public Administration at the University of Rajasthan. India. Her works have appeared in various publications of National and International repute. Her research interests include E-governance, Ethics, and Socio-psychological experimentation. Her basic inclination is towards constructing the conceptual frameworks that are high in normative contents. She has authored a book on Organization Change. The edited volume by her relates to the Transformative Pathways with collections from scholars around the globe on the prognosis of the future society. Her innovativeness to analyze various aspects of Governance from interdisciplinary perspective reflects scientific aptitude. Her conceptual frameworks have been well acknowledged and she has been invited to deliver keynote addresses on her conceptual constructs at various professional forums.

Michael J. Smith is Professor emeritus. He received his Ph.D. degree in Industrial Psychology from the University of Wisconsin-Madison in 1973. Dr. Smith directed a research program on human factors and safety at the US National Institute for Occupational Safety and Health from1974-1984. Professor Smith received the US Public Health Service Superior Service Award for his research on applying human factors methods to reduce occupational injuries, and two special awards for his research on the health effects of using computers at work, and for research on the causes of occupational injuries. Dr. Smith was a professor of Industrial Engineering at the University of Wisconsin from 1984-2007 where he received many teaching awards. He is currently professor emeritus. Professor Smith has published many journal articles and refereed book chapters dealing with human factors and ergonomics, and has edited 22 books. He has been the editor-in-chief for the two scientific journals, the *International Journal on Human-Computer Interaction*, and *Cognitive Ergonomics*. He has served on the editorial boards of several scientific journals. Professor Smith is a Certified Professional Ergonomist (CPE) and a licensed psychologist. Professor Smith is a Fellow of the International Ergonomics Association.

Jacques Steyn is the Head of the School of IT at the South African campus of Monash University. In 2006 he established IDIA (International Development Informatics Association - www.developmentin-formatics.org) which serves as a network for researchers and practitioners in the field of ICT for Developing Countries (ICT4D). He is Editor-in-Chief of a book set in the field of Development Informatics, and Editor of a book on Music Informatics. He holds a multidisciplinary PhD and received an award for excellence in science from the South African Association for the Advancement of Science (S2A3). His present research interest is in the relationship between humans and technology. He lectured and served as Senior Advisor at UNISA until 1995, after which he was a self-employed information and knowledge consultant for a bout a decade, operating in the fields of New Media, such as Web Technologies and Multimedia. He was Associate Professor in Multimedia at the School of Information Technology of the University of Pretoria. In 1999 he developed the first XML-based general music markup language (http://www.musicmarkup.info). He was the South African representative at the international ISO/MPEG-7 standards workgroup on metadata for interactive-TV and Multimedia. He was also member of the ISO/MPEG-4 extension workgroup for music notation (i.e. symbolic music representation).

Larry Stillman, PhD is a Senior Research Fellow at the Centre for Community Networking Research (CCNR) within the Faculty of Information Technology at Monash University, Melbourne. His most recent research activity has included a comprehensive study of ICT cultures in welfare organisations in the State of Victoria Australia as well as social-technical issues around the development of the Digital Doorway project, project for deprived communities, based in South Africa. He is also interested in theoretical issues about the relationship between community informatics and Information Systems, as well as broader issues concerned with theory development, rigour, and methodology in technology field work where the emphasis is upon community engagement and development. He has been key to the Community Informatics conferences held at the Monash Centre, Prato, Italy.

Myra Strober is a labor economist at Stanford University where she is Emerita Professor of Education and Emerita Professor of Economics at the Graduate School of Business (by courtesy). She was the founding director of Stanford's Center for Research on Women (now the Clayman Institute for Research on Gender). Dr. Strober has a Ph.D. in economics from MIT. Her research has focused on gender issues at work and she has written numerous articles as well as the book, *The Road Winds Uphill all the Way: Gender, Work, and Family in the United States and Japan. Her newest book, Challenging Habits of Thought: Conversations Across the Disciplines, will be published in 2010 by Stanford University Press.*

Dagny Stuedahl, PhD and postdoc at Department of Media and Communication, University of Oslo, has a background in ethnology, history and theatre studies. Her design research focus is related to socio-cultural aspects of participatory design, digital design, communication design – and especially related to design with and for youths. Her background in ethnology brings a concentration on performative interactions between individuals and the collective in media spaces, in which technological artefacts play an important role. Her current research focuses on the interchange between narratives, proximity-based social and personal media and digital environments related to youths' engagement with digital cultural heritage.

Anna Ståhlbröst PhD, is a researcher and project manager at Luleå University of Technology, Sweden. Her research interests are process-based methods, which include various stakeholders, to appreciate opportunities for innovative technology development in Living Lab environments. These methods specifically focus on generating user needs from different real-world use situations and assessing users' experience of specific IT artefacts. Anna's research objective is to contribute to the design process to assure that innovative technologies will represent user needs and thereby give the users an added value. Anna has participated in several international and national innovation projects and her research is related to Botnia Living Lab and to establishing networks of Living Labs, both on European and Nordic levels.

Margaret Tan is Associate Professor at the Wee Kim Wee School of Communication and Information and Deputy Director, Singapore Internet Research Centre at Nanyang Technological University. Her research interests include the building of online trust and security, data protection and privacy, e-payment, Internet policies and governance, and the digital societies. With many scholarly publications and 2 books: "The Virtual Workplace" and "e-Payment: The Digital Exchange", Margaret has also spoken at international conferences as well as serving numerous editorial boards of international journals. She has taught senior executives in areas ranging from information technology planning and strategies, change management and process redesign as well as knowledge management.

Sebastian Vetter studied psychology at the universities of Maastricht, Netherlands, and Aachen, Germany. He received the Dipl.-psych. degree from RWTH Aachen University in 2007. Since then, he is a research assistant and Ph.D. candidate at the Institute of Industrial Engineering and Ergonomics at RWTH Aachen University. His research interests include ergonomics and human-computer interaction.

Diane Whitehouse is a founding partner of the UK-based business partnership, The Castlegate Consultancy. She was previously a European Commission (EC) official, where her foci were eHealth and eInclusion. She has also worked in the domains of action research, academic, civic and human rights, and publishing. As a social scientist, her interests lie in the social, organisational, and ethical aspects of ICT and she has written widely on these subjects. A longstanding member of the International Federation for Information Processing (IFIP), she has recently been appointed as the next Chair of IFIP Working Group 9.2 (Computers and Social Accountability). Diane met Professor Gunilla Bradley at the first IFIP summer school on social citizenship and ICT two decades ago. Their friendship and fruitful academic interactions have continued ever since.

Karin Danielsson Öberg, is a PhD-student at the Department of Informatics, Umeå University, Sweden. Her main areas of interest in research are user participation in design of edutainment games. Karin has worked within the research projects User-Centred Development of Collaborative Learning supported by Personal Technologies, Entertainment Services, and Cross-Media Design. She is one of the organizers for the Distributed Participatory Design workshop series. Her dissertation is scheduled for summer 2010. Karin's personal web site may be reached through: http://www.informatik.umu.se/~kdson/

Index